Advances in Treatment of Hepatitis C and B
http://dx.doi.org/10.5772/62815
Edited by Naglaa Allam

Contributors

Valeriu Gheorghita, Florin Alexandru Căruntu, Imran Shahid, Mohammed AlRabia, Waleed Almalki, Muhammad Ahmed, Muhammad Hassan Hafeez, Sanaa Kamal, Mohamed Hassany, Aisha Elsharkawy, Chih-Wen Lin, Hussien Elsiesy, Liang-Tzung Lin, Damjan Glavac, Mateja M. Jelen, Mankgopo Kgatle, Gizem Dinler-Doganay, Seyma Katrinli, H. Levent Doganay, Kamil Ozdil, Andrew Dargan, Hie-Won Hann, Costin Teodor Teodor Streba, Letitia Adela Maria Streba, Waleed Al-Hamoudi, Yong-Yuan Zhang, John Boletis, Yang Chang Qing, Naglaa Allam

Published by InTech
Janeza Trdine 9, 51000 Rijeka, Croatia

Publishing Process Manager Edi Lipovic
Technical Editor SPi Global
Cover InTech Design team

First published March, 2017
Printed in Croatia
Legal deposit, Croatia: National and University Library in Zagreb

Additional hard copies can be obtained from orders@intechopen.com

Advances in Treatment of Hepatitis C and B, Edited by Naglaa Allam
p. cm.
Print ISBN 978-953-51-2993-6
Online ISBN 978-953-51-2994-3

For EU product safety concerns:
IN TECH d.o.o., Prolaz Marije Krucifikse Kozulić 3, 51000 Rijeka, Croatia,
info@intechopen.com or visit our website at intechopen.com.

Meet the editor

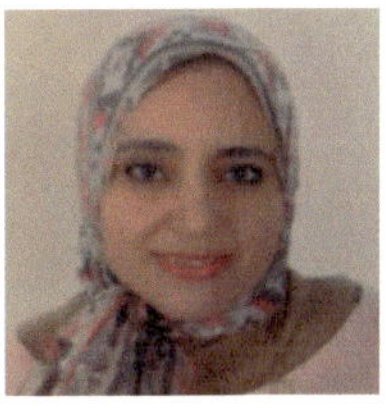

Dr. Naglaa Allam is a professor of hepatology at the National Liver Institute (NLI) Menoufia University in Egypt. The NLI is a leading medical institution in the Middle East dedicated for the management of liver diseases as well as advanced training and research in hepatology and liver transplantation. Dr. Naglaa Allam was trained at the Northern General Hospital, UK, and Hospital of the University of Pennsylvania in the USA. She is an editorial board member and reviewer in many medical journals and has several publications in eminent journals as well as books in the field of hepatology and liver transplantation.

Contents

Preface

One of the greatest breakthroughs in medicine is our current capability to cure nearly everyone with chronic hepatitis C virus infection. With the emergence of direct-acting antiviral agents, hepatitis C virus infection has entered a new era. On the other hand, hepatitis B viral replication can be suppressed by potent antiviral drugs, but strategies to enhance the eradication rates of HBV infection are still needed on the horizon. Treatment of viral hepatitis is a rapidly evolving field that will continue to grow and maintain excitement over the next few years.

"Advances in Treatment of Hepatitis C and Hepatitis B" book is divided into two parts. The first part provides a comprehensive overview on the current state of knowledge and latest advances in hepatitis C and hepatitis B therapeutics. The chapters include management in special conditions during pregnancy and in kidney transplantation. The second part attempts to provide a conceptual framework of emerging and investigational treatment strategies.

This book is addressed to researchers, practicing physicians in hepatology, medical students, residents, and fellows seeking a broader understanding of updates in the treatment of viral hepatitis. The authors are bright internationally renowned experts from four continents across the globe (Africa, Asia, Europe, and the United States of America). We sincerely thank the authors for their time and expertise, and we hope the readers find their chapters useful.

I am also grateful to all my seniors and colleagues at the National Liver Institute whose zeal and dedication make the institute a vibrant, exciting place to work at.

Finally, I dedicate this book to the soul of my father, Dr. Allam, who always invested a great deal of love in supporting my work. He was excited about this book project but did not live to witness its emergence. I also acknowledge my wonderful husband, Prof. Hesham Abdeldayem, for his love, encouragement, and support.

Naglaa Allam
National Liver Institute,
Menoufia University,
Egypt

Section 1

Introduction

Introductory Chapter: Treatment of Viral Hepatitis - Current Challenges and Future Perspectives

Naglaa Allam and Imam Waked

Additional information is available at the end of the chapter

http://dx.doi.org/10.5772/67420

1. Hepatitis C therapy

Cure of hepatitis C has come true!

Clinical care for patients with hepatitis C (HCV) has advanced remarkably during the last two decades, as a result of better understanding of the pathophysiology of the disease, and because of developments in diagnostic procedures and improvements in therapy and prevention. With the introduction of genotype 1 effective directly acting antiviral agents (DAAs) in 2011, the management of HCV infection started to change. By 2013, second-generation pangenotypic DAAs became available, and the biggest problem was solved: interferon (IFN) became no longer necessary.

Unlike IFN regimens, which rely on upregulating the patients' own immune system, these DAAs block different stages of viral replication. There are four major groups of DAAs namely: NS5B nucleotide inhibitors, NS5B nonnucleoside inhibitors, NS5A replication complex inhibitors, and NS3/4A protease inhibitors [1]. Specific treatment regimens vary, depending on factors such as HCV genotype, and may include multiple drugs [2]. Multiple regimens have been approved and several new regimens with high potencies, less resistance, and better safety profile are in the process of approval. Prof. Kamal elegantly describes them in detail in Chapter 2.

Sustained virological response (SVR) rates achieved in phase III clinical trials generally exceeded 90% (although real-world rates may be lower) along with reduction in treatment duration to 12 weeks or less and with fewer adverse events. An SVR is generally associated with normalization of liver enzymes and amelioration or disappearance of liver necroinflammation and fibrosis in noncirrhotic patients [3]. The use of DAAs in patients with cirrhosis, as discussed in Chapter 4, has also shown excellent results with good safety profile. SVR also improves HCV-induced portal hypertension [4]. DAAs have also begun to change the landscape of management of the HCV transplant candidate on the waiting list. Prof. Al-Hamoudi provides an update on this in Chapter 5. Even patients with HCV infection and advanced kidney disease now have alternative treatment options.

Thus, the era of HCV eradication and cure has begun. And in 2017, hepatologists can treat *all* patients irrespective of fibrosis score—but the job is not over yet. Real-world experience has revealed several challenges and unmet needs!

1.1. Challenges:

(a) Limited or absent access to therapy in the majority of infected patients

Unfortunately, the very high cost of the new DAA drugs is creating a barrier for introduction of treatment in most limited resource settings and may prove an obstacle on the path for elimination of HCV infection worldwide. Of course, successful treatment should prevent many late HCV complications, but even if treatment actually proves cost saving in the long run, it is too expensive and infeasible to treat all patients immediately [5].

Hence hepatitis C treatment prioritization, as the European Association for the Study of the Liver states, is necessary when resources are limited [6]. However, new data suggest that this approach may be suboptimal, if not carefully executed. Treatment prioritization is complex and may not be fair. Treating first those with the most need makes sense. But, those who need it most may also be those who benefit the least because of issues as extensive liver damage, comorbid illness, older age, or have already developed hepatocellular carcinoma? Targeting populations with high HCV prevalence like drug users, prisoners, and migrants also makes sense since they are most likely to spread infection to others. But, those most likely to transmit to others often have low disease stage. Besides they are most likely to abrogate the personal benefits of treatment by being reinfected. Treating those who have the most symptoms also makes sense, but unfortunately symptoms do not always improve with cure. And there is another major issue: who should decide whom to prioritize? [7]. Health care providers often impose socioeconomic and racial biases when prioritizing treatments [8]. Moreover, health care providers prefer not to be the barrier between patients and life-saving therapies.

While *not* all patients require immediate treatment, an ideal strategy should treat patients before they progress toward end-stage liver disease when even highly effective treatments can confer only marginal benefit. In response, many countries have instituted coverage policies that authorize treatment only for the advanced patients, putting off therapy for less severely ill patients [5].

Aggressive action is warranted to see progress toward HCV elimination. Only if we use *efficacious therapy* in a *significant* proportion of patients will we *significantly* decrease the burden of the disease. So efforts should be made to make DAAs cost effective in all clinical scenarios and accessible to all patients. In places like Egypt and India, generic versions of the DAAs sofosbuvir and daclatasvir are being mass produced for <1% of the current US retail price and are available for a higher proportion of patients.

Another solution to reduce treatment cost is by shortening the duration of treatment without affecting efficacy. A study in China demonstrated 100% SVR with triple DAAs for only 3 weeks if the patient without cirrhosis achieved ultra-rapid virological response (HCV-RNA < 500 IU 48 hours after starting treatment) [9]. By shortening the duration of therapy from the currently recommended 12 to 3 weeks, the cost of therapy could be markedly reduced as well as the rate of adverse events. Large clinical trials should further study the application of this response-guided treatment approach in patients with different ethnic backgrounds and with different genotypes.

(b) Emergence of drug resistance and DAA failure

Despite improved SVR rates with DAA-based combination regimens, treatment fails to eradicate HCV infection in 5–15%, dependening on the treatment regimen and treated population. Treatment failure is generally associated with the selection of HCV resistant-associated substitution (RAS) (or resistant-associated variant (RAV)), that is, viral molecular substitutions or variants that have reduced susceptibility to the DAA(s) administered. NS5A inhibitors have a low barrier to resistance, and the variants they select confer cross-resistance across all members of the drug class. Thus, NS5A resistance currently appears as the principal challenge of IFN-free, DAA-based therapy and they tend to persist for several years after treatment failure. In contrast, RASs selected by NS3/4A protease inhibitors persist for a much shorter time and are progressively replaced by wild-type virus within a few months posttherapy. Additionally, RASs selected by the NS5B polymerase inhibitor sofosbuvir have poor viral fitness; thus, they rarely emerge in the presence of the drug and tend to rapidly disappear if selected [10]. The utility of HCV resistance testing, i.e., the determination of the sequence of the DAA target region prior to retreatment in patients who failed on any of the DAA-containing regimens is unknown. Chapter 6 summarizes the retreatment in case of drug failures.

(c) HCV eradication and the risk of hepatocellular carcinoma (HCC): issues with direct acting antiviral (DAA) therapy?

Several recent publications raise concerns about unexpected high rate of HCC recurrence after undergoing direct-acting antiviral therapy. Reig et al. showed early tumor "recurrence" in patients with HCV-related hepatocellular carcinoma (HCC) [11]. Conti et al. showed that in patients with HCV-related cirrhosis, DAA-induced resolution of HCV infection does *not* reduce recurrence of HCC, and patients previously treated for HCC have still a high risk of tumor recurrence, in the short term [12]. Kozbial et al. showed an unexpected high "occurrence" in patients with advanced liver diseases after SVR [13].

In contrast, Cheung et al. found that DAA therapy in patients with decompensated cirrhosis led to sustained improvement in liver function, with no evidence of increase in HCC development in Chinese patients [14]. Also, the French ANRS study analyzed more than 6000 DAA-treated patients who underwent curative therapies for HCC and they found no increased risk of HCC [15].

Altogether these studies convey a strong message that great attention is needed to address the issue of HCC recurrence/occurrence. There is an urgent need for large prospective studies evaluating the impact of DAA therapy on the risk of HCC in patients with HCV-related cirrhosis. For the time being, the risk of HCC development justifies HCC screening after viral clearance in patients with HCV-related cirrhosis.

(d) There is no vaccine yet. Is a prophylactic vaccine still necessary?

Obviously, therapy is not enough to surmount the burden of HCV. Is it technically possible to have vaccine? If HCV vaccines are available in the future, then vaccination program in high-risk populations would probably have a great impact on preventing and eradicating HCV infection. An experimental protective vaccine, as shown in Chapter 14, demonstrated promise in preliminary human safety trials, and a phase II clinical trial is under way to further determine the efficacy of the vaccine.

1.2. Future perspectives:

Therefore, although the DAAs have opened up new horizons for HCV cure, challenges persist in the real-world setting. It is becoming clear that developing therapeutic strategies with different modes of action would be necessary to address the various limitations of current DAAs. Third generation pangenotypic antivirals are currently in final phases of development: voxilaprevir [16], glecaprevir [17] (both NS3/NS4 protease inhibitors) and pibrentasvir (NS5A inhibitor) [17]. Antivirals with alternate mechanism of action, such as by restricting viral entry or cell-to-cell spread could help expand the scope of antiviral strategies for the management of hepatitis C. Chapters 14 and 15 describe some of the new paradigms in antiviral strategies to preclude HCV entry, such as through monoclonal antibodies and small molecules.

With these strategies, it is foreseeable, in a not too distant future, that they will help provide a better management of hepatitis C.

2. Hepatitis B therapy

An overview of the six currently approved treatments is presented in Chapter 7. The advent of anti-HBV treatment drugs has made *significant progress* in improving the health and life expectancy of patients with HBV.

But there is no cure for Hepatitis B till now!

Chronic hepatitis B remains a difficult to treat disease because at this time no treatment provides both an optimal virological and immunological control. There is a high rate of relapse following any antiviral therapy. In addition, there are no approved therapy stopping rules, especially in HBeAg negative patients treated with nucleoside and nucleotide analogs. An early stopping rule using the combination of serum HBsAg and HBV DNA was proposed and is discussed in Chapter 9.

While there have been significant advances in the management of hepatitis B with available nucleos(t)ide analogues, there remains much work to be done to prevent HCC. Viral suppression alone has proven not effective for the absolute prevention of HCC.

Additionally, the required long-term therapy imposes not only financial burden but also may put patients at risk for potential drug resistance and unknown toxicity. Therefore, more effective treatment regimens aiming for HBV cure are urgently needed. New investigational therapies are in the pipeline as discussed in Chapter 17. With multiple new therapies in the pipeline,

http://dx.doi.org/10.5772/67420

the future of treating hepatitis B is an exciting one, and there is hope that it will become a disease of the past but this will not be too soon! The new therapy will not be available soon.

Another challenge is a demand for screening pregnant females and newborns for HBV. Pregnancy screening for HBV is very defective in most countries; it is not practiced except on individual basis. Chapter 10 reviews current management strategies for hepatitis B in the pregnancy and the postpartum.

Conclusion

So, in conclusion, the highly effective and well-tolerated direct-acting antiviral drugs (DAAs) for the treatment of the hepatitis C virus have revolutionized therapy for HCV. Several novel therapeutic strategies for each of HBV and HCV are under development. But until the developing antiviral strategies are available, there is much more that can be done.

The public health burden posed by viral hepatitis should be recognized as a priority. The leading professional organizations in liver disease, the American Association for the Study of Liver Diseases (AASLD), the European Association for the Study of the Liver (EASL), and the Asian Pacific Association for the Study of the Liver (APASL) urge governments, health care organizations, and nongovernmental organizations to adopt recommendations for immunization, screening, diagnosis and treatment and to make them available and affordable for public health programs [18].

Overall, the achievements and improvements in the field of HCV and HBV care predict that the future of HCV and HBV therapeutics is becoming brighter every day.

Author details

Naglaa Allam* and Imam Waked

*Address all correspondence to: naglaaallam@yahoo.com

Hepatology, National Liver Institute, Menoufeya University, Egypt

References

[1] Rupp D, Bartenschlager R. Targets for antiviral therapy of hepatitis C. Semin Liver Dis 2014;34:9–21.

[2] Chung Raymond T et al. Hepatitis C guidance: AASLD-IDSA recommendationsfor testing, managing, and treating adults infected with hepatitis C virus. Hepatology 2015;62:932–54.

[3] Pinzani M. Liver fibrosis in the Post-HCV Era. Semin Liver Dis 2015;35:157–65.

[4] Mandorfer M, Kozbial K, Schwabl P, Clarissa Freissmuth C, Schwarzer R, Stern R, Chromy D Stättermayer AF, Reiberger T, Beinhardt S, Sieghart W, Trauner M, Hofer H, Ferlitsch A, Ferenci P, Markus Peck-Radosavljevic M. Sustained virologic response to interferon-free therapies ameliorates HCV-induced portal hypertension. J Hepatol 2016;65:692–99.

[5] Fox S, McCombs J. Optimizing HCV treatment – Moving beyond the cost conundrum. J Hepatol 2016;65:222–25.

[6] World Health Organization guidelines for the screening care and treatment of chronic hepatitis C infection; 2016. Update. http://www.who.int/hiv/pub/hepatitis/hepatitis-cguidelines/en/

[7] Mehta SH, David L, Thomas DL. Doing the math on hepatitis C virus treatmentJ Hepatol 2016;65:5–6.

[8] Institute of Medicine Committee on U, Eliminating R, Ethnic Disparities in Health C. In: Smedley BD, Stith AY, Nelson AR, editors. Unequal treatment: confronting racial and ethnic disparities in health care. Washington (DC): National Academies Press (US); 2003.

[9] Lau G, Benhamou Y, Chen G, Li J, Shao Q, Ji D, Li F, Li B, Liu J, Hou J, Jian Sun J, Wang C, Chen J, Wu V, Wong A, Wong C, Tsang S, Wang Y, Bassit L, Tao S, Jiang Y, Hsiao H, Ke R, Perelson A, Schinazi R. Efficacy and safety of 3-week response-guided triple direct-acting antiviral therapy for chronic hepatitis Cinfection: a phase 2, open-label, proof-of-concept study. Lancet Gastroenterol Hepatol 2016;1(2):97–104.

[10] Pawlotsky JM. Hepatitis C virus resistance to direct-acting antiviral drugs in interferon-free regimens. Gastroenterology 2016;151(1):70–86.

[11] Reig M, Mariño Z, Perelló C, Iñarrairaegui M, Ribeiro A, Lens S, Díaz A, Vilana R, Darnell A, Varela M, Sangro B, Calleja JL, Forns X, Bruix J. Unexpected high rate of early tumor recurrence in patients with HCV-related HCC undergoing interferon-free therapy. J Hepatol 2016;65:719–26.

[12] Conti F, Buonfiglioli F, Scuteri A, Crespi C, Bolondi L, Caraceni P, Foschi FG, Lenzi M, Mazzella G, Verucchi G, Andreone P, Brillanti S. Early occurrence and recurrence of hepatocellular carcinoma in HCV-related cirrhosis treated with direct acting antivirals. J Hepatol 2016;65:727–33.

[13] Kozbial K, Moser S, Schwarzer R, Laferl H, Al-Zoairy R, Stauber R, Stättermayer AF, Beinhardt S, Graziadei I, Freissmuth C, Maieron A, Gschwantler M, Strasser M, Peck-Radosalvjevic M, Trauner M, Hofer H, Ferenci P. Unexpected high incidence of hepatocellular carcinoma in cirrhotic patients with SVR following IFN-free DAA treatment. J Hepatol 2016;65:856–8.

[14] Cheung MC, Walker AJ, Hudson BE, Verma S, McLauchlan J, Mutimer DJ, Brown A, Gelson WT, MacDonald DC, Agarwal K, Foster GR, Irving WL; HCV Research UK. Outcomes after successful direct-acting antiviral therapy for patients with chronic hepatitis C and decompensated cirrhosis. J Hepatol 2016;65(4):741–7.

http://dx.doi.org/10.5772/67420

[15] ANRS collaborative study group on hepatocellular carcinoma (ANRS CO22 HEPATHER, CO12 CirVir and CO23 CUPILT cohorts). Lack of evidence of an effect of direct-acting antivirals on the recurrence of hepatocellular carcinoma: data from three ANRS cohorts. J Hepatol 2016;65(4):734–40.

[16] Jacobson IM, Asselah T, Nahass R, Bhandari BR, Tran A, Hyland RH, Stamm LH, Dvory-Sobol H, Zhu Y, Brainard DM, Subramanian M, McHutchison JG, Shafran S, Davis M, Stedman CA, Lawitz E, Gane J. POLARIS-2: A Randomized Phase 3 Trial of Sofosbuvir/Velpatasvir/Voxilaprevir for 8 Weeks Compared to Sofosbuvir/Velpatasvir for 12 Weeks in DAA-Naïve Genotype 1-6 HCV-Infected Patients: The POLARIS-2 Study. Abstract LB-12. Presented at: The Liver Meeting; Nov. 11–15, 2016; Boston.

[17] Gane E, Poordad F, Wang S, Asatryan A, Kwo PY, Lalezari J, Wyles DL, Hassanein T, Aguilar H, Maliakkal B, Liu R, Lin CW, Ng TI, Kort J, Mensa FJ. High Efficacy of ABT-493 and ABT-530 treatment in patients with HCV Genotype 1 or 3 infection and compensated cirrhosis. Gastroenterology 2016;151(4):651–659.e1. Epub 2016 Jul 25.

[18] Brahm J, Castera L, Hou J, Lindor K. Joint society statement for the elimination of viral hepatitis. J Hepatol 2016;65;661–2.

Section 2

Currently Available Therapies

Chapter 2

Advances in Treatment of Hepatitis C

Sanaa M. Kamal

Additional information is available at the end of the chapter

http://dx.doi.org/10.5772/66719

Abstract

Hepatitis C infection (HCV) is a major cause of chronic hepatitis and cirrhosis worldwide. Interferon-based regimen has been the sole therapy to eradicate HCV infection for decades. However, this interferon and ribavirin combination is associated with several serious adverse events and the sustained virologic response rate was suboptimal. The recent discovery of oral direct-acting antiviral agents (DAAs) heralded a revolution in the treatment of chronic HCV. This breakthrough in HCV resulted in high rates of HCV eradication with sustained virologic response rates ranging between 90 and 100% across different genotypes. New therapies were administered orally for 12 or 24 months and this resulted in better compliance and few adverse events. DAAs are categorized into four major groups namely: NS5B nucleotide inhibitors, NS5B nonnucleoside inhibitors, NS5A replication complex inhibitors, and NS3/4A protease inhibitors (PI). Several interferon-free regimens have been approved and adequately assessed and several new regimens with high potencies, less cross-resistance, and better safety profile are in the process of approval. Thus, the era of HCV eradication and cure has begun.

Keywords: hepatitis C, direct-acting antivirals, interferon-free regimen

1. Introduction

Hepatitis C virus (HCV) is a major cause of liver cirrhosis, end-stage liver disease, and liver transplantation throughout the world [1]. Approximately 170–200 million people equating to 3% of the world's population are infected with HCV [2]. The prevalence of HCV varies in different geographic regions. The prevalence of HCV infection is greater in Africa and Asia, with infection rates exceeding 5% [3–5]. Egypt has the highest prevalence of hepatitis C in the world, with 15% of the population affected [6–8]. In the USA, nearly 2% of the population is infected [9, 10]. In Europe, the prevalence ranges from 0.1% in northern European countries and 1% in countries on the Mediterranean [10, 11]. The immigration crisis may increase HCV prevalence in Europe given that immigrants originate from countries with high rates of HCV [12].

2. Natural history and outcome of HCV infection

Acute HCV infection is mostly asymptomatic and rarely recognized clinically. Spontaneous viral clearance (SVC) occurs in approximately 25% of patients [13, 14]. The striking feature of HCV infection is its tendency to persist and evolve to chronic hepatitis. In some patients, chronic HCV progresses to liver cirrhosis and hepatocellular carcinoma (HCC) [14, 15].

The outcome of HCV infection depends largely on several host, viral and environmental factors. During an early stage, HCV infection triggers viral-associated molecular pattern (PAMP) receptors resulting in induction of an antiviral state through several pathways such as limiting cellular, modifying and degrading viral RNA, altering cellular vesicle trafficking and probably other not yet discovered antiviral mechanisms [15–17]. Clearance of HCV is associated with the development of robust and multispecific $CD4^+$ and $CD8^+$T-cell responses in blood and liver that can be maintained for years after recovery from acute disease [18–20]. In contrast, individuals who progress to chronic infection fail to mount such a response or may have inadequate production of the cytokines essential to control viral replication. Incomplete control of viral replication by $CD8^+$ T cells in the absence of sufficient memory $CD4^+$T cells leads to viral persistence and emergence of CTL escape mutants [21–24].

Acute resolving hepatitis has been shown to be associated with HCV homogeneity, whereas progressing hepatitis correlated with genetic diversity, presumably reflecting greater immune pressure during acute spontaneous clearance [25]. Polymorphisms of genes involved in innate immunity as well as those in genes encoding cytokines and other immunologic mediators may explain spontaneous recovery from acute HCV and influence the strength and nature of immune defense. Genes encoding the inhibitory NK cell receptor *KIR2DL3* and its human leukocyte antigen C group 1 (*HLA-C1*) ligand influenced spontaneous resolution of HCV infection suggesting that inhibitory NK cell interactions are critical for antiviral immunity [26, 27].

To date, there are no reliable methods to predict who will resolve acute HCV spontaneously and who will develop chronic HCV. Similarly, no reliable indicators exist for distinguishing chronic hepatitis C patients who may develop cirrhosis or HCC. Thus, early effective treatment of patients with HCV is necessary for prevention of progression of liver disease to cirrhosis, hepatocellular carcinoma. In the absence of a vaccine against HCV, efficient treatment is important for prevention of transmission along with adoption of infection control measures.

3. Evolution of HCV therapy

The ultimate goal of hepatitis C treatment is to reduce the occurrence of end-stage liver disease and its complications including decompensated cirrhosis, liver transplantation, and

HCC. Treatment success is assessed by sustained virologic response (SVR), defined undetectable HCV RNA in blood several months after completing a course of treatment [28].

For two decades, the standard of care (SOC) for hepatitis C infection was interferon based. IFNα has potent antiviral activity due to its ability to induce IFN-stimulated genes (ISGs) that encode proteins which inhibit various stages of viral replication [29]. Type I IFNs bind a unique ubiquitous heterodimeric receptor consisting of interferon-alpha receptor 1/2 (IFNAR1/IFNAR2), resulting in the activation of signaling pathways and induction of a large number of IFN-stimulated genes (ISGs). ISG-encoded proteins mediate the antiviral and other effects of interferons [29]. IFNAR1 and IFNAR2 are associated with the Janus-activated kinases (JAKs) tyrosine kinase 2 (TYK2) and JAK1, respectively. Binding of type I IFNs to their heterodimeric receptors leads to activation of JAKs, which results in tyrosine phosphorylation of signal transducer and activator of transcription 2 (STAT2) and STAT1; STAT1/STAT2 migrates into the nucleus and associates with the IFN regulatory factor 9 (IRF9) to form the STAT1-STAT2-IRF9 complex. This complex then binds IFN-stimulated response elements (ISREs) inside DNA to initiate the transcription of hundreds of different ISGs [30, 31]. IFN regulatory genes (IRGs) facilitate both clearance of virus from infected cells and protection of neighboring uninfected cells from incoming viral progeny. The antiviral-associated protein kinase R (PKR) plays an important role in restricting HCV 1a replication through regulating the NF-κB pathway [32, 33].

Initially, chronic hepatitis C was treated by conventional interferon (IFN) monotherapy which yielded very poor response rates. Addition of the guano sine analog, ribavirin, to conventional interferon was associated with slight improvement in sustained virologic response (SVR) although the improvement was far from satisfactory particularly in HCV genotypes 1 and 4. Pegylation of the interferon molecule resulted in modification of the pharmacokinetic profile of IFN-α-2. Both PEG-IFN-α-2a and PEG-IFN-α-2b have slower absorption, more reduced distribution and lower elimination rate than the nonpegylated IFN-α. The maintained concentrations of PEG-IFNα allowed longer periods of viral inhibition with once a week dosing. Pegylated interferon and ribavirin therapy resulted in improved sustained virologic response (SVR), defined as undetectable HCV RNA 24 weeks after completion of treatment. With pegylated interferon alpha-2 and ribavirin (RBV) combination, response rates in genotypes 2 and 3 range between 70 and 80%. However, SVR rates in chronic HCV genotypes 1 and 4 infection are suboptimal. Adverse events are common with interferon-based regimen and include fatigue, flu-like symptoms, anxiety, skin rash, and gastrointestinal symptoms such as nausea and diarrhea. Hemolytic anemia is frequent due to the use of ribavirin. Some patients treated with PEG-IFN and RBV may develop cardiac arrhythmias or severe neuropsychiatric adverse events depression and suicidal tendency. The various adverse effects, the long duration of therapy and the need to inject interferon reduce compliance and treatment adherence. These factors have driven the urgent need to develop new treatments that are safer and more effective (**Figure 1**). The discovery of direct-acting antiviral agents (DAAs) heralded the dawn of a new era of HCV cure which was a dream.

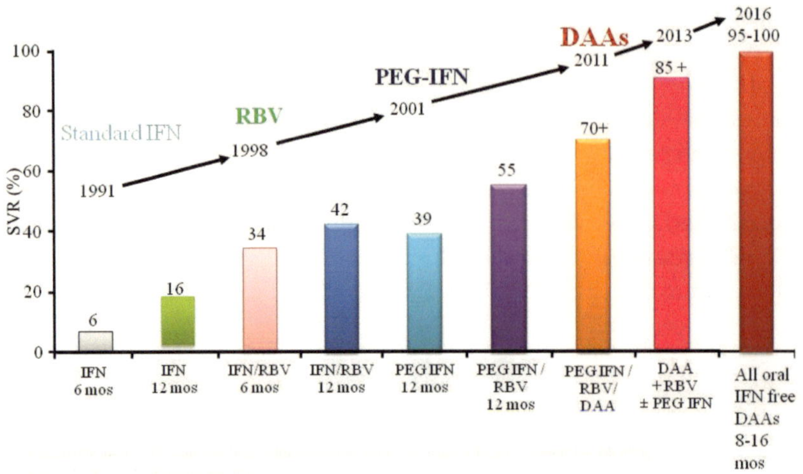

Figure 1. Evolution of HCV therapy.

4. Direct-acting antiviral agents (DAAs)

Direct-acting antiviral agents (DAAs) represent a revolution in HCV drug discovery. DAAs were developed to improve the SVR rates, reduce adverse events, and improve adherence to therapy among HCV patients. DAAs were initially introduced as add-ons to the previous standard of care (SOC) consisting of pegylated interferon alpha plus ribavirin (PR). Recently, a breakthrough in HCV therapy has been achieved with the introduction of interferon-free all-oral DAAs, with SVR rates now in excess of 90% after 12 weeks of therapy for genotype 1 patients.

DAAs target specific steps within the HCV life cycle and disrupt viral replication in an attempt to terminate that cycle before its completion (**Figure 2**) [34]. The first step in the life cycle of the virus is cell attachment and entry of HCV RNA through hepatocyte surface receptors. The HCV RNA is then translated to one polyprotein of 3010 amino acids that is subsequently cleaved by protease. It is then processed into four structural proteins (namely Core, E1, E2, and P7) as well as the nonstructural proteins (NS2-3 and NS3-4A proteases, NS3 helicase, and NS5B RdRp). All of these enzymes are essential for the replication of the virus and are potential drug discovery targets [35–37].

4.1. Goals of HCV and endpoints of treatment with DAAs

The goal of therapy is to eradicate HCV infection to prevent hepatic cirrhosis, decompensation of cirrhosis, HCC, and severe extrahepatic manifestations. The endpoint of therapy is undetectable HCV RNA in blood by a sensitive assay (with the lower limit of detection <15 IU/ml) 12 weeks (SVR-12) and/or 24 weeks (SVR-24) after the completion of treatment. Undetectable HCV core antigen (HCV c Ag) 12 or 24 weeks after the completion of therapy can be an alternative to HCVRNA testing to assess the SVR12 or the SVR24, respectively [38]. In patients with advanced fibrosis and cirrhosis, HCV eradication reduces the rate of

http://dx.doi.org/10.5772/66719

decompensation and will reduce, albeit not abolish the risk of HCC. In these patients surveillance for HCC should be continued.

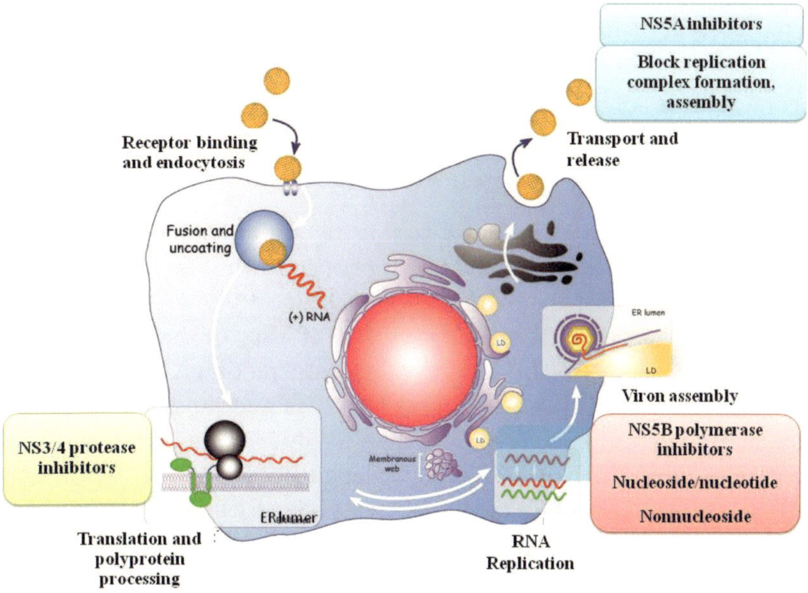

Figure 2. Hepatitis C life cycle and the targets of direct-acting antiviral agents.

4.2. Classes of DAAs

There are four classes of DAAs, which are defined by their mechanism of action and therapeutic target. DAAs include NS5B nucleotide inhibitors, NS5B nonnucleoside inhibitors, NS5A replication complex inhibitors, and NS3/4A protease inhibitors (PI) (**Figure 3**).

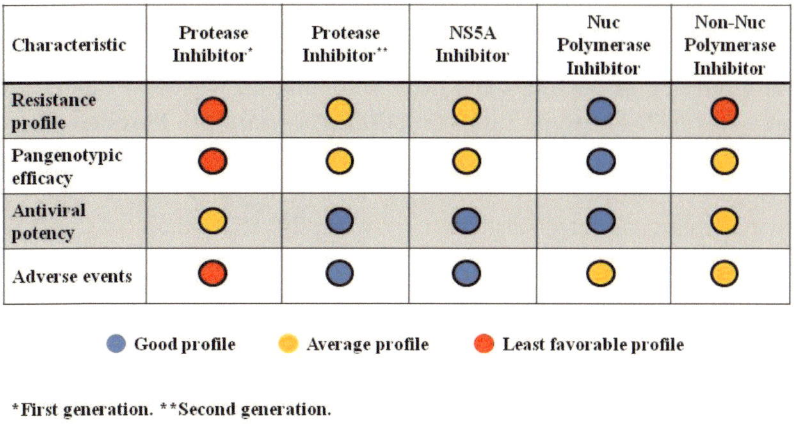

Figure 3. Resistance patterns in different direct-acting antiviral agents (DAAs).

4.2.1. NS3/4A protease inhibitors (PIs)

PIs block the activity NS3/4A serine protease, an enzyme which inhibits TRIF-mediated Toll-like receptor signaling and Cardif-mediated retinoic acid–inducible gene 1 (RIG-1) signaling resulting in impaired induction of interferons and blocking viral elimination [39, 40]. PIs have been grouped according to their resistance profile into first- and second-generation agents and into separate waves according to dosing, safety, and tolerability characteristics.

4.2.1.1. First-generation PIs

Telaprevir and boceprevir were the first direct-acting antivirals for treatment of HCV and represented the first generation of PIs. Telaprevir or boceprevir was used in combination with peginterferon and ribavirin for the treatment of genotype 1 [40, 41]. Although telaprevir or boceprevir regimen enhanced SVR rates; the clinical efficacy of the triple regimen was limited by narrow genotype specificity, low barrier to resistance, and drug-drug interactions. This regimen also increased adverse events such as rash and moderate to severe anemia to an extent that might require the reduction of the RBV dose. Patient adherence and tolerability to triple therapy with BOC or TPV is a challenging issue as the two DAAs should be given three times daily with food. Triple therapy was not very effective in previous PEG-IFN/RBV dual therapy, no responders. From an economic perspective, the triple therapy dramatically increased the costs of HCV treatment which are originally prohibitive. Thus, the clinical importance of these agents diminished substantially with the discovery of subsequent-generation protease inhibitors.

4.2.1.2. Second-wave, first-generation protease inhibitors

The second wave of PIs for HCV includes agents such as simeprevir, asunaprevir, danoprevir, faldaprevir, and vaniprevir [42, 43]. Simeprevir (*Olysio*) is a NS3/4A HCV PI. Simeprevir is a macrocyclic compound that noncovalently binds to and inhibits the NS3/4A HCV protease, a protein that is responsible for cleaving and processing the HCV-encoded polyprotein, a critical step in HCV viral life cycle [42, 43]. Simeprevir shows enhanced binding affinity and specificity to NS3/4A when compared with the first-generation PIs, TPV, and BOC.

The safety and efficacy of SIM/PEG-IFN/RBV combination was investigated in treatment-naïve patients with HCV genotype 1 infection (PILLAR trial) [44]. Enrolled patients received different SIM doses administered once-daily (QD) with pegylated interferon (Peg-IFN)-α-2a and ribavirin (RBV). According to response-guided therapy (RGT) criteria, 79.2–86.1% of SMV-treated patients completed treatment by week 24; 85.2–95.6% of these subsequently achieved SVR. The safety profile of triple therapy with SIM was found to be comparable to that of PEG-IFN/RBV combination therapy [44]. In the QUEST 1 and QUEST 2 studies [45, 46], conducted on treatment-naïve genotype 1, patients were randomized to receive either triple therapy with simeprevir plus PEG-IFN and RBV using a response-guided therapy (RGT) approach or standard of care (48 weeks of PEG-IFN and RBV with placebo control). SVR12 rates were 81% in the simeprevir arm versus 50% in the control arm. The majority of simeprevir-treated patients met the RGT and received 24 weeks of treatment and 86% of these patients achieved an SVR12.

Simeprevir also enhanced SVR in treatment-experienced patients. In the ASPIRE trial [47] treatment-experienced patients (with prior failure to PEG/RBV) were randomized to receive placebo plus PEG/RBV, or one of six regimens consisting of SMV plus PEG-IFN-α-2a plus ribavirin. In the SMV-treated patients, the SVR 24 rates ranged from 61 to 80% (according to the regimen used), which was significantly higher than the 23% SVR in patients treated with PEG-IFN/RBV. The safety profile observed among patients in the simeprevir arm was similar to the safety profile for patients in the placebo arm. These results were supported by those of another clinical trial conducted on treatment-experienced HCV genotype 1 patients with a history of viral relapse. The overall SVR12 in patients treated with SIM/PEG-IFN/RBV was of 79% compared to 36% for the peginterferon plus ribavirin arm. Patients with advanced fibrosis (F3-F4 by METAVIR) also had superior SVR12 rates with the addition of simeprevir (73% SVR12 compared with 24% in control arm) [48].

The efficacy of SIM/PEG-IFN/RBV in treatment-naïve and treatment-experienced patients with chronic HCV genotype 4 was evaluated in the RESTORE trial. Overall, 65.4% of the patients achieved an SRV12. The SVR12 rates varied with treatment group being 83% in treatment-naïve, 86% in treatment-experienced with prior relapse, 60% in prior partial responders, and 40% in prior null responders [49].

These trials showed that simeprevir-based/PEG-IFN/RBV triple therapy was effective, well-tolerated, and safe. However, the fast-paced HCV drug discovery paved the way to new interferon-free combinations which combine efficacy, safety, and convenience. Thus, SMV was included with other DAAs such as sofosbuvir to form one of the earliest interferon-free combinations (discussed later).

Danoprevir (DNV) is a highly selective and potent second-wave inhibitor of HCV NS3/4A protease. Coadministration of 100 mg of ritonavir with DNV has been shown to optimize the pharmacokinetics of DNV, allowing for lower dosing and better antiviral activity The DAUPHINE trial [50] evaluated three different dosages of DNV/r: 50, 100, and 200 mg danoprevir, boosted with 100 mg ritonavir, consumed twice a day for 24 weeks. A study arm also explored danoprevir/r 100/100 mg, in a response-guided therapy (RGT) algorithm, in which patients reaching an RVR received a total of 12 weeks of treatment. Overall, the better SVR rates were achieved in higher dosage arms compared to lower dosage arms. SVR rates decreased with decreasing dosage of danoprevir/r as follows: 89.1, 78.5, and 69.1% [50]. Faldaprevir was evaluated in IFN-free regimen in combination with deleobuvir, an NS5B no nucleoside polymerase inhibitor and ribavirin, in HCV-1b patients. The combination was highly efficacious, with 95% achieving SVR12 including patients with compensated cirrhosis [51].

Taken together, the second-wave, first-generation protease inhibitors offer several benefits over the first-generation PIs, TVR, and BOC in terms of less side effect profile and more convenient dosing. However, these preparations still have low genetic barrier to resistance particularly for HCV-1a.

4.2.1.3. Second-generation protease inhibitors

Recent second-generation PIs such as the macrocyclic compound grazoprevir offer several benefits over earlier protease inhibitors, including fewer drug-drug interactions, improved dosing schedules, and less frequent and less severe side effects. Grazoprevir is distinct from earlier-generation protease inhibitors in potency against a broader array of HCV genotypes, as well as its activity against some of the major resistance-associated variants (R155K and D168Y) resulting from failure with first-generation protease inhibitors. Grazoprevir is available in combination with the NS5A inhibitor elbasvir. Elbasvir/grazoprevir (Zepatier) [52] is available as fixed dose tablets (50/100 mg) are prescribed as one tablet orally once daily, with or without food. The treatment duration and whether to take with or without ribavirin are dependent on genotypes and other patient variables [53].

The C-EDGE treatment-naïve trial assessed the safety and efficacy of the fixed-dose combination of elbasvir-grazoprevir (50/100 mg) in patients with genotype 1, 4, or 6 hepatitis C infection, with or without compensated cirrhosis. The overall SVR12 rate was 95%, with rates of 92% for genotype 1a, 99% for genotype 1b, 100% for genotype 4, and 80% for genotype 6. No statistically significant difference in SVR12 was found between cirrhotic and noncirrhotic patients [54]. The C-EDGE CO-STAR trial enrolled treatment-naïve patients who inject drugs and were infected with chronic HCV genotype 1, 4, or 6. In this difficult to treat cohort, the SVR12 were 95% [55].

Treatment-naïve patients with compensated cirrhosis and treatment-experienced patients with a prior null response to PEG plus RBV were randomized to receive elbasvir plus grazoprevir, with or without ribavirin, for 12 or 18 weeks. The SVR12 rates ranged between 90 and 97% in cirrhotics and 94% in null responder cirrhotic patients. The SVR12 was 100% for genotype 1b. No additional benefit was achieved by adding ribavirin to elbasvir plus grazoprevir in a subset of patients [56]. Treatment-experienced patients with genotype 1 HCV with previous failure of peg interferon/ribavirin (PR) and an earlier-generation protease inhibitor (BOC, TPV, or SIM) achieved SVR 24 of 96% when treated with elbasvir plus grazoprevir and RBV [57].

In the C-EDGE coinfection trial, patients with chronic hepatitis C genotype 1, 4, or 6 and HIV coinfection received elbasvir-grazoprevir once daily for 12 weeks. Patients were on antiretroviral therapy with HIV viral suppression and the median CD4 cell count was 568 cells/mm^3. The overall SVR12 rate was 96, with the breakdown by genotype SVR12 rates were 96.5, 95.5, and 96.4% for genotypes 1a, 1b, and 4, respectively. All cirrhotic patients achieved an SVR12 [58].

Thus, zepatier is active against a broad array of HCV genotypes including genotypes 1, 4, 6, as well as some of the major resistance-associated variants (R155K and D168Y) resulting from failure with first-generation protease inhibitors. Elbasvir/grazoprevir is generally well tolerated; however, the adverse effects reported include headache, nausea, fatigue, decreased appetite, anemia, pyrexia, and elevations of ALT.

4.2.2. NS5B nucleoside polymerase inhibitors (NPIs)

NS5B is an RNA-dependent RNA polymerase (RdRp) involved in posttranslational processing which is vital for HCV replication. NPIs are analogs of natural substrates that bind the active site of NS5B and terminate viral RNA chain generation. Given that the structure of NS5B is highly conserved across all HCV genotypes, NPIs are effective against all genotypes. NPIs show high antiviral activities in all genotypes and provide a high genetic barrier to resistance. Thus, NPIs are included in several efficacious all-oral combination therapies. Polymerase inhibitors are categorized according to their mode of action and specificity into NPIs and NNPIs. These two classes generally differ in specificity. Nucleoside inhibitors (NIs) bind to the catalytic site of the RNA polymerase causing chain termination. Nonnucleoside inhibitors bind to a less conserved site resulting in a conformational change that distorts the positioning of residues binding RNA resulting in inhibition of polymerization [59, 60].

4.2.2.1. Sofosbuvir (sovaldi)

Sofosbuvir is a nucleoside analog inhibitor of hepatitis C virus NS5B polymerase. The triphosphate form of sofosbuvir mimics the natural cellular uridine nucleotide and is incorporated by the HCV RNA polymerase into the elongating RNA primer strand, resulting in viral chain termination. Sofosbuvir is a prodrug which is rapidly converted after oral intake to GS-331007 which is taken up by hepatocytes. The cellular kinases convert GS-331007 to its pharmacologically active uridine analog 5′-triphosphate form (GS-461203) that is incorporated by the HCV RNA polymerase into the elongating RNA primer strand, resulting in chain termination. Sofosbuvir is a potent pangenotypic NS5B polymerase inhibitor with a high barrier to resistance. It is available as 400 mg tablets administered once a day with or without food. The discovery of sofosbuvir has been a breakthrough in HCV treatment. Currently, SOF represents the backbone of several interferon-free regimens for the treatment of chronic hepatitis caused by various HCV genotypes. Excretion of sofosbuvir is through the kidney (80%) [58, 59, 61].

4.2.3. Efficacy of sofosbuvir plus peginterferon and ribavirin

The ATOMIC and ELECTRON (Arms 1-8 studies) [62, 63] established the effectiveness of a 12-week course of sofosbuvir plus peginterferon and ribavirin in treatment-naïve patients with HCVgenotype-1 with SVR rates ranging between 87 and 100%. In genotypes 3, the SVR 12 rates were 71% with the 16-week SOF plus RBV regimen, 84% with 24 weeks of SOV plus RBV, and 93% with 12 weeks of SOF plus RBV plus PEG-IFN. For the patients with genotype 2 infections, the SVR 12 rates were 87% with the 16-week SOF plus RBV regimen, 100% with 24 weeks of SOF plus RBV, and 94% with 12 weeks of SOF plus RBV plus PEG-IFN [64].

4.2.4. Efficacy of interferon-free sofosbuvir regimen

4.2.4.1. Sofosbuvir (SOF) and simeprevir (SIM) combination (Olysio)

This combination is the earliest interferon-free regimen that reached optimal results in terms of SVR. Trials showed efficacy and safety of this drug combination in treatment-naïve and treatment-experienced patients across several genotypes. The OPTIMIST-1 trial evaluated the efficacy of sofosbuvir plus simeprevir for 8 or 12 weeks in treatment naive or experienced patients with chronic HCV genotype 1 infection without cirrhosis. The sustained response rates were 97% in patients treated for 12 weeks and the SVR was 83% in patients treated for 8 weeks. These findings were further confirmed in the OPTIMIST-2 trial which demonstrated that 12-week regimen of SOF plus SIM is effective in treatment-naïve and treatment-experienced patients with cirrhosis and HCV genotype 1 infection, with the exception that patients with genotype 1a and the baseline Q80K mutation have SVR rates of only 74% [66].

A large cohort prospective study in genotype 1 patients treated with SOF plus SIM for 12–16 weeks showed that the overall SVR rate was 84%. Model-adjusted estimates demonstrated that patients with cirrhosis, prior decompensation, and previous protease inhibitor treatments were less likely to achieve an SVR. Addition of ribavirin enhances SVR rates in such patients [67].

Taken together, several clinical trials demonstrate that all-oral 12-week regimen of simeprevir plus sofosbuvir is effective and well tolerated in treatment-naïve and treatment-experienced HCV genotype 1 patients without and with cirrhosis. Ribavirin may be needed in patients with decompensation, and previous protease inhibitor treatment failure. The frequent adverse events include fatigue, headache, nausea, rashes, and insomnia. Serious adverse events and treatment discontinuation occur in only 3% of patients.

4.2.4.2. Sofosbuvir with the NS5A inhibitor ledipasvir (Harvoni)

- Treatment-naïve and treatment-experienced genotype 1 patients

Gane et al. [68] evaluated an all-oral regimen comprising sofosbuvir with ledipasvir or the NS5B nonnucleoside inhibitor GS-9669 in patients with genotype 1 HCV infection. Sofosbuvir (400 mg once daily) and ledipasvir (90 mg once daily) plus ribavirin were given for 12 weeks to treatment-naïve patients and prior null responders. Sofosbuvir and GS-9669 (500 mg once daily) plus ribavirin were given for 12 weeks to treatment-naïve patients and prior null responders. Additionally, prior null responders with cirrhosis were randomly assigned to groups given a fixed-dose combination of sofosbuvir and ledipasvir, with ribavirin or without ribavirin and a group of treatment-naïve patients received sofosbuvir, ledipasvir, and ribavirin for 6 weeks. SVR12 was 100, 92, and 68% in treatment-naïve patients receiving sofosbuvir, those receiving SOV, ledipasvir, ribavirin, GS-9669, and ribavirin and patients receiving 6 weeks of sofosbuvir, ledipasvir, and ribavirin, respectively. All noncirrhotic prior null responders receiving 12 weeks of sofosbuvir along with another DAA plus RBV achieved SVR12 of 100%.

In the NIAID SYNERGY (genotype 1 study) [69], treatment-naïve patients with genotype 1 chronic HCV were randomized to receive either ledipasvir-sofosbuvir for 12 weeks; or ledipasvir-sofosbuvir (90-400 mg) plus the nonnucleoside NS5B inhibitor GS-9669 (500 mg once daily) for 6 weeks, or ledipasvir-sofosbuvir (90-400 mg) plus the NS3/4A protease inhibitor GS-9451 (80 mg once daily) for 6 weeks. Patients in the 12-week ledipasvir-sofosbuvir arm with any stage of fibrosis could be enrolled in the study. The SVR12 rates were 100, 95, and 95% in the ledipasvir-sofosbuvir arm, the ledipasvir-sofosbuvir plus GS-9669 group, and the ledipasvir-sofosbuvir plus GS-9451 group, respectively.

A trial [70] evaluated 8- and 12-week courses of the fixed-dose combination of ledipasvir (90 mg) and sofosbuvir (400 mg), with or without ribavirin in treatment-naïve and treatment-experienced patients with chronic HCV genotype 1 infection. In all of the five study arms,

SVR12 was achieved in 95–100% of patients. The regimen of ledipasvir-sofosbuvir was well tolerated; only one patient had a serious adverse event of anemia, thought to be related to ribavirin. A recent large study that enrolled 4365 genotype 1, treatment-naïve, HCV-infected patients treated with LDV/SOF±RBV demonstrated SVR rates of 91.3 and 92.0% (3191/3495) for LDV/SOF and LDV/SOF+RBV, respectively [71].

Thus, the combination of ledipasvir-sofosbuvir with or without ribavirin is highly effective in treatment-naïve and treatment-experienced patients with chronic HCV genotype 1.

- Sofosbuvir- ledipasvir in HCV nongenotype 1 patients

Patients with genotype 3 and 6 achieved good SVR rates when treated with ledipasvir-sofosbuvir. The SVR 12 responses in treatment-naïve patients with genotype 3 were superior in the regimen with ribavirin (100%) than without ribavirin (64%). Among the treatment-experienced patients, 82% of treated ledipasvir-sofosbuvir plus ribavirin achieved an SVR 12 and the SVR 12 rate was 96% in the patients with genotype 6 [72].

The NIAID SYNERGY (Genotype 4) trial enrolled treatment-naïve and treatment-experienced patients with genotype 4 chronic HCV to receive ledipasvir-sofosbuvir for 12 weeks. Patients with compensated cirrhosis were allowed to enroll in the study. Overall, in the intent-to-treat SVR was 95% [73]. A recent study that enrolled treatment-naïve and -experienced patients with chronic HCV genotype 4 revealed SVR12 of 78% in patients treated with ledipasvir-sofosbuvir for 12 weeks and SVR 12 in patients treated with 24 weeks [74]. These findings suggest that further studies are still needed to optimize ledipasvir-sofosbuvir therapy in patients with different stages of chronic HCV genotype 4. To date, the efficacy and duration of DAAs in HCV genotype 4 have not been adequately studied and further trials are required to optimize therapy in this genotype.

A clinical trial assessed response to ledipasvir-sofosbuvir in 41 patients with chronic HCV genotype 5 (21 treatment-naïve and 20 treatment-experienced). The overall SVR12 was 95% in treatment-naïve and treatment-experienced patients, while the SVR12 was 97% in patients without cirrhosis and 89% in patients with cirrhosis [75].

- HCV and HIV coinfected patients

The ERADICATE trial investigated the safety and efficacy of a 12-week regimen of ledipasvir-sofosbuvir in HCV treatment-naïve patients with genotype 1 chronic hepatitis C who are coinfected with HIV. Patients on antiretroviral therapy were allowed to receive tenofovir-emtricitabine plus either efavirenz, raltegravir, rilpivirine, rilpivirine plus raltegravir, or efavirenz plus raltegravir. In patients taking antiretroviral therapy, SVR12 was 97% [76]. The SVR12 was 96.4% in German HIV-HCV coinfected patients [77]. A study investigated the efficacy and safety of ledipasvir/sofosbuvir plus ribavirin for 24 weeks in HCV/HIV-coinfected patients who relapsed after receiving 12 weeks of ledipasvir/sofosbuvir therapy. The SVR12 was 89% suggesting that ledipasvir/sofosbuvir can be an effective salvage therapy for patients for whom direct-acting antiviral treatment has failed [78].

Thus, ledipasvir-sofosbuvir is well tolerated and effective in patients with genotype 1 HCV and HIV coinfection. However, more studies are required to investigate the efficacy and safety of ledipasvir/sofosbuvir in treatment of HIV patients infected with various HCV genotypes.

Importantly the drug-drug interactions between ledipasvir/sofosbuvir and antiretroviral therapy need extensive investigations on large cohorts.

-Retreatment of sofosbuvir failures

In the NIAID retreatment of sofosbuvir failures trial [79], patients with genotype 1 HCV who previously had failed a 24-week course of sofosbuvir plus ribavirin achieved SVR12 ranged between 98 and 100% when retreated with fixed-dose combination of ledipasvir-sofosbuvir for 12 weeks. Despite the small sample size in this study, the trial showed that 12-week regimen of ledipasvir-sofosbuvir without or with ribavirin was well tolerated and shows promise as a treatment option for patients with prior sofosbuvir failure.

4.2.4.3. Sofosbuvir/velpatasvir (Epclusa)

Sofosbuvir-velpatasvir (sofosbuvir 400 mg plus velpatasvir 100 mg) is an oral fixed-dose combination of sofosbuvir, and the novel NS5A replication complex inhibitor, velapatasvir. Velpatasvir (formerly GS-5816) has potent *in vitro* anti-HCV activity across all genotypes at the picomolar level. The combination of sofosbuvir-velpatasvir is the first once-daily single-tablet regimen with pangenotypic activity. Sofosbuvir-velpatasvir is indicated for patients with chronic HCV genotype 1 through 6 [80]. A clinical trial [81] assessed the efficacy and safety of the combination of the nucleotide polymerase inhibitor sofosbuvir, the NS5A inhibitor velpatasvir, and the NS3/4A protease inhibitor GS-9857 in patients with hepatitis C virus (HCV) genotype 1 infection. Among treatment-naïve patients without cirrhosis, the SVR rates were 71 and 100% after 6 and 8 weeks of treatment, respectively. Among treatment-naïve patients with cirrhosis, 94% achieved SVR12 after 8 weeks therapy and 81% after 8 weeks of treatment with ribavirin. The SVR12 rates were 100% in DAA-experienced patients without cirrhosis and with cirrhosis, respectively.

Sofosbuvir-velpatasvir showed high efficacy in non-1 genotypes. ASTRAL-2 study demonstrated that the SVR12 was 99% treatment-naïve and treatment-experienced patients infected with HCV genotype 2 [82]. Among HCV with chronic HCV genotype 3 treated with sofosbuvir-velpatasvir, the ASTRAL-3 trial showed that the SVR12 rate were 93% for treatment-naïve and 89% for treatment-experienced patients [83]. SVR12 was 100% in patients with chronic HCV genotype 4 [84]. The ASTRAL-4 studies [82] demonstrated that sofosbuvir/velpatasvir plus ribavirin were effective in achieving a high SVR12 rate in patients with decompensated cirrhosis [85].

The ASTRAL-5 study investigated the safety and efficacy of 12 weeks sofosbuvir-velpatasvir in patients with HIV and HCV coinfection. Enrolled patients were infected with genotype 1, 2, 3, 4, or 6 HCV infection; 18% had compensated cirrhosis and 29% were treatment-experienced. The mean CD4 count was 583 cells/mm^3 and all patients had HIV viral suppression. The antiretroviral regimens included tenofovir disoproxil fumarate (DF). The overall SVR12 rate was 95%. The presence of cirrhosis or treatment experience did not negatively influence treatment response [86].

4.2.5. Nonstructural protein 5A (NS5A) inhibitors

The NS5A protein is essential for replication and assembly of HCV. Inhibitors of NS5A block viral production at an early stage of assembly, so that no viral RNA or nucleocapsid protein is released [87]. Therefore, agents that block NS5B activity (polymerase inhibitors) inhibit the virus's RdRp [87]. Nucleoside inhibitors (NIs) bind to RdRp's active site, whereas the non-nucleoside inhibitors (NNIs) bind to the enzyme outside the active site, inducing conformational changes that downregulated RdRp's activity. As a result of mechanistic and potency differences, the NIs tend to have broad potency against multiple HCV genotypes and are less likely to select for resistant strains than are the NNIs [88]. Cyclophilin is a host protein that interacts with NS5B and appears to promote the HCV protein's ability to bind.

4.2.5.1. Daclatasvir (Daklinza)

Daclatasvir HCV is first-in-class inhibitor of the nonstructural viral protein 5A (NS5A), a phosphoprotein that plays an important role in hepatitis C replication. The exact mechanism by which daclatasvir inhibits the NS5A replication complex is unclear, but it is believed that daclatasvir inhibits viral RNA replication and virion assembly. It may also inhibit phosphorylation of the NS4A, and therefore the formation and activation of the HCV replication complex. Based on *in vitro* data, daclatasvir has shown activity against HCV genotypes 1 through 6, with EC50 values ranging from picomolar to low nanomolar against wild-type HCV [89].

When used in combination with sofosbuvir, with or without ribavirin, daclatasvir showed high efficacy in pangenotypic all-oral regimen. According to the results of the AI444040 and ALLY-3 trials [90, 91], a 12-week regimen of daclatasvir plus sofosbuvir in patients with chronic HCV genotype 1 or 3 infection without cirrhosis resulted in high SVR12 rates, regardless of prior treatment experience. The ALLY-3 [91] trial demonstrated high SVR12 rates with a 12- or 16-week regimen of daclatasvir plus sofosbuvir and ribavirin in patients with chronic HCV genotype 3 infections and advanced fibrosis or compensated cirrhosis. A daclatasvir plus sofosbuvir-based regimen demonstrated efficacy in patients with chronic HCV genotype 1, 3, or 4 infection and advanced cirrhosis or posttransplant recurrence in the ALLY-1 trial [92], and in patients coinfected with HCV genotype 1, 3, or 4 and HIV-1 in the ALLY-2 trial [93].

Daclatasvir plus sofosbuvir with or without ribavirin was generally well tolerated. Fatigue, headache, nausea, and diarrhea were the adverse events reported in some patients treated with daclatasvir [91–93]. Daclatasvir and sofosbuvir combination can potentially cause serious bradycardia when coadministered with amiodarone. Given that daclatasvir is a substrate of CYP3A, it is contraindicated for use with drugs that are strong inducers of CYP3A, including phenytoin, carbamazepine, and rifampin [94].

Data from clinical trials showed resistance-associated substitutions in the *NS5A* gene [95]. Thus, the AASLD/IDSA HCV Guidance Panel recommends testing for these substitutions when NS5A inhibitors fail [96]. Baseline NS5A polymorphisms may also impact the emergence of NS5A resistance [96].

Taken together, daclatasvir plus sofosbuvir with or without ribavirin is an important option for use in treatment-naïve or treatment-experienced patients with chronic HCV genotype 1, 3, or 4 infections, including patients with advanced liver disease, posttransplant recurrence, and HIV-1 coinfection. Daclatasvir with sofosbuvir is a particularly useful ribavirin-free oral option for genotype 3 patients. Testing for the presence of NS5A polymorphisms is recommended at baseline for patients with HCV genotype 1a prior to initiation of treatment with in patients with genotype 1a and cirrhosis prior to sofosbuvir plus daclatasvir treatment.

4.2.5.2. Liedipasvir

Ledipasvir is a potent inhibitor of HCV NS5A, a viral phosphoprotein that plays a critical role in viral replication, assembly, and secretion [97]. The results of clinical trials assessing ledipasvir combinations with SOF have been discussed previously.

Coadministration of amiodarone and ledipasvir-sofosbuvir is not recommended given that severe cases of symptomatic bradycardia have been reported. Ledipasvir-sofosbuvir has significant drug-drug interactions with P-gp inducers such as rifampin that may cause a significant reduction in levels of ledipasvir and sofosbuvir and reduced efficacy of ledipasvir-sofosbuvir [97].

4.2.6. Ombitasvir-paitaprevir-ritonavir-dasabuvir (Viekira Pak)

The four medications: ombitasvir, paritaprevir, ritonavir, and dasabuvir are combined as a fixed-dose tablet and the dasabuvir is a separate tablet. Ombitasvir is an NS5A inhibitor with potent pangenotypic picomolar antiviral activity, paritaprevir is an inhibitor of the NS3/4A serine protease, and dasabuvir is a nonnucleoside NS5B polymerase inhibitor. Ritonavir is a potent inhibitor of CYP3A4 enzymes and is used as a pharmacologic booster for paritaprevir—it significantly increases peak and trough paritaprevir plasma concentrations, as well as the area under the curve of paritaprevir [98].

PEARL III trial demonstrated the SVR12 rate of 99.5% in treatment-naïve patients with chronic HCV genotype 1b treated with ombitasvir-paritaprevir-ritonavir and dasabuvir plus ribavirin group and 99% in patients who received ombitasvir-paritaprevir-ritonavir and dasabuvir without ribavirin [99]. The TURQUOISE trial assessed the efficacy and safety of ombitasvir, paritaprevir, ritonavir, and dasabuvir plus RBV in HCV/HIV-1 coinfected patients for 12 or 24 weeks. The study enrolled HCV treatment-naïve or PEG-IFN/RBV-experienced patients, with or without Child-Pugh A cirrhosis. Patients with CD4+ count ≥200 cells/mm3 or CD4+ % ≥14%, and plasma HIV-1 RNA suppressed on a stable atazanavir- or raltegravir-inclusive antiretroviral (ART) regimen were included. Among patients treated with 3D+RBV for 12 weeks, 93.5% achieved SVR12. Among patients receiving 24 weeks of treatment, 96.9% achieved EOTR; the most common AEs were fatigue, insomnia, and nausea. Elevation in total bilirubin was the most common laboratory abnormality, occurring predominantly in patients receiving atazanavir.

This combination was effective liver transplant recipients who have recurrent hepatitis C genotype 1 infection [101]. In patients with stage 4 or 5 renal disease and patients on dialysis treated with ombitasvir-paritaprevir-ritonavir and dasabuvir., EOT response was 100% and SVR12 response was achieved in 85% of patients with genotype 1b [102].

5. Treatment of different HCV genotypes

According to the 2016 HCV treatment guidelines of the American Association for the Study of Liver Diseases (AASLD) and the Infectious Diseases Society of America (IDSA) [96] and European Association of Study of Liver Diseases (EASL) [99], chronic HCV due to any genotype can be efficiently treated using all-oral DAA interferon-free regimens.

http://dx.doi.org/10.5772/66719

5.1. HCV genotype 1 (Figure 4)

Optimizing the regimen of therapy for chronic HCV genotype 1 depends on several factors such as whether the patient is treatment naïve or experienced and the previous therapies provided and the status of resistance in some cases. Given the high cost of IFN-free regimen and difficulties in access to this therapy in various countries, it is necessary to tailor therapy according to the patient population treated and the available therapies.

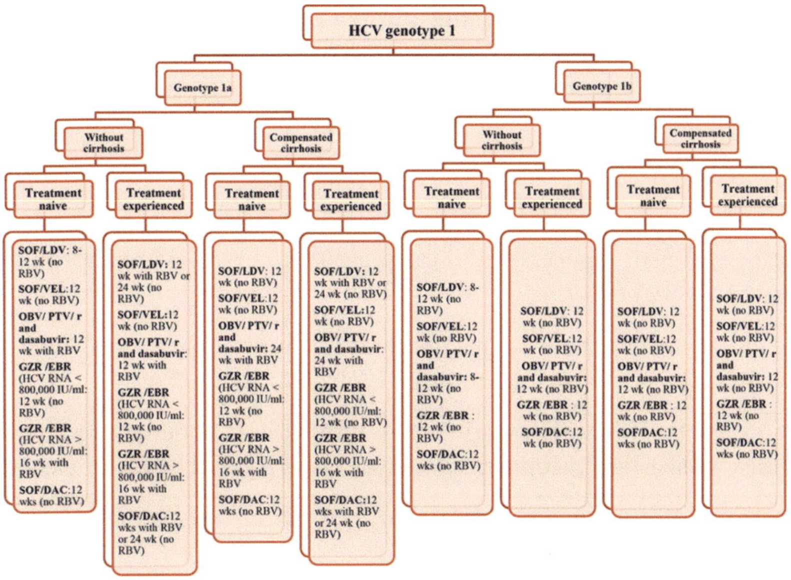

Figure 4. Treatment of HCV genotype 1.

5.2. Ledipasvir-sofosbuvir combination

- Treatment-naïve patients with or without compensated cirrhosis patients are treated with a fixed-dose combination of sofosbuvir and ledipasvir for 12 weeks.
- Therapy may be shortened to 8 weeks in patients with a viral load <6 million IU/ml.
- Treatment-experienced, DAA-naïve patients infected with genotype 1b with or without compensated cirrhosis are treated with the fixed-dose combination of sofosbuvir and ledipasvir for 12 weeks without ribavirin.
- Treatment-experienced, DAA-naïve patients infected with genotype 1a with or without compensated cirrhosis are treated with the fixed-dose combination of sofosbuvir and ledipasvir for 12 weeks with daily weight-based ribavirin (1000 or 1200 mg in patients <75 kg or =75 kg, respectively).
- If there is a contraindication to ribavirin, the treatment-experienced, DAA-naïve patients are treated with Harvoni for 24 weeks.

- Treatment-experienced, DAA-naïve patients infected with genotype 1a with or without compensated cirrhosis who have NS5A RASs and resistance to ledipasvir (M28A/G/T, Q30E/G/H/K/R, L31M/V, P32L/S, H58D, and/or Y93C/H/N/S) are treated with the fixed-dose combination of sofosbuvir and ledipasvir for 12 weeks with ribavirin.

5.3. Sofosbuvir-velpatasvir

- Genotype 1a, regardless of the presence of cirrhosis: sofosbuvir-velpatasvir is prescribed for 12 weeks without ribavirin in treatment naïve or treatment experienced.
- Genotype 1b, regardless of the presence of cirrhosis: sofosbuvir-velpatasvir is prescribed for 12 weeks without ribavirin in treatment naïve or treatment experienced.

5.4. Elbasvir-grazoprevir

Elbasvir-grazoprevir (50 mg/100 mg) therapy in chronic hepatitis C genotypes 1 is tailored according prior treatment experience and the presence of baseline polymorphisms at amino acid positions 28, 30, 31, or 93.

- Genotype 1a, treatment-naïve or peginterferon/ribavirin-experienced with no baseline NS5A polymorphisms: elbasvir-grazoprevir is given for 12 weeks.
- Genotype 1a, treatment-naïve or peginterferon/ribavirin-experienced with baseline NS5A polymorphisms: elbasvir-grazoprevir plus ribavirin is prescribed for 16 weeks.
- Genotype 1b, treatment-naïve or peginterferon/ribavirin-experienced: elbasvir-grazoprevir is given for 12 weeks.
- Genotype 1a or 1b, peginterferon/ribavirin/protease inhibitor-experienced: elbasvir-grazoprevir plus ribavirin is given for 12 weeks.

5.4.1. Sofosbuvir and daclatasvir

In genotype 1 infections, sofosbuvir and daclatasvir are used with or without ribavirin depending on the patient population

- Genotype 1, without cirrhosis: daclatasvir plus sofosbuvir are prescribed for 12 weeks.
- Genotype 1 with compensated cirrhosis: daclatasvir plus sofosbuvir are given for 12 weeks.
- Genotype 1 with decompensated (Child-Pugh B or C) cirrhosis: daclatasvir plus sofosbuvir plus ribavirin are given for 12 weeks.

5.4.2. Ombitasvir-paritaprevir-ritonavir-dasabuvir

In regions where this combination is available, the therapeutic strategy is recommended as follows:

- Genotype 1a, without cirrhosis: ombitasvir-paritaprevir-ritonavir and dasabuvir plus ribavirin are prescribed for 12 weeks.

- Genotype 1a, with cirrhosis: ombitasvir-paritaprevir-ritonavir and dasabuvir plus ribavirin are prescribed for 24 weeks.
- Genotype 1b, without cirrhosis: ombitasvir-paritaprevir-ritonavir and dasabuvir are prescribed for 12 weeks.
- Genotype 1b, with cirrhosis: ombitasvir-paritaprevir-ritonavir and dasabuvir plus ribavirin are prescribed for 12 weeks

Thus, Viekira Pak prescribed with ribavirin except in patients without cirrhosis

*Genotype 2 (***Figure 5***)*

Chronic HCV genotype 2 treatment-naïve or treatment-experienced patients are treated with either with aofosbuvir/velpatasvir for 12 weeks without ribavirin or sofosbuvir and daclatasvir without ribavirin.

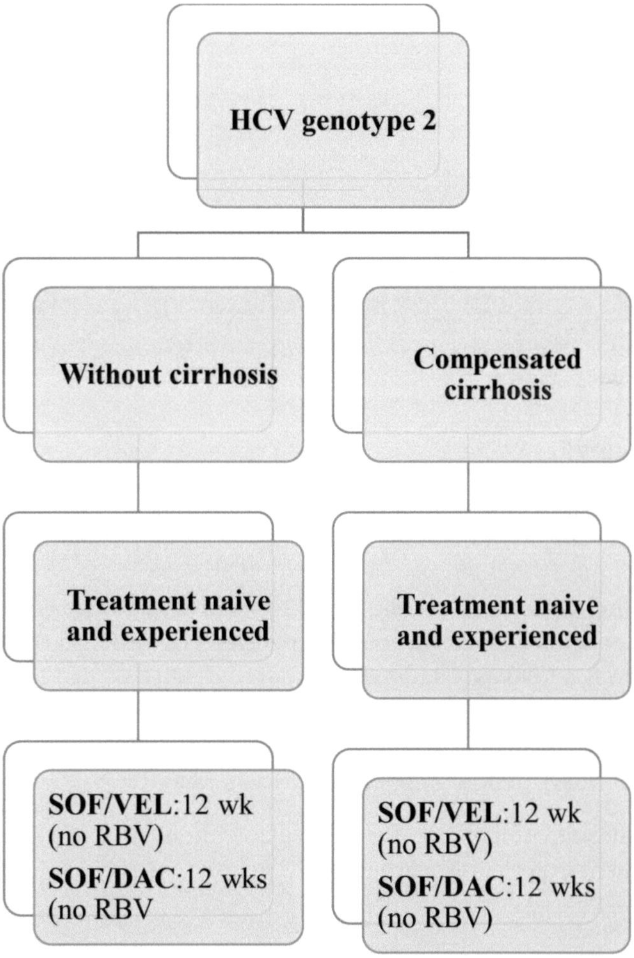

Figure 5. Treatment of HCV genotype 2.

HCV genotype 3 (**Figure 6**)

Chronic HCV genotype 2 treatment-naïve patients are treated with either sofosbuvir/velpatasvir for 12 weeks without ribavirin or sofosbuvir and daclatasvir without ribavirin. Ribavirin is added for the therapy of treatment-experienced patients.

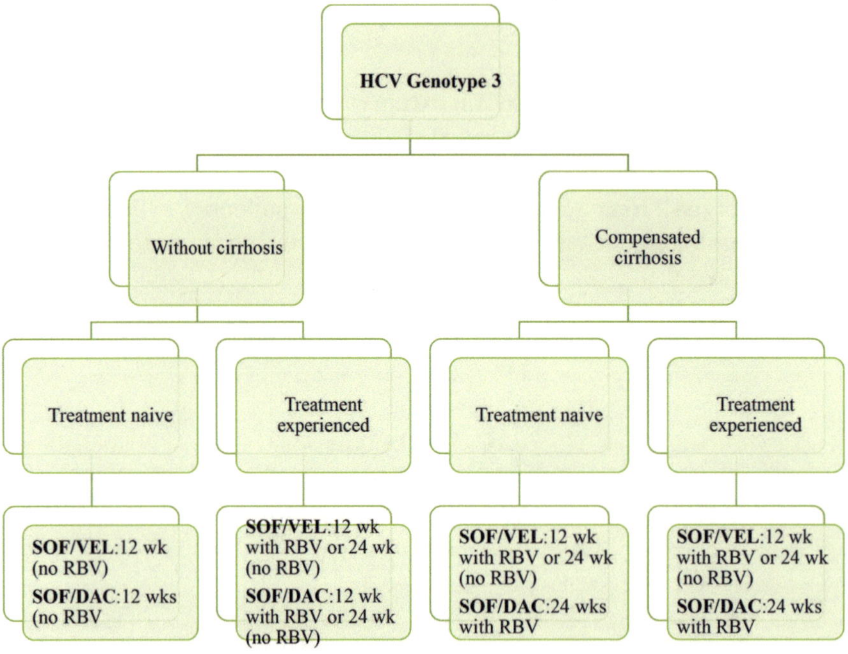

Figure 6. Treatment of HCV genotype 3.

HCV genotype 4 (**Figure 7**)

Treatment-naïve patients with chronic hepatitis C genotype 4 can be treated by one of the following regimen according to availability:

- Sofosbuvir (400 mg)/ledipasvir (90 mg) for 12 weeks without ribavirin is prescribed for treatment-naïve patients with or without compensated cirrhosis. In treatment-experienced patients, ribavirin is added as a daily weight-based dose (1000 or 1200 mg in patients <75 kg or =75 kg, respectively). Sofosbuvir and ledipasvir for 24 weeks is recommended for treatment-experienced patients with or without compensated cirrhosis with contraindications to the use of ribavirin or with poor tolerance to ribavirin.
- Sofosbuvir/velpatasvir combination for 12 weeks without ribavirin is given to treatment-naïve and treatment-experienced chronic HCV genotype 4 patients with or without compensated cirrhosis.
- Ombitasvir (12.5 mg), paritaprevir (75 mg), and ritonavir (50 mg) is given as two tablets once daily without dasabuvir to patients infected with HCV genotype 4 with and without compensated cirrhosis.

http://dx.doi.org/10.5772/66719

- Grazoprevir (100 mg) and elbasvir (50 mg) without ribavirin is prescribed as one tablet daily to treatment-naïve patients infected with genotype 4 with or without compensated cirrhosis. In treatment-experienced patients infected with genotype 4 with or without compensated cirrhosis with an HCV RNA level at baseline >800,000 IU/ml are treated with grazoprevir and elbasvir for 16 weeks with daily weight-based ribavirin (1000 or 1200 mg in patients <75 kg or =75 kg, respectively).

- Sofosbuvir (400 mg) and daclatasvir (60 mg) is given to treatment-naïve patients with or without cirrhosis should be treated with the combination of sofosbuvir and daclatasvir for 12 weeks without ribavirin. Ribavirin (1000 or 1200 mg in patients <75 kg or =75 kg) is added for treatment-experienced patients with or without compensated cirrhosis.

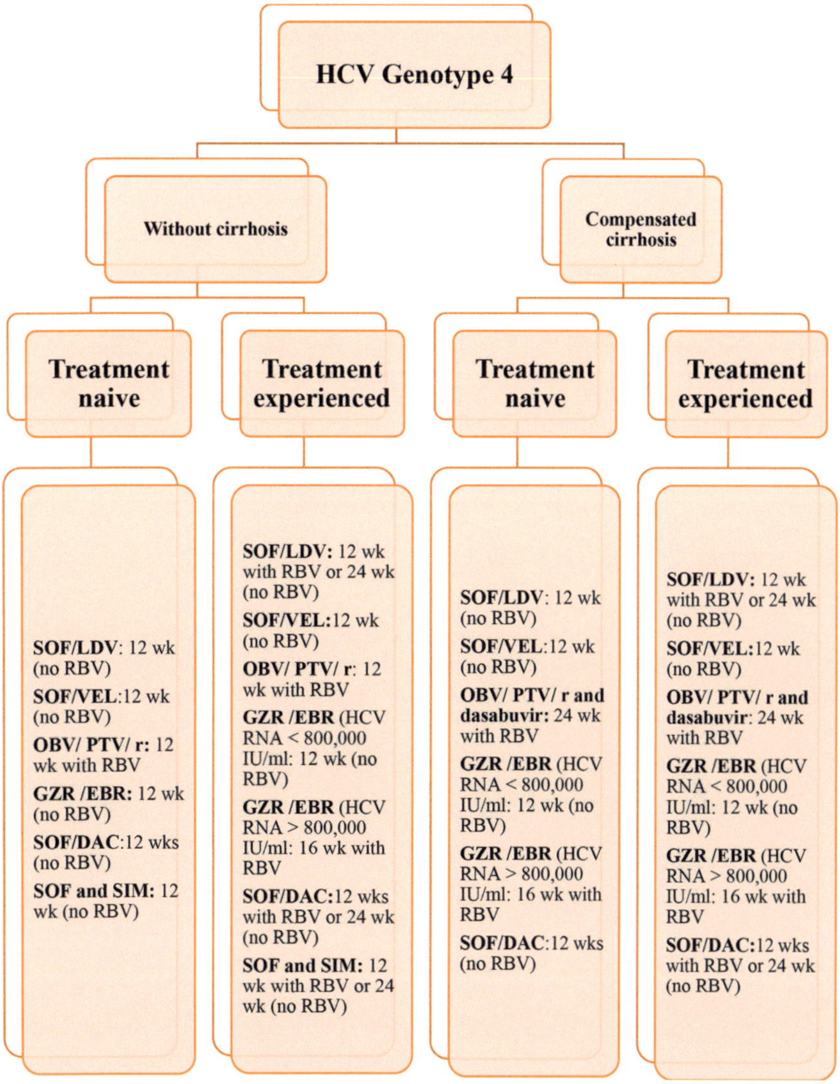

Figure 7. Treatment of HCV genotype 4.

*HCV genotype 5 or 6 (***Figure 8***)*

Treatment-naïve patients with or without compensated cirrhosis patients with chronic HCV genotype 5 or 6 are treated with sofosbuvir and ledipasvir for 12 weeks without ribavirin. Treatment-experienced patients with or without compensated cirrhosis are treated with the combination of sofosbuvir and ledipasvir for 12 weeks with daily weight-based ribavirin (1000 or 1200 mg in patients <75 kg or =75 kg, respectively. Treatment-naïve and treatment-experienced patients with or without compensated cirrhosis are treated with the fixed-dose combination of sofosbuvir and velpatasvir for 12 weeks without ribavirin, and ribavirin is added in patients with treatment-experienced patients.

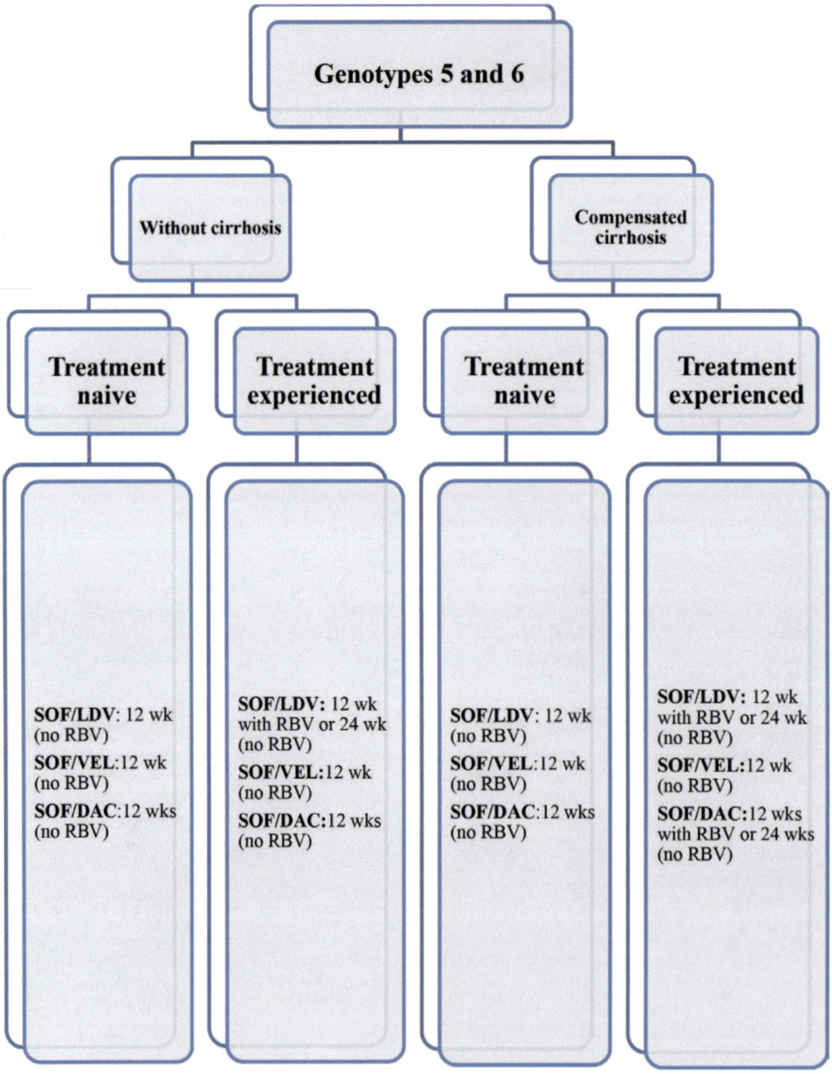

Figure 8. Treatment of HCV genotype 5, 6. *Note*: Ledipasvir: LDV; Sofosbuvir: SOF; Ribavirin: RBV; Simeprevir: SIM, Velpatasvir: VEL; Elbasvir: EBR; Grazoprevir: GZR; Daclatasvir: DAC; Ombitasvir: OBV; Paritaprevir: PTV; Rintonavir: r.

http://dx.doi.org/10.5772/66719

6. Patients with HCV and HIV coinfection

Patients with HCV and HIV coinfection are treated according to genotype and prior treatment status as follows [96, 99, 100, 101]:

(1) Genotype 1a, treatment-naïve patients may be treated with any of the following regimen:

   a. Sofosbuvir/ledipasvir for 12 weeks without ribavirin

   b. Sofosbuvir/velpatasvir for 12 weeks without ribavirin

   c. Ombitasvir/paritaprevir/ritonavir and dasabuvir for 12 weeks with ribavirin

   d. Grazoprevir/elbasvir for 12 weeks without ribavirin if HCV RNA=800,000 IU/ml or 16 weeks with ribavirin if HCV RNA >800,000 IU/ml

   e. Sofosbuvir/daclatasvir for 12 weeks without ribavirin

   Genotype 1a, treatment-experienced patients may be treated with any of the following regimen:

   a. Sofosbuvir/ledipasvir for 12 weeks with ribavirin or 24 weeks without ribavirin

   b. Sofosbuvir/velpatasvir for 12 weeks without ribavirin

   c. Ombitasvir/paritaprevir/ritonavir and dasabuvir for 12 weeks with ribavirin

   d. Grazoprevir/elbasvir for 12 weeks without ribavirin if HCV RNA=800,000 IU/ml or 16 weeks with ribavirin if HCV RNA >800,000 IU/ml

   e. Sofosbuvir/daclatasvir for 12 weeks with ribavirin or 24 weeks without ribavirin

(2) Genotype 1b, treatment-naïve and treatment-experienced patients may be treated with any of the following regimen:

   a. Sofosbuvir/ledipasvir for 12 weeks without ribavirin

   b. Sofosbuvir/velpatasvir for 12 weeks without ribavirin

   c. Ombitasvir/paritaprevir/ritonavir and dasabuvir for 12 weeks with ribavirin

   d. Grazoprevir/elbasvir for 12 weeks without ribavirin

   e. Sofosbuvir/daclatasvir for 12 weeks without ribavirin

(3) Genotype 2, treatment-naïve and treatment-experienced patients may be treated with any of the following regimen:

   a. Sofosbuvir/velpatasvir for 12 weeks without ribavirin

   b. Sofosbuvir/daclatasvir for 12 weeks without ribavirin

(4) Genotype 3, treatment-naïve and treatment-experienced patients may be treated with any of the following regimen:

a. Sofosbuvir/velpatasvir for 12 weeks with ribavirin or 24 weeks without ribavirin

b. Sofosbuvir/daclatasvir for 12 weeks with ribavirin

(5) Genotype 4 treatment-naïve patients may be treated with any of the following regimen:

a. Sofosbuvir/ledipasvir for 12 weeks without ribavirin

b. Sofosbuvir/velpatasvir for 12 weeks without ribavirin

c. Ombitasvir/paritaprevir/ritonavir with ribavirin for 12 weeks

d. Grazoprevir/elbasvir for 12 weeks without ribavirin

e. Sofosbuvir/daclatasvir for 12 weeks without ribavirin

f. Sofosbuvir and simeprevir for 12 weeks without ribavirin

Genotype 4 treatment-experienced patients may be treated with any of the following regimen:

g. Sofosbuvir/ledipasvir for 12 weeks with ribavirin and 24 weeks with ribavirin

h. Sofosbuvir/velpatasvir for 12 weeks without ribavirin

i. Ombitasvir/paritaprevir/ritonavir with ribavirin for 12 weeks

j. Grazoprevir/elbasvir for 12 weeks without ribavirin if HCV RNA =800,000 or 16 weeks with ribavirin if HCV RNA >800,000 IU/ml

k. Sofosbuvir/daclatasvir for 12 weeks with ribavirin or 24 weeks without ribavirin

l. Sofosbuvir and simeprevir for 12 weeks with ribavirin or 24 weeks without ribavirin

Daclatasvir, dose requirement is needed with ritonavir-boosted atazanavir and efavirenz or etravirine. Simeprevir should be used with antiretroviral drugs with which it does not have clinically significant interactions. In addition, it is recommended daily fixed doses of combined sofosbuvir (400 mg)/velpatasvir (100 mg) and of ledipasvir (90 mg)/sofosbuvir (400 mg). For combinations expected to increase tenofovir levels, baseline and ongoing assessment for tenofovir nephrotoxicity is recommended. Regarding HCV/HIV individuals, they should be treated and retreated the same as persons without HIV infection, after recognizing and managing interactions with antiretroviral medications [100, 101].

6.1. Treatment of patients with decompensated cirrhosis

Patients with decompensated cirrhosis and those awaiting liver transplantation are managed according to the HCV genotype. Patients with genotypes 1 and 4 are treated with daily fixed-dose combination of ledipasvir (90 mg)/sofosbuvir (400 mg) with low initial dose of ribavirin (600 mg, increased as tolerated) for 12 weeks. Another regimen is a daily fixed-dose combination of sofosbuvir (400 mg)/velpatasvir (100 mg) with weight-based ribavirin for 12 weeks. Finally, daily doses of daclatasvir (60 mg) plus sofosbuvir (400 mg) with low initial dose of ribavirin (600 mg, increased as tolerated) are given for 12 weeks. For patients who are ribavirin ineligible, the recommended regime is a daily fixed dose combination of sofosbuvir (400 mg)/velpatasvir (100 mg) for 24 weeks. Another regime is a combination of ledipasvir (90 mg)/sofosbuvir (400 mg) for 24 weeks. Patients who previously failed sofosbuvir-based treatment are given a combination of ledipasvir (90 mg)/sofosbuvir (400 mg) with low initial dose of ribavirin (600 mg, increased as tolerated) for 24 weeks [96, 99, 102]. Patients with HCV genotype 2 or 3 infection and decompensated cirrhosis are treated with daily fixed-dose combination sofosbuvir (400 mg)/velpatasvir (100 mg) with weight-based ribavirin for 12 weeks [96, 99, 102].

6.2. Patients with HCV recurrence after liver transplantation

Patients who develop HCV after transplantation and with compensated cirrhosis are treated with daily fixed-dose combination of ledipasvir (90 mg)/sofosbuvir (400 mg) with weight-based ribavirin for 12 weeks. Treatment-naïve patients with HCV genotype 1 or 4 infection in the allograft and with compensated liver disease and who are ribavirin ineligible can be treated by a daily fixed-dose combination of ledipasvir (90 mg)/sofosbuvir (400 mg) for 24 weeks [96, 99, 103]. Patients with HCV genotype 1 infection in the allograft, including those with compensated cirrhosis can receive daily simeprevir (150 mg) plus sofosbuvir (400 mg) with or without weight-based ribavirin for 12 weeks. For those with early stage fibrosis, the recommended regimen is daily fixed-dose combination of paritaprevir (150 mg)/ritonavir (100 mg)/ombitasvir (25 mg) plus twice-daily dosed dasabuvir (250 mg) with weight-based ribavirin for 24 weeks. Treatment-naïve and -experienced patients with HCV genotype 2 infection in the allograft, including those with compensated cirrhosis, are treated with daclatasvir (60 mg) plus sofosbuvir (400 mg), with low initial dose of ribavirin (600 mg, increased as tolerated) for 12 weeks [92, 96, 99].

7. Patients with HCV and renal impairment

In patients with mild to moderate renal impairment, no dosage adjustment is required when using daclatasvir (60mg), fixed-dose combination of ledipasvir (90 mg)/sofosbuvir (400 mg), fixed-dose combination of sofosbuvir (400mg)/velpatasvir (100mg), or fixed-dose combination of paritaprevir (150 mg)/ritonavir (100 mg)/ombitasvir (25 mg) with (or without for HCV genotype 4 infection) twice-daily dosed dasabuvir (250 mg), simeprevir (150 mg), or sofosbuvir (400 mg) to treat or retreat HCV infection in patients with appropriate genotypes [96, 99, 104].

For patients with severe renal impairment or end stage renal disease and patients with genotype 1a, or 1b, or 4 infection and CrCl below 30 ml/min, for whom treatment has been elected before kidney transplantation, the recommended daily fixed-dose combination of elbasvir (50 mg)/grazoprevir (100mg) for 12 weeks. Genotype 1b infection patients and CrCl below 30 ml/min for whom the urgency to treat is high and treatment has been elected before kidney transplantation, daily fixed-dose combination of paritaprevir (150 mg)/ritonavir (100 mg)/ombitasvir (25 mg) plus twice-daily dosed dasabuvir (250 mg) for 12 weeks. For patients with HCV genotype 2, 3, 5, or 6 infection and CrCl below 30 ml/min for whom the urgency to treat is high and treatment has been elected before kidney transplantation, PEG-IFN and dose-adjusted ribavirin (200 mg daily) [104–107].

8. Retreatment of patients who failed prior therapy [57, 96, 99, 108, 109]

Patients who failed PEG-IFN-α, ribavirin, and DAA or all DAA regimens are retreated according to the previous therapies and genotype as follows:

- Patients infected with HCV genotype 1 who failed after a triple combination regimen of PEG-IFN-α, ribavirin and telaprevir, boceprevir or simeprevir are treated with combination of sofosbuvir and ledipasvir or sofosbuvir and velpatasvir, or sofosbuvir and daclatasvir, with ribavirin for 12 weeks.
- Patients who failed on sofosbuvir alone or sofosbuvir plus ribavirin or sofosbuvir plus pegylated IFN- α and ribavirin can be retreated with any of the following:
    - Genotypes 1, 4, 5, or 6 can be treated with sofosbuvir and ledipasvir
    - All genotypes can be treated with sofosbuvir and velpatasvir
    - Genotype 1 may be treated with ritonavir-boosted paritaprevir, ombitasvir, and dasabuvir
    - Genotype 4 is treated with ritonavir boosted, paritaprevir and ombitasvir or sofosbuvir plus simeprevir
    - Genotypes 1 or 4 are treated with grazoprevir and elbasvir for 24 weeks in F0-F2 patients with HCV RNA >800,000 IU/ml)
    - All genotypes may be treated with sofosbuvir plus daclatasvir

9. Treatment of HCV and HBV coinfection

The goal of therapy in HBV and HCV coinfection is to eradicate HCV infection and inhibit HBV replication. Evaluation of liver disease progression, predominance of one virus over another, and comorbidities are essential for optimal antiviral regimens. For patients with active hepatitis C, the same regimens following the same rules as for monoinfected patients should be applied based on AASLD and EASL recommendations [96, 99]. For patients with active hepatitis B before, during or after HCV clearance or with established cirrhosis, nucleoside or nucleotide analog (NA), tenofovir or entecavir is indicated [110, 111]. Concurrent HBV nucleoside/nucleotide analog therapy is indicated either if there is a potential risk of HBV reactivation during or after HCV clearance or if HBV replication is detectable at a significant level before initiation of HCV treatment [112].

Patients should be carefully investigated for the replicative status of both HBV and HCV, and hepatitis delta virus infection prior selecting the treatment strategy. When HCV is replicating and causes liver disease, it should be treated following the same rules as applied to HCV monoinfected patients. There is a potential risk of HBV reactivation during or after HCV clearance. Prior initiating DAA-based treatment for hepatitis C, patients should be tested for HBs antigen, anti-HBc antibodies and anti-HBs antibodies. If HBs antigen is present or if HBV DNA is detectable in HBs antigen-negative, anti-HBc antibody-positive patients ("occult" hepatitis B), concurrent HBV nucleoside/nucleotide analog therapy is indicated [96, 99].

9.1. DAA resistance

Despite the great efficacy of the interferon-free DAA regimen, real-life experience revealed that approximately 5–10% of patients end up with virologic failure. Treatment failure raised the issue of resistance and occurrence of mutations. To date, the impact of such mutations on the treatment outcome is not clarified. It is not clear if the presence of mutations at baseline may independently lead to relapse [113]. HCV resistance-associated variants (RAVS) remain a challenging issue in HCV therapy. The prevalence of NS5A RAVs at baseline was shown to vary considerably across genotypes 1a, 1b, 3 and 4. Some studies showed that virologic failure tended to be more frequent when an NS5A Y93H substitution was present at baseline. Resistance-associated substitutions (RASs) have been reported both in treatment-naïve patients and following treatment with protease (NS3), phosphoprotein (NS5A) and polymerase (NS5B) inhibitors [113].

The different next-generation sequencing (NGS) technologies for (HCV) are critical for identification of both viral genotype and resistance genetic motifs in the era of DAA therapies. A study [114] compared the ability of high-throughput NGS methods to generate full-length, deep, HCV sequence data sets and evaluated their utility for diagnostics and clinical assessment. The study showed that the consensus sequences generated by different NGS methods were generally concordant, and majority RAVs were consistently detected. However, methods differed in their ability to detect minor populations of RAVs. NGS provided a rapid, inexpensive method for generating whole HCV genomes to define infecting genotypes, RAVs, comprehensive viral strain analysis and quasispecies diversity. Enrichment methods are particularly suited for high-throughput analysis while providing the genotype and information on potential DAA resistance [114].

In conclusion, discovery of short duration, safe and highly effective regimens has opened up new horizons for HCV cure. However, real-life experience demonstrated some challenges such as emergence of mutations and management of special patient populations. Despite the optimism for the near future and the excellent efficacy, the prohibitive cost of such regimen is a great obstacle that interferes with accessibility of patients in countries with high HCV prevalence to the new IFN-free regimens. Thus, more efforts should be made to make IFN-free cost-effective in all clinical scenarios and accessible to all patients.

Abbreviations

HCV	hepatitis C
HCC	hepatocellular carcinoma

PEG IFN	peginterferon
RBV	ribavirin
DAA	direct-acting antiviral
GT	genotype
NNI	nonnucleotide polymerase inhibitor
NS5A	nonstructural protein 5A
Nuc	nucleotide polymerase inhibitor
PI	protease inhibitor
RAV	resistance-associated variant
TPV	telaprevir
BOC	boceprevir
RGT	response-guided therapy
RdRp	RNA-dependent RNA polymerase
SIM	simeprevir
DNV	danoprevir
EBR-GZR	elbasvir-grazoprevir
SOF	sofosbuvir
VEL	velpatasvir
EOTR	ombitasvir/paritaprevir/ritonavir + dasabuvir
GT	genotype
HCV	hepatitis C virus
OMV, RTV	ritonavir
ART	antiretroviral

Author details

Sanaa M. Kamal

Address all correspondence to: sanaakamal@ainshamsmedicine.net

Department of Gastroenterology and Hepatology, Ain Shams Faculty of Medicine, Cairo, Egypt

References

[1] World Health Organization. Hepatitis C. WHO fact sheet 164. Geneva, Switzerland: World Health Organization; 2000. Available from: http://www.who.int/mediacentre/factsheets/fs164/en/. Accessed August 28, 2016.

[2] Lavanchy D. The Global Burden of Hepatitis C. Liver Int. 2009; 29 (Suppl. 1): 74–81.

[3] Shepard CW, Finelli L, Alter MJ. Global Epidemiology of Hepatitis C Virus Infection. Lancet Infect Dis. 2005; 5: 558–567.

[4] Gower E, Estes C, Blach S, Razavi-Shearer K, Razavi H. Global Epidemiology and Genotype Distribution of the Hepatitis C Virus Infection. J Hepatol. 2014; 61(Suppl. 1): S45–S57.

[5] D. Lavanchy. Evolving Epidemiology of Hepatitis C Virus. Clin Microbiol Infect. 2011; 17: 107–115

[6] Egyptian Ministry of Health. Annual Report 2007. Available from: http://www.mohp.gov.eg/Main.asp. Accessed August 13, 2016.

[7] Lehman EM, Wilson ML. Epidemic Hepatitis C Virus Infection in Egypt: Estimates of Past Incidence and Future Morbidity and Mortality. J Viral Hepat. 2009; 16(9): 650–658.

[8] Guerra J, Garenne M, Mohamed MK, Fontanet A. HCV Burden of Infection in Egypt: Results from a Nationwide Survey. J Viral Hepat. 2012; 19: 560–567.

[9] Armstrong GL, Wasley A, Simard EP, et al. The Prevalence of Hepatitis C Virus Infection in the United States, 1999 through 2002. Ann Intern Med. 2006; 144(10): 705–714.

[10] Hanafiah KM, Groeger J, Flaxman AD, Wiersma ST. Global Epidemiology of Hepatitis C Virus Infection: New Estimates of Age-Specific Antibody to HCV Seroprevalence. Hepatology 2013; 57; 1333–1342.

[11] Desenclos JC. The Challenge of Hepatitis C Surveillance in Europe. Euro Surveill. 2003; 8(5): 99–110.

[12] Sharma S, Carballo M, Feld JJ, Janssen HLA. Immigration and Viral Hepatitis. J Hepatol. 2015; 63(2): 515–522.

[13] Micallef JM, Kaldor JM, Dore GJ. Spontaneous Viral Clearance Following Acute Hepatitis C Infection: A Systematic Review of Longitudinal Studies. J Viral Hepat. 2006; 13(1): 34–41.

[14] Hoofnagle JH. Course and Outcome of Hepatitis C. Hepatology. 2002; 36(5 Suppl 1): S21–S29.

[15] Seeff LB. The Natural History of Chronic Hepatitis C Virus Infection. Clin Liver Dis. 1997; 1(3): 587–602.

[16] Stone AE, Giugliano S, Schnell G, Cheng L, Leahy A, Golden-Mason L, Gale M, Rosen HR. Hepatitis C virus Pathogen Associated Molecular Pattern (PAMP) Triggers Production

of Lambda-Interferons by Human Plasmacytoiddendritic Cells. PLoS Pathol. 2013; 9(4): e1003316.

[17] Kell A, Stoddard M, Li H, Marcotrigiano J, Shaw JM Gale MM Jr. Pathogen-Associated Molecular Pattern Recognition of Hepatitis C Virus Transmitted/Founder Variants by RIG-I Is Dependent on U-Core Length. J Virol. 2015; 89(21): 11056–11068.

[18] Thimme R, Oldach D, Chang KM, et al. Determinants of Viral Clearance and Persistence During Acute Hepatitis C Virus Infection. J Exp Med. 2001; 194: 1395–1406.

[19] Kamal SM, Kassim SK, Ahmed AI, Mahmoud S, Bahnasy KA, Hafez TA, Aziz IA, Fathelbab IF, Mansour HM. Host and Viral Determinants of the Outcome of Exposure to HCV Infection Genotype 4: A Large Longitudinal Study. Am J Gastroenterol. 2014 Feb; 109(2): 199–211.

[20] Keoshkerian E, Hunter M, Cameron B, Nguyen N, Sugden P, Bull R, Zekry A, Maher L, Seddiki N, Zaunders J, Kelleher A, Lloyd AR. HITS-p and HITS-c Investigators. Hepatitis C-Specific Effector and Regulatory CD4 T-Cell Responses are Associated with the Outcomes of Primary Infection. J Viral Hepat. 2016 Aug 25. J Viral Hepat. 2016 Dec;23(12):985–993

[21] Goh CC, Roggerson KM, Lee HC, Golden-Mason L, Rosen HR, Hahn YS. Hepatitis C virus-induced myeloid-derived suppressor cells suppress NK cell IFN-γ production by altering Cellular metabolism via Arginase-1. J Immunol. 2016 Mar 1; 196(5): 2283–2292.

[22] Morishima C, Di Bisceglie AM, Rothman AL, Bonkovsky HL, Lindsay KL, Lee WM, Koziel MJ, Fontana RJ, Kim HY, Wright EC. HALT-C Trial Group. Antigen-specific T Lymphocyte Proliferation Decreases over Time in Advanced Chronic Hepatitis C. J Viral Hepat. 2012 Jun; 19(6): 404–413.

[23] Kang W, Sung PS, Park SH, Yoon S, Chang DY, Kim S, Han KH, Kim JK, Rehermann B, Chwae YJ, Shin EC. Hepatitis C Virus Attenuates Interferon-Induced Major Histocompatibility Complex Class I Expression and Decreases CD8+ T Cell Effector Functions. Gastroenterology. 2014 May; 146(5): 1351–60.

[24] Park SH, Rehermann B. Immune Responses to HCV and Other Hepatitis Viruses. Immunity. 2014 Jan 16; 40(1): 13–24.

[25] Farci P. New Insights into the HCV Quasispecies and Compartmentalization. Semin Liver Dis. 2011 Nov; 31(4): 356–374.

[26] Lunemann S, Martrus G, Hölzemer A, Chapel A, Ziegler M, Körner C, Garcia Beltran W, Carrington M, Wedemeyer H, Altfeld M. Sequence Variations in HCV Core-Derived Epitopes Alter Binding of KIR2DL3 to HLA-C*03:04 and Modulate NK Cell Function. J Hepatol. 2016 Aug; 65(2): 252–258.

[27] Suppiah V, Gaudieri S, Armstrong NJ, O'Connor KS, Berg T, Weltman M, Abate ML, Spengler U, Bassendine M, Dore GJ, Irving WL, Powell E, Hellard M, Riordan S, Matthews G, Sheridan D, Nattermann J, Smedile A, Müller T, Hammond E, Dunn D,

Negro F, Bochud PY, Mallal S, Ahlenstiel G, Stewart GJ, George J, Booth DR. International Hepatitis C Genetics Consortium (IHCGC). L28B, HLA-C, and KIR variants Additively Predict Response to Therapy in Chronic Hepatitis C Virus Infection in a European Cohort: A Cross-Sectional Study. PLoS Med. 2011 Sep; 8(9):e1001092.

[28] Singal, AG, M Volk, D Jensen, et al. A Sustained Viral Response is Associated with Reduced Liver Related Morbidity and Mortality in Patients with Hepatitis C Virus, Clin Gastroenterol Hepatol. 2010; 8: 280–288.

[29] Takaoka A, Yanai H. Interferon Signalling Network in Innate Defence. Cell Microbiol. 2006; 8: 907–922.

[30] Fensterl, G.C. Sen. Interferons and Viral Infections. Biofactors 2009: 35: 14–20.

[31] deWeerd NA, Samarajiwa SA, Hertzog PJ. Type I Interferon Receptors: Biochemistry and Biological Functions. J Biol Chem 2007; 282: 20053–20057.

[32] Zhao W, Lee C, Piganis R, Plumlee C, de Weerd N, Hertzog PJ, et al. A Conserved IFN-α Receptor Tyrosine Motif Directs the Biological Response to Type I IFNs. J Immunol. 2008; 180: 5483–5489.

[33] Zhang L, Alter HJ, Wang H, Jia S, Wang E, Marincola FM, et al. The Modulation of Hepatitis C Virus 1a Replication by PKR is Dependent on NF-κB Mediated Interferon *B* response in Huh7.5.1 Cells. Virology 2013; 438: 28–36.

[34] Pokers P. New Direct-Acting Antivirals in the Development for Hepatitis C Virus Infection. Therap Adv Gastroenterol. 2010 May; 3(3): 191–202.

[35] Kim CW, Mi Chang K. Hepatitis C Virus: Virology and Life Cycle. Clin Mol Hepatol. 2013 Mar; 19(1): 17–25.

[36] Bartenschlager R, Penin F, Lohmann V, Andre P. Assembly of infectious hepatitis C virus particles. Trends Microbiol. 2011; 19: 95–103.

[37] Moradpour D, Penin F, Rice CM. Replication of Hepatitis C Virus. Nat Rev Microbiol. 2007; 5(6): 453–463.

[38] Liang TJ, Ghany MG. Current and Future Therapies for Hepatitis C Virus Infection. N Engl J Med. 2013; 368: 1907–1917.

[39] Rupp D, Bartenschlager R. Targets for antiviral therapy of hepatitis C. Semin. Liver Dis 2014; 34: 9–21.

[40] Chang MH, Gordon LA, Fung HB. Boceprevir: A Protease Inhibitor for the Treatment of Hepatitis C. Clin Ther. 2012 Oct; 34(10): 2021–2038.

[41] Matthews SJ, Lancaster JW. Telaprevir: A Hepatitis C NS3/4A Protease Inhibitor. ClinTher. 2012 Sep; 34(9): 1857–1882.

[42] Asselah T, Marcellin P. Second-wave IFN-Based Triple Therapy for HCV Genotype 1 Infection: Simeprevir, Faldaprevir and Sofosbuvir. Liver Int. 2014; 34 (Suppl. 1): 60–68.

[43] Clark VC, Peter JA, Nelson DR. New Therapeutic Strategies in HCV: Second-Generation Protease Inhibitors. Liver Int. 2013; 33 (Suppl. 1): 80–84.

[44] Fried MW, Buti M, Dore GJ, et al. Once-Daily Simeprevir (TMC435) With Pegylated Interferon and Ribavirin in Treatment-Naïve Genotype 1 Hepatitis C: The Randomized PILLAR Study. Hepatology. 2013 Dec; 58(6): 1918–1929.

[45] Jacobson IM, Dore GJ, Foster GR, et al. Simeprevir with Pegylated Interferon Alfa 2a Plus Ribavirin in Treatment-Naive Patients with Chronic Hepatitis C Virus Genotype 1 Infection (QUEST-1): A Phase 3, Randomised, Double-Blind, Placebo-Controlled Trial. Lancet. 2014; 384: 403–413.

[46] Manns M, Marcellin P, Poordad F, et al. Simeprevir with Pegylated Interferon Alfa 2a or 2b Plus Ribavirin in Treatment-Naive Patients with Chronic Hepatitis C Virus Genotype 1 Infection (QUEST-2): A Randomised, Double-Blind, Placebo-Controlled Phase 3 Trial. Lancet. 2014; 384: 414–426.

[47] Zeuzem S, Berg T, Gane E, et al. Simeprevir Increases Rate of Sustained Virologic Response Among Treatment-Experienced Patients with HCV Genotype-1 Infection: A Phase IIb Trial. Gastroenterology. 2014; 146: 430–441.

[48] Forns X, Lawitz E, Zeuzem S, et al. Simeprevir with Peginterferon and Ribavirin leads to High Rates of SVR in Patients with HCV Genotype 1 Who Relapsed after Previous Therapy: A Phase 3 trial. Gastroenterology. 2014; 146: 1669–1679.

[49] Moreno C, Hezode C, Marcellin P, et al. Efficacy and Safety of Simeprevir with PegIFN/Ribavirin in Naïve or Experienced Patients Infected with Chronic HCV Genotype 4. J Hepatol. 2015; 62: 1047–1055.

[50] Everson G, Cooper C, Hézode C, Shiffman ML, Yoshida E, Beltran-Jaramillo T, Andreone P, Bruno S, Ferenci P, Zeuzem S, Brunda M, Le Pogam S, Nájera I, Zhou J, Navarro MT, Voulgari A, Shulman NS, Yetzer ES. DAUPHINE: A Randomized Phase II Study of Danoprevir/Ritonavir Plus Peginterferon Alpha-2a/Ribavirin in HCV Genotypes 1 or 4. Liver Int. 2015 Jan; 35(1): 108–119.

[51] Zeuzem S, Dufour JF, Buti M, Soriano V, Buynak RJ, Mantry P, Taunk J, Stern JO, Vinisko R, Gallivan JP, Böcher W, Mensa FJ. SOUND-C3 Study Group. Interferon-Free Treatment of Chronic Hepatitis C with Faldaprevir, Deleobuvir and Ribavirin: SOUND-C3, a Phase 2b study. Liver Int. 2015 Feb; 35(2): 417–421.

[52] Keating GM. Elbasvir/Grazoprevir: First Global Approval. Drugs. 2016 Apr; 76(5): 617–624.

[53] Sperl J, Horvath G, Halota W, Ruiz-Tapiador JA, Streinu-Cercel A, Jancoriene L, Werling K, Kileng H, Koklu S, Gerstoft J, Urbanek P, Flisiak R, Leiva R, Kazenaite E, Prinzing R, Patel S, Qiu J, Asante-Appiah E, Wahl J, Nguyen BY, Barr E, Platt HL. Efficacy and Safety of Elbasvir/Grazoprevir and Sofosbuvir/Pegylated Interferon/Ribavirin: A Phase III Randomized Controlled Trial. J Hepatol. 2016: S0168–8278(16)30429-9.

[54] Zeuzem S, Ghalib R, Reddy KR, et al. Grazoprevir-Elbasvir Combination Therapy for Treatment-Naive Cirrhotic and Noncirrhotic Patients with Chronic Hepatitis C Virus Genotype 1, 4, or 6 Infection: A Randomized Trial. Ann Int Med. 2015; 163(1): 1–13.

[55] Dore G, Altice F, Litwin AH, et al. C-EDGE CO-STAR: Efficacy of Grazoprevir and Elbasvir in Persons Who Inject Drugs (PWID) Receiving Opioid Agonist Therapy. Presented at the 2015 Annual Meeting of the American Association for the Study of Liver Diseases, San Francisco; November 13–17, 2015.

[56] Lawitz E, Gane E, Pearlman B, et al. Efficacy and Safety of 12 Weeks Versus 18 Weeks of Treatment with Grazoprevir (MK-5172) and Elbasvir (MK-8742) with or without Ribavirin for Hepatitis C virus Genotype 1 Infection in Previously Untreated Patients with Cirrhosis and Patients with Previous Null Response with or without Cirrhosis (C-WORTHY): a Randomised, Open-Label Phase 2 Trial. Lancet. 2015; 385: 1075–1086.

[57] Buti M, Gordon SC, Zuckerman E, et al. Grazoprevir, Elbasvir, and Ribavirin for Chronic Hepatitis C Virus Genotype 1 Infection After Failure of Pegylated Interferon and Ribavirin With an Earlier-Generation Protease Inhibitor: Final 24-Week Results from C-SALVAGE. Clin Infect Dis. 2016; 62: 32–36.

[58] Rockstroh JK, Nelson M, Katlama C, et al. Efficacy and Safety of Grazoprevir (MK-5172) and Elbasvir (MK-8742) in Patients with Hepatitis C Virus and HIV Co-Infection (C-EDGE CO-INFECTION): A Non-Randomised, Open-Label Trial. Lancet HIV. 2015; 2:e319–27.

[59] Soriano V, Vispo E, de Mendoza C, Labarga P, Fernandez-Montero JV, Poveda E, Treviño A, Barreiro P. Hepatitis C Therapy with HCV NS5B Polymerase Inhibitors. Expert Opin Pharmacother. 2013; 14(9): 1161–1170.

[60] Marascio N, Torti C, Liberto M, Focà A. Update on Different Aspects of HCV Variability: Focus on NS5B polymerase. BMC Infect Dis. 2014; 14 Suppl 5:S1.

[61] Bhatia HK, Singh H, Grewal N, Natt NK. Sofosbuvir: A Novel Treatment Option for Chronic Hepatitis C Infection. J Pharmacol Pharmacother. 2014; 5(4): 278–284.

[62] Kowdley KV, Lawitz E, Crespo I, et al. Sofosbuvir with Pegylated Interferon Alfa-2a and Ribavirin for Treatment-Naive Patients with Hepatitis C Genotype-1 Infection (ATOMIC): An Open-Label, Randomised, Multicentre Phase 2 Trial. Lancet 2013 Jun 15; 381(9883): 2100–21007.

[63] Gane EJ, Stedman CA, Hyland RH, Ding X, Svarovskaia E, Symonds WT, Hindes RG, Berrey MM. Nucleotide Polymerase Inhibitor Sofosbuvir Plus Ribavirin for Hepatitis C. N Engl J Med. 2013 Jan 3; 368(1): 34–44.

[64] Foster GR, Pianko S, Brown A, et al. Efficacy of Sofosbuvir Plus Ribavirin with or without Peginterferon-Alfa in Patients with Hepatitis C Virus Genotype 3 Infection and Treatment-Experienced Patients with Cirrhosis and Hepatitis C Virus Genotype 2 Infection. Gastroenterology. 2015; 149: 1462–1470.

[65] Kwo P, Gitlin N, Nahass R, Bernstein D, Etzkorn K, Rojter S, Schiff E, Davis M, Ruane P, Younes Z, Kalmeijer R, Sinha R, Peeters M, Lenz O, Fevery B, De La Rosa G, Scott J, Witek J. Simeprevir Plus Sofosbuvir (12 and 8 weeks) in Hepatitis C Virus Genotype 1-Infected Patients without Cirrhosis: OPTIMIST-1, a Phase 3, Randomized Study. Hepatology. 2016 Aug; 64(2): 370–380.

[66] Lawitz E, Matusow G, DeJesus E, Yoshida EM, Felizarta F, Ghalib R, Godofsky E, Herring RW, Poleynard G, Sheikh A, Tobias H, Kugelmas M, Kalmeijer R, Peeters M, Lenz O, Fevery B, De La Rosa G, Scott J, Sinha R, Witek J. Simeprevir Plus Sofosbuvir in Patients with Chronic Hepatitis C Virus Genotype 1 Infection and Cirrhosis: A Phase 3 Study (OPTIMIST-2). Hepatology. 2016 Aug; 64(2): 360–369.

[67] Sulkowski MS, Vargas HE, Di Bisceglie AM, Kuo A, Reddy KR, Lim JK, Morelli G, Darling JM, Feld JJ, Brown RS, Frazier LM, Stewart TG, Fried MW, Nelson DR, Jacobson IM, HCV-TARGET Study Group. Effectiveness of Simeprevir Plus Sofosbuvir, with or without Ribavirin, in Real-World Patients with HCV Genotype 1 Infection. Gastroenterology. 2016 Feb; 150(2): 419–429.

[68] Gane EJ, Stedman CA, Hyland RH, et al. Efficacy of Nucleotide Polymerase Inhibitor Sofosbuvir plus the NS5A Inhibitor Ledipasvir or the NS5B Non-Nucleoside Inhibitor GS-9669 against HCV Genotype 1 Infection. Gastroenterology. 2013: S0016-5085(13)01653-3.

[69] Kohli A, Osinusi A, Sims Z, et al. Virological Response after 6 Week Triple-Drug Regimens for Hepatitis C: A Proof-Of-Concept Phase 2A Cohort Study. Lancet. 2015; 385: 1107.

[70] Lawitz E, Poordad FF, Pang PS, Hyland RH, Ding X, Mo H, Symonds WT, McHutchison JG, Membreno FE. Sofosbuvir and Ledipasvir Fixed-Dose Combination with and without Ribavirin in Treatment-Naive and Previously Treated Patients with Genotype 1 Hepatitis C Virus Infection (LONESTAR): An Open-Label, Randomised, Phase 2 Trial. Lancet 2014. 8; 383(9916): 515–523.

[71] Backus LI, Belperio PS, Shahoumian TA, Loomis TP, Mole LA. Real-world effectiveness of Ledipasvir/Sofosbuvir in 4,365 Treatment-Naive, Genotype 1 Hepatitis C-Infected Patients. Hepatology. 2016; 64(2): 405–414.

[72] Gane EJ, Hyland RH, An D, et al. Efficacy of Ledipasvir and Sofosbuvir, with or without Ribavirin, for 12 Weeks in Patients with HCV Genotype 3 or 6 Infection. Gastroenterology. 2015; 149: 1454–1461.

[73] Kohli A, Kapoor R, Sims Z, et al. Ledipasvir and Sofosbuvir for Hepatitis C Genotype 4: A Proof-Of-Concept, Single-Centre, Open-Label Phase 2a Cohort Study. Lancet Infect Dis. 2015; 15: 1049–1054.

[74] Manns M, Samuel D, Gane EJ, Mutimer D, McCaughan G, Buti M, Prieto M, Calleja JL, Peck-Radosavljevic M, Müllhaupt B, Agarwal K, Angus P, Yoshida EM, Colombo M, Rizzetto M, Dvory-Sobol H, Denning J, Arterburn S, Pang PS, Brainard D, McHutchison

JG, Dufour JF, Van Vlierberghe H, van Hoek B, Forns X, SOLAR-2 investigators. Ledipasvir and Sofosbuvir Plus Ribavirin in Patients with Genotype 1 or 4 Hepatitis C Virus Infection and Advanced Liver Disease: A Multicentre, Open-Label, Randomised, Phase 2 Trial. Lancet Infect Dis. 2016; 16(6): 685–697.

[75] Abergel A, Asselah T, Metivier S, et al. Ledipasvir-Sofosbuvir in Patients with Hepatitis C Virus Genotype 5 Infection: An Open-Label, Multicentre, Single-Arm, Phase 2 Study. Lancet Infect Dis. 2016; 16: 459–464.

[76] Osinusi A, Townsend K, Kohli A, et al. Virologic Response Following Combined Ledipasvir and Sofosbuvir Administration in Patients with HCV Genotype 1 and HIV Co-infection. JAMA. 2015; 313: 1232–1239.

[77] Ingiliz P, Christensen S, Kimhofer T, Hueppe D, Lutz T, Schewe K, Busch H, Schmutz G, Wehmeyer MH, Boesecke C, Simon KG, Berger F, Rockstroh JK, Schulze Zur Wiesch J, Baumgarten A, Mauss S. Sofosbuvir and Ledipasvir for 8 Weeks for the Treatment of Chronic Hepatitis C Virus Infection in HCV-Mono-Infected and HIV-HCV Co-Infected Individuals—Results from the German Hepatitis C Cohort (GECCO-01). Clin Infect Dis. 2016 Aug 17. Clin Infect Dis. 2016 15;63(10):1320–1324

[78] Rosenthal ES, Kottilil S, Polis MA. Sofosbuvir and Ledipasvir for HIV/HCV Co-infected patients. Expert Opin Pharmacother. 2016; 17(5): 743–749.

[79] Osinusi A, Kohli A, Marti MM, et al. Re-Treatment of Chronic Hepatitis C Virus Genotype 1 Infection after Relapse: An Open-Label Pilot Study. Ann Intern Med. 2014; 161: 634–638.

[80] Chahine EB, Sucher AJ, Hemstreet BA. Sofosbuvir/Velpatasvir: The First Pangenotypic Direct-Acting Antiviral Combination for Hepatitis C. Ann Pharmacother. 2016 Sep 8. Annals of Pharmacotherapy 2016; 51 (1): 44–53

[81] Lawitz E, Reau N, Hinestrosa F, Rabinovitz M, Schiff E, Sheikh A, Younes Z, Herring R Jr., Reddy KR, Tran T, Bennett M, Nahass R, Yang JC, Lu S, Dvory-Sobol H, Stamm LM, Brainard DM, McHutchison JG, Pearlman B, Shiffman M, Hawkins T, Curry M, Jacobson I. Efficacy of Sofosbuvir, Velpatasvir, and GS-9857 in Patients with Genotype 1 Hepatitis C Virus Infection in an Open-label, Phase 2 Trial. Gastroenterology. 2016 Jul 30.

[82] Feld JJ, Jacobson IM, Hézode C, et al. Sofosbuvir and Velpatasvir for HCV Genotype 1, 2, 4, 5, and 6 Infection. N Engl J Med. 2015; 373: 2599–2607.

[83] Foster GR, Afdhal N, Roberts SK, et al. Sofosbuvir and Velpatasvir for HCV Genotype 2 and 3 Infection. N Engl J Med. 2015; 373: 2608–2617.

[84] Gane E, Kowdley KV, Pound D, Stedman CA, Davis M, Etzkorn K, Gordon SC, Bernstein D, Everson G, Rodriguez-Torres M, Tsai N, Khalid O, Yang JC, Lu S, Dvory-Sobol H, Stamm LM, Brainard DM, McHutchison JG, Tong M, Chung RT, Beavers K, Poulos JE, Kwo PY, Nguyen MH. Efficacy of Sofosbuvir, Velpatasvir, and GS-9857 in Patients with

HCV Genotype 2, 3, 4, or 6 Infections in an Open-label, Phase 2 Trial. Gastroenterology. 2016 Jul 30. Gastroenterology. 2016;151(5):902–909.

[85] Curry MP, O'Leary JG, Bzowej N, et al. Sofosbuvir and Velpatasvir for HCV in Patients with Decompensated Cirrhosis. N Engl J Med. 2015; 373: 2618–28.

[86] Wyles D, Brau N, Kottilil S, et al. Sofosbuvir/Velpatasvir Fixed Dose Combination for 12 Weeks in Patients Co-Infected with HCV and HIV-1: The Phase 3 ASTRAL-5 Study. Presented at the 51st Annual Meeting of the European Association for the Study of the Liver, Barcelona, April 13–17, 2016.

[87] Gao M, Nettles RE, Belema M, Snyder LB, Nguyen VN, R. Fridell A, et al. Chemical Genetics Strategy Identifies an HCV NS5A Inhibitor with a Potent Clinical Effect. Nature 2010, 465: 96–100.

[88] Schinazi R, Halfon P, Marcellin P, Asselah T. HCV Direct-Acting Antiviral Agents: The Best Interferon-Free Combinations. Liver Int. 2014; 34: 69–78.

[89] Gao M. O'Boyle DR 2nd, Roberts S. HCV NS5A Replication Complex Inhibitors. Curr Opin Pharmacol. 2016 Sep 16; 30: 151–157.

[90] Sulkowski MS, Gardiner DF, Rodriguez-Torres M, et al. Daclatasvir plus Sofosbuvir for Previously Treated or Untreated Chronic HCV Infection. N Engl J Med. 2014; 370: 211–221.

[91] Nelson DR, Cooper JN, Lalezari JP, et al. All-Oral 12-Week Treatment with Daclatasvir plus Sofosbuvir in Patients with Hepatitis C Virus Genotype 3 Infection: ALLY-3 Phase III Study. Hepatology. 2015; 61: 1127–1135.

[92] Poordad F, Schiff ER, Vierling JM, Landis C, Fontana RJ, Yang R, McPhee F, Hughes EA, Noviello S, Swenson ES. Daclatasvir with sofosbuvir and ribavirin for hepatitis C virus infection with advanced cirrhosis or post-liver transplantation recurrence. Hepatology. 2016 May;63(5):1493-505

[93] Wyles DL, Ruane PJ, Sulkowski MS, et al. Daclatasvir plus Sofosbuvir for HCV in Patients Coinfected with HIV-1. N Engl J Med. 2015; 373: 714–725.

[94] DAKLINZA ™ [package insert]. Bristol-Myers Squibb Corp; 2016.

[95] Lontok E, Harrington P, Howe A, et al. Hepatitis C Virus Drug Resistance-Associated Substitutions: State of the Art Summary. Hepatology. 2015; 62: 1623–1632.

[96] American Association for the Study of Liver Diseases (AASLD) and Infectious Diseases Society of America (IDSA). Recommendations for Testing, Managing, and Treating Hepatitis C. Available from: http://www.hcvguidelines.org/full-report-view. Accessed August 29, 2016.

[97] Harvoni® [package insert]. Foster City, CA: Gilead Sciences, Inc., 2015.

[98] Deeks ED. Ombitasvir/Paritaprevir/Ritonavir plus Dasabuvir: A Review in Chronic HCV Genotype 1 Infection. Drugs. 2015 Jun; 75(9): 1027–1038.

[99] EASL Recommendations on Treatment of Hepatitis C 2016. [Internet]. Available from: http://www.easl.eu/medias/cpg/HCV2016/English-report.pdf. Accessed September 23, 2016.

[100] Cotte L, Pugliese P, Valantin MA, Cuzin L, Billaud E, Duvivier C, Naqvi A, Cheret A, Rey D, Pradat P, Poizot-Martin I. Dat'AIDS Study Group. Hepatitis C Treatment Initiation in HIV-HCV Coinfected Patients. BMC Infect Dis. 2016 Jul 22; 16: 345.

[101] Wyles DL, Sulkowski MS, Dieterich D. Management of Hepatitis C/HIV Coinfection in the Era of Highly Effective Hepatitis C Virus Direct-Acting Antiviral Therapy. Clin Infect Dis. 2016 Jul 15; 63 (Suppl 1): S3–S11.

[102] Foster GR, Irving WL, Cheung MC, Walker AJ, Hudson BE, Verma S, McLauchlan J, Mutimer DJ, Brown A, Gelson WT, MacDonald DC, Agarwal K; HCV Research, UK. Impact of Direct Acting Antiviral Therapy in Patients with Chronic Hepatitis C and Decompensated Cirrhosis. J Hepatol. 2016 Jun; 64(6): 1224–1231.

[103] Gane EG, Agarwal K. Directly Acting Antivirals (DAAs) for the Treatment of Chronic Hepatitis C Virus Infection in Liver Transplant Patients: "A Flood of Opportunity". Am J Transplantation 2014; 14: 994–1002.

[104] Khatri A, Dutta S, Marbury TC, Preston RA, Rodrigues L Jr., Wang H, Awni WM, Menon RM. Pharmacokinetics and Tolerability of Anti-Hepatitis C Virus Treatment with Ombitasvir, Paritaprevir, Ritonavir, with or without Dasabuvir, in Subjects with Renal Impairment. Clin Pharmacokinet. 2016 Jul 7. Clin Pharmacokinet. 2017 Feb;56(2):153–163.

[105] European Journal of Drug Metabolism and Pharmacokinetics May, 2016 [Interne]. Available at: http://link.springer.com/search?query=Ombitasvir%2C+Paritaprevir%2C+Ritonavir%2C+Dasabuvir

[106] Smolders EJ, de Kanter CT, van Hoek B, Arends JE, Drenth JP, Burger DM. Pharmacokinetics, Efficacy, and Safety of Hepatitis C Virus Drugs in Patients with Liver and/or Renal Impairment. Drug Saf. 2016 Jul; 39(7): 589–611.

[107] Sorbera MA, Friedman ML, Cope R. New and Emerging Evidence on the Use of Second-Generation Direct Acting Antivirals for the Treatment of Hepatitis C Virus in Renal Impairment. J Pharm Pract. 2016 Feb 22.

[108] Wilson EM, Kattakuzhy S, Sidharthan S, Sims Z, Tang L, McLaughlin M, Price A, Nelson A, Silk R, Gross C, Akoth E, Mo H, Subramanian GM, Pang PS, McHutchison JG, Osinusi A, Masur H, Kohli A, Kottilil S. Successful Retreatment of Chronic HCV Genotype-1 Infection with Ledipasvir and Sofosbuvir after Initial Short Course Therapy with Direct-Acting Antiviral Regimens. Clin Infect Dis. 2016 Feb 1; 62(3): 280–288.

[109] Ray K. Therapy: Retreatment of HCV Infection in DAA Nonresponders. Nat Rev Gastroenterol Hepatol. 2015 May; 12(5): 252.

[110] European Association for the Study of the Liver. EASL Clinical Practice Guidelines: Management of Chronic Hepatitis B Virus Infection. J. Hepatol. 2012; 57: 167–185.

[111] Liaw YF, Kao JH, Piratvisuth T et al. Asian-Pacific Consensus Statement on the Management of Chronic Hepatitis B: A 2012 Update. Hepatol. Int. 2012; 6: 531–561.

[112] Potthoff A, Berg T, Wedemeyer H. Late Hepatitis B Virus Relapse in Patients Coinfected with Hepatitis B Virus and Hepatitis C Virus after Antiviral Treatment with Pegylated Interferon-A2b and Ribavirin. Scand J Gastroenterol. 2009; 44: 1487–1490.

[113] Pawlotsky JM. Hepatitis C Virus Resistance to Direct-Acting Antiviral Drugs in interferon-Free Regimens. Gastroenterology 2016; 151(1): 70–86.

[114] Thomson E, Ip CL, Badhan A, Christiansen MT, Adamson W, Ansari MA, Bibby D, Breuer J, Brown A, Bowden R, Bryant J, Bonsall D, Da Silva Filipe A, Hinds C, Hudson E, Klenerman P, Lythgow K, Mbisa JL, McLauchlan J, Myers R, Piazza P, Roy S, Trebes A, Sreenu VB, Witteveldt J, STOP-HCV Consortium, Barnes E, Simmonds P. Comparison of Next-Generation Sequencing Technologies for Comprehensive Assessment of Full-Length Hepatitis C Viral Genomes. J Clin Microbiol. 2016 Oct; 54(10): 2470–2484.

Chapter 3

Comparative Study of IFN-Based Versus IFN-Free Regimens and Their Efficacy in Treatment of Chronic Hepatitis C Infections

Ramesh Rana, Yizhong Chang, Jing Li,

ShengLan Wang, Li Yang and ChangQing Yang

Additional information is available at the end of the chapter

http://dx.doi.org/10.5772/67214

Abstract

The hepatitis C viral (HCV) infection is a global health burden, WHO estimates 130–150 million people chronically infected with hepatitis C virus worldwide. Additional 3–4 million people become newly infected annually and more than 350,000 people die each year of HCV-related liver diseases. HCV infection exhibits higher genetic diversity with regional variations in genotypic prevalence resulting big challenges on disease management. Introduction of DAAs revolutionised the new era of all oral therapy in treatment of chronic hepatitis C infection and is the regimens of choice in present days. However, IFN-based combination therapy with sofosbuvir has promising efficacy in genotypes 3, 4, 5 or 6 infections compared to genotypes 1 and 2 infections. So, these regimens could be an option in DAAs regimen failure cases. The poor availability of data on recent DAAs (IFN-free) regimens questioned on regular use and cost effectiveness is the another challenge with DAAs regimens. So phase III trials (sofosbuvir and velpatasvir) of recent DAAs with pangenotypic actions and better tolerability in HCV infected patients are the future advances in treatment of chronic hepatitis C. After all those recent combination therapies with better SVR, the combination of pegylated interferon with ribavirin is the only option available where unavailability of other regimens still exists.

Keywords: hepatitis C virus, HCV genotypes, pegylated interferon, direct-acting antivirals, sustained virological response

1. Introduction

Hepatitis C virus (HCV) is a global public health problem causing progressive liver disease. The World Health Organization (WHO) estimates 130–150 million people chronically infected worldwide, which corresponds to 2–2.5% of world's total population. Additional 3–4 million people becoming newly infected annually and more than 350,000 people die each year due to HCV-related diseases. Primary HCV infection causes acute hepatitis (AHC), asymptomatic in majorities; however, it can progress to chronicity in about 55–85% cases and spontaneous remission within 6 months without treatment in 15–45% [1–3]. Chronic hepatitis C (CHC) frequently presents with complications such as liver cirrhosis, liver failure, and hepatocellular carcinoma (HCC). In CHC, 15–30% have risk of cirrhosis of liver within 20 years and risk of HCC in cirrhotic is approximately 2–4% per year. Decompensated cirrhosis leads to death in 50–70% of cases without liver transplantation after 5 years. Difficulties occur in determining number of new HCV infections, as most of the acute cases are not detected clinically. Less than 25% of acute cases of hepatitis C are only clinically apparent [1, 4–6].

Hepatitis C virus (HCV) is an envelope, single-stranded RNA virus of genus hepacivirus within the Flaviviridae family. HCV has seven genotypes (GT 1–7) with 67 subtypes and 20 provisional subtypes [7]. Each genotype of HCV has its own geographical variation. GT-1 is the most prevalent worldwide, one third in East Asia followed by GT-3; GT-2, 4, and 6; and GT-5 is the least prevalent [8]. The prevalence of HCV GT-1 and 3 dominate in most of the countries irrespective of economic status while HCV GT-4 and 5 are prevalent largely in countries with lower income [7, 8]. HCV subtypes 1a and 1b are the most common genotypes in the United States and also in Europe while subtype 1b is predominant in Japan [9]. HCV subtypes 2a and 2b are relatively common in North America, Europe, and Japan, subtype 2c is common in Northern Italy. Although, GT-3 has endemic strain in South Asia, 3a is especially prevalent in intravenous drug abusers in Europe and in the United States. GT-4 is prevalent in North Africa and Middle East; GT-5 seems to be confined to South Africa and GT-6 in Southeast Asia. A newly identified GT-7 isolated from a Central African (Congolese) immigrant in Canada [9]. The increased risk of HCV is highest among persons who inject drugs (PWID), global prevalence of HCV among PWID is 67%; HIV infected person, men who have sex with men (MSM); unsafe medical procedures-recipients of infected blood products or invasive procedures in health care facilities with inadequate infection control practice. Vertical or perinatal transmission of HCV occurs in up to 4–8% of cases, and transmission risk among mothers of HIV infection is estimated 17–25% [9–11].

The HCV infection is the public health problem and global burden, and the early diagnosis and treatment are necessary. The treatment of HCV infection was begun with the approval of interferon (IFN) by the Food and Drug Administration (FDA) in 1991, followed by combined IFN with ribavirin (RBV) in 1998 and then directly acting antiviral agents (**Table 1**). Until approval of directly acting antiviral agents, combination of pegylated interferon alfa (PegIFN

Year	Generic	Genotypes (SVR)
1991	Interferon-alfa-2b	
1996	Interferon-alfa-2a	
1997	Consensus interferon	
	All standard interferon SVR rates (approximately)	Genotype 1 (9%) Genotypes 2, 3 (30%)
1998	Interferon-alfa plus ribavirin	Genotype 1 (29%) Genotypes 2, 3 (62%)
2001	PegInterferon-alfa-2b	Genotype 1 (14%) Genotypes 2, 3 (47%)
2001	PegInterferon-alfa-2b/ribavirin	Genotype 1 (47%) Genotypes 2–6 (75%)
2002	PegInterferon-alfa-2a	Genotype 1 (28%) Genotypes 2, 3 (56%)
2003	Pegylated alfa-2a/ribavirin	Genotype 1 (51%) Genotypes 2–6 (70%) Genotypes 2, 3 (82%)
2011	Boceprevir/PEG/RBV	Genotype 1 (66%)
2011	Telaprevir/PEG/RBV	Genotype 1 (79%)
2013	Simeprevir/PEG/RBV	Genotype 1 (up to 80%)
2013	Sofosbuvir/PEG/RBV	Genotype 1 (up to 92%) Genotype 4 (92%)
2013	Sofosbuvir/RBV	Genotype 2 (up to 100%) Genotype 3 (up to 92%)
2014	Sofosbuvir/simeprevir/RBV	Genotype 1 (up to 92%)
2014	Sofosbuvir/ledipasvir	Genotypes 1, 4, 5, 6 (up to 100%)
2014	Ombitasvir/paritaprevir/ritonavir/dasabuvir with/without RBV	Genotype 1 (up to 100)
2015	Daclatasvir for use with sofosbuvir	Genotype 3 (up to 98%)
2015	Ombitasvir, paritaprevir and ritonavir plus RBV	Genotype 4 (up to 100%)

PEG, pegylated interferon by injection; RBV, ribavirin (pills), HCV inhibitors are pills; SVR, sustained virological response, SVR 12, 24-viral cure.

Reference: http://hcvadvocate.org/treatment/drug-pipeline/#Quick

Table 1. FDA approved medications for treatment of Hepatitis C infections.

alfa) and ribavirin (RBV) was the standard treatment for all genotypic infections (**Figure 1**) [4, 12]. Over the past few years, the treatment options of HCV have exponentially grown. The development of directly acting antiviral (DAA) therapy, targeting non-structural proteins involved in replication of HCV revolutionised in the treatment of HCV infection. The combination of DAAs with or without PegIFN alfa regimens is assessed in different studies, and their efficacies in treatment of different HCV genotypes are evaluated individually. Recently, the combination of IFN-free DAAs regimens with or without ribavirin is evaluated as "All oral regimens" for treatment of HCV infection in different genotypes with better efficacy and tolerability [13]. The current treatment strategies for HCV are based on HCV genotyping; and HCV RNA load determination before, during, and after antiviral therapy; then selection of agents that are active against the isolated specific HCV genotype [4, 12, 14]. The aim of this review is to compare the efficacy of IFN-based and IFN-free regimens (DAAs combination therapy) on the basis of sustained virological response (SVR) rates in HCV genotypic infections.

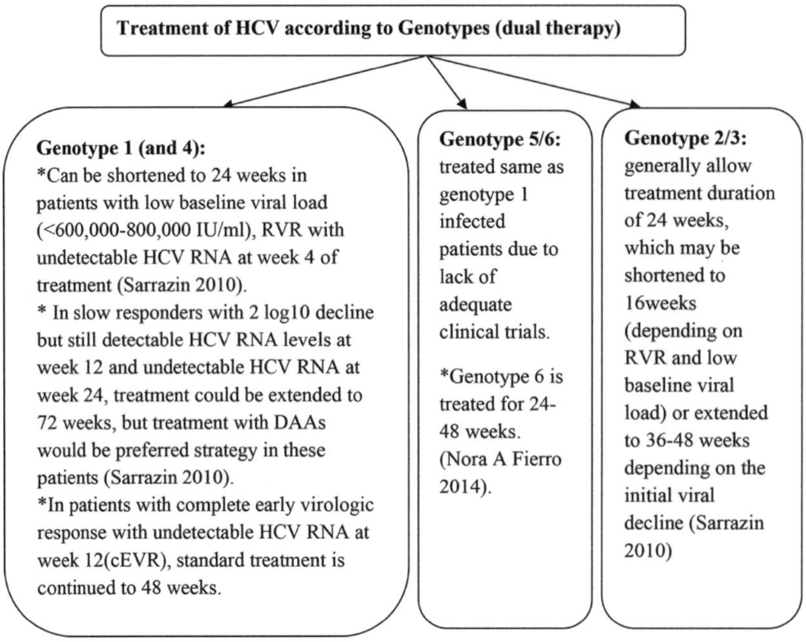

Figure 1. Combination of PegIFN-alfa and ribavirin for the treatment of HCV infections according to genotypes [4]. HCV, hepatitis C virus; RNA, ribonucleic acid; RVR, rapid virological response; DAAs, directly acting antivirals; cEVR, complete early virological response.

2. Treatment

The primary goal of HCV treatment is to cure the infection. The obtaining sustained virological response (SVR) is defined as undetectable HCV RNA in 12 weeks (SVR 12) or 24 weeks (SVR 24) after treatment completion. Cure rate, which achieves SVR, is more than 99%. SVR is generally associated with resolution of liver disease in patient without cirrhosis, but the patient with cirrhosis remains risk of life-threatening complications. However, the hepatic fibrosis may regress, and risk of complications like hepatic failure and portal hypertension is reduced. The risk of HCC and all causes of mortality are significantly reduced, nevertheless, not eliminated in cirrhotic patients who clear HCV compared to untreated patients and non-sustained

http://dx.doi.org/10.5772/67214

virological responders [4, 15–17]. The endpoint of therapy is an SVR after therapy as assessed by sensitive molecular method with the lower limit of HCV RNA detection ≤15 International Units/ml (IU/ml) [4, 12, 14].

2.1. Efficacy of IFN-based versus IFN-free regimens for treatment of HCV genotype 1 infections

HCV genotype 1 infection is the most prevalent genotype among all genotypes [8]. So, the drug trials are also largely assessed on this genotype. Previously, the combination of PegIFN alfa with ribavirin was widely used. However, after the introduction of directly acting antiviral (DAA) agents, either they were used in combination with PegIFN and ribavirin or they were used in combination with themselves as two DAAs or four DAAs regimen. The efficacy and tolerability were superior to the previously standard regimen (PegIFN alfa and ribavirin) and also duration was significantly reduced from 24–72 to 12–24 weeks. The IFN-free regimens were better preferred due to higher efficacy rate and fewer adverse effects compared to combination of PegIFN regimens. However, we cannot exclude the fact that PegIFN and ribavirin remain the ultimate option in setting where no other options are available [4, 12, 14]. The different regimens and their efficacy for treatment of genotype 1 infection are given in **Table 2**.

Treatment regimens	Naïve (SVR)	Treatment-experienced (SVR)	Partial responders	Null responders	Relapsers
PegIFN alfa/ ribavirin	SVR 24/48: 42–46% SVR: 49% in North America and 50% Western Europe	–	–	–	–
PegIFN/RBV + boceprevir	SVR 24/44wks (NB): 67–68% (B): 42–53%	SVR32: 59–66% SVR44: 88%	–	–	–
PegIFN/RBV + telaprevir (in previously untreated patients)	T12PR: 75% T8PR: 69% T12PR24: 61% T12PR48: 67% PWID: 71% Non-PWID: 72%	–	68%	46%	–
PegIFN alfa/RBV + simeprevir	**SVR12**: 80% (overall) (1a–71% 1b–90%) NCN: 81%	–	**SVR 24**: 48–86% (1a-56% 1b-88%) C: 82% NCN: 70%	**SVR 24**: 38–59% (1a-42% 1b-58%) C: 31% NCN: 44%	**SVR24**: 77–89% C: 73% NCN: 79.2%
PegIFN alfa/RBV + sofosbuvir	**SVR12**: 89% (overall) (1a-92%, 1b-82%) C: 80% **SVR4**: 85% (overall) NC: 90% C: 70%	**SVR 12**: NC: 77% C: 62%	–	–	–

Treatment regimens	Naïve (SVR)	Treatment-experienced (SVR)	Partial responders	Null responders	Relapsers
Sofosbuvir+ simeprevir	**SVR12:** 91% (+RBV) 95% (−RBV) **SVR12**: 88% (NC) 75% (C)	SVR12: 87% (NC) 76% (C)	–	Non-responders 91%	–
Sofosbuvir + ledipasvir	**SVR8 (NC)**: 94% (−RBV) 93% (+RBV) 95%(+RBV* 12wks) **SVR12:** 99% (−RBV) 97% (+RBV) **SVR24:** 98% (−RBV) 99% (+RBV)	**SVR12 (overall)**: 94% (−RBV) 96% (+RBV) **SVR24:** 99% (−RBV) 99% (+RBV)	–	–	–
Sofosbuvir+ daclatasvir	**NC:** 100% (±RBV) **Cirrhotic**: SVR12: 84.9% SVR24: 93.4%	–	–	**NC**: 100% (−RBV) 95% (+RBV)	–
Sofosbuvir + velpatasvir	–	**SVR12 (overall)**: 98% (1a) 99% (1b)	–	–	–
Ritonavir-boosted paritaprevir, ombitasvir, dasabuvir ± RBV	**SVR12-1a (NC)**: 95–97% (+RBV) 90% (−RBV) 91% (+HIV) **SVR12-1b (NC)**: 98–100% (−RBV) 97–100% (+RBV) **SVR12 (C)**: 92% (1a) 99% (1b)	**SVR12 (NC)**: 96% (1a) 97% (1b) CC: SVR12: 92% SVR24: 96%	NC: 100%	NC: 95%	NC: 95%

PegIFN alfa-pegylated interferon-alfa; RBV-ribavirin; T12PR-telaprevir, pegylated interferon-alfa and ribavirin for 12 weeks; T12PR24-telaprevir, pegylated interferon-alfa and ribavirin for 12 weeks, then pegylated interferon-alfa and ribavirin for remaining 12 weeks (total 24 weeks); T12PR48-telaprevir, pegylated interferon-alfa and ribavirin for 12 weeks then pegylated interferon alfa and ribavirin for remaining 36 weeks (total 48 weeks); NCN, non-cirrhotic naïve; C, cirrhotic; CC, compensated cirrhosis; NB, non-black patients; B, Black patients; PWID, people who inject drugs; SVR 4/8/12/24/48, sustained virological response at 4 weeks, 8 weeks, 12 weeks, 24 weeks or 48 weeks; (+) RBV, with ribavirin; (−)RBV, without ribavirin; (±) RBV, with or without ribavirin

Table 2. Efficacy of IFN-based vs. IFN-free regimens for treatment of HCV genotype 1 infections.

2.1.1. *Pegylated interferon alpha and ribavirin*

The combination of pegylated interferon alpha and ribavirin was a standard regimen previously in treatment of hepatitis C genotype 1 infection. The main drawback with this regimen was longer duration of treatment course, that is, 24–72 weeks. With this regimen, HCV genotype 1 infected patient had SVR rates of approximately 40% in North America and 50% in Western Europe [18]. The SVR rate was comparatively lower in genotype 1 than other genotypes. The previous studies showed SVR of 42–46% infected with genotype 1, treated for 24 or 48 weeks [18, 19]. The HIV co-infected patients had SVR of 40% with this regimen [20]. This regimen is contraindicated in patients with uncontrolled depression, psychosis, or epilepsy, pregnant women or couples unwilling to comply with adequate contraception, severe concurrent medical diseases and co-morbidities including retinal disease, autoimmune thyroid disease, and decompensated liver disease. In patient with hepatitis B co-infection, this regimen is used as monoinfected patients, although there is a potential risk of hepatitis B infection reactivation during HCV clearance [12].

2.1.2. *Boceprevir in combination with pegylated interferon alfa and ribavirin*

Boceprevir is a first generation NS3/4A protease inhibitors (PIs) approved by FDA in 2011. Introduction of PIs constituted a milestone in treating CHC infection, achieved SVR rates of up to 75% in naïve and 29–88% in treatment-experienced patients with GT-1 infection [21, 22]. However, low genetic barrier to resistance is the main limitation. Introduction of newer DAAs replaced the choice of this regimen. The phase 1 and 2 double blind studies carried out for untreated HCV genotype 1 infection in non-black and black populations who were treated for 24–44 weeks showed SVR of 67–68 and 42–53%, respectively [23]. Another study of 403 patients previously treated with PegIFN alfa/RBV regimen, the triple therapy with boceprevir for 32–44 weeks showed SVR of 59–66%. Among patients with an undetectable HCV RNA level at week 8, SVR was 86 and 88% after 32 and 44 weeks of triple therapy, respectively [24]. A study done in 179 cases who inject drugs (PWID) versus non-PWID with this regimen showed SVR of 71 and 72%, respectively. Among them, 53% were advanced stage (F3–4) and 44% were on antiviral therapy [25]. The main side effect of this regimen was anaemia 21–46% for which erythropoietin has to be used or treatment had to discontinue 1–2% [24].

2.1.3. *Telaprevir in combination with pegylated interferon alfa and ribavirin*

Telaprevir is a first generation NS3/4A protease inhibitors (PIs) approved by FDA in 2011. Telaprevir, a protease inhibitor specific to the HCV non-structural 3/4A serine protease, rapidly reduced HCV RNA levels in early studies. A study with this regimen grouped into Telaprevir/PegIFN alfa/RBV (TPR) 12 weeks; T12PR24; and T12PR48 showed sustained virological response of 35, 61 and 67%, respectively [26]. In phase 3 trial with triple therapy in previously untreated genotype 1 infected cases showed T12PR and T8PR SVR of 75 and 69%, respectively [27]. Previously in non-responders and partial responders, the SVR of 44 and 70%, respectively, was achieved [28]. A study done in 179 cases who inject drugs (PWID) versus non-PWID with this regimen showed SVR of 71 and 72%, respectively. Among them, 53% were advanced in stage F3–4 and 44% were on antiviral therapy [25]. The main adverse effect 10–21% with telaprevir was anaemia, gastrointestinal side effect, and skin rash. Rash was the most common reason for discontinuation of therapy [26, 27].

2.1.4. *Simeprevir in combination with pegylated interferon alfa and ribavirin*

Simeprevir (TMC435) is an oral HCV NS3/4A protease inhibitor used in combination with PegIFN alfa and ribavirin to treat HCV genotype 1 infected patients. This combination is generally well tolerated with potent antiviral activity and pharmacokinetic profile. In ASPIRE phase IIb trial done in previously treated patients with PegIFN and ribavirin, the SVR at 24 weeks was 38–59% (1a-42 and 1b-58%) in prior null responders, 48–86% (1a-56 and 1b-88%) in prior partial responders, and 77–89% (no difference) in prior relapsed cases. There were same SVR rates in patient with or without Q80k polymorphism at baseline 60.9%. In patients with cirrhosis (METAVIR score F4), combination therapy with 150 mg of simeprevir had SVR rate at 24 weeks was 73% in prior relapsers, 82% in prior partial responders, and 31% in prior null responders [29]. Another phase 3 trial on partials and null responders showed SVR of 70 and 44%, respectively [28]. According to QUEST 1 & 2 phase 3 study, overall SVR 12 in previously untreated and treated naïve patients was 81 (209/257) and 80% (1a-71 and 1b-90%). On subtype analysis, SVR rates on with or without Q80K polymorphism at baseline in 1a were 52–75 and 80–85%, respectively, and 82% in 1b. The SVR rates were comparatively higher in F0–2 83–85% than F3–4 66–70% [30, 31]. In patients who relapsed on previous therapy, the SVR 12 was 79.2%. Among them, 92.7% were enabled to shorten therapy with PR at 24 weeks [32]. The cause of treatment failure with this regimen was viral breakthrough in 10.6–13%. The main side effects were fatigue, headache, pruritus, and influenza like illness and anaemia. Skin rash and photosensitivity were also very common with simeprevir [29–32].

2.1.5. Sofosbuvir in combination with pegylated interferon alfa and ribavirin

Sofosbuvir is a nucleotide analogue HCV NS5B polymerase inhibitor with similar *in vitro* activity against pan-HCV genotypes. This therapy is used for HCV pan-genotype infections (1–6 genotypes) treatment-naïve patients with or without cirrhosis but no evidence on treatment-experienced patients. In the NEUTRINO phase III trial in treatment-naïve patients, the overall SVR rate was 89% (259/291), 92% (207/225) for subtype 1a and 82% (54/66) for subtype 1b. Cirrhotic patients had a lower SVR rate than non-cirrhotic patients (80 vs. 92%, respectively) [33]. According to two large-scale US real-life studies, the overall SVR4 rate was 85% (140/164, treatment-naïve—55% and treatment-experienced—45%). SVR4 rate was 90% (114/127) in non-cirrhotic compared to 70% (26/37) in cirrhotic patients [34]. In TRIO real-life study including treatment-naïve (58%) and treatment-experienced (42%), SVR12 was 81 (112/138) and 81% (25/31) in non-cirrhotic and cirrhotic treatment-naïve patients, respectively, and 77% (30/39) in non-cirrhotic treatment-experienced and 62% (53/85) in cirrhotic treatment-experienced patients [21].

2.1.6. Sofosbuvir and simeprevir plus ribavirin

In COSMOS study, the combination of sofosbuvir and simeprevir with or without ribavirin for 12 or 24 weeks was assessed in naïve or null responders infected with genotype 1 patient without severe fibrosis. SVR12 was achieved in 91% (98/108) with ribavirin vs. 95% (56/59) of those who did not. SVR rates were similar by treatment status, treatment-naïve 95% (38/40) vs. previous non-responders 91% (116/127) or treatment duration 94% (77/82) after 12 weeks vs. 91% (77/85) after 24 weeks. Neither ribavirin nor treatment duration had clear effect on sustained virological response in HCV-infected patients with Gln80Lys polymorphism at baseline [22]. In TRIO real-life study, SVR12 achieved in 88% (68/88) of non-cirrhotic treatment-naïve and

75% (41/55) of cirrhotic treatment-naïve patients, whereas 87 (64/74) and 76% (53/70) in non-cirrhotic and cirrhotic treatment-experienced patients, respectively [21].

2.1.7. Sofosbuvir and ledipasvir plus ribavirin

Three phase III trials ION-1-3 have assessed the combination of sofosbuvir with ledipasvir, an NS5A inhibitor with or without ribavirin in genotype 1 infected populations. In naïve patients, including 16% compensated cirrhotic populations in ION-1 showed SVR12 in 99 (211/214) and 97% (211/217) patients after 12 weeks combination therapy without or with RBV, respectively. The SVR12 rate was 98% (212/217) in without RBV and 99% (215/217) in with RBV after 24 weeks [35]. In ION-3, non-cirrhotic treatment-naïve patients, SVR12 was 94% (202/215) without RBV for 8 weeks, 93% (201/216) with RBV for 8 weeks, and 95% (205/216) without RBV for 12 weeks. However, relapse rates were higher in 8 weeks compared to 12 weeks therapy [36]. In ION-2, in treatment-experienced patients including 20% cirrhotic patients, overall SVR12 rates were 94 (102/109) and 96% (107/111) without or with RBV, respectively. The SVR rates were 99 (108/109) and 99% (110/111) without or with RBV after 24 weeks, respectively [37]. The different phase III studies were not powered to compare responses to regimens with or without RBV or to 12 weeks or 24 weeks of treatment [38].

2.1.8. Sofosbuvir and daclatasvir

Daclatasvir is a potent, pan-genotypic NS5A inhibitor with antiviral activity against HCV genotypes 1–6 *in vitro* [39], combined with sofosbuvir for treatment of hepatitis C. In phase IIb trial in patient without cirrhosis, the 24 weeks of therapy achieved SVR rates of 100% (14/14 and 15/15) without or with ribavirin, respectively, in treatment-naïve patients, and 100% (21/21) without ribavirin and 95% (19/21) with ribavirin non-responders to combination therapy of PegIFN alfa, ribavirin, and either telaprevir or boceprevir. Whereas SVR rates were achieved in 98% (40/41) of treatment-naïve without ribavirin after 12 weeks of therapy [40]. In phase II clinical trial, the efficacy of sofosbuvir plus daclatasvir with or without ribavirin for 12 or 24 weeks has been evaluated in large real-life cohort including genotype 1 cirrhotic patients. The SVR12 rates were 84.9% after weeks and 93.4% after 24 weeks of treatment. However, majority of analyses performed on data available after 4 weeks of follow up showed SVR4 rates of 85.2% with 12 weeks and 95.1% with 24 weeks of treatment without RBV, whereas 100% with 12 weeks and 98.7% with 24 weeks treatment with RBV [41]. In cirrhosis, the addition of RBV improved SVR, SVR4 of 76.5% with 12 weeks vs. 94% with 24 weeks without RBV treatment, which rose to 100 and 98.3%, respectively, with RBV. In non-cirrhotic patients, SVR4 achieved in all regardless of use of RBV or treatment duration. Without RBV, SVR4 in treatment-naïve after 12 or 24 weeks was 87.1 vs. 88.7%; however, rates increased to 100% (for both duration) with addition of RBV. In treatment-experienced patients, SVR4 without or with RBV after 12 weeks was 82.6 vs. 100%, and after 24 weeks 96.7 vs. 98.5% [41].

2.1.9. Sofosbuvir and velpatasvir

Velpatasvir is a new pangenotypic HCV NS5A inhibitor with antiviral activity against HCV replicons in genotype 1–6 infections. The combination of sofosbuvir and velpatasvir for

12 weeks has been assessed in ASTRAL phase 3 trial in previously treatment-experienced patients (PegIFN/RBV with PIs) including cirrhosis, relapsed cases, patients who had detectable HCV RNA after PegIFN and ribavirin treatment. The overall sustained virological response rate was 98% in subtype 1a and 99% in subtype 1b infected patients [42]. In phase II trial in treatment-experienced patients including 50% cirrhosis and treatment failure, the combination of sofosbuvir and velpatasvir with or without ribavirin was assessed. The SVR showed 100% in without ribavirin and 96% in with ribavirin treatment patients [43]. The overall relapse rate was very low, and this regimen was well tolerated in treatment-experienced patient including cirrhosis [42, 43].

2.1.10. Ritonavir boosted paritaprevir, ombitasvir, and dasabuvir

In seven phase III trials, in non-cirrhotic treatment-naïve patients, SAPPHIRE-I trial with combination therapy with RBV for 12 weeks showed SVR of 95% (307/322) in subtype 1a and 98% (148/151) in subtype 1b infected patients [44]. In PEARL-IV trial, the combination therapy without or with RBV showed SVR of 90 (185/205) vs. 97% (197/100) in subtype 1a treatment-naïve patients, respectively [45]. In PEARL-III trial in non-cirrhotic treatment-naïve of subtype 1b patients, SVR12 rates were 99% (207/209) without RBV vs. 99% (209/210) with RBV [45]. TURQUOISE-I study in non-cirrhotic treatment-naïve patients co-infected with HIV-1 (stable on antiviral treatment – atazanavir or raltegravir), SVR12 rates were 93% (29/31) after 12 weeks vs. 91% (29/32) after 24 weeks of treatment. The SVR12 rates based on subtypes 1a and 1b were 91 (51/56) and 100% (7/7), respectively [46]. In SAPPHIRE-II trial, non-cirrhotic treatment-experienced patients (PegIFN-alfa and RBV failures) were treated with this regimen in combination with RBC for 12 weeks. The SVR12 rates were 96% (166/173) in subtype 1a vs. 97% (119/123) in subtype 1b. The overall SVR12 rates were 95% (82/86) in prior relapsers, 100% (65/65) in partial responders, and 95% (139/146) in null responders [47]. In PEARL-II trial, SVR12 achieved in 100% (91/91) without RBV vs. 97% (85/88) with RBV in subtype 1b infected patients [48]. In compensated cirrhotic treatment-naïve and treatment-experienced patients, the SVR rates were 92% (191/208) after 12 weeks vs. 96% (165/172) after 24 weeks of treatment with RBV in TURQUISE-II trial. The SVR12 rates were 92% (239/261) in subtype 1a vs. 99% (118/119) in subtype 1b infected patients [49].

2.2. Efficacy of IFN-based versus IFN-free regimens for treatment of HCV genotype 2 infections

HCV genotype 2 is the third most prevalent genotype worldwide [8]. Although PegIFN alfa with ribavirin used previously, IFN-free combination of sofosbuvir with ribavirin is the best first line treatment option in genotype 2 infection [12]. Other regimens, IFN-based or IFN-free could be an option in cases who fail with this regimen (**Table 3**). The combination of PegIFN alfa and ribavirin remains acceptable when all other options are not available [12, 14].

2.2.1. Pegylated interferon alfa and ribavirin

The initial treatment of HCV genotype 2 began with PegIFN alfa alone or combination of PegIFN alfa and ribavirin. Although sustained virological response rate was lower than recent newer regimens, this regimen remains acceptable for treatment of genotype 2 where other options are not available [12]. In randomised study, the sustained virological response rates were 62% (232/372) in 16 weeks vs. 75% (268/356) in 24 weeks treatment course. The chances of relapse rates were higher among 16 weeks than 24 weeks [50]. In phase IV single arm study, 24 weeks therapy with this regimen in previously untreated naïve patients showed end of treatment (EOT) and SVR of 100 and 93%, respectively [51]. In phase III multicenter study in prior relapsers who were retreated for 24–48 weeks showed a sustained virological response rates of 53–81% in 48 weeks retreated patients vs. 75% in 24 weeks retreated patients [52].

Treatment regimens	Naïve	Treatment-experienced	Partial responders	Null responders	Relapsers
PegIFN alfa/ ribavirin	**SVR 24**: 62% (16 weeks) 75% (24 weeks) **24 weeks therapy**: SVR: 93% EOT: 100%	SVR24:75% SVR48: 53–81% (48 weeks)	–	–	–
PegIFN/RBV + sofosbuvir	SVR12: 92%	SVR12: 96% (overall)	–	–	–
Sofosbuvir + ribavirin	**SVR12**: 93–100% (overall) 93–97%(NC) 83–100%(C) **SVR12**: 82% (NC) 60% (C) **SVR16**: 89% (NC) 78% (C)	**SVR12**: 91% (NC) 88% (C) **SVR12**: 94% (overall)	-	-	-
Sofosbuvir + daclatasvir	SVR12: 92%	–	–	–	–
Sofosbuvir + velpatasvir	–	**SVR12**: 99% (overall)	–	–	–

PegIFN, pegylated interferon-alfa; RBV, ribavirin; EOT, end of treatment; SVR-12/16/24, sustained virological response at 12 weeks, 16 weeks and 24 weeks; NC, non-cirrhotic; C, cirrhotic.

Table 3. Efficacy of IFN-based vs. IFN-free regimens for treatment of HCV genotype 2 infections.

2.2.2. *Pegylated interferon alfa and ribavirin plus sofosbuvir*

In LONESTAR-2 phase IIb study, in treatment-experienced patients infected with HCV genotype 2 patients including 14 with cirrhosis received therapy for 12 weeks, the sustained virological response rates were 96% [53]. Another study showed that the relapsed cases of sofosbuvir and ribavirin regimen treated for 12 weeks were retreated with this regimen for 12 weeks, achieved SVR [54]. In phase II study in previously untreated naïve patients, the sustained virological responses in 12 or 24 weeks treatment were 92% (23/25) [55]. The main side effects with this regimen were fatigue, headache, nausea, pain, and insomnia [55].

2.2.3. Sofosbuvir and ribavirin

This IFN-free combination therapy is the best first-line treatment option in HCV genotype 2 infected patients [12]. In FISSION trial in treatment-naïve patients who were treated for 12 weeks, the SVR was 95% (69/73). The virological response rate was higher in non-cirrhotic patients, 97 vs. 83% in cirrhotic patients [33]. In POSITRON trial, who were intolerant or ineligible to IFN, treated for 12 weeks, SVR was 93% (101/109) [56]. The 12 vs. 16 weeks therapy was in FUSION trial showed SVR of 82 (32/39) vs. 89% (31/35) in non-cirrhotic and 60 (6/10) vs. 78% (7/9) in cirrhotic cases, respectively. The longer than 12 weeks therapy was beneficial in cirrhotic population [56]. In VALENCE trial, the treatment was given for 12 weeks in treatment-naïve and treatment-experienced patients with or without cirrhosis. In treatment-naïve patients, the SVR rates were 97% (29/30) in without cirrhosis and 100% (2/2) in with cirrhosis. In treatment-experienced patients, SVR rates were 91 (30/33) vs. 88% (7/8) in without cirrhosis and with cirrhosis, respectively [57]. This combination therapy was well tolerated, and no virological breakthroughs were observed in treatment adherent patients [12].

2.2.4. Sofosbuvir and daclatasvir

Daclatasvir, NS5A replication complex inhibitor, is active against HCV genotype 2 *in vitro*. The combination of sofosbuvir with daclatasvir therapy was observed in phase II trial showed sustained virological response of 92% (24/26) after 12 weeks of therapy and overall 93% after 24 weeks of therapy [40]. Based on data with other, 12 weeks is probably sufficient to treat more difficult-to-cure HCV genotypes. This regimen should be kept reserved for patients who failed with other options in HCV genotype 2 infections [12, 40].

2.2.5. Sofosbuvir and velpatasvir

In 2 phase III trial (open label studies), the combination of sofosbuvir (400 mg) and velpatasvir (100 mg) was assessed in patients infected with HCV genotype 2 who previously received treatment and who did not received previous treatment including compensated cirrhosis. The sustained virological response was achieved in 99% of cases with this regimen [58]. In ASTRAL phase III double blind trial in treatment-experienced patients including cirrhosis, treatment relapsed, and detectable HCV RNA under PegIFN and ribavirin therapy, the SVR12 was 100% in genotype 2 infected patients [42]. From the data available, this regimen was well tolerated with higher SVR in treatment of genotype 2 infection. However, these data have to be compared with the blind trials or studies.

2.3. Efficacy of IFN-based versus IFN-free regimens for treatment of HCV genotype 3 infections

There are four treatment options available for treatment of hepatitis C genotype 3 infection including one phase III trial drug (**Table 4**). The IFN-based combination therapy-PegIFN alfa and ribavirin regimen remains acceptable only in settings where none other options are available [12]. The triple combination of PegIFN alfa, ribavirin and sofosbuvir appears to be valuable even in, who failed on sofosbuvir and ribavirin combinations. However, it has to be done in larger population infected with HCV genotype 3 patients [54]. The IFN-free combination therapy—sofosbuvir and ribavirin—appears to be suboptimal particularly in cirrhotic HCV genotype 3 infected patients, although it is the best first line treatment option for genotype 2 infection [12]. Sofosbuvir and daclatasvir with or without ribavirin are a new attractive option for patients infected with genotype 3. Ledipasvir is considerably less potent against genotype 3 *in vitro* than daclatasvir. In clinical trials, the combination of ledipasvir with sofosbuvir or other agents is not recommended in patients infected with HCV genotype 3 [12, 14].

Treatment regimens	Naïve	Treatment-experienced	Partial responders	Null responders	Relapsers
PegIFN alfa/ ribavirin	24 weeks: SVR-79% EOT-93%	–	–	–	–
PegIFN/RBV + sofosbuvir	–	SVR12: 83% (+C)	–	–	SVR12: 91%
Sofosbuvir and ribavirin	**SVR12**: 56–61% (overall) 61% (NC) 34% (C) **SVR12 vs. SVR16**: 30 vs. 62% (NC) 19 vs. 61% (C) **SVR24**: 94%(NC) 92%(C)	**SVR24**: 80% (overall) 87% (NC) 60% (C)	–	–	**SVR24**: 63%
Sofosbuvir and daclatasvir	**SVR24**: 89% (NC) **SVR12 (–RBV)**: 97% (NC) 58% (C)	**SVR12 (–RBV)**: 94% (NC) 69% (C)	–	–	–
Sofosbuvir and velpatasvir		**SVR12 (overall)**: 95% **SVR12 (NC)**: 100% (±RBV) **SVR12 (C)**: 88% (–RBV) 96% (+RBV)	–	–	–

PegIFN, pegylated interferon-alfa; RBV, ribavirin; SVR 12/24, sustained virological response at 12 weeks and 24 weeks; EOT, end of treatment; NC, non-cirrhotic; C, cirrhotic.

Table 4. Efficacy of IFN-based vs. IFN-free regimens for treatment of HCV genotype 3 infections.

2.3.1. Pegylated interferon alfa and ribavirin

This combination therapy remained acceptable for treatment of genotype 3 infections until the development of other regimens with higher sustained virological response and also in setting where other options are not available [12]. In this regimen, the treatment is given for 24 weeks in genotype 3 infected patients. In phase 4 single arm study in 182 HCV genotype 3 infected population and treatment was given with this regimen for 24 weeks; the overall sustained virological response rate was observed and also at end of treatment (EOT). It showed EOT and SVR were of 93 and 79%, respectively [51]. Baseline viremia, treatment duration >16 weeks, and steatosis were independent predictors of SVR. The relapsed rate were higher among male and older age >55 years [51].

2.3.2. Pegylated interferon alfa and ribavirin plus sofosbuvir

In LONESTAR-2 phase IIb trial, in treatment-experienced patients infected with HCV genotype 3, the sustained virological response rate was 83% (20/24) including (10/12) patients with cirrhosis [53]. However, pangenotypic activity of sofosbuvir together with higher SVR in other genotypes 89% (overall in genotype 1, 4 or 6) indicates this regimen can be safely used in patients with genotype 3 infections [53]. In phase 2 trial, in non-cirrhotic treatment-naïve patients were treated for 12 weeks, the sustained virological response was achieved in 92% (23/25) cases [55]. In another study, patients who relapsed after treatment with sofosbuvir and ribavirin regimens were retreated with this triple combination therapy for 12 weeks, and the SVR was achieved in 91% (20/22) cases [54].

2.3.3. Sofosbuvir and ribavirin

The combination of sofosbuvir with daily fixed dose ribavirin is used for treatment of genotype 3 infection for 24 weeks. In FISSION trial, in treatment-naïve patients who were treated for 12 weeks, the SVR rate was 56% (102/183). The non-cirrhotic patients had better SVR of 61 vs. 34% in cirrhotic patients [33]. In POSITRON trial, patients were also treated for 12 weeks with this regimen who were ineligible or intolerant to interferon. The SVR rate was 61% (60/98) of cases. In FUSION trial, the 12 vs. 16 weeks treatment was compared. The SVR rate was significantly higher, 62% in non-cirrhotic and 61% in cirrhotic patients with 16 weeks treatment compared to 30% in non-cirrhotic and 19% in cirrhotic patient with 12 weeks treatment [56]. In VALENCE trial, treatment was given for 24 weeks in both treatment-naïve and treatment-experienced without or with cirrhosis. In treatment- naïve, the SVR24 was 94% (86/92) in non-cirrhotic and 92% (12/13) in cirrhotic patients. Whereas, in treatment-experienced, SVR 24 was 87% (87/100) in non-cirrhotic and 60% (27/45) in cirrhotic patients [57]. So based on these studies, 24 weeks treatment is appropriate for the HCV genotype 3 infected patients. Another study, in relapsed cases with sofosbuvir and ribavirin, patients were retreated for 24 weeks, achieved SVR only of 63% (24/38) of cases, indicating the regimen is suboptimal in such patients with HCV genotype 3 infection [54].

2.3.4. Sofosbuvir and daclatasvir

In treatment of HCV genotype 3 infected patients, this regimen is given for 12 weeks in non-cirrhotic patients and 24 weeks with daily weight-based ribavirin for 24 weeks in cirrhotic patients. In phase IIb trial, after 24 weeks of combination therapy, SVR rate was 89% (16/18) in treatment-naïve without cirrhosis [40]. In ALLY-3 phase III trial, after 12 weeks of combination therapy without ribavirin, SVR12 was 97% (73/75) in non-cirrhotic and 58% (11/19) in cirrhotic treatment-naïve patients, whereas SVR12 was 94 (32/34) and 69% (9/13) in treatment-experienced patients without or with cirrhosis, respectively [59]. This regimen was well tolerated with rare adverse events, and none of them discontinued treatment [12].

2.3.5. Sofosbuvir and velpatasvir

In phase II trial, the combination of sofosbuvir (400 mg) and velpatasvir (100 mg) with or without daily fixed dose ribavirin for 12 weeks was assessed in treatment-experienced patients with or without cirrhosis infected with HCV genotype 3. The sustained virological response was achieved 100% with or without ribavirin in non-cirrhotic patients. However, SVR of 88% without ribavirin and 96% with ribavirin was achieved in compensated cirrhotic patients [43]. In another 2 phase III trial (open label studies), in patients infected with genotype 3 who have previously received treatment and who did not receive treatment including compensated cirrhosis, 12 weeks of this regimen without ribavirin achieved SVR of 95% [58]. Based on these studies, this regimen was well tolerated in treatment of HCV genotype 3 infections.

2.4. Efficacy of IFN-based versus IFN-free regimens for treatment of HCV genotype 4 infections

There are seven treatment options available for treatment of hepatitis C genotype 4 infections, including two IFN-based regimens and four IFN-free regimens (**Table 5**). The combination of PegIFN alfa and ribavirin remains acceptable only in that case where other options are not available [12].

Treatment regimens	Naïve	Treatment-experienced	Partial responders	Null responders	Relapsers
PegIFN alfa/ ribavirin	SVR24: 29% SVR36: 66% SVR48: 69%				
PegIFN/RBV + simeprevir	SVR24: 93%	–	SVR48: 60%	SVR48: 40%	SVR24: 86%
PegIFN/RBV + sofosbuvir	SVR 12: 96%	–	–	–	–
Sofosbuvir + simeprevir	SVR12: >98% (F1–2) 80–97.7% (F3–4)	SVR12: 98–100% (F1–2) 88–94.7% (F3–4)	–	–	–
Sofosbuvir+ ledipasvir	SVR12: 95% (–RBV)	–	–	–	–
Sofosbuvir+ daclatasvir	–	–	–	-	-
Sofosbuvir and velpatasvir	–	SVR12 (overall): 100% (+C/R)	–	–	–
Ritonavir boosted paritaprevir, ombitasvir	SVR12: 100% (+RBV) 90.9% (–RBV)	SVR12 (+RBV): 100%	–	–	–

PegIFN, pegylated interferon-alfa; RBV, ribavirin; SVR 12/24/36/48, sustained virological response at 12 weeks, 24 weeks, 36 weeks and 48 weeks; (+)C/R, with cirrhosis and relapse; (–)RBV, with ribavirin; (+) RBV, with ribavirin.

Table 5. Efficacy of IFN-based vs. IFN-free regimens for treatment of HCV genotype 4 infections.

2.4.1. *Pegylated interferon alfa and ribavirin*

The combination of PegIFN alfa and ribavirin is still the option for treatment of HCV genotype 4 when other options are not available [12]. In prospective randomise controlled trial, the combination of PegIFN alfa and ribavirin was used for 24–48 weeks. The sustained virological response rates were 29 vs. 66 vs. 69% in 24 vs. 36 vs. 48 weeks of treatment, respectively [60].

2.4.2. *Pegylated interferon alfa and ribavirin plus simeprevir*

Simeprevir is active against HCV genotype 4 *in vitro*. So, this combination therapy can be used in genotype 4 infection. However, the duration of therapy is 24 weeks (SPR 12 + PR 12 weeks) in treatment-naïve or prior relapsers including cirrhosis and 48 weeks (SPR12 + PR 36 weeks) in prior partial or null responders including cirrhosis. In phase III study, SVR12 was achieved in 83% (29/35) in treatment-naïve patients, 86% (19/22) in prior relapsers, 60% (6/10) in prior partial responders, and 40% (16/40) in prior null responders. This regimen was effective in treatment-naïve and prior relapsers, however, suboptimal in prior partial and null responders [61].

2.4.3. *Pegylated interferon alfa and ribavirin plus sofosbuvir*

In NEUTRINO phase III in treatment-naïve patients, this combination therapy for 12 weeks was evaluated. The SVR rate was 96% (27/28) in HCV genotype 4 infected patients [33]. Those who failed in this combination therapy did not select HCV variants resistant to sofosbuvir. No data were available in treatment-experienced or HIV-coinfected patients [12].

2.4.4. *Sofosbuvir and ledipasvir*

Sofosbuvir in combination with ledipasvir is used in treatment-naïve and treatment-experienced patients with or without cirrhosis for 12 weeks. Addition of ribavirin to this therapy has beneficial effect in cirrhotic individuals. In SYNERGY trial, efficacy and safety of combination of sofosbuvir and ledipasvir without ribavirin are assessed in patient with genotype 4 infection. The sustained virological response was achieved in 95% (20/21) of cases [62]. The shorter 8 weeks treatment duration as in patients infected with genotype 1 infections is not clear due to lack of data in genotype 4 infected cases [12].

2.4.5. *Sofosbuvir and simeprevir*

The unavailability of data on treatment of HCV genotype 4 infection had questioned the use of this IFN-free regimen (sofosbuvir plus simeprevir) as an option previously, however, according to a very recently published two studies, sofosbuvir (SOF) plus simeprevir (SIM) regimen with or without ribavirin, can be a good option in treating HCV genotype 4 infected cases [12, 63, 64]. A retrospective multicentre observational study in 53 patients (naïve or experienced patients) including advanced liver fibrosis or liver cirrhosis treated with SOF and SIM with or without ribavirin showed a SVR12 of 92% (49/53). In this study, treatment failures were observed in those who didn't receive ribavirin and interferon non-responders except one naïve patient [63]. Another multicentre observational study in 583 patients infected with HCV genotype 4 showed the overall SVR rates of 95.7% (558/583) with SOF/SIM regimen. Based on fibrosis stages in naïve patients, mild fibrosis score had better SVR12 of 98.9% (94/95) in F1 and 98.1% (105/107) in F2 stage than severe fibrosis score with SVR12 of 97.7% (86/88) in F3 and 80.8% (42/52) in F4 stage. While in treatment-experienced patients with severe fibrosis score, SVR12 was 94.7% (72/76) in F3 and 88.9% (40/45) in F4 stage. In addition, patients who were previously treated with interferon had SVR of 100% (45/45) in F1 and 98.7% (74/75) in F2 mild fibrosis score [64]. Therefore, this regimen can be efficacious and well tolerated in treatment-naïve and experienced patients including severe fibrosis score or liver cirrhosis. Furthermore, the addition of ribavirin could be considered especially in treatment-experienced and advanced cirrhosis patients as recommended by recent AASL and EASL guidelines [12, 14, 63, 64].

2.4.6. *Sofosbuvir and daclatasvir*

Daclatasvir has its antiviral activity against genotype 4 *in vitro*. The combination of sofosbuvir and daclatasvir with or without ribavirin is effective in treating patients infected with HCV genotype 4. However, there is no data available with this combination in treatment of this genotype. Nevertheless, both sofosbuvir and daclatasvir have antiviral effectiveness against genotype 4 *in vitro*. So, the results in patients infected with genotype 1 can be extrapolated [12].

2.4.7. *Sofosbuvir and velpatasvir*

Velpatasvir and sofosbuvir have a pangenotypic action for treatment of HCV genotype 1–6 infections. The combination of sofosbuvir and velpatasvir assessed in ASTRAL phase 3 trial in previously treatment-experienced patients (PegIFN/RBV with PIs) including cirrhosis, relapsed cases, patients who had detectable HCV RNA after PegIFN and ribavirin treatment. The overall sustained virological response rate was 100% in genotype 4 infected patients. The overall relapse rate was very low, and this regimen was well tolerated in treatment-experienced patient including cirrhosis [42].

2.4.8. *Ritonavir-boosted paritaprevir and ombitasvir*

A fixed dose ritonavir, paritaprevir, and ombitasvir with or without ribavirin treatment for 12–24 weeks were assessed in treatment-naïve and treatment-experienced patients with or without compensated cirrhosis infected with HCV genotype 4. According to PEARL-I trial in non-cirrhotic chronic HCV genotype 4 infected patients, sustained virological response rates were 100% in treatment-naïve (42/42) and treatment-experienced patients (49/49) with ribavirin regimen, whereas 90.9% (40/44) in treatment-naïve patients without ribavirin regimen for 12 weeks [65]. In AGATE-I trial with a fixed dose ritonavir, paritaprevir, and ombitasvir plus ribavirin in chronic HCV genotype 4 infected treatment-naïve and treatment-experienced patients including compensated cirrhosis, post-treatment sustained virological response rates were 97% (57/59) in 12 weeks and 98% (60/61) in 16 weeks group [66]. In addition, AGATE-II trial in Egyptian patients, SVR12 was 94% (94/100) in patients without cirrhosis, whereas SVR12 of 97% (30/31) and SVR24 of 93% (27/29) in patients with cirrhosis [67]. Extension of this treatment regimen beyond 12 weeks (16 and 24 weeks) for HCV genotype 4 infected patients with compensated cirrhosis seemed to have no additional benefits [66, 67]. This regimen was generally well tolerated by chronic HCV genotype 4 infected patients with or without compensated cirrhosis in clinical trials, so this regimen is a valuable option, although having postmarking reports of hepatic decompensation and hepatic failure mainly in patients with advanced cirrhosis [68].

2.5. Efficacy of IFN-based versus IFN-free regimens for treatment of HCV genotypes 5 or 6 infections

HCV genotype 5 is the least prevalent worldwide and then genotype 6 infection [8]. The treatment options for these genotypes are one IFN-based triple combination of PegIFN alfa, ribavirin, and sofosbuvir; and three IFN-free combination therapy: sofosbuvir and ledipasvir, sofosbuvir and daclatasvir, and sofosbuvir and velpatasvir (**Table 6**). IFN-based combination of PegIFN-alfa and ribavirin remains acceptable in setting where other treatment options are not available [12].

Treatment Regimens	Naïve	Treatment-experienced	Partial responders	Null responders	Relapsers
PegIFN/RBV + sofosbuvir	SVR12: 90%	–	–	–	–
Sofosbuvir and ledipasvir	SVR (GT-5): 95% SVR12 (TN+TE): 96% (overall)	SVR (GT-5): 95%	–	–	–
Sofosbuvir and daclatasvir	–	–	–	–	–
Sofosbuvir and velpatasvir	SVR12 (overall): 96%	SVR12 (overall): 97% (GT-5) 100% (GT-6)	–	–	–

PegIFN, pegylated interferon alfa; RBV, ribavirin; GT-5, genotype 5; GT-6, genotype 6; SVR12, sustained virological response at 12 weeks; TN+TE, treatment-naïve and treatment-experienced.

Table 6. Efficacy of IFN-based vs. IFN-free regimens for treatment of HCV genotype 5 or 6 infections.

2.5.1. Pegylated interferon alfa and ribavirin plus sofosbuvir

In NEUTRINO phase III trial, this combination therapy has been evaluated in treatment-naïve patients. There were total seven patients (one infected genotype 5 and six infected with genotype 6), all patients achieved sustained virological response [33]. However, no data have been presented with this regimen in treatment-experienced patients. So, it is not clear whether longer duration of treatment is needed [12].

2.5.2. Sofosbuvir and ledipasvir

Ledipasvir is active against both genotype 5 or 6 *in vitro*. The combination of sofosbuvir and ledipasvir is used in treatment of these genotypes. Those patients without cirrhosis, including treatment-naïve and treatment-experienced should be treated for 12 weeks without ribavirin. Addition of ribavirin is recommended in cirrhotic cases. However, 24 weeks combination of sofosbuvir and ledipasvir is recommended, when ribavirin is contraindicated or with poor tolerance [12]. In multicentre open label phase II trial, in treatment-naïve and treatment-experienced patients infected with genotype 5 including cirrhosis, the overall SVR was 95% (39/42). The SVR was 95% (20/21) in treatment-naïve and 95% (19/20) in treatment-experienced patients. However, SVR was 97% (31/32) in non-cirrhotic vs. 89% (8/9) in cirrhotic patients [69]. In phase 2 clinical trial, in treatment-naïve and treatment-experienced patients infected with HCV genotype 6, the 12 weeks treatment with this regimen without ribavirin had a sustained virological response of 96% (24/25) [12, 70].

2.5.3. Sofosbuvir and daclatasvir

Daclatasvir and sofosbuvir are active against genotype 5 or 6 *in vitro*. This regimen is given for 12 weeks with or without ribavirin in these genotypes. However, in cirrhotic patients with contraindications or intolerance to ribavirin, combination therapy can be extended to 24 weeks. There were no data available with this regimen for these rare genotypes [12].

2.5.4. Sofosbuvir and velpatasvir

The combination of sofosbuvir (400 mg) and velpatasvir (100 mg) for 12 weeks was assessed in ASTRAL phase III trial for treatment of genotypes 5 and 6. In this double blind, placebo controlled trial, patients were previously treatment-experienced (PegIFN and ribavirin or PegIFN, ribavirin and protease inhibitors), relapsed cases, and who had persistent detectable HCV RNA on PegIFN alfa and ribavirin therapy. The sustained virological response achieved in patients infected with genotypes 5 and 6 were 97 and 100%, respectively. This regimen was well tolerated, with very low failure rate in treatment of HCV genotype 5 and 6 infections [42]. In another randomised trial, the overall sustained virological response was 95% in treatment-naïve patients [71].

3. Discussion

The development of DAAs was the milestone in the treatment of chronic hepatitis C, and their combination therapy became the first option for almost all genotypes. However, the IFN-based combination therapies have their own role in treatment of chronic hepatitis C infections when DAAs combination regimens are unavailable or fails [12]. In genotype 1 infections, the IFN-based combination therapy: PegIFN alfa, RBV, and simeprevir, and PegIFN, RBV, and sofosbuvir combination had higher overall SVR of 60–90% including relapsers or partial/null responders compared to other three regimens. In IFN-free regimens, all the DAAs combination regimens (2/4 DAAs ± RBV) have overall SVR of above 90% [12, 14]. The combination of sofosbuvir with ledipasvir or daclatasvir velpatasvir or 4DAAs (ritonavir, paritaprevir, ombitasvir, & dasabuvir) had superior SVR rates compared to IFN-based regimens [35, 36, 40, 42, 44]. In HCV genotype 2 infections, though PegIFN alfa with RBV and sofosbuvir has higher SVR >90%, the combination of sofosbuvir and ribavirin is the first line regimen for its treatment [33]. Although combination of sofosbuvir with daclatasvir or velpatasvir has SVR > 90%, they are reserved for treatment failed options with first line drugs [40–43]. In genotype 3 infections, the combination of sofosbuvir and ribavirin is suboptimal [54], so IFN-based PegIFN/RBV/SOF regimen or IFN-free combination of SOF and daclatasvir becomes the choice of treatment [40, 54, 59]. The phase 3 trials, sofosbuvir and velpatasvir have higher SVR, so it might be the choice of regimen in future [43, 58]. In genotype 4 infections, IFN-based PegIFN, RBV with simeprevir or sofosbuvir have SVR > 90% in treatment-naïve cases. However, SVR in partial or null responders is suboptimal [33, 61]. The IFN-free two DAAs or three DAAs with or without RBV has overall SVR > 90%, although no data available for partial or null responders or relapsers cases [42, 62, 65, 72]. In genotype 5 or 6 infections, IFN-based PegIFN/RBV/SOF has SVR of 90% in treatment-naïve [33]. However, two DAAs combinations have better SVR of > 95% [12, 43, 69, 70]. In this review, it showed that IFN-free DAAs regimens have better SVR and well tolerated compared to IFN-based regimen. The combination of DAAs with or without ribavirin has almost replaced the IFN-based combination therapy in present context. Nevertheless, we cannot exclude the fact that the combination of PegIFN alfa and ribavirin still leaves us an ultimate option in setting where all other options are not available [12, 14].

4. Conclusion

The combination of IFN-free DAAs regimens has superior in their efficacy and tolerability compared to IFN-based regimens in case of treatment of chronic hepatitis C in all genotypes. However, in genotypes 3, 4, 5 or 6, the IFN-based combination of pegylated interferon alfa, ribavirin, and sofosbuvir can be an option in case of treatment failure with DAAs first line regimens. Nevertheless, this is not mentioned in the retreatment guidelines, and this is just an assumed recommendation that needs to be evaluated in trials.

Authors' contributions

All the authors have equally contributed to research design, editing, and finalising of this chapter.

Conflict of interest statement

The authors declared that there is no conflict of interest regarding the publication of this chapter.

Acknowledgements

This study was supported by the grants from the National Natural Science Foundation of China (No. 81370559), Shanghai major joint project for important diseases (2014ZYJB0201), and Shanghai joint project with advanced technology (SHDC12014122).

http://dx.doi.org/10.5772/67214

Abbreviations

HCV	hepatitis C virus
WHO	World Health Organisation
DAA	directly acting antivirals
IFN	interferon
SVR	sustained virological response
CHC	chronic hepatitis C
AHC	acute hepatitis C
HCC	hepatocellular carcinoma
GT	genotype
PWID	persons who inject drugs
MSM	men who have sex with men
HIV	human immunodeficiency virus
RBV	ribavirin
SVR12/24/48	sustained virological response at 12, 24, and 48 weeks
PegIFN alfa	pegylated interferon alfa
PIs	protease inhibitors
TPR	telaprevir/pegylated interferon alfa/ribavirin
EOT	end of treatment

Author details

Ramesh Rana, Yizhong Chang, Jing Li, ShengLan Wang, Li Yang and ChangQing Yang*

*Address all correspondence to: cqyang@tongji.edu.cn

Division of Gastroenterology and Hepatology, Digestive Disease Institute, Tongji Hospital, Tongji University School of Medicine, Shanghai, PR China

References

[1] World Health Organization. WHO Guidelines Approved by the Guidelines Review Committee. In: Guidelines for the Screening Care and Treatment of Persons with Chronic Hepatitis C Infection: Updated Version. Edn. Geneva: World Health Organization. 2016. PMID: 27227200.

[2] Chopp S, Vanderwall R, HUIT A, Klepser M: Simeprevir and sofosbuvir for treatment of hepatitis C infection. Am J Health Syst Pharm 2015, 72(17), p1445–1455. DOI: 10.214/ajhp140290

[3] Thomson EC, Fleming VM, Main J, Klenerman P, Weber J, Eliahoo J, Smith J, McClure MO, Karayiannis P: Predicting spontaneous clearance of acute hepatitis C virus in a large cohort of HIV-1-infected men. Gut 2010:gut. 2010, 60(6): 837–845. DOI: 10.1136/gut.2010.217166

[4] Mauss S, Berg T, Rockstroh J, Sarrazin C, Wedemeyer H: Hepatology – A Clinical Textbook 2016, 356. http://www.hepatologytextbook.com/download/hepatology2016.pdf.

[5] Coppola N, Pisaturo M, Zampino R, Macera M, Sagnelli C, Sagnelli E: Hepatitis C virus markers in infection by hepatitis C virus: In the era of directly acting antivirals. World J Gastroenterol 2015, 21(38):10749. DOI: 10.3748/wjg.v21.i38.10749

[6] Thein HH, Yi Q, Dore GJ, Krahn MD: Estimation of stage-specific fibrosis progression rates in chronic hepatitis C virus infection: A meta-analysis and meta-regression. Hepatology 2008, 48(2):418–431. DOI: 10.1002/hep.22375

[7] Smith DB, Bukh J, Kuiken C, Muerhoff AS, Rice CM, Stapleton JT, Simmonds P: Expanded classification of hepatitis C virus into 7 genotypes and 67 subtypes: Updated criteria and genotype assignment web resource. Hepatology 2014, 59(1):318–327. DOI: 10.1002/hep.26744

[8] Messina JP, Humphreys I, Flaxman A, Brown A, Cooke GS, Pybus OG, Barnes E: Global distribution and prevalence of hepatitis C virus genotypes. Hepatology 2015, 61(1):77–87. DOI: 10.1002/hep.27259

[9] Wasitthankasem R, Vongpunsawad S, Siripon N, Suya C, Chulothok P, Chaiear K, Rujirojindakul P, Kanjana S, Theamboonlers A, Tangkijvanich P: Genotypic distribution of hepatitis C virus in Thailand and Southeast Asia. PLoS One 2015, 10(5):e0126764. DOI: 10.1002/hep.27259

[10] Magiorkinis G, Magiorkinis E, Paraskevis D, Ho SY, Shapiro B, Pybus OG, Allain J-P, Hatzakis A: The global spread of hepatitis C virus 1a and 1b: A phylodynamic and phylogeographic analysis. PLoS Med 2009, 6(12):e1000198. DOI: 10.1371/journal.pmed.1000198

[11] Murphy DG, Sablon E, Chamberland J, Fournier E, Dandavino R, Tremblay CL: Hepatitis C virus genotype 7, a new genotype originating from Central Africa. J Clin Microbiol 2015, 53(3):967–972. DOI: 10.1128/JCM.02831

[12] European Association for Study of L: EASL recommendations on treatment of hepatitis C 2015. J Hepatol 2015, 63(1):199–236. DOI: 10.1016/j.jhep.2015.03.025

[13] Hézode C, Bronowicki J-P: Ideal oral combinations to eradicate HCV: The role of ribavirin. J Hepatol 2016, 64(1):215–225. DOI: 10.1016/j.jhep.2015.09009

[14] Panel A: Hepatitis C guidance: AASLD-IDSA recommendations for testing, managing, and treating adults infected with hepatitis C virus. Hepatology 2015, 62:932–954. DOI: 10.1002/hep.27950

[15] Solbach P, Wedemeyer H: The new era of interferon-free treatment of chronic hepatitis C. Viszeralmedizin 2015, 31(4):290–296. DOI: 10.1159/000433594

[16] Arase Y, Kobayashi M, Suzuki F, Suzuki Y, Kawamura Y, Akuta N, Kobayashi M, Sezaki H, Saito S, Hosaka T, et al.: Effect of type 2 diabetes on risk for malignancies includes hepatocellular carcinoma in chronic hepatitis C. Hepatology 2013, 57(3):964–973. DOI: 10.1002/hep.26087

[17] van der Meer AJ, Veldt BJ, Feld JJ, Wedemeyer H, Dufour J-F, Lammert F, Duarte-Rojo A, Heathcote EJ, Manns MP, Kuske L: Association between sustained virological response and all-cause mortality among patients with chronic hepatitis C and advanced hepatic fibrosis. JAMA 2012, 308(24):2584–2593. DOI: 10.1001/jama.2012.144878

[18] Manns MP, McHutchison JG, Gordon SC, Rustgi VK, Shiffman M, Reindollar R, Goodman ZD, Koury K, Ling M-H, Albrecht JK: Peginterferon alfa-2b plus ribavirin compared with interferon alfa-2b plus ribavirin for initial treatment of chronic hepatitis C: A randomised trial. Lancet 2001, 358(9286):958–965. DOI: 10.1016/S0140-6736(01)06102-5

[19] Fried MW, Shiffman ML, Reddy KR, Smith C, Marinos G, Gonçales FL, Häussinger D, Diago M, Carosi G, Dhumeaux D, et al.: Peginterferon alfa-2a plus ribavirin for chronic hepatitis C virus infection. N Engl J Med 2002, 347(13):975–982. DOI: 10.1056/NEJMoa020047

[20] Torriani FJ, Rodriguez-Torres M, Rockstroh JK, Lissen E, Gonzalez-García J, Lazzarin A, Carosi G, Sasadeusz J, Katlama C, Montaner J, et al.: Peginterferon alfa-2a plus ribavirin for chronic hepatitis C virus infection in HIV-infected patients. N Engl J Med 2004, 351(5):438–450. DOI: 10.1056/NEJMoa040842

[21] Dieterich D, Bacon BR, Flamm SL, Kowdley KV, Milligan S, Tsai N, Younossi Z, Lawitz E: Evaluation of sofosbuvir and simeprevir-based regimens in the TRIO network: Academic and community treatment of a real-world, heterogeneous population. Hepatology 2014, 2014 (60): 220A.

[22] Lawitz E, Sulkowski MS, Ghalib R, Rodriguez-Torres M, Younossi ZM, Corregidor A, DeJesus E, Pearlman B, Rabinovitz M, Gitlin N: Simeprevir plus sofosbuvir, with or without ribavirin, to treat chronic infection with hepatitis C virus genotype 1 in non-responders to pegylated interferon and ribavirin and treatment-naive patients: The COSMOS randomised study. Lancet 2014, 384(9956):1756–1765. DOI: 10.1016/S0140-6736(14)61036

[23] Poordad F, McCone J, Bacon BR, Bruno S, Manns MP, Sulkowski MS, Jacobson IM, Reddy KR, Goodman ZD, Boparai N, et al.: Boceprevir for untreated chronic HCV genotype 1 infection. N Engl J Med 2011, 364(13):1195–1206. DOI: 10.1056/NEJMoa1010494

[24] Bacon BR, Gordon SC, Lawitz E, Marcellin P, Vierling JM, Zeuzem S, Poordad F, Goodman ZD, Sings HL, Boparai N, et al.: Boceprevir for previously treated chronic HCV genotype 1 infection. N Engl J Med 2011, 364(13):1207–1217. DOI: 10.1056/NEJMoa1009482

[25] Arain A, Bourgeois S, de Galocsy C, Henrion J, Deltenre P, d'Heygere F, George C, Bastens B, Van Overbeke L, Verrando R, et al.: Belgian experience with triple therapy with boceprevir and telaprevir in genotype 1 infected patients who inject drugs. J Med Virol 2016, 88(1):94–99. DOI: 10.1002/jmv.24308

[26] McHutchison JG, Everson GT, Gordon SC, Jacobson IM, Sulkowski M, Kauffman R, McNair L, Alam J, Muir AJ: Telaprevir with peginterferon and ribavirin for chronic HCV genotype 1 infection. N Engl J Med 2009, 360(18):1827–1838. DOI: 10.1056/NEJMoa0806104

[27] Jacobson IM, McHutchison JG, Dusheiko G, Di Bisceglie AM, Reddy KR, Bzowej NH, Marcellin P, Muir AJ, Ferenci P, Flisiak R, et al.: Telaprevir for previously untreated chronic hepatitis C virus infection. N Engl J Med 2011, 364(25):2405–2416. DOI: 10.1056/NEJMoa1012912

[28] Reddy KR, Zeuzem S, Zoulim F, Weiland O, Horban A, Stanciu C, Villamil FG, Andreone P, George J, Dammers E, et al.: Simeprevir versus telaprevir with peginterferon and ribavirin in previous null or partial responders with chronic hepatitis C virus genotype 1 infection (ATTAIN): A randomised, double-blind, non-inferiority phase 3 trial. Lancet Infect Dis 2015, 15(1):27–35. DOI: 10.1016/S1473-3099(14)71002

[29] Zeuzem S, Berg T, Gane E, Ferenci P, Foster GR, Fried MW, Hezode C, Hirschfield GM, Jacobson I, Nikitin I: Simeprevir increases rate of sustained virologic response among treatment-experienced patients with HCV genotype-1 infection: A phase IIb trial. Gastroenterology 2014, 146(2):430–441.e436. DOI: 10.1053/j.gastro.2013.10.058

[30] Manns M, Marcellin P, Poordad F, de Araujo ESA, Buti M, Horsmans Y, Janczewska E, Villamil F, Scott J, Peeters M: Simeprevir with pegylated interferon alfa 2a or 2b plus ribavirin in treatment-naive patients with chronic hepatitis C virus genotype 1 infection (QUEST-2): A randomised, double-blind, placebo-controlled phase 3 trial. Lancet 2014, 384(9941):414–426. DOI: 10.1016/S0140-6736(14)60538

[31] Jacobson IM, Dore GJ, Foster GR, Fried MW, Radu M, Rafalsky VV, Moroz L, Craxi A, Peeters M, Lenz O: Simeprevir with pegylated interferon alfa 2a plus ribavirin in treatment-naive patients with chronic hepatitis C virus genotype 1 infection (QUEST-1): A phase 3, randomised, double-blind, placebo-controlled trial. Lancet 2014, 384(9941):403–413. DOI: 10.1016/S0140-6736(14)60494-3

[32] Forns X, Lawitz E, Zeuzem S, Gane E, Bronowicki JP, Andreone P, Horban A, Brown A, Peeters M, Lenz O: Simeprevir with peginterferon and ribavirin leads to high rates of SVR in patients with HCV genotype 1 who relapsed after previous therapy: A phase 3 trial. Gastroenterology 2014, 146(7):1669–1679.e1663. DOI: 10.1053/j.gastro.2014.01.051

[33] Lawitz E, Mangia A, Wyles D, Rodriguez-Torres M, Hassanein T, Gordon SC, Schultz M, Davis MN, Kayali Z, Reddy KR: Sofosbuvir for previously untreated chronic hepatitis C infection. N Engl J Med 2013, 368(20):1878–1887. DOI: 10.1056/NEJMoa1214853

[34] Jensen DM, O'Leary JG, Pockros PJ, Sherman KE, Kwo PY, Mailliard ME, Kowdley KV, Muir AJ, Dickson RC, Ramani A: Safety and efficacy of sofosbuvir-containing regimens for hepatitis C: Real-world experience in a diverse, longitudinal observational cohort. Hepatology 2014, 2014:219A–220A.

[35] Afdhal N, Zeuzem S, Kwo P, Chojkier M, Gitlin N, Puoti M, Romero-Gomez M, Zarski J-P, Agarwal K, Buggisch P: Ledipasvir and sofosbuvir for untreated HCV genotype 1 infection. N Engl J Med 2014, 370(20):1889–1898. DOI: 10.1056/NEJMoa1402454

[36] Kowdley KV, Gordon SC, Reddy KR, Rossaro L, Bernstein DE, Lawitz E, Shiffman ML, Schiff E, Ghalib R, Ryan M: Ledipasvir and sofosbuvir for 8 or 12 weeks for chronic HCV without cirrhosis. N Engl J Med 2014, 370(20):1879–1888. DOI: 10.1056/NEJMoa1402555

[37] Townsend KS, Osinusi A, Nelson AK, Kohli A, Gross C, Polis MA, Pang PS, Sajadi MM, Subramanian M, McHutchison JG: High efficacy of sofosbuvir/ledipasvir for the treatment of HCV genotype 1 in patients coinfected with HIV on or off antiretroviral therapy: results from the NIAID ERADICATE trial. Hepatology 2014, 2014:240A–241A.

[38] Bourliere M, Sulkowski MS, Omata M, Zeuzem S, Feld JJ, Lawitz E, Marcellin P, Hyland RH, Ding X, Yang JC: An integrated safety and efficacy analysis of >500 patients with compensated cirrhosis treated with ledipasvir/sofosbuvir with or without ribavirin. Hepatology 2014, 2014 (60): 239A.

[39] Gao M: Antiviral activity and resistance of HCV NS5A replication complex inhibitors. Curr Opin Virol 2013, 3(5):514–520. DOI: 10.1016/j.coviro.2013.06.014

[40] Sulkowski MS, Gardiner DF, Rodriguez-Torres M, Reddy KR, Hassanein T, Jacobson I, Lawitz E, Lok AS, Hinestrosa F, Thuluvath PJ: Daclatasvir plus sofosbuvir for previously treated or untreated chronic HCV infection. N Engl J Med 2014, 370(3):211–221. DOI: 10.1056/NEJMoa1306218

[41] Pol S, Bourliere M, Lucier S, De Ledinghen V, Zoulim F, Dorival-Mouly C, Métivier S, Larrey D, Tran A, Hezode C: Safety and efficacy of the combination daclatasvir-sofosbuvir in HCV genotype 1-mono-infected patients from the French observational cohort ANRS CO22 HEPATHER. J Hepatol 2015, 62(Suppl 2):S258.

[42] Feld JJ, Jacobson IM, Hézode C, Asselah T, Ruane PJ, Gruener N, Abergel A, Mangia A, Lai C-L, Chan HLY, et al.: Sofosbuvir and velpatasvir for HCV genotype 1, 2, 4, 5, and 6 infection. N Engl J Med 2015, 373(27):2599–2607. DOI: 10.1056/NEJMoa1512610

[43] Pianko S, Flamm SL, Shiffman ML, Kumar S, Strasser SI, Dore GJ, McNally J, Brainard DM, Han LL, Doehle B, et al.: Sofosbuvir plus velpatasvir combination therapy for treatment-experienced patients with genotype 1 or 3 hepatitis C virus infection a randomized trial. Ann Intern Med 2015, 163(11):11. DOI: 10.7326/M15-1014

[44] Feld JJ, Kowdley KV, Coakley E, Sigal S, Nelson DR, Crawford D, Weiland O, Aguilar H, Xiong J, Pilot-Matias T: Treatment of HCV with ABT-450/r–ombitasvir and dasabuvir with ribavirin. N Engl J Med 2014, 370(17):1594–1603. DOI: 10.1056/NEJMoa1315722

[45] Ferenci P, Bernstein D, Lalezari J, Cohen D, Luo Y, Cooper C, Tam E, Marinho RT, Tsai N, Nyberg A: ABT-450/r–ombitasvir and dasabuvir with or without ribavirin for HCV. N Engl J Med 2014, 370(21):1983–1992. DOI: 10.1056/NEJMoa1402338

[46] Wyles DL, Sulkowski MS, Eron JJ, Trinh R, Lalezari J, Slim J, Gathe JC, Wang CC, Elion R, Bredeek F: TURQUOISE-I: 94% SVR12 in HCV/HIV-1 coinfected patients treated with ABT-450/r/ombitasvir, dasabuvir and ribavirin. Hepatology 2014, 2014:1136A–1137A.

[47] Zeuzem S, Jacobson IM, Baykal T, Marinho RT, Poordad F, Bourliere M, Sulkowski MS, Wedemeyer H, Tam E, Desmond P, et al.: Retreatment of HCV with ABT-450/r-ombitasvir and dasabuvir with ribavirin. N Engl J Med 2014, 370(17):1604–1614. DOI: 10.1056/NEJMoa1401561

[48] Andreone P, Colombo MG, Enejosa JV, Koksal I, Ferenci P, Maieron A, Mullhaupt B, Horsmans Y, Weiland O, Reesink HW, et al.: ABT-450, ritonavir, ombitasvir, and dasabuvir achieves 97% and 100% sustained virologic response with or without ribavirin in treatment-experienced patients with HCV genotype 1b infection. Gastroenterology 2014, 147(2):359.e1. DOI: 10.1053/j.gastro.2014.04.045

[49] Poordad F, Hezode C, Trinh R, Kowdley KV, Zeuzem S, Agarwal K, Shiffman ML, Wedemeyer H, Berg T, Yoshida EM: ABT-450/r–ombitasvir and dasabuvir with ribavirin for hepatitis C with cirrhosis. N Engl J Med 2014, 370(21):1973–1982. DOI: 10.1056/NEJMoa1402869

[50] Shiffman ML, Suter F, Bacon BR, Nelson D, Harley H, Sola R, Shafran SD, Barange K, Lin A, Soman A, et al.: Peginterferon alfa-2a and ribavirin for 16 or 24 weeks in HCV genotype 2 or 3. N Engl J Med 2007, 357(2):124–134. DOI: 10.1056/NEJMoa066403

[51] Zeuzem S, Hultcrantz R, Bourliere M, Goeser T, Marcellin P, Sanchez-Tapias J, Sarrazin C, Harvey J, Brass C, Albrecht J: Peginterferon alfa-2b plus ribavirin for treatment of chronic hepatitis C in previously untreated patients infected with HCV genotypes 2 or 3. J Hepatol 2004, 40(6):993–999. DOI: 10.1016/j.jhep.2004.02.007

[52] Lagging M, Rembeck K, Rauning Buhl M, Christensen P, Dalgard O, Farkkila M, Hellstrand K, Langeland N, Lindh M, Westin J, et al.: Retreatment with peg-interferon and ribavirin in patients with chronic hepatitis C virus genotype 2 or 3 infection with prior relapse. Scand J Gastroenterol 2013, 48(7):839–847. DOI: 10.3109/00365521.2013.793389

[53] Lawitz E, Poordad F, Brainard DM, Hyland RH, An D, Symonds WT, McHutchison JG, Membreno FE: Sofosbuvir in combination with pegIFN and ribavirin for 12 weeks provides high SVR rates in HCV-infected genotype 2 or 3 treatment experienced patients with and without compensated cirrhosis: Results from the LONESTAR-2 study. Hepatology 2013, 58(Suppl 1):1380A.

[54] Esteban R, Nyberg L, Lalezari J, Ni L, Doehle B, Kanwar B, Brainard D, Subramanian M, Symonds W, McHutchison J: O8 successful retreatment with sofosbuvir-containing regimens for HCV genotype 2 or 3 infected patients who failed prior sofosbuvir plus ribavirin therapy. J Hepatol 2014, 1(60):S4–S5. DOI: 10.1016/S0168-8278(14)60010-6

[55] Lawitz E, Lalezari JP, Hassanein T, Kowdley KV, Poordad FF, Sheikh AM, Afdhal NH, Bernstein DE, DeJesus E, Freilich B, et al.: Sofosbuvir in combination with peginterferon alfa-2a and ribavirin for non-cirrhotic, treatment-naive patients with genotypes 1, 2, and 3 hepatitis C infection: A randomised, double-blind, phase 2 trial. Lancet Infect Dis. 2013; 13(5):401–408. DOI: 10.1016/S1473-3099(13)70033-1

[56] Jacobson IM, Gordon SC, Kowdley KV, Yoshida EM, Rodriguez-Torres M, Sulkowski MS, Shiffman ML, Lawitz E, Everson G, Bennett M: Sofosbuvir for hepatitis C genotype 2 or 3 in patients without treatment options. N Engl J Med 2013, 368(20):1867–1877. DOI: 10.1056/NEJMoa1214854

[57] Zeuzem S, Dusheiko GM, Salupere R, Mangia A, Flisiak R, Hyland RH, Illeperuma A, Svarovskaia E, Brainard DM, Symonds WT: Sofosbuvir and ribavirin in HCV genotypes 2 and 3. N Engl J Med 2014, 370(21):1993–2001. DOI: 10.1056/NEJMoa1316145

[58] Foster GR, Afdhal N, Roberts SK, Bräu N, Gane EJ, Pianko S, Lawitz E, Thompson A, Shiffman ML, Cooper C: Sofosbuvir and velpatasvir for HCV genotype 2 and 3 infection. N Engl J Med 2015; 373 (27): 2608–2617. DOI: 10.1056/NEJMoa1512612

[59] Nelson DR, Cooper JN, Lalezari JP, Lawitz E, Pockros PJ, Gitlin N, Freilich BF, Younes ZH, Harlan W, Ghalib R, et al.: All-oral 12-week treatment with daclatasvir plus sofosbuvir in patients with hepatitis C virus genotype 3 infection: ALLY-3 phase III study. Hepatology 2015, 61(4):1127–1135. DOI: 10.1002/hep.27726

[60] Kamal S, El Tawil A, Nakano T, He Q, Rasenack J, Hakam S, Saleh W, Ismail A, Aziz A, Madwar MA: Peginterferon α-2b and ribavirin therapy in chronic hepatitis C genotype 4: Impact of treatment duration and viral kinetics on sustained virological response. Gut 2005, 54(6):858–866. DOI: 10.1136/gut.2004.057182

[61] Moreno C, Hezode C, Marcellin P, Bourgeois S, Francque S, Samuel D, Zoulim F, Grange J-D, Shukla U, Lenz O: Efficacy and safety of simeprevir with PegIFN/ribavirin in naïve or experienced patients infected with chronic HCV genotype 4. J Hepatol 2015, 62(5):1047–1055. DOI: 10.1016/j.jhep.2014.12.031

[62] Kapoor R, Kohli A, Sidharthan S, Sims Z, Petersen TL, Osinusi A, Nelson AK, Silk R, Kotb C, Sugarman K: All oral treatment for genotype 4 chronic hepatitis C infection with sofosbuvir and ledipasvir: Interim results from the NIAID SYNERGY trial. Hepatology. 2014, 60: 321A.

[63] Willemse S, Baak L, Kuiken S, Sluys Veer A, Lettinga K, Meer J, Depla A, Tuynman H, Nieuwkerk C, Schinkel C: Sofosbuvir plus simeprevir for the treatment of HCV genotype 4 patients with advanced fibrosis or compensated cirrhosis is highly efficacious in real life. J Viral Hepat 2016; 23 (12): 950–954. DOI: 10.1111/jvh.12567

[64] El-Khayat HR, Fouad YM, Maher M, El-Amin H, Muhammed H: Efficacy and safety of sofosbuvir plus simeprevir therapy in Egyptian patients with chronic hepatitis C: A real-world experience. Gut 2016: gutjnl-2016. DOI: 10.1136/gutjnl-2016-312012

[65] Hézode C, Asselah T, Reddy KR, Hassanein T, Berenguer M, Fleischer-Stepniewska K, Marcellin P, Hall C, Schnell G, Pilot-Matias T, et al.: Ombitasvir plus paritaprevir plus ritonavir with or without ribavirin in treatment-naive and treatment-experienced patients with genotype 4 chronic hepatitis C virus infection (PEARL-I): A randomised, open-label trial. Lancet. 2015; 385(9986):2502–2509. DOI: 10.1016/S0140-6736(15)60159-3

[66] Asselah T, Hézode C, Qaqish RB, ElKhashab M, Hassanein T, Papatheodoridis G, Feld JJ, Moreno C, Zeuzem S, Ferenci P: Ombitasvir, paritaprevir, and ritonavir plus ribavirin in adults with hepatitis C virus genotype 4 infection and cirrhosis (AGATE-I): A multicentre, phase 3, randomised open-label trial. Lancet Gastroenterol Hepatol 2016, 1(1):25–35. DOI: 10.1016/S2468-1253(16)30001-2

[67] Waked I, Shiha G, Qaqish RB, Esmat G, Yosry A, Hassany M, Soliman R, Mohey MA, Allam N, Zayed N: Ombitasvir, paritaprevir, and ritonavir plus ribavirin for chronic hepatitis C virus genotype 4 infection in Egyptian patients with or without compensated cirrhosis (AGATE-II): A multicentre, phase 3, partly randomised open-label trial. Lancet Gastroenterol Hepatol 2016, 1(1):36–44. DOI: 10.1016/S2468-1253(16)30002-4

[68] Keating GM: Ombitasvir/paritaprevir/ritonavir: A review in chronic HCV genotype 4 infection. Drugs 2016, 76(12):1203–1211. DOI: 10.1007/s40265-016-0612-1

[69] Abergel A, Asselah T, Metivier S, Kersey K, Jiang D, Mo H, Pang PS, Samuel D, Loustaud-Ratti V: Ledipasvir-sofosbuvir in patients with hepatitis C virus genotype 5 infection: An open-label, multicentre, single-arm, phase 2 study. Lancet Infect Dis. 2016; 16 (4): 459–464. DOI: 10.1016/S1473-3099(15)00529-0

[70] Gane EJ, Hyland RH, An D, Svarovskaia E, Pang PS, Brainard D, Stedman CA: Efficacy of ledipasvir and sofosbuvir, with or without ribavirin, for 12 weeks in patients with HCV genotype 3 or 6 infection. Gastroenterology 2015, 149(6):1454-e1. DOI: 10.1053/j.gastro.2015.07.063

[71] Everson GT, Towner WJ, Davis MN, Wyles DL, Nahass RG, Thuluvath PJ, Etzkorn K, Hinestrosa F, Tong M, Rabinovitz M, et al.: Sofosbuvir with velpatasvir in treatment-naive noncirrhotic patients with genotype 1 to 6 hepatitis C virus infection a randomized trial. Ann Intern Med 2015, 163(11):818–826. DOI: 10.7326/M15-1000

[72] Pol S, Reddy KR, Baykal T, Hezode C, Hassanein T, Marcellin P, Berenguer M, Fleischer-Stepniewska KM, Hall C, Collins C: Interferon-free regimens of ombitasvir and ABT-450/r with or without ribavirin in patients with HCV genotype 4 infection: PEARL-I study results. Hepatology 2014, 2014:1129A–1130A.

Chapter 4

Management of Hepatitis C Virus Infection in Patients with Cirrhosis

Aziza Ajlan and Hussien Elsiesy

Additional information is available at the end of the chapter

http://dx.doi.org/10.5772/66096

Abstract

In this chapter, we review the history of HCV infection in patients with liver cirrhosis. Selection of appropriate regimens for HCV-infected patients with cirrhosis, consistent with approved indications, practice guidelines, and emerging data is presented. Finally, this chapter explains individualization of therapy to maximize SVR rates in HCV-infected patients with cirrhosis and to critically appraise the role of newer agents and regimens in the management of HCV-infected patients with cirrhosis.

Keywords: HCV, liver cirrhosis, treatment

1. Introduction

Hepatitis C virus (HCV) is the leading cause of liver cirrhosis and hepatocellular carcinoma (HCC) [1]. It remains the main indication for liver transplantation in North America and Europe [2]. The indication for liver transplantation has changed in the past two decades where NASH surpasses HBV to become the second most common cause of liver transplantation but HCV remains unchanged.

Chronic hepatitis C infection in patients with cirrhosis escalates the chances of developing severe liver-related complications, including hepatic decompensation, hepatocellular cancer and subsequently, death. It is been a matter of large debate whether to treat cirrhotic patients and what could be the potential benefit as cirrhosis is irreversible. However, multiple studies have shown that successful treatment of hepatitis C in patients with compensated cirrhosis will decrease subsequent cirrhosis-related complications.

HCV causes increased mortality compared to any other infection; therefore, both the American Association for the Study of the Liver (AASLD) and European Association for the Study of the Liver (EASL) guidelines recommend that treatment be indicated for all HCV-infected patients. However, due to outrageously high cost of the new directly acting antivirals (DAA), treating every HCV-infected patient is not practical even in countries with strong economy.

Given the high cost of the medications for HCV, both AASLD and EASL guidelines prioritize the treatment for specific population with liver cirrhosis among the top list.

The goal of HCV treatment in patients with liver cirrhosis depends on the stage of disease. For Child's class A compensated liver cirrhosis, the goal of treatment is to prevent progression or to reverse cirrhosis [3] and to decrease the prevalence of HCC [4–6].

The goal in decompensated liver cirrhosis is to reverse decompensation, delisting from the liver transplant waiting list or preventing the disease recurrence after liver transplantation [7–9]. More importantly, achieving sustained virological response (SVR) was associated with reduced all-cause mortality in patients with advanced fibrosis related to HCV [6].

Several studies have shown reversal of cirrhosis, delisting from liver transplant waiting liver, improvement of liver function and decrease the risk of HCC in patients who achieved SVR. Decrease in model for end-stage liver disease (MELD) due to biochemical improvement without resolution of ascites may delay the liver transplantation by lowering the patient's rank on the liver transplant waiting list.

There are also studies showing prevention of disease recurrence after liver transplantation on those who achieved SVR before liver transplantation.

We predict NASH to be the leading cause of liver transplant in the next decade, not only because of the growing obesity epidemic and increasing rate of diabetes, but because of the predicted long-term effect of HCV treatment.

The HCV treatment has evolved since the introduction of Interferon monotherapy in early 1990 until having several options of highly effective interferon-free DAA.

The first randomized multicentre trial comparing interferon alfa-2b versus no treatment in compensated HCV cirrhosis did not show benefit, whoever, it was small in number, have high drop-out rate and did not evaluate the patients who achieved sustained virological response (SVR) well but established safety [10]. In the same year, a study showed that patients with chronic hepatitis C who have an SVR to IFN therapy, there is a dramatic effect on normalization of ALT levels, improvement of histological activity and slowing of fibrosis progression [11].

From 2000 to 2011, the combination of PEG-IFN/RBV became the standard of care for HCV treatment, the overall SVR is 40–50% in genotypes 1 and 4 and 70–80% in genotypes 2 and 3; however, the SVR rate was significantly lower in patients with liver cirrhosis, about 22% for genotypes 1 and 4, and 55% for genotypes 2 and 3 [12–14].

Treating patients with decompensated HCV cirrhosis was challenging, it is associated with poor tolerance, higher side effect profile, and lower SVR rate. Everson and co-workers reported the results of a low-accelerating dose regimen of IFN or PEG-IFN with RBV in 124 patients with decompensated cirrhosis. The SVR was 24%, it was significantly lower in patients with genotype 1 (13%) than in those with non-1 genotype (50%); ($P < 0.0001$). SVR was highly predictive of maintaining viral clearance after liver transplant [8].

Forns et al. evaluated the treatment with IFN a-2b/RBV in 30 patients awaiting Orthotopic liver transplant (OLT) [9]. A virological response was observed in nine patients (30%). After LT, six of them (20%) remained negative after liver transplantation.

The study by Carrion et al. evaluated PEG-IFN/RBV therapy in 51 patients with HCV and cirrhosis awaiting LT matched with 51 untreated controls [15]. The aim of this study is to evaluate both the prevention of post-transplantation recurrent HCV and the risk of bacterial infections during therapy. Only 15 patients (29%) were HCV RNA-negative at transplantation and 10 (20%) achieved an SVR after transplantation.

There is major safety concern of PEG-IFN therapy in patients with decompensated cirrhosis. The haematological side effect includes neutropenia (50–60%), thrombocytopaenia (30–50%), and anaemia (30–60%). There is an increased risk of infection (4–13%) or hepatic decompensation during therapy (11–20%) [8, 9]. Carrion et al. reported high incidence of episodes of bacterial infection, mostly spontaneous bacterial peritonitis in treated patients (25%) compared to controls (6%) ($P = 0.01$) [15]. Variables independently associated with the occurrence of bacterial infections were antiviral treatment and a Child-Pugh score of B–C. The adverse effect of this therapy increase as the child score increase, where child C patients has very high complication rate with extremely low response. We reported the safety and efficacy of PEG-IFN and ribavirin therapy in 90 patients with liver cirrhosis, 18% required dose reduction, 33% stopped treatment because of adverse effects, 9% had deterioration of liver function, 7% died and13% of patients SVR. The rate of serious complications was 16.3% in child's class A, 48% in B, and 100% in C ($P = 0.005$). Serum albumin was a significant predictor for worsening liver function ($P = 0.007$), none of the child C patients achieved SVR [16].

2. New direct acting antivirals (DAAs)

Accordingly, the AASLD-IDSA guidelines consider any patient with chronic hepatitis C infection who is diagnosed with compensated cirrhosis highest priority for hepatitis C treatment [4].

For HCV-infected patients with decompensated cirrhosis or hepatocellular cancer, treatment of HCV may provide benefit, but the treatment plans and goals may need modifying if the patient is planning to undergo liver transplantation.

2.1. Patients with compensated cirrhosis

For patients with compensated cirrhosis (Child-Turcotte-Pugh Class A), including those with hepatocellular carcinoma, the AASLD/IDSA/IAS-USA guidance [4] recommends using the same general treatment approach as used for patients without cirrhosis, with several key exceptions primarily related to duration of therapy or inclusion of ribavirin.

2.1.1. *Genotype 1*

2.1.1.1. *Ledipasvir/sofosbuvir*

Ledipasvir (90 mg) and sofosbuvir (400 mg) are a fixed-dose combination (Harvoni®) of two direct-acting antiviral agents that were initially studied in the ION-1 trial. The trial that included 865 treatment-naïve patients, looked at the length of treatment (12 weeks versus 24 weeks) as well as the need for RBV [5]. SVR12 rates exceeded 97%, with no added benefit observed with longer treatment duration, the addition of RBV length of treatment, nor HCV genotype 1 subtype. In the study, 16% of the included patients had cirrhosis. The presence of cirrhosis did not affect SVR12 rates compared with those without cirrhosis (97%) versus (98%) [5].

2.1.1.2. *Paritaprevir/ritonavir/ombitasvir + dasabuvir (PrOD)*

The 3D combination was studied in the TURQUOISE-II and TURQUOISE-III trials. The trail included 261, HCV genotype 1a and CTP class A, the patients were both treatment-naïve and -experienced. The study compared 12 weeks or 24 weeks of PrOD regimen with the addition of RBV. SVR12 rates were higher in patients who received 24 weeks arm (89% vs. 95%) [6]. Factors that may have contributed to these differences could be the inclusion of patients who failed previous PEG-IFN/RBV therapy. Overall, treatment-naïve patient had slightly better response to therapy (92% vs. 95%). Interestingly, in patients with HCV genotype 1b patient, the SVR12 rates reached 98.5% in the 12-week arm [6]. Subsequently, the TURQUOISE-III trail questioned the role of RBV with the 3D regimen for 12 weeks in patients with HCV genotype 1b and compensated cirrhosis. Among the 60 patients included, more than 50% of the patients had negative predictors of response as follows: 55% treatment-experienced, 83% with IL28B non-CC genotype, 22% had platelet counts of greater than 90×10^9 L^{-1}, and 17% had albumin levels greater than 3.5 g/dL). SVR12 rates were 100%. Hence, this regimen was approved for HCV genotype 1b for 12 weeks irrespective of previous treatment history or the presence or of cirrhosis [7].

The PrOD regimen, however, carries FDA warning [8]. In October 2015, the US FDA announced that the PrOD and PrO are contraindicated in patients with Child-Turcotte-Pugh (CTP) class B or C cirrhosis. This was based on reports by the manufacturer of accelerated liver injury in patients who were receiving PrOD or PrO. The onset of liver harm and decompensating incidents were observed mainly during the first month of therapy and mainly involved a quick rise in total and direct bilirubin, as well as a concomitant increase in liver transaminases. Timely recognition and termination of PrOD or PrO resulted in resolution of injury, death was reported in two cases with compensated cirrhosis. If the decision is made to initiate treatment with PrOD or PrO, patients should be made aware of the risks associated with such therapy in addition to adequate monitoring.

2.1.1.3. Simeprevir + sofosbuvir

Simiprevir + sofosbuvir regimen were studied in the OPTIMIST-2 trial. The single armed, open-label trial looked at 12 weeks of simeprevir plus sofosbuvir in 103 cirrhotic patients [9]. SVR12 rates were 88% (44/50) of treatment-naïve and 79% (42/53) of treatment-experienced patients with the total SVR12 rate was 83% (86/103). Furthermore, both genotype 1a and the presence of Q80K mutation negatively affected SVR12 (genotype 1 and 1b 84% [26/31] and 92% [35/38], respectively. And 74% [25/34] with Q80K mutation. Currently, there is no data that proves that extending treatment, with or without the addition of RBV, will increase efficacy of these two groups. Hence, until further data proves otherwise, this regimen should be avoided in patients with genotype 1a or in the case Q80K mutation is present.

2.1.1.4. Daclatasvir + sofosbuvir

Cirrhotic patients tend to take advantage from extension of therapy with daclatasvir and sofosbuvir to 24 weeks, with or without RBV [10, 11]. The data from ALLY-1 trial investigated daclatasvir and sofosbuvir with RBV dosed at 600 mg, in 60 patients with advanced cirrhosis [12]. Only 76% of patients with HCV genotype 1a (n = 34) and 100% of patients with HCV genotype 1b (n = 11) achieved an SVR at 12 weeks (SVR12). It is unclear how many treatment failures were among treatment-naïve patient was 54% or those with CTP class A cirrhosis. SVR was significantly lower in CTP class C cirrhosis (54%) when compared with CTP classes A and B 92% and 94% (see **Table 1**).

	SVR12 rates in patients with Child Pugh A cirrhosis					
	GT1a	**GT1b**	**GT2**	**GT3**	**GT4**	**GT5/6**
SOF +SIM 12 weeks	83% (9)&	NA	NA	NA	NA	NA
SOF+DAC 12 weeks	76%(12)	100%(12)	NA	85.9%^(27)	NA	NA
SOF+DAC 24 weeks		NA	NA	NA	NA	NA
SOF+LED+RBV 12 weeks	97–98%(5)	NA	NA	NA	100%	NA
SOF+LED 24 weeks	NA	NA	NA	NA	NA	NA
PrOD 12 weeks	98.5%^(6)	100%^(6)	NA	NA	NA	NA
PrO 12 weeks			NA	NA	96$(30)	NA
SOF+VEL 12	99%	95%	100%	100%	100%	100%
GRZ+ELB 12	97%*(13, 14)	99%	NA	NA	NA	NA
GRZ+ELB 16	100%(15)	NA	NA	NA	NA	NA

&With 88% (44/50) of treatment-naïve and 79% (42/53) of treatment-experienced patients.
^With ribavirin.
$100% SVR12 rates achieved with extending the duration to 16 weeks.
*Treatment naïve. SOF: sofosbuvir, SIM: simiprevir, DAC: daclatasvir LED: ledipasvir, PrOD: paritaprevir, ritonavir, ombitasvir and dasabuvir. PrO: paritaprevir, ritonavir, ombitasvir. VEL: velpatasvir, GRZ: grazoprevir, ELB: elbasvir.

Table 1. SVR12 rates among HCV-infected patients with compensated cirrhosis.

2.1.1.5. Elbasvir/grazoprevir

For genotype 1a, recommendations for cirrhotic patients are based on 92 (22%) patients in the phase III C-EDGE trial that had Metavir F4 disease [13]. SVR 12 was 97% in the subgroup of cirrhotic patients. A similar 97% (28/29) SVR 12 rate had previously been demonstrated in genotype 1 cirrhotic treatment-naïve patients treated with 12 weeks of elbasvir/grazoprevir without ribavirin in the open-label phase II C-WORTHY trial [14]. The presence or absence of compensated cirrhosis does not appear to alter the efficacy of the elbasvir/grazoprevir regimen [13, 14].

The presence of NS5A resistance-associated variants (RAVs) at baseline was found to be associated with reduced efficacy in patients with genotype 1a, and was not apparent with genotype 1b [13]. In this phase III open-label trial of elbasvir/grazoprevir that enrolled treatment-experienced patients; among 58 genotype 1a patients who received 16 weeks of therapy with elbasvir/grazoprevir plus ribavirin, there were no virologic failures and the SVR12 rates were 100% [15–17].

2.1.1.6. Sofosbuvir/velpatasvir

The use of this combination in patients with decompensated cirrhosis was investigated in the ASTRAL-4 trial. The study was multicentre, open-label patients were randomly assigned in a 1:1:1 ratio to receive a fixed-dose combination tablet containing 400 mg of sofosbuvir and 100 mg of velpatasvir, administered orally once daily for 12 weeks; sofosbuvir-velpatasvir plus ribavirin once daily for 12 weeks; or sofosbuvir-velpatasvir once daily for 24 weeks. Ribavirin was administered orally with food twice daily, with the dose determined according to body weight (1000 mg daily in patients with a body weight of greater than 75 kg and 1200 mg daily in patients with a body weight ≥75 kg). The overall SVR12 rates in the three groups were 83, 94 and 86%, respectively. The study highlights a potential role of RBV in such population [18]. Nineteen percent of the patients included in the ASTRAL-1 study had cirrhosis and observed SVR12 rates of 99% when received sofosbuvir/velpatasvir for 12 weeks [19].

2.1.2. Genotype 2

Sofosbuvir (400 mg daily) was combined with weight-based RBV for treatment-naïve patients with HCV genotype 2 infection in three clinical trials, each of which enrolled patients with HCV genotype 2 or 3: FISSION, POSITRON and VALENCE with very high SVR12 rates [20–22]. However, patients with cirrhosis have lower response rates that were seen in treatment-naïve patients with cirrhosis compared to in those without cirrhosis [23]. One may consider extending treatment duration when cirrhosis is present despite the lack of data to support such extension, as longer treatment duration is known to improve SVR in treatment-experienced patients with cirrhosis [22, 24]. Due to the small numbers of patients with HCV genotype 2 infection and cirrhosis enrolled in the registration trials, several phase III b studies are ongoing to specifically determine the appropriate length of treatment for this subgroup of patients (see **Table 1**).

2.1.3. Genotype 3

2.1.3.1. Sofosbuvir/daclatasvir

ALLY-3 is a phase III study of the once-daily NS5A inhibitor daclatasvir plus sofosbuvir for 12 weeks; the study included 101 treatment-naïve patients and demonstrated an SVR12 rate of 90%. Cirrhotic patients (Metavir F4), 58% achieved SVR12 [25]. Hence extension of therapy may be considered in such cases. European compassionate use program has supported these recommendations in cohort studies, which reported and improvement in rates of up to 70% versus 86% when daclatasvir and sofosbuvir was used for 12 weeks and 24 weeks. RBV did not seem to have a big impact on SVR12 (85.9% without RBV compared to 81.3% with RBV). SVR12 rates were also higher in those with compensated Child-Pugh A cirrhosis (85–90% compared to 70.6% in child B/C). Previous data suggested that SVR 12 rates were higher in treatment-naïve patients (91–100%) compared to experienced (81–82%) [26].

2.1.4. Genotype 4

2.1.4.1. Ledipasvir/sofosbuvir

The SYNERGY trial was an open-label study evaluating 12 weeks of ledipasvir/sofosbuvir in 21 HCV genotype 4-infected patients, Among that 60% were treatment-naïve and 43% had advanced fibrosis (Metavir stage F3 or F4) [27]. All patients achieved an SVR12. Note that the study used an assay by ROCH with lower limit of quantitation (LLOQ) of 43 IU/ml, while the AASLD guidelines recommended to use an assay with LLOQ of 25 IU/ml. However, this had no impact on SVR12 results [28].

2.1.4.2. Paritaprevir/ritonavir/ombitasvir (PrO)

Pro regimen has interesting SVR12 rates according to the AGATE-I trial. The trial randomized 120 subjects with genotype 4 HCV and compensated cirrhosis to 12 weeks or 16 weeks of paritaprevir/ritonavir/ombitasvir (PrO) in addition to weight-based ribavirin. The SVR12 rates were 96% and 100% in the 12 week and 16 week arms, respectively [29]. On the other hand, the AGATE-II trial randomized 60 patients with compensated (1:1) to Pro for either 12 weeks or 24 weeks. SVR12 rates in the 12 weeks group were 97% versus 93% in the 24 week group [30].

2.1.4.3. Sofosbuvir/simiprevir

In a study by Moreno et al., the combination was studied in patients with advanced fibrosis/cirrhosis. All patients achieved end of treatment response but SVR12 data were not available [31]. In another study by Kayali et al., the combination was found to achieve SVR12 rates of 77% MELD scores remain unchanged. Interestingly, black gender and BMI were identified as independent negative predictors of response in univariate regression analysis (see **Table 1**) [32].

3. Patients with decompensated cirrhosis

3.1. Sofosbuvir/ledipasvir

The SOLAR-1 study was a multicentre, randomized controlled trial of 108 patients with HCV genotype 1 and 4 who had decompensated cirrhosis, of whom 59 were classified as CTP class B and 49 classified as CTP class C cirrhosis. Subjects were randomly assigned to receive daily fixed dose combination ledipasvir/sofosbuvir and RBV (initial dose of 600 mg, increased as tolerated) for 12 or 24 weeks. Extension of treatment in cirrhotic patients did not seem to affect SVR rates much. For CTP B patients, SVR rates were 87% versus 89% in subjects who received 12 versus 24 weeks, respectively. Likewise, the rates of SVR CTP class C subjects were 86 and 87%, respectively, with 12 and 24 weeks of antiviral therapy [33]. During the study, only one patient with CTP class C cirrhosis died.

The SOLAR-2 study was a multicentre randomized controlled trial of 108 subjects with decompensated cirrhosis secondary to HCV genotypes 1 and 4. Some of the patients were treatment-experienced, with CTP class B cirrhosis or CTP class C cirrhosis. The patients were randomly assigned to receive daily fixed-dose combination ledipasvir/sofosbuvir and RBV (initial dose of 600 mg, increased as tolerated) for 12 weeks or 24 weeks. Sustained virologic response (SVR) was achieved in 87% of those given the 12-week treatment course and 89% of those given the 24-week treatment course. On the 4th week of treatment, the total bilirubin and serum albumin levels improved compared with baseline in all patients. Despite the fact that some patients experienced worsening of hepatic function, baseline CTP and model for end-stage liver disease (MELD) scores improved in more than 50% of the treated patients. Five patients died during the study period but none of the death occurred was attributed to the study medication. Adverse events were more common in the 24-week arm (34%) than in the 12-week arm (15%). These results indicate that a 12-week course of ledipasvir/sofosbuvir and RBV (initial dose of 600 mg, increased as tolerated) is an appropriate regimen for patients with decompensated cirrhosis who are infected with HCV genotype 1 or 4. Such therapy may lead to objective improvements in hepatic function and reduce the likelihood of recurrent HCV infection after subsequent transplantation [33].

3.2. Sofosbuvir/daclatasvir

Patients with advanced cirrhosis (Child-Turcotte-Pugh [CTP] class B and C; $n = 60$) were particularly investigated in the ALLY-1 study [34]. The study found the use of daclatasvir (60 mg daily) with sofosbuvir (400 mg) and low initial dose of RBV (600 mg) for 12 weeks to treatment-naïve and -experienced patients with HCV genotype 1 infection. The overall SVR12 rate was 83% among those with advanced cirrhosis. The SVR12 rate was slightly lower in patients with genotype 1a compared with patients with genotype 1b (76 and 100%, respectively). Response rates were also affected by severity of disease among those with advanced cirrhosis (94% SVR12 rates in patients with CTP class B and 56% in patients with CTP class C). Patients with genotype 3 had also lower SVR12 rates 83%.

In another real-world study by Foster et al., involving 235 genotype 1 patients with decompensated cirrhosis, the SVR rates were comparable in the genotype 1 subjects ($n = 235$) receiving SOF/LDV/RBV or SOF/LDV (86% vs. 81%) and those receiving SOF/DCV/RBV or SOF/DCV therapy (82–60%). In this study, 91% of the patients received ribavirin with 20% requiring a RBV dose reduction and only 6% discontinued RBV. Improvement in MELD scores was observed in 42% of treated patients and worsening occurred in 11%. Moreover, 14 deaths occurred with relatively higher incidence of SAE (26%) but none were attributed to study medication.

3.3. Genotype 2 and 3

A multicentre, compassionate use study included 101 genotype 3 patients to be treated with daclatasvir (60 mg), sofosbuvir (400 mg) ± RBV for 24 weeks [35]. Of those, 81% had CTP class B cirrhosis, the MELD score was higher than15 in 16%, and 7% were post-liver transplant. The reported SVR 12 data has demonstrated an SVR of 85–100%. Two patients died while 22 patients had an SAE and therapy was discontinued in five subjects. Summary of SVR in Child B and C (**Table 2**).

	SVR12 rates in patients with Child Pugh B and/or C cirrhosis					
	GT1a	**GT1b**	**GT2**	**GT3**	**GT4**	**GT5/6**
SOF +SIM 12 weeks	NA	NA	NA	NA	NA	NA
SOF+DAC 12 weeks	76%*(35)	100%(35)	NA	83%(35)	NA	NA
SOF+DAC 24 weeks	NA	NA	85% (36)		NA	NA
SOF+LED+RBV 12 weeks	87%(34)	NA	NA	NA	NA	NA
SOF+LED +RBV 24 weeks	89%(34)	NA	NA	NA	NA	NA
SOF+VEL 12	88	89	100	50	100	NA
SOF+VEL+RBV 12	94	100	100	85	100	NA
SOF+VEL 24	93	88	75	50	100	100

*SVR12 rate was 94% among patients with CTP class B cirrhosis but only 56% among patients with CTP class C cirrhosis.
SOF: sofosbuvir, SIM: simiprevir, DAC: daclatasvir, LED: ledipasvir, PrOD: paritaprevir, ritonavir, ombitasvir and dasabuvir. PrO: paritaprevir, ritonavir, ombitasvir. VEL: velpatasvir, GRZ: grazoprevir, ELB: elbasvir.

Table 2. SVR12 rates in patients with Child Pugh B and/or C cirrhosis.

4. Summary

There is a remarkable advance in treatment of HCV in the recent few years allowing an excellent result in difficult to treat patients with liver cirrhosis with good safety profile.

Treating HCV in patients with liver cirrhosis is a high priority to prevent decompensation and prevent HCV recurrence after liver transplantation.

Author details

Aziza Ajlan[1] and Hussien Elsiesy[2,3*]

*Address all correspondence to: helsiesy@gmail.com

1 Department of Pharmacy, King Faisal Specialist Hospital & Research Center, Riyadh, Saudi Arabia

2 Department of Liver Transplantation and Hepatobiliary Surgery, King Faisal Specialist Hospital & Research Center, Riyadh, Saudi Arabia

3 Department of Medicine, Alfaisal, Riyadh, Saudi Arabia

References

[1] Seeff LB. The natural history of chronic hepatitis C virus infection. Clinical Liver Disease. 1997;1(3):587–602.

[2] Wise M, Bialek S, Finelli L, Bell BP, Sorvillo F. Changing trends in hepatitis C-related mortality in the United States, 1995–2004. Hepatology. 2008;47(4):1128–1135.

[3] D'Ambrosio R, Aghemo A, Rumi MG, Ronchi G, Donato MF, Paradis V, et al. A morphometric and immunohistochemical study to assess the benefit of a sustained virological response in hepatitis C virus patients with cirrhosis. Hepatology. 2012;56(2): 532–543.

[4] AASLD-IDSA. Recommendations for testing, managing, and treating hepatitis C. Available from: http://www.hcvguidelines.org. [cited 30/4/2016].

[5] Afdhal N, Zeuzem S, Kwo P, Chojkier M, Gitlin N, Puoti M, et al. Ledipasvir and sofosbuvir for untreated HCV genotype 1 infection. The New England Journal of Medicine. 2014;370(20):1889–1898.

[6] Poordad F, Hezode C, Trinh R, Kowdley KV, Zeuzem S, Agarwal K, et al. ABT-450/r-ombitasvir and dasabuvir with ribavirin for hepatitis C with cirrhosis. The New England Journal of Medicine. 2014;370(21):1973–1982.

[7] Feld JJ MC, Trinh R, et al. Sustained virologic response of 100% in HCV genotype 1b patients with cirrhosis receiving ombitasvir/paritaprevir/r and dasabuvir for 12weeks. Journal of Hepatology. 2016;64(2):301–307.

[8] FDA Drug Safety Communication: FDA warns of serious liver injury risk with hepatitis C treatments Viekira Pak and Technivie [updated 10-22-2015 cited 2015 10-22-2015]. Available from: http://www.fda.gov/Drugs/DrugSafety/ucm468634.htm

[9] Forns X, Garcia-Retortillo M, Serrano, T Feliu A, Suarez F, de la Mata M, Garcia-Valdecasas JC, Navasa M, Rimola A, Rodes J. Antiviral therapy of patients with decompensated cirrhosis to prevent recurrence of hepatitis C after liver transplantation. J Hepatol 2003;39:389–396

[10] Welzel TM HK, Ferenci P, et al. Daclatasvir plus sofosbuvir with or without ribavirin for the treatment of HCV in patients with severe liver disease: interim results of a multicenter compassionate use program. [Abstract P0072.] 50th Annual Meeting of the European Association for the Study of the Liver (EASL). April 22–26, 2015;S619; Vienna, Austria.

[11] de Ledinghen V FH, Dorival C, et al. Safety and efficacy of sofosbuvir-containing regimens in the French obervational cohort ANRS C022 hepather. [Abstract P0795.] 50th Annual Meeting of the European Association for the Study of the Liver (EASL). April 22–26, 2015;S631; Vienna, Austria.

[12] Poordad F SE, Vierling JM, et al. Daclatasvir with sofosbuvir and ribavirin for HCV infection with advanced cirrhosis or post-liver transplant recurrence. Hepatology. 2016;63(5):1493–505 DOI: 10.1002/hep.28446. [Epub ahead of print].

[13] Zeuzem S, Ghalib R, Reddy KR, Pockros PJ, Ben Ari Z, Zhao Y, et al. Grazoprevir-Elbasvir combination therapy for treatment-naive cirrhotic and noncirrhotic patients with chronic hepatitis C Virus Genotype 1, 4, or 6 infection: a randomized trial. Annals of Internal Medicine 2015;163(1):1–13.

[14] Lawitz E GE, Pearlman B, Tam E, Ghesquiere W, Guyader D, Alric L, Bronowicki JP, Lester L, Sievert W, Ghalib R, Balart L, Sund F, Lagging M, Dutko F, Shaughnessy M, Hwang P, Howe AY, Wahl J, Robertson M, Barr E, Haber B. Efficacy and safety of 12 weeks versus 18 weeks of treatment with grazoprevir (MK-5172) and elbasvir (MK-8742) with or without ribavirin for hepatitis C virus genotype 1 infection in previously untreated patients with cirrhosis and patients with previous null response with or without cirrhosis (C-WORTHY): a randomised, open-label phase 2 trial. Lancet. 2015;385(9973):1075–1086..

[15] Carrion JA, Martinez-Bauer E, Crespo G, et al. Antiviral therapy increases the risk of bacterial infections in HCVinfected cirrhotic patients awaiting liver transplantation: a retrospective study. J Hepatol 2009; 50: 719–28.

[16] Jacobson IM A-AE, Wong P, et al. Prevalence and Impact of Baseline NSA Resistance Associated Variants (RAVs) on the Efficacy of Elbasvir/Grazoprevir (EBR/GZR) Against GT1a Infection [Abstract LB-22]. 66th Annual Meeting of the American Association for the Study of Liver Diseases (AASLD). November 13–17, 2015; San Francisco, CA.

[17] Thompson A ZS, Rockstroh J, Kwo P, Roth D, Lawitz E, Sulkowski M, Forns X, Wahl J, Nguyen B, Barr E, Howe A, Miller M, Hwang P, Robertson M. The Combination of

Grazoprevir and Elbasvir + RBV is highly effective for the treatment of GT1a-Infected patients. American Association for the Study of Liver Diseases. The Liver Meeting 2015, San Francisco, Abstract 703, 2015.

[18] Curry MP, O'Leary JG, Bzowej N, Muir AJ, Korenblat KM, Fenkel JM, et al. Sofosbuvir and velpatasvir for HCV in patients with decompensated cirrhosis. The New England Journal of Medicine. 2015;373(27):2618–2628.

[19] Feld JJ, Jacobson IM, Hezode C, Asselah T, Ruane PJ, Gruener N, et al. Sofosbuvir and velpatasvir for HCV genotype 1, 2, 4, 5, and 6 infection. The New England Journal of Medicine. 2015;373(27):2599–2607.

[20] Lawitz E, Mangia A, Wyles D, Rodriguez-Torres M, Hassanein T, Gordon SC, et al. Sofosbuvir for previously untreated chronic hepatitis C infection. The New England Journal of Medicine. 2013;368(20):1878–1887.

[21] Jacobson IM, Gordon SC, Kowdley KV, Yoshida EM, Rodriguez-Torres M, Sulkowski MS, et al. Sofosbuvir for hepatitis C genotype 2 or 3 in patients without treatment options. The New England Journal of Medicine. 2013;368(20):1867–1877.

[22] Zeuzem S, Dusheiko GM, Salupere R, Mangia A, Flisiak R, Hyland RH, et al. Sofosbuvir and ribavirin in HCV genotypes 2 and 3. The New England journal of Medicine. 2014;370(21):1993–2001.

[23] Dieterich D BB, Flamm SL, et al. Evaluation of sofosbuvir and simeprevir-based regimens in the TRIO network: academic and community treatment of a real-world, heterogeneous population. [Abstract 46.] 65th Annual Meeting of the American Association for the Study of Liver Diseases (AASLD). November 7–11, 2014; 220A; Boston, MA.

[24] Foster GR, Pianko S, Brown A, Forton D, Nahass RG, George J, et al. Efficacy of sofosbuvir plus ribavirin with or without peginterferon-alfa in patients with hepatitis C virus genotype 3 infection and treatment-experienced patients with cirrhosis and hepatitis C virus genotype 2 infection. Gastroenterology. 2015;149(6):1462–1470.

[25] Nelson DR, Cooper JN, Lalezari JP, Lawitz E, Pockros PJ, Gitlin N, et al. All-oral 12-week treatment with daclatasvir plus sofosbuvir in patients with hepatitis C virus genotype 3 infection: ALLY-3 phase III study. Hepatology. 2015;61(4):1127–1135.

[26] Hezode C LV, Fontaine H, et al. Daclatasvir plus sofosbuvir with or without ribavirin in genotype 3 patients from a large French multicenter compassionate use program [Abstract 206]. 66th Annual Meeting of the American Association for the Study of Liver Diseases (AASLD). November 13–17, 2015; San Francisco, CA.

[27] Kohli A, Kapoor R, Sims Z, Nelson A, Sidharthan S, Lam B, et al. Ledipasvir and sofosbuvir for hepatitis C genotype 4: a proof-of-concept, single-centre, open-label phase 2a cohort study. Lancet Infectious Diseases. 2015;15(9):1049–1054.

[28] Smith MA, Mohammad RA. Ledipasvir-sofosbuvir for hepatitis C genotype 4 infection. Lancet Infectious Diseases. 2015;15(9):993–995.

[29] Asselah T HT, Qaqish RB, et al. Efficacy and safety of ombitasvir/paritaprevir/ritonavir co-administered with ribavirin in adults with genotype 4 chronic hepatitis C infection and cirrhosis (AGATE-I) [Abstract 714]. 66th Annual Meeting of the American Association for the Study of Liver Diseases (AASLD). November 13–17, 2015; San Francisco, CA.

[30] Waked I, Shiha G, Qaqish RB, Esmat G, Yosry A, Hassany M, et al. Ombitasvir, paritaprevir, and ritonavir plus ribavirin for chronic hepatitis C virus genotype 4 infection in Egyptian patients with or without compensated cirrhosis (AGATE-II): a multicentre, phase 3, partly randomised open-label trial. The Lancet Gastroenterology & Hepatology. 1(1):36–44.

[31] Moreno C, Lasser L, Delwaide J, et al. Sofosbuvir in combination with simeprevir +/- ribavirin in genotype 4 hepatitis C patients with advanced fibrosis or cirrhosis: real-life experience from Belgium. AASLD: Boston, 2015.

[32] Kayali Z, Amador C, Lowe A, et al. Prospective study for the efficacy of sofosbuvir and simeprevir ± ribavirin in hepatitis C genotype 1 and 4 compensated cirrhotic patients. Single Center Study and Real Life Experience. AASLD: Boston, USA, 2015.

[33] Charlton M, Everson GT, Flamm SL, Kumar P, Landis C, Brown RS, Jr., et al. Ledipasvir and sofosbuvir plus ribavirin for treatment of HCV infection in patients with advanced liver disease. Gastroenterology. 2015;149(3):649–659.

[34] Poordad F, Schiff ER, Vierling JM, Landis C, Fontana RJ, Yang R, et al. Daclatasvir with sofosbuvir and ribavirin for hepatitis C virus infection with advanced cirrhosis or post-liver transplantation recurrence. Hepatology. 2016;63(5):1493–1505.

[35] Welzel TM ZS, Petersen J, et al. Safety and efficacy of daclatasvir plus sofosbuvir with or without ribavirin for the treatment of chronic HCV genotype 3 infection: Interim results of a multicenter European compassionate use program [Abstract 37]. 66th Annual Meeting of the American Association for the Study of Liver Diseases (AASLD). November 13–17, 2015; San Francisco, CA.

Chapter 5

Management of Hepaitits C Virus Genotype 4 in the Liver Transplant Setting

Waleed K. Al-Hamoudi

Additional information is available at the end of the chapter

http://dx.doi.org/10.5772/65473

Abstract

End-stage liver disease secondary to hepatitis C virus (HCV) infection is the major indication for orthotopic liver transplantation (OLT) worldwide. It also has a negative impact on patient and graft survival leading to an inferior transplant outcome when compared to other liver transplant indications. The percentage of HCV patients infected with genotype 4 (G4) among recipients of OLT varies depending on geographic location. In the Middle East G4 infection is the most common genotype among transplant recipients. Direct antiviral agents (DAAs) have revolutionized the management of HCV infection in the pre- and post-transplant setting. Recent clinical trials have shown high sustained virologic response rates, shorter durations of treatment, and decreased adverse events when compared with the previous treatment of pegylated interferon (PEG-IFN)-based therapy. However, most of these studies were performed in HCV-G1-infected patients. Due to the low prevalence of HCV-G4 in Europe and the USA, this genotype has not been adequately studied in prospective trials evaluating treatment outcomes. The aim of this chapter is to summarize the natural history and treatment outcome of HCV-G4 in the liver transplant setting, with particular attention to new HCV therapies.

Keywords: cirrhosis, direct antiviral agents, genotype 4, hepatitis C, liver transplantation

1. Introduction

Hepatitis C virus (HCV) infection is the leading indication for liver transplantation (LT) and is a major cause of liver-related mortality [1, 2]. It also has a negative impact on patient and graft survival leading to an inferior transplant outcome when compared with other indications [3, 4].

HCV eradication prior to LT will likely improve the outcome by eliminating the risk of post transplant recurrence. In the absence of an effective HCV vaccine to prevent infection and with therapy until very recently limited to interferon (IFN)-based regimens, most HCV-infected candidates for LT patients remained untreated.

Hepatitis C genotype 4 (HCV-G4) is the most prevalent genotype in the Middle East and Northern Africa [5–8]. The frequency of infection with HCV-G4 is also increasing in European countries, particularly among intravenous drug users [9–12]. The most common genotype in Europe and the USA is genotype 1; therefore, HCV-G4 has not been adequately studied in prospective trials evaluating treatment outcomes and remains the least studied variant.

The impact of HCV-G4 on treatment outcomes in the general nontransplant population has been evaluated [13–18]. Studies from the Middle East suggest a higher rate of spontaneous resolution after acute HCV-G4 infection [19, 20]. Other studies suggest that HCV-G4 infection is associated with significant steatosis. These observations suggest that specific features of HCV-G4 infection may contribute to the natural history and treatment outcomes of the disease [21, 22].

The percentage of HCV-G4 patients among recipients of orthotopic liver transplantation (OLT) varies depending on the geographic location. HCV-G4 represents more than 90% of indications for liver transplantation in Egypt [23]. In Saudi Arabia, hepatitis C represents ~29% of indications for liver transplantation, ~60% of which are secondary to HCV-G4 [24]. On the other hand, HCV-G4 is a relatively uncommon indication for liver transplantation in Europe and North America [25, 26].

Until recently, interferon-based therapy was the only treatment for HCV. However, this treatment has its own drawbacks given its prolonged therapeutic course (24–48 weeks), numerous side effects, low barrier to resistance, and reduced efficacy in prior null responders or cirrhotic patient. Direct antiviral agents (DAAs) represent a breakthrough in the management of HCV. First generation DAAs (telaprevir, boceprevir) in post-liver transplant patients resulted in sustained virological response (SVR) of up to 60% with telaprevir in HCV-G1. However, significant side effects including severe anemia, skin complications and significant drug interactions resulted in major concerns [27]. These agents are currently contraindicated and are not used anymore. Second line direct-acting antiviral DAAs have emerged with better safety and efficacy profiles, leading to dramatic changes in the practice of HCV management. Multiple clinical studies have shown superiority of sofosbuvir (SOF)-based therapy when compared with the current standard of care in both treatment naïve and treatment experienced patients and across all HCV genotypes [28–34]. Because of its favorable pharmacologic profile and its reasonable drug–drug interactions, sofosbuvir has become the cornerstone in the management of HCV infection [35]. Furthermore, data are emerging on the outcome of multiple newer agents. The, aim of this chapter is to examine the natural history and treatment outcomes of HCV-G4 following liver transplantation. This review includes all published studies and abstracts involving HCV-G4 patients.

2. Hepatitis C genotype influences post-liver transplantation

Campos-Varela et al. evaluated the role of the various HCV genotypes on the progression and outcome of liver transplantation. Among 745 recipients, 81% had genotype 1 (G1), 7% had genotype 2 (G2), and 12% had genotype 3 (G3). Patients were followed for a median of 3.1 years (range 2–8 years). The risk of advanced fibrosis and graft rejection was significantly higher among those infected with G1 compared with other genotypes [36]. In another multicentre European study involving 652 liver recipients, genotype 1b, age, and absence of pretransplantation coinfection by HBV are risk factors for recurrent HCV. However, graft and patient survival was comparable to other genotypes [37]. Similarly, in another prospective study involving 60 liver transplant recipients, HCV 1b was associated with more aggressive recurrent liver disease than other genotypes [38]. Gordon et al. assessed the relationship between hepatitis C genotype on posttransplant frequency of recurrent hepatitis, histologic severity of recurrence, and progression to cirrhosis. They concluded that histologic evidence of recurrent hepatitis C is seen in 90% of liver allografts; however, genotype 1b was associated with more severe histologic disease recurrence and was more likely to progress to cirrhosis when compared to non-1b genotypes [39].

By contrast, some large studies have observed no difference in the rate or degree of hepatitis or in graft or patient survival between G1 and other genotypes [40, 41]. Therefore, the impact of various genotypes on the outcome of liver transplantation remains controversial. Due to the low prevalence of HCV G-4 in western countries, these studies neglected evaluating the impact of this particular genotype.

3. Natural history of HCV-G4 after liver transplantation

Re-infection of the graft is universal after liver transplantation regardless of genotype, leading to an accelerated course of liver injury in many cases [42]. Most studies of disease recurrence worldwide have investigated HCV-G1, HCV-G2, and HCV-G3, and there are few reports on post-OLT recurrence of HCV-G4.

Zekry et al. analyzed factors that predicted outcome of HCV-liver transplant recipients in the Australian and New Zealand communities. The following variables were evaluated demographic factors, coexistent pathology at the time of transplantation, HCV genotype, and donor age. In this analysis, 182 patients were transplanted for HCV including 16 patients infected with genotype 4 and the median follow-up was 4 years. Among many factors studied in univariate and multivariate analyses, HCV-G4 was associated with an increased risk of re-transplantation and death. Additionally, patients infected with HCV-G4 were more likely to progress to advanced stages of fibrosis [43]. Patients infected with G2 and G3 had better post-transplant outcomes. Whether this difference in outcomes was related to the pathogenicity of HCV-G4 or to other factors not examined in this study, including donor age, immunosuppression, and compliance with medications, is not clear (**Table 1**). Furthermore, patients infected with HCV-G4 in this study were older and more likely to have coexisting hepatocellular carcinoma. Gane et al. investigated the impact of persistent HCV infection after liver transplantation on patient and graft survival and the effects of the HCV genotype on the severity of recurrent hepatitis. A group of 149 patients with HCV infection who received liver transplants were followed for a median of 36 months; 623 patients without HCV infection who underwent liver transplantation for end-stage chronic liver disease were used as a control group. Among the patient population, 14 patients were infected with HCV-G4. Approximately 50% of these patients had progressive liver disease (moderate hepatitis or cirrhosis) during the follow-up period [44]. In the same study, patients infected with G1b had the worst outcome, whereas patients infected with G2 and G3 had less severe disease recurrence. The authors speculated that patients infected with G1b had an increased replicative potential and an increased expression of viral antigen in liver tissue. A more detailed study from the UK aimed at studying the impact of HCV-G4 on transplant outcome. The study group included 128 patients who underwent transplantation for HCV infection: 28 patients, genotype 1; 11 patients, genotype 2; 19 patients, genotype 3; and 32 patients, genotype 4 [45]. A significantly higher fibrosis progression rate was observed in HCV-G4 patients compared with non-G4 patients, although their rates of survival were similar. The 5-year cumulative rates for the development of cirrhosis or severe fibrosis were 84% in HCV-G4-infected patients and 24% in patients infected with other genotypes. The HCV-G4 groups were predominantly Egyptian patients who received organs from older donors. Furthermore, the majority of these patients were placed on an alternative waiting list to be offered organs that were suitable for transplantation but unsuitable or not needed for citizens of the UK. This policy may have led to the selection of inferior grafts for the HCV-G4 patients, who were predominantly non-UK citizens, leading to inferior results in these patients.

Factors affecting transplant outcome
Viral load
Genotype
Coinfections
Alcohol
Compliance
Steatosis
Donor age
Immunosuppression
Rejection

Table 1. Factors affecting the outcome of HCV-related transplantation.

On the other hand, studies from the Middle East show a more favorable outcome. According to reports from Saudi Arabia and Egypt, overall graft and patient survival for HCV-G4 are comparable to rates reported in the international literature. Reports from Saudi Arabia reveal an overall 3-year graft and patient survival rates of 90 and 80%, respectively [24, 46–50]. Similarly, in Egypt, where many active living-related liver transplant programs exist and HCV-G4 represents more than 90% of cases, graft and patient survival rates are ~86% [23].

Multiple recent studies from the Middle East evaluated the natural history of HCV-G4 following liver transplantation. Mudawi et al. conducted a study to determine the epidemiological, clinical and virological characteristics of patients with biopsy-proven recurrent HCV infection and analyzed the factors that influence recurrent disease severity. They also compared disease recurrence and outcomes between HCV-4 and other genotypes [51]. Of 116 patients who underwent OLT for hepatitis C, 46 (39.7%) patients satisfied the criteria of recurrent hepatitis C. Twenty-nine (63%) patients were infected with HCV genotype 4. Among many factors included in that analysis, the only factor predictive of an advanced histological score was the HCV RNA level at the time of biopsy. The conclusion was that HCV recurrence following OLT in HCV-4 patients is not significantly different from its recurrence for other genotypes.

In studies published from Egypt reporting on living donor related liver (LDLT) transplantation of HCV-G4 patients, similar favorable outcomes were observed. In a recent Egyptian study 74 adult hepatitis C virus positive subjects were monitored for 36 months after living-donor liver transplant and demographic and laboratory data for the recipients and donors were evaluated. HCV clinical recurrence was observed in 31% of patients and was mostly mild; 91% of patients had fibrosis scores less than F2. And during the study period 91% of patients were alive with excellent graft function. Similar to the study from Saudi Arabia, recurrent HCV was associated with a high pre- and post-transplant viral load and the presence of antibodies to hepatitis B core antigen [52]. In another study, the outcome of LDLT was evaluated in Egyptian patients with HCV-G4-related cirrhosis. Recurrence of HCV was studied in 38 of 53 adult patients who underwent LDLT. Recipient and graft survivals were 86.6% at the end of the 16 ± 8.18 months (range, 4–35 months) follow-up period. Clinical HCV recurrence was observed in 10/38 patients (26.3%). None of the recipients developed allograft cirrhosis during the follow-up period [23]. In a recent study, Allam et al. compared the outcomes of Saudi and Egyptian patients who received liver transplantation either in China or locally in Saudi Arabia (~30% infected with HCV-G4), respective 1- and 3-year cumulative survival rates were 81 and 59% in patients transplanted in China compared with 90 and 84% for patients transplanted locally. They attributed the poorer outcomes in patients transplanted in China to liberal selection criteria, the use of donations after cardiac death, and to the limited post-transplant care [53].

The role of HCV-G4 in the natural history of this disease requires further study. Furthermore, HCV-G4 exhibits significant genetic diversity, and there are a number of viral subtypes. The impacts of the various subtypes have been demonstrated in recent studies; for example, HCV G1 subtype 1b patients were more likely to achieve a rapid virological response (RVR) compared with subtype 1a [54]. Studies performed in Egypt, where HCV-G4 subtypes 4a and 4b predominate, have consistently indicated higher rates of virological response to therapy (69–76%) compared with Saudi Arabia, where response rates are substantially lower (44–50%) [55–57]. In a retrospective analysis of HCV-G4 patients, Roulot et al. reported better sustained virological response (SVR) in 4a subtype-compared with 4d subtype-infected individuals [58]. The majority of patients involved in these European/Australian studies are Egyptians, who are likely older, have coexisting HCC and have received marginal donor grafts. Co-morbidities, such as infection with schistosomiasis, and other nonstudied variables may also have affected outcomes in these patients, leading to an impression that HCV-G4 is an aggressive virus. However, more recent studies originating from the Middle East, where HCV-G4 predominates have revealed no significant difference in outcomes between G1 and G4.

4. Treatment prior to transplantation

4.1. Pegylated interferon and ribavirin

Viral eradication or suppression prior to liver transplantation reduces post-transplant recurrence rates [59]. Until recently, the only available treatment regimens were interferon-based and were therefore contraindicated in patients with advanced cirrhosis [60–62].

Everson et al. evaluated the effectiveness, tolerability, and outcome of a low accelerating dose regimen (LADR) of pegylated interferon (PEG-IFN) therapy in the treatment of patients with advanced HCV. One hundred twenty-four patients were treated with LADR. Sixty-three percent had clinical complications of cirrhosis (ascites, spontaneous bacterial peritonitis, varices, variceal hemorrhage, encephalopathy). Forty-six percent were HCV RNA-negative at end of treatment, and 24% were HCV RNA-negative at last follow-up. Twelve of 15 patients who were HCV RNA-negative before transplantation remained HCV RNA-negative 6 months or more after transplantation. They concluded that LADR may result in viral eradication, stabilize clinical course, and prevent posttransplantation recurrence [61]. In a more recent study patients with various genotypes were randomized 2:1 to treatment ($n = 31$) or untreated control ($n = 16$). Of the 30 patients who were treated, 23 underwent liver transplantation, and 22% achieved a post-transplantation virological response. Although pre-transplant treatment prevented post-transplant recurrence of HCV infection in 25% of cases, including patients infected with HCV-G4, this approach was poorly tolerated and resulted in life-threatening complications [63].

5. Treatment of advanced disease in the new era

The treatment of HCV patients is rapidly evolving. New oral DAAs have emerged with better safety and efficacy profiles, leading to dramatic changes in the practice of HCV management. These choices include sofosbuvir plus weight-adjusted ribavirin (RBV), ledipasvir/sofosbuvir with or without RBV, sofosbuvir/daclatasvir with or without RBV, daclatasvir/simeprevir/sofosbuvir, ombitasvir/paritaprevir/ritonavir with weight-adjusted RBV, elbasvir-grazoprevir with or without RBV. The choice between them depends primarily on potential for drug interactions, availability, and cost. Data on the use of these new agents in cirrhotic G4 patients awaiting liver transplantation are limited. Up-to-date studies evaluating the safety and efficacy of these agents in HCV-G4 patients are summarized below.

5.1. Sofosbuvir and ribavirin

Sofosbuvir (SOF) is a novel pangenotypic nucleotide analog inhibitor that inhibits HCV RNA replication. SOF is administered orally and inhibits the HCV NS5B polymerase. SOF exerts potent antiviral activity against all HCV genotypes [28–30, 32, 64].

In a recently published open-label study, 61 patients with HCV of any genotype awaiting liver transplantation for hepatocellular carcinoma were included. The primary end point was the proportion of patients with HCV-RNA levels <25 IU/ml at 12 weeks after transplantation among patients with this HCVRNA level at their last measurement before transplantation. Patients received up to 48 weeks of SOF/RBV before liver transplantation. Of 46 patients who were transplanted, 43 had HCV-RNA levels of <25 IU/ml at the time of transplantation. Of these 43 patients, 30 (70%) exhibited a post-transplantation virological response at 12 weeks [65]. A recently published study evaluated the efficacy and safety of SOF in combination with RBV in HCV-G4 patients in patients of Egyptian ancestry. Thirty treatment-naive and thirty previously treated patients were enrolled and treated for 12 weeks (n = 31) or 24 weeks (n = 29). Overall, 23% of patients had cirrhosis. SVR12 was achieved by 68% of patients in the 12-week group, and by 93% of patients in the 24-week group. No patient discontinued treatment due to an adverse event [66]. In another Egyptian study, 103 patients' studies were treated with a combination of SOF and weight-adjusted RBV. Seventeen percentage of the study population were cirrhotic. Patients with cirrhosis at baseline had lower rates of SVR12 (63% at 12 weeks, 78% at 24 weeks) than those without cirrhosis (80% at 12 weeks, 93% at 24 weeks). However, the treatment was safe and well tolerated, with no serious drug-related adverse events [67].

However, with the emergence of other treatment options, this combination is not considered the best treatment option.

5.2. Ledipasvir/sofosbuvir and ribavirin

A recently published phase 2, open-label study (Solar-1) assessed treatment with ledipasvir (LDV), SOF, and RBV in patients infected with HCV-G1 or HCV-G4. This study included a cohort of patients with cirrhosis who had not undergone liver transplantation and another cohort of patients who had undergone liver transplantation. In the nontransplant cirrhotic group, SVR12 was achieved in 86–89% of patients. There were no differences in response rates in the 12- and 24-week groups [68]. In another study, 20 (95%) of 21 patients infected with HCV-4 completed 12 weeks of treatment and achieved SVR12 including seven patients with cirrhosis. One patient was non-adherent to study drugs and withdrew from the study but was included in the intention-to-treat analysis [69].

5.3. Sofosbuvir/daclatasvir/ribavirin

The ALLY-1 study evaluated daclatasvir (DCV) + SOF + RBV in patients with advanced cirrhosis or post-transplant HCV recurrence of all genotypes, including G4. DCV is a pangenotypic NS5A inhibitor with a very low potential for drug interaction and a favorable safety profile. All patients with advanced cirrhosis were treated with a combination of DCV 60 mg +

SOF 400 mg + RBV (adjusted dose) for 12 weeks. Overall, 83% of the advanced cirrhosis patients achieved SVR12. SVR12 rates were higher in patients with Child-Pugh class A or B, 93%, versus class C, 56%. The response rate of cirrhotic patients infected with HCV-G4 (4 patients) was 100%. Treatment was well tolerated, with no adverse events or drug-drug interactions [70].

5.4. Simeprevir/daclatasvir/sofosbuvir

The interim results of the IMPACT study indicated favorable responses to this combination in cirrhotic patients infected with G1 and G4. Simeprevir (SIM) is a NS3/4A protease inhibitor with antiviral activity against G1, G2, G4, G5, and G6. All cirrhotic patients (100%) 28/28 achieved SVR4. The treatment was safe and well tolerated, with no major adverse effects. The study is ongoing, and final results will be reported later [71]. A recent report from Qatar has examined the efficacy and safety of Sofosbuvir/daclatasvir and Sofosbuvir/Simeprevir on 85 patients. SVR4 was achieved in 96% of the study population [72].

5.5. Ombitasvir, ritonavir and paritaprevir

The combination of ombitasvir, ritonavir and paritaprevir was evaluated in a large cohort of non cirrhotic genotype-4 patients. After 12 weeks of treatment, 100% of naïve patient who had RBV containing regimen achieved SVR compared to 90.9% in the RBV free regimen. Furthermore, all treatment experienced patients achieved SVR [73]. This combination when used with RBV was also found very effective in HCV genotype-4 with compensated (child A) cirrhosis. Twelve and 16 weeks of treatment resulted in SVR12 of 97 and 100%, respectively [74]. This regimen in addition to dasabuvir was also effective in cirrhotic genotype 1b patient. SVR 12 was 100% in 60 compensated cirrhotic patients [75]. The regimen is contraindicated in Child Pugh classes B and C cirrhosis. More recently, an open-label, partly randomised trial in patients with chronic HCV genotype 4 infection was conducted in Egypt. One hundred and sixty patients were included; 100 patients were assessed as not having cirrhosis and were given 12 weeks of treatment, and 60 patients assessed as having cirrhosis were randomly assigned to the 12-week treatment group (n = 31) or the 24-week treatment group (n = 29). Ninety-four (94%) of 100 patients in the without cirrhosis group, 30 (97%) of 31 patients in the cirrhosis 12-week treatment group, and 27 (93%) of 29 patients in the cirrhosis 24-week treatment group achieved SVR12. Adverse events were predominantly mild or moderate in severity, and laboratory abnormalities were not clinically meaningful. No patients discontinued treatment because of an adverse event [76].

5.6. Elbasvir/grazoprevir

In a recent study, an SVR rate of 96% was achieved in 56 treatment-naïve patients receiving 12 weeks of elbasvir-grazoprevir. In contrast, SVR rates were lower with only 12 weeks among a small number of treatment-experienced patients (78% in 9 patients) but were higher with the addition of ribavirin and treatment extension to 16 weeks (100% in 8 patients). SVR rates were similar in patients with and without cirrhosis. However, this regimen is contraindicated in Child Pugh classes B and C cirrhosis [77].

5.7. Sofosbuvir/velpatasvir

Sofosbuvir and velpatasvir (NS5A inhibitor) is a pangenotypic combination that was recently evaluated in the ASTRAL-1 trial that included 624 naïve and treatment experienced patients, of whom 116 (19%) were genotype-4. Patients with compensated cirrhosis (19%) were included and all genotype-4 patients achieved SVR (100%) after 12 weeks of RBV-free treatment [78]. A phase 3 open-label study involving patients infected with HCV genotypes 1 through 6 who had decompensated cirrhosis was recently conducted. Patients were randomly assigned in a 1:1:1 ratio to receive sofosbuvir and velpatasvir once daily for 12 weeks, sofosbuvir-velpatasvir plus ribavirin for 12 weeks, or sofosbuvir-velpatasvir for 24 weeks. Overall rates of sustained virologic response were 83% among patients who received 12 weeks of sofosbuvir-velpatasvir, 94% among those who received 12 weeks of sofosbuvir-velpatasvir plus ribavirin, and 86% among those who received 24 weeks of sofosbuvir-velpatasvir [79].

6. Treatment after liver transplantation

Earlier studies on preemptive treatment prior to established disease recurrence were disappointing. The conclusion of these studies was that the outcome of preemptive treatment was similar to that of controls in terms of histological recurrence, graft loss, and death [80, 81]. Treatment regimens in these studies were interferon based which resulted in poor tolerability, renal impairment, cytopenias, and drug interactions. DAAs have revolutionized the management of HCV infection in the posttransplant setting. Recent clinical trials have shown high sustained virologic response rates, shorter durations of treatment, and decreased adverse events when compared with the previous PEG-INF based therapy. However, most of these studies were performed in HCV-G1-infected patients. Data on treating HCV-G4 recurrence following liver transplantation are limited (**Table 2**).

6.1. Pegylated interferon and ribavirin

Reported SVR rates for pegylated interferon combination therapy following liver transplantation are lower than those in the nontransplant population. Treatment regimens have been hindered by a high incidence of adverse effects, leading to treatment withdrawal.

Dabbous et al. evaluated 243 patients transplanted for HCV-G4-related cirrhosis. All patients had a protocol biopsy 6 months post-transplant. Patients received PEG-IFN and ribavirin in case of histological recurrence. Repeated liver biopsies were performed at 3, 6, and 12 months during treatment for the detection of immune-mediated rejection induced by interferon. Fifty-six (23%) patients had evidence of histopathological disease recurrence, and 42 patients completed the treatment. Five patients were excluded due to fibrosing cholestatic hepatitis (FCH); therefore, 37 patients were included in the study. The patients received treatment in the form of combined PEG-IFN and RBV. Erythropoietin and granulocyte colony-stimulating factor were used in 70% of patients. SVR was achieved in 29 (78%) patients. The high SVR rate in this study was attributed to several factors, including the early treatment protocol, exclusion of patients with fibrosing cholestatic hepatitis and aggressive treatment of hematological

Study	Sample size	Genotypes	SVR	Treatment protocol
Ajlan [88]	36	4	91.6%	SOF + RBV + PEG − INF for 12 weeks or SOF + RBV for 24 weeks
Dabbous [27]	39	4	76%	SOF + RBV for 24 weeks
Charlton [89]	40	All (1 genotype 4)	70%	SOF + RBV for 24 weeks
Forns [90]	104	1, 2, 3, 4	59%	SOF + RBV for 24–48 weeks
Abergel [91]	44	4	93%	SOF + LDV for 12 weeks
Charlton [68]	108	1 and 4	96–98% in compe nsated cirrhosis 85–88% in cirrhosis with mild hepatic dysfunction 60–75% in cirrhosis with se- vere hepatic dysfunction	SOF + LDV + RBV for 12–24 weeks
Manns [92]	227	1(200) and 4(27)	92.5% of genotype 4 pa- tients	SOF + LDV + RBV for 12–24 weeks
Dumortier [94]	125	All (11 genotype 4)	92%	Predominant SOF/daclatasvir ± RBV
Coilly [95]	137	All (12 genotype 4)	96%	SOF + daclatasvir (DAC)
Leroy [97]	23 (all with FCH)	All	96%	SOF + DCV for 24 weeks

SVR = sustained virological response,
SOF = sofosbuvir,
RBV = ribavirin,
LDV = ledipsavir,
DCV = daclatasvir,
SIM = simeprevir,
FCH = fibrosing cholestatic hepatitis,
PEG-INF = pegylated interferon.

Table 2. Prospective studies that included HCV-G4 patients following liver transplantation.

complications [82]. Conversely, in the largest series reported from Europe, Ponziani et al. evaluated treatment responses in 17 Italian patients with HCV-G4 recurrence following liver transplantation. The observed overall survival after LT was 100% at 1 year and 83.3% at 5 years. Thirty-five percent of patients achieved SVR. However, this retrospective study included patients treated in the 1990s with conventional interferon; the drug tolerability, the lack of aggressive management of hematological side effects and the inclusion of patients with advanced liver disease contributed to the low response rate [83]. In a recent study from Saudi Arabia, 25 patients infected with HCV-G4 were treated with PEG-IFN alpha-2a and RBV [84].

Pretreatment liver biopsies were obtained from all patients. Biochemical and virological markers were assessed before, during, and after treatment. Five patients had advanced pretreatment liver fibrosis. Eighty-eight percent achieved an early virological response; of those, 15 (60%) and 14 (56%) patients achieved end of treatment virological response and SVR, respectively. The most common adverse effects were flu-like symptoms and cytopenia. Eighteen patients (72%) required erythropoietin alpha and/or granulocyte-colony stimulating factor as a supportive measure. One patient developed severe rejection complicated by sepsis, renal failure, and death. Other adverse effects included depression, mild rejection, impotence, itching, and vitiligo. The relatively high response rate in this study may have been due to the treatment-naïve status of the patients, the use of growth factors that allowed patients to complete their course of therapy, the low treatment-withdrawal rate, and the reduction in immunosuppressive therapy during treatment.

The results of these studies suggest that post-transplant treatment outcomes for HCV-G4 are likely better than for G1 and less favorable than for G2 and G3. This response pattern among the different genotypes parallels the response pattern in the immunocompetent population. The availability of newer treatment options with better safety profiles is drawing attention away from PEG-IFN and RBV.

7. HCV treatment in the new antiviral era

7.1. Telaprevir and boceprevir

Following the approval of telaprevir (Incivek™) and boceprevir (Victrelis™) for G1 treatment outcomes improved [85, 86]. Treatment regimens for chronic HCV-G1 infection include a combination of either of these protease inhibitors three times daily with once-weekly subcutaneous injections of PEG-IFN and twice-daily oral RBV. These new combinations increased SVR to 80% and 63–66%, respectively, in nontransplant patients. Some studies have reported poor clinical outcomes of the use of telaprevir and PEG-IFN in patients with HCV-G4 [87]. Burton et al. conducted a retrospective cohort study of 81 patients with genotype 1 HCV treated with boceprevir (10%) or telaprevir (90%) plus PEG-IFN and RBV at six US transplant centers (53% stage 3–4/4 fibrosis, 57% treatment experienced). The intent-to-treat SVR12 rate was 63%. Adverse effects were common; 21% of patients developed anemia (hemoglobin < 8 g/dl) and 57% required blood transfusions during the first 16 weeks. Twenty-seven percent were hospitalized and 9% died; all were liver-related [88]. Although the use of these two DAAs in post–liver transplant patients resulted in SVR up to 60% with telaprevir, nonresponders were observed in the boceprevir treatment, and it was associated with severe side effects, including severe anemia that required erythropoietin, RBV dose reduction and red blood cell transfusions. Significant drug interactions also occurred with immunosuppressants, requiring average cyclosporine dose reductions of 50–84% after telaprevir initiation and 33% after boceprevir initiation. Tacrolimus doses were reduced by 95% with telaprevir [27]. These significant side effects coupled with the introduction of safer antiviral drugs have shifted HCV treatment away from these agents; in fact, these agents are contraindicated by many liver association.

7.2. Sofosbuvir and ribavirin

SOF has become a cornerstone of the management of HCV infection because of its favorable pharmacological and drug interaction profiles. However, there are very limited data on the use of SOF in patients with HCV recurrence post–liver transplant, particularly G4. Ajlan et al. conducted an open label prospective cohort study at a tertiary care hospital in Saudi Arabia. The primary endpoint was SVR12 in patients treated with sofosbuvir-based therapy in post-liver transplant patients with genotype 4 HCV recurrence. Thirty-six treatment-experienced liver transplant patients with HCV recurrence received sofosbuvir and ribavirin with or without PEG-INF. The majority of patients had ≥stage 2 fibrosis. Twenty-eight patients were treated with PEG-IFN and RBV in addition to SOF for 12 weeks and the remaining were treated with SOF and RBV only for 24 weeks. By week 4, only four (11.1%) patients had detectable HCV RNA. Of the 36 patients, two (5.5%) relapsed and one died (2.75%) [89]. Another recent study evaluated the efficacy, safety, and tolerability of SOF and RBV in LDLT recipients with recurrent HCV-4. In this study Thirty-nine Egyptian LDLT recipients were treated for recurrent HCV after LDLT with SOV and RBV without PEG-IFN for 6 months. Thirty eight patients completed 24 weeks of treatment and were followed for 12 weeks after end of treatment. One patient died during the first week of treatment. SVR was achieved by 76% (29/38) of recipients. SVR was significantly higher in treatment-naïve patients and in recipients with a low stage of fibrosis. Only two patients developed severe side effects wile on treatment in the form of severe pancytopenia and acute renal failure [90]. A recent prospective multicenter study enrolled 40 patients with compensated recurrent HCV infection of any genotype after a primary or secondary liver transplantation. All patients received 24 weeks of SOF 400 mg daily and RBV. Of the 40 patients enrolled and treated, 40% had biopsy proven cirrhosis, and 88% had been previously treated with interferon. SVR12 was achieved by 28 of 40 patients. Relapse accounted for all cases of virological failure, including the only patient with HCV-G4. The most common adverse events were fatigue (30%), diarrhea (28%), and headache (25%). In addition, 20% of the subjects experienced anemia. No deaths, graft losses, or episodes of rejection occurred. No interactions with any concomitant immunosuppressive agents were reported [91]. A recent post-transplantation study was conducted in which SOF and RBV were provided on a compassionate-use basis to patients with severe recurrent HCV, including those with fibrosing cholestatic hepatitis (FCH) and decompensated liver cirrhosis with a life expectancy of <1 year. Data from the first 104 patients who completed or prematurely discontinued treatment were included. All patients received SOF and RBV for 24–48 weeks. Investigators were allowed to add PEG-IFN to the regimen at their discretion. The study population included patients infected with HCV- G4. The overall SVR rate was 59% and was higher (73%) in those with early severe recurrence. At the end of the study, 57% of patients displayed clinical improvement, 22% were unchanged, 3% had worsened clinical status, and 13% had died. Overall, 123 serious adverse events occurred in 49 patients (47%). Serious adverse events associated with hepatic decompensation were the most frequent, with 26 adverse events occurring in 19 patients (18%) [92].

7.3. Sofosbuvir/ledipasvir with or without ribavirin

Abergel evaluated the efficacy and safety of therapy with LDV and SOF in patients with HCV genotype 4. Forty-four patients (22 treatment naïve and 22 treatment experienced) received a fixed-dose combination tablet of 90 mg LDV and 400 mg SOV orally once daily for 12 weeks. Among study participants, HCV genotype 4 subtypes were well represented (4a, $n = 25$; 4d, $n = 10$; other subtypes, $n = 9$). Ten patients (23%) had compensated cirrhosis. All 44 patients completed the full 12 weeks of treatment. The SVR12 rate was 93% and was similar in treatment-naïve (95%, 21/22) and treatment-experienced (91%, 20/22) patients. The three patients who did not achieve SVR12 had virological relapse within 4 weeks of the end of treatment; all three had a high baseline HCV RNA, a non-CC IL-28B genotype, and pretreatment NS5A resistance-associated variants. None of the patients experienced a serious adverse event [93].

Cohort B (of the previously described Solar-1 study) enrolled patients who had undergone liver transplantation and included patients with various degrees of disease severity. Patients were randomly assigned to receive a fixed-dose combination tablet containing LDV and SOF plus RBV for 12 or 24 weeks. The cohort included 108 post-transplant patients. SVR12 was achieved in 96–98% of patients without cirrhosis or with compensated cirrhosis, in 85–88% of patients with moderate hepatic impairment, in 60–75% of patients with severe hepatic impairment, and in all six patients with FCH. Response rates were also similar in the 12- and 24-week groups [68]. An open-label study at 34 sites in Europe, Canada, Australia, and New Zealand recruited two groups of patients, cohort A included patients with Child-Turcotte-Pugh class B (CTP-B) or CTP-C cirrhosis who had not undergone liver transplantation. Cohort B included post-transplantation patients who had either no cirrhosis; CTP-A, CTP-B, or CTP-C cirrhosis; or fibrosing cholestatic hepatitis. Patients in each group were randomly assigned (1:1) using a computer-generated randomisation sequence to receive 12 or 24 weeks of LDV (90 mg) and SOF (400 mg) once daily, plus ribavirin (600–1200 mg daily). Of 333 patients who received treatment, 296 had genotype 1 HCV and 37 had genotype 4 HCV. Among all patients with genotype 4 HCV, SVR12 was achieved by 14 of 18 (78%) patients (12 weeks treatment) and 16 of 17 (94%) patients (24 weeks treatment). Of the five patients who did not achieve SVR12, three—all receiving 12 weeks of treatment—had virological relapse, and two died (one post-transplantation CTP-A on 12 weeks of treatment, and one untransplanted CTP-C on 24 weeks of treatment) and were not included in the analysis. Twenty five of twenty seven HCV-G4 in cohort B of the study achieved SVR the only two relapsers were cirrhotics [94]. Despite including G1 and G4 in these studies, the number of HCV-G4 infected patients was relatively small, limiting solid conclusions on the response of HCV-G4.

The safety profile of LVD/SOF with RBV was evaluated in a pooled analysis of two large multicenter studies (Solar-1 and -2). The patients involved were either cirrhotic or post–liver transplantation patients (616 G1 and 42 G4) and were randomized to 12 or 24 weeks of treatment. Of 134 SAEs, only 20 were related to treatment. RBV-associated anemia was the most common adverse effect, representing 11/20 (55%) of reported drug-related adverse events [95].

7.4. Sofosbuvir/daclatasvir

Data on the use of DCV in the post-transplant setting for HCV-G4-infected patients are limited. A prospective multicenter cohort including patients with HCV-recurrence following LT treated with second generation direct antivirals was conducted. The aim of the t study was to assess efficacy and tolerance of sofosbuvir (SOF)-based regimens for the treatment of HCV recurrence in patients with severe fibrosis after LT. A SOF-based regimen was administered to 125 patients including patients infected with HCV-G4 (11 patients). The main combination regimen was SOF/DCV (73.6%). SVR12 was 92.8% (on an intent-to-treat basis); seven cases of virological failure were observed including 1 HCV-G4 patient treated with SOF/daclatasvir (DAC) combination [96]. In another multicenter prospective study137 patients with HCV recurrence receiving SOF and DCV, were included whatever the genotype or fibrosis stage. This cohort included 12 patients infected with HCV-G4. The primary efficacy end point was a sustained virological response 12 weeks after the end of treatment. The SVR rate 12 weeks after completing treatment was 96% under the intention-to treat analysis and 99% when excluding non-virological failures. Only two patients experienced a virological failure. The serious adverse event rate reached 17.5%. Four patients (3%) stopped their treatment prematurely because of adverse events. Anaemia was the most common adverse event, with significantly more cases in the RBV group. No clinically relevant drug–drug interactions were noted, but 52% of patients required a change to the dosage of immunosuppressive drugs [97]. Fontana et al. in a retrospective multicenter study evaluated daclatasvir (DAC)/SOF combination post liver transplantation in established HCV recurrence including HCV-4 patients. Eighty seven percent of patients achieved SVR and the treatment was well tolerated [98]. Leroy et al. analyzed data from 23 patients with FCH who participated in a prospective cohort study in France and Belgium to assess the effects of antiviral agents in patients with recurrence of HCV infection after liver transplantation. Three patients with G4 infection were included in this study (one patient was treated with SOF/RBV, and two were treated with SOF/DCV). All patients survived without re-transplantation. Rapid and dramatic improvements in clinical status were observed. The patients' median bilirubin concentration decreased from 122 μmol/L at baseline to a normal value at week 12 of treatment. Twenty-two patients (96%) had a complete clinical response at week 36, and 22 patients (96%) achieved SVR12, including all 3 patients infected with G4 [99].

7.5. Sofosbuvir and simeprevir

Data on the use of SIM for HCV-G4 recurrence following liver transplantation are limited to a small number of case reports and case series. In a recent report, three patients with HCV-G4 recurrence following liver transplantation were treated with SOF and SIM for 12–24 weeks. All three had high pretreatment viral loads, and one patient had established cirrhosis. SVR12 was achieved in all three patients, with no significant adverse effects or drug interactions [100]. Obed A et al. reported a patient with a recurring HCV-G4 infection and fibrosing cholestatic hepatitis following liver retransplantation, who was successfully treated with a combination therapy of SIM and SOF without PEG-INF/RBV [101].

8. Timing of treatment for patients on the transplant list

The management of hepatitis C virus (HCV) infection in patients with decompensated cirrhosis has evolved dramatically. DAAs have shown to be safe and effective in patients with decompensated cirrhosis with high SVR rates. However it is still debatable on when to initiate treatment in patients with advanced liver disease (**Figure 1**). Many factors may contribute to and affect the approach on an individual basis; for example, it may be better to defer treatment in extremely ill patients. Belli et al. assessed the impact of DAAs on patients awaiting liver transplant. They evaluated whether patients can be first inactivated due to clinicall improvement and subsequently delisted in a real life setting. They included 103 consecutive listed patients without hepatocellular carcinoma who were treated with different DAA combinations in 11 European centers. Treated patient had a significant improvement in the median model for end-stage liver disease (MELD) and Child Pugh score. They concluded that all oral DAAs were able to reverse liver dysfunction and favoured the inactivation and delisting of about one patient out-of-three and one patient out of- five in 60 weeks, respectively. Patients with lower MELD scores had higher chances to be delisted. However, the longer term benefits of therapy need to be ascertained [102]. Similarly Afdhal et al. evaluated the outcome of treatment with SOF and RBV in compensated and decompensated cirrhotic patients. They also monitored the clinical picture and measured the hepatic venous pressure gradient before and after treatment. They observed a clinically meaningful improvement in portal hypertension in addition to improvements in liver biochemistry, Child–Pugh score and model for end-stage liver disease scores [103]. The potential benefits of treating patients on the waiting list include potential improvements in overall clinical status that may salvage these patients from liver transplan-

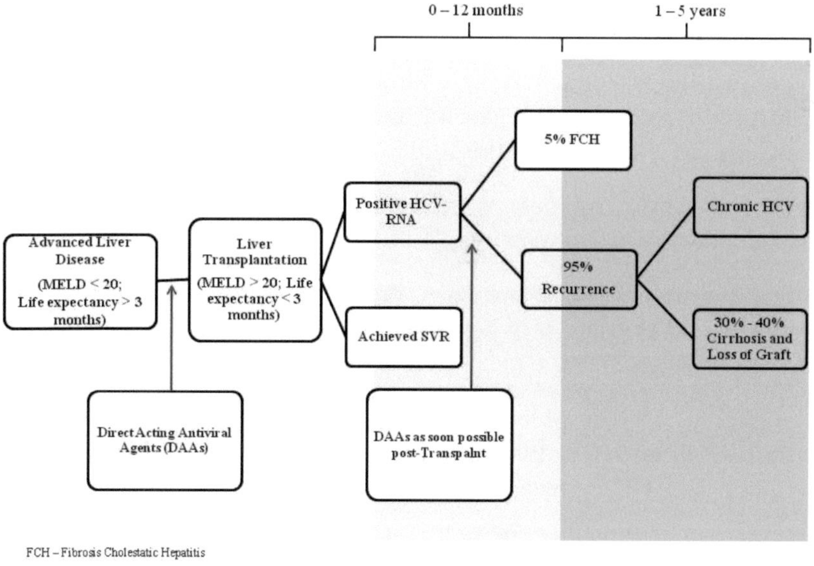

Figure 1. Post transplant natural history of HCV recurrence with potential treatment strategies.

tation; reducing post-transplant recurrence; and avoiding possible post-transplant drug–drug interactions. One concern is that treating these patients may lower their MELD scores and drive them down the transplant list, thus delaying transplantation despite persistent portal hypertensive complications. The decision to treat HCV in patients with decompensated cirrhosis should be individualized till short and long term outcome data become available.

Author details

Waleed K. Al-Hamoudi

Address all correspondence to: walhamoudi@gmail.com

Department of Medicine, Gastroenterology and Hepatology Unit, College of Medicine, King Saud University, Riyadh, Saudi Arabia

References

[1] Kim WR. The burden of hepatitis C in the United States. Hepatology. 2002; 36: S30–S34. doi:10.1002/hep.1840360705

[2] Wiesner RH, Sorrell M, Villamil F. Report of the first International Liver Transplantation Society expert panel consensus conference on liver transplantation and hepatitis C. Liver Transpl. 2003; 9: S1–S9. doi:10.1053/jlts.2003.50268

[3] Garcia-Retortillo M, Forns X, Feliu A, Moitinho E, Costa J, Navasa M, Rimola A, Rodes J. Hepatitis C virus kinetics during and immediately after liver transplantation. Hepatology. 2002; 35: 680–687. doi:10.1053/jhep.2002.31773

[4] Vinaixa C, Rubín A, Aguilera V, Berenguer M. Recurrence of hepatitis C after liver transplantation. Ann Gastroenterol. 2013; 26: 304–313.

[5] Messina JP, Humphreys I, Flaxman A, Brown A, Cooke GS, Pybus OG, et al. Global distribution and prevalence of hepatitis C virus genotypes. Hepatology. 2015; 61: 77–87. doi:10.1002/hep.27259

[6] Abdel-Aziz F, Habib M, Mohamed MK, Abdel-Hamid M, Gamil F, Madkour S, et al. Hepatitis C virus (HCV) infection in a community in the Nile Delta: population description and HCV prevalence. Hepatology. 2000; 32: 111–115. doi:10.1053/jhep.2000.8438

[7] Al Traif I, Al Balwi MA, Abdulkarim I, Handoo FA, Alqhamdi HS, Alotaibi M, et al. HCV genotypes among 1013 Saudi nationals: a multicenter study. Ann Saudi Med. 2013; 33: 10–12.

[8] Xu LZ, Larzul D, Delaporte E, Bréchot C, Kremsdorf D. Hepatitis C virus genotype 4 is highly prevalent in central Africa (Gabon). J Gen Virol. 1994; 75: 2393–2398. doi: 10.1099/0022-1317-75-9-2393

[9] Katsoulidou A, Sypsa V, Tassopoulos NC, Boletis J, Karafoulidou A, Ketikoglou I, et al. Molecular epidemiology of hepatitis C virus (HCV) in Greece: temporal trends in HCV genotype-specific incidence and molecular characterization of genotype 4 isolates. J Viral Hepat. 2006; 13: 19–27. doi:10.1111/j.1365-2893.2005.00649.x

[10] Ansaldi F, Bruzzone B, Salamaso S, Rota MC, Durando P, Gasparini R, et al. Different seroprelavence and molecular epidemiology pattern of hepatitis C virus infection in Italy. J Med Virol. 2005; 76: 327–332. doi:10.1002/jmv.20376

[11] Fernández-Arcás N, López-Siles J, Trapero S, Ferraro A, Ibá-ez A, Orihuela F, et al. High prevalence of hepatitis C virus subtypes 4c and 4d in Malaga (Spain): phylogenetic and epidemiological analyses. J Med Virol. 2006; 78: 1429–1435. doi:10.1002/jmv.20706

[12] Nicot F, Legrand-Abravanel F, Sandres-Saune K, Boulestin A, Dubois M, Alric L, et al. Heterogeneity of hepatitis C virus genotype 4 strains circulating in south-western France. J Gen Virol. 2005; 86: 107–114. doi:10.1099/vir.0.80409-0

[13] Dahlan Y, Ather HM, Al-Ahmadi M, Batwa F, Al-Hamoudi W. Sustained virological response in a predominantly hepatitis C virus genotype 4 infected population. World J Gastroenterol. 2009; 15: 4429–4433. doi:10.3748/wjg.15.4429

[14] Al Ashgar H, Helmy A, Khan MQ, Al Kahtani K, Al Quaiz M, Rezeig M, et al. Predictors of sustained virological response to a 48-week course of pegylated interferon alfa-2a and ribavirin in patients infected with hepatitis C virus genotype 4. Ann Saudi Med. 2009; 29: 4–14. doi:10.4103/0256-4947.51816

[15] Derbala MF, El Dweik NZ, Al Kaabi SR, Al-Marri AD, Pasic F, Bener AB, et al. Viral kinetic of HCV genotype-4 during pegylated interferon alpha 2a: ribavirin therapy. J Viral Hepat. 2008; 15: 591–599. doi:10.1111/j.1365-2893.2008.00988.x

[16] El Khayat HR, Fouad YM, El Amin H, Rizk A. A randomized trial of 24 versus 48 weeks of peginterferon alpha-2a plus ribavirin in Egyptian patients with hepatitis C virus genotype 4 and rapid viral response. Trop Gastroenterol. 2012; 33: 112–117. doi:10.7869/tg.2012.27

[17] Kamal SM, El Kamary SS, Shardell MD, Hashem M, Ahmed IN, Muhammadi M, et al. Pegylated interferon alpha-2b plus ribavirin in patients with genotype 4 chronic hepatitis C: the role of rapid and early virologic response. Hepatology. 2007; 46: 1732–1740. doi:10.1002/hep.21917

[18] Kamal SM. Hepatitis C genotype 4 therapy: increasing options and improving outcomes. Liver Int. 2009; 29(Suppl 1): 39–48. doi:10.1111/j.1478-3231.2008.01930.x

[19] Kamal SM, Fouly AE, Kamel RR, Hockenjos B, Al Tawil A, Khalifa KE, et al. Peginterferon alfa-2b therapy in acute hepatitis C: impact of onset of therapy on sustained

virologic response. Gastroenterology 2006; 130: 632–638. doi:10.1053/j.gastro.2006.01.034

[20] Kamal SM, Moustafa KN, Chen J, Fehr J, Abdel Moneim A, Khalifa KE, et al. Duration of peginterferon therapy in acute hepatitis C: a randomized trial. Hepatology. 2006; 43: 923–931. doi:10.1002/hep.21197

[21] Kamal S, Nasser I. Hepatitis C genotype 4: what we know and what we don't yet know. Hepatology. 2008; 47: 1371–1383. doi:10.1002/hep.22127

[22] AlQaraawi AM, Sanai FM, Al-Husseini H, Albenmousa A, AlSheikh A, Ahmed LR, et al. Prevalence and impact of hepatic steatosis on the response to antiviral therapy in Saudi patients with genotypes 1 and 4 chronic hepatitis C. Dig Dis Sci. 2011; 56: 1222–1228. doi:10.1007/s10620-010-1417-9

[23] Yosry A, Esmat G, El-Serafy M, Omar A, Doss W, Said M, et al. Outcome of living donor liver transplantation for Egyptian patients with hepatitis c (genotype 4)-related cirrhosis. Transplant Proc. 2008; 40: 1481–1484. doi:10.1016/j.transproceed.2008.03.085

[24] Al-Sebayel M, Khalaf H, Al-Sofayan M, Al-Saghier M, Abdo A, Al-Bahili H, et al. Experience with 122 consecutive liver transplant procedures at King Faisal Specialist Hospital and Research Center. Ann Saudi Med. 2007; 27: 333–338. doi:10.4103/0256-4947.51468

[25] Rustgi VK. The epidemiology of hepatitis C infection in the United States. J Gastroenterol. 2007; 42: 513–521. doi:10.1007/s00535-007-2064-6

[26] Roche B, Samuel D. Risk factors for hepatitis C recurrence after liver transplantation. J Viral Hepat. 2007; 14(Suppl 1): 89–96. doi:10.1111/j.1365-2893.2007.00920.x

[27] Antonini TM, Furlan V, Teicher E, Haim-Boukobza S, Sebagh M, Coilly A, Bonhomme-Faivre L, et al. Therapy with boceprevir or telaprevir in HIV/hepatitis C virus co-infected patients to treat recurrence of hepatitis C virus infection after liver transplantation. AIDS 2015 Jan 2; 29(1): 53–58. doi:10.1097/QAD.0000000000000516

[28] Gane EJ, Stedman CA, Hyland RH, Ding X, Svarovskaia E, Symonds WT, Hindes RG, et al. Nucleotide polymerase inhibitor sofosbuvir plus ribavirin for hepatitis C. N Engl J Med. 2013; 368: 34–44. doi:10.1056/NEJMoa1208953

[29] Kowdley KV, Lawitz E, Crespo I, Hassanein T, Davis MN, DeMicco M, Bernstein DE, et al. Sofosbuvir with pegylated interferon alfa-2a and ribavirin for treatment-naive patients with hepatitis C genotype-1 infection (ATOMIC): an open-label, randomised, multicentre phase 2 trial. Lancet. 2013; 381: 2100–2107. doi:10.1016/S0140-6736(13)60247-0

[30] Lawitz E, Lalezari JP, Hassanein T, Kowdley KV, Poordad FF, Sheikh AM, Afdhal NH, et al. Sofosbuvir in combination with peginterferon alfa-2a and

ribavirin for non-cirrhotic, treatment-naive patients with genotypes 1, 2, and 3 hepatitis C infection: a randomised, double-blind, phase 2 trial. Lancet Infect Dis. 2013; 13: 401–408. doi:10.1016/S1473-3099(13)70033-1

[31] Lalezari JP, Nelson DR, Hyland RH. Once daily sofosbuvir plus ribavirin for 12 and 24 weeks in treatment-naïve patients with HCV infection: the QUANTUM study. J Hepatol. 2013; 58: S236. doi:10.1016/S0168-8278(13)60847-8

[32] Lawitz E, Mangia A, Wyles D, Rodriguez-Torres M, Hassanein T, Gordon SC, Schultz M, et al. Sofosbuvir for previously untreated chronic hepatitis C infection. N Engl J Med. 2013; 368: 1878–1887. doi:10.1056/NEJMoa1214853

[33] Jacobson IM, Gordon SC, Kowdley KV, Yoshida EM, Rodriguez-Torres M, Sulkowski MS, Shiffman ML, et al. Sofosbuvir for hepatitis C genotype 2 or 3 in patients without treatment options. N Engl J Med. 2013; 368: 1867–1877. doi:10.1056/NEJMoa1214854

[34] Osinusi A, Meissner EG, Lee YJ, Bon D, Heytens L, Nelson A, Sneller M, et al. Sofosbuvir and ribavirin for hepatitis C genotype 1 in patients with unfavorable treatment characteristics: a randomized clinical trial. JAMA. 2013; 310: 804–811. doi:10.1001/jama.2013.109309

[35] AASLD/IDSA HCV Guidance Panel. Hepatitis C guidance: AASLD-IDSA recommendations for testing, managing, and treating adults infected with hepatitis C virus. Hepatology. 2015; 62(3): 932–954. doi:10.1002/hep.27950

[36] Campos-Varela I, Lai JC, Verna EC, O'Leary JG, Todd Stravitz R, Forman LM, et al. Consortium to Study Health Outcomes in HCV Liver Transplant Recipients (CRUSH-C). Hepatitis C genotype influences post-liver transplant outcomes. Transplantation. 2015; 99: 835–840. doi:10.1097/TP.0000000000000413

[37] Féray C, Caccamo L, Alexander GJ, et al. European collaborative study on factors influencing outcome after liver transplantation for hepatitis C. European Concerted Action on Viral Hepatitis (EUROHEP) Group. Gastroenterology. 1999; 117: 619. doi:10.1016/S0016-5085(99)70454-3

[38] Féray C, Gigou M, Samuel D, et al. Influence of the genotypes of hepatitis C virus on the severity of recurrent liver disease after liver transplantation. Gastroenterology. 1995; 108: 1088. doi:10.1016/0016-5085(95)90207-4

[39] Gordon FD, Poterucha JJ, Germer J, et al. Relationship between hepatitis C genotype and severity of recurrent hepatitis C after liver transplantation. Transplantation. 1997; 63: 1419. doi:10.1097/00007890-199705270-00009

[40] Zhou S, Terrault NA, Ferrell L, Hahn JA, Lau JY, Simmonds P, et al. Severity of liver disease in liver transplant ation recipients with hepatitis C virus infection: relationship to genotype and level of viremia. Hepatology. 1996; 24: 1041–1046. doi:10.1002/hep.510240510

[41] Vargas HE, Laskus T, Wang LF, Radkowski M, Poutous A, Lee R, et al. The influence of hepatitis C virus genotypes on the outcome of liver transplantation. Liver Transpl Surg. 1998; 4: 22–27. doi:10.1002/lt.500040103

[42] Berenguer M, Prieto M, Rayón JM, Mora J, Pastor M, Ortiz V, et al. Natural history of clinically compensated hepatitis C virus-related graft cirrhosis after liver transplantation. Hepatology. 2000; 32: 852–858. doi:10.1053/jhep.2000.17924

[43] Zekry A, Whiting P, Crawford DH, Angus PW, Jeffrey GP, Padbury RT, et al. Australian and New Zealand Liver Transplant Clinical Study Group. Liver transplantation for HCV-associated liver cirrhosis: predictors of outcomes in a population with significant genotype 3 and 4 distribution. Liver Transpl. 2003; 9: 339–347. doi:10.1053/jlts.2003.50063

[44] Gane EJ, Portmann BC, Naoumov NV, Smith HM, Underhill JA, Donaldson PT, et al. Long-term outcome of hepatitis C infection after liver transplantation. N Engl J Med. 1996; 334: 815–820. doi:10.1056/NEJM199603283341302

[45] Wali MH, Heydtmann M, Harrison RF, Gunson BK, Mutimer DJ. Outcome of liver transplantation for patients infected by hepatitis C, including those infected by genotype 4. Liver Transpl. 2003; 9: 796–804. doi:10.1053/jlts.2003.50164

[46] Al-Sebayel M. Survival after liver transplantation: experience with 89 cases. Ann Saudi Med. 1999; 19: 216–218.

[47] Kizilisik TA, Al-Sebayel M, Hammad A, Al-Traif I, Ramirez CG, Abdulla A. Hepatitis C recurrence in liver transplant recipients. Transplant Proc. 1997; 29: 2875–2877. doi:10.1016/S0041-1345(97)00715-X

[48] Al Sebayel M, Kizilisik AT, Ramirez C, Altraif I, Hammad AQ, Littlejohn W, et al. Liver transplantation: experience at King Fahad National Guard Hospital, Riyadh, Saudi Arabia. Transplant Proc. 1997; 29: 2870–2871. doi:10.1016/S0041-1345(97)00713-6

[49] Al Sebayel M. Liver transplantation: five-year experience in Saudi Arabia. Transplant Proc. 1999; 31: 3157. doi:10.1016/S0041-1345(99)00765-4

[50] Al Sebayel MS, Ramirez CB, Abou Ella K. The first 100 liver transplants in Saudi Arabia. Transplant Proc. 2001; 33: 2709. doi:10.1016/S0041-1345(01)02155-8

[51] Mudawi H, Helmy A, Kamel Y, Al Saghier M, Al Sofayan M, Al Sebayel M, et al. Recurrence of hepatitis C virus genotype-4 infection following liver transplantation: natural history and predictors of outcome. Ann Saudi Med. 2009; 29: 91–97. doi:10.4103/0256-4947.51796

[52] Yosry A, Abdel-Rahman M, Esmat G, El-Serafy M, Omar A, Doss W, et al. Recurrence of hepatitis c virus (genotype 4) infection after living-donor liver transplant in Egyptian patients. Exp Clin Transplant. 2009; 7: 157–163.

[53] Allam N, Al Saghier M, El Sheikh Y, Al Sofayan M, Khalaf H, Al Sebayel M, et al. Clinical outcomes for Saudi and Egyptian patients receiving deceased donor liver transplanta-

tion in China. Am J Transplant. 2010; 10: 1834–1841. doi:10.1111/j.1600-6143.2010.03088.x

[54] Jensen DM, Morgan TR, Marcellin P, Pockros PJ, Reddy KR, Hadziyannis SJ, *et al*. Early identification of HCV genotype 1 patients responding to 24 weeks peginterferon alpha-2a (40 kd)/ribavirin therapy. Hepatology 2006;43:954–60.

[55] Alfaleh FZ, Hadad Q, Khuroo MS, Aljumah A, Algamedi A, Alashgar H, et al. Peginterferon alpha-2b plus ribavirin compared with interferon alpha-2b plus ribavirin for initial treatment of chronic hepatitis C in Saudi patients commonly infected with genotype 4. Liver Int. 2004; 24: 568–574. doi:10.1111/j.1478-3231.2004.0976.x

[56] Khuroo MS, Khuroo MS, Dahab ST. Meta-analysis: a randomized trial of peginterferon plus ribavirin for the initial treatment of chronic hepatitis C genotype 4. Aliment Pharmacol Ther. 2004; 20: 931–938. doi:10.1111/j.1365-2036.2004.02208.x

[57] Kamal SM, El Tawil AA, Nakano T, He Q, Rasenack J, Hakam SA, et al. Peginterferon {alpha}-2b and ribavirin therapy in chronic hepatitis C genotype 4: impact of treatment duration and viral kinetics on sustained virological response. Gut. 2005; 54: 858–866. doi:10.1136/gut.2004.057182

[58] Roulot D, Bourcier V, Grando V, Deny P, Baazia Y, Fontaine H, et al. Observational VHC4 Study Group. Epidemiological characteristics and response to peginterferon plus ribavirin treatment of hepatitis C virus genotype 4 infection. J Viral Hepat. 2007; 14: 460–467. doi:10.1111/j.1365-2893.2006.00823.x

[59] Fortune BE, Martinez-Camacho A, Kreidler S, Gralla J, Everson GT. Post-transplant survival is improved for hepatitis C recipients who are RNA negative at time of liver transplantation. Transpl Int. 2015; 28: 980–989. doi:10.1111/tri.12568

[60] Everson GT. Treatment of hepatitis C in the patient with decompensated cirrhosis. Clin Gastroenterol Hepatol. 2005; 3(Suppl 2): S106–S112. doi:10.1016/S1542-3565(05)00699-3

[61] Everson GT, Trotter J, Forman L, Kugelmas M, Halprin A, Fey B, et al. Treatment of advanced hepatitis C with a low accelerating dosage regimen of antiviral therapy. Hepatology. 2005; 42: 255–262. doi:10.1002/hep.20793

[62] Crippin JS, McCashland T, Terrault N, Sheiner P, Charlton MR. A pilot study of the tolerability and efficacy of antiviral therapy in hepatitis C virus-infected patients awaiting liver transplantation. Liver Transpl. 2002; 8: 350–355. doi:10.1053/jlts.2002.31748

[63] Everson GT, Terrault NA, Lok AS, Rodrigo del R, Brown RS Jr, Saab S, et al. Adult-to-Adult Living Donor Liver Transplantation Cohort Study. A randomized controlled trial of pretransplant antiviral therapy to prevent recurrence of hepatitis C after liver transplantation. Hepatology. 2013; 57: 1752–1762. doi:10.1002/hep.25976

[64] Pawlotsky JM. Treatment of chronic hepatitis C: current and future. Curr Top Microbiol Immunol. 2013; 369: 321–342. doi:10.1007/978-3-642-27340-7_13

[65] Curry MP, Forns X, Chung RT, Terrault NA, Brown R Jr, Fenkel JM, et al. Sofosbuvir and ribavirin prevent recurrence of HCV infection after liver transplantation: an open-label study. Gastroenterology. 2015; 148: 100–107.e1. doi:10.1053/j.gastro.2014.09.023

[66] Ruane PJ, Ain D, Stryker R, Meshrekey R, Soliman M, Wolfe PR, et al. Sofosbuvir plus ribavirin for the treatment of chronic genotype 4 hepatitis C virus infection in patients of Egyptian ancestry. J Hepatol. 2015; 62(5): 1040.

[67] Doss W, Shiha G, Hassany M, Soliman R, Fouad R, Khairy M, et al. Sofosbuvir plus ribavirin for treating Egyptian patients with hepatitis c genotype 4. J Hepatol. 2015. doi: 10.1016/j.jhep.2015.04.023 [Epub ahead of print]

[68] Charlton M, Everson GT, Flamm SL, Kumar P, Landis C, Brown RS Jr, et al. Ledipasvir and sofosbuvir plus ribavirin for treatment of HCV infection in patients with advanced liver disease. Gastroenterology. 2015 Sep; 149(3): 649–659. doi:10.1053/j.gastro.2015.05.010

[69] Kohli A, Kapoor R, Sims Z, Nelson A, Sidharthan S, Lam B, et al. Ledipasvir and sofosbuvir for hepatitis C genotype 4: a proof-of-concept, single-centre, open-label phase 2a cohort study. Lancet Infect Dis. 2015; 15(9): 1049. doi:10.1016/S1473-3099(15)00157-7

[70] Poordad F, Schiff ER, Vierling JM, Landis C, Fontana RJ, Yang R, et al. Daclatasvir, sofosbuvir, and ribavirin combination for HCV patients with advanced cirrhosis or post-transplant recurrence: ALLY-1 phase 3 study. Hepatology. 2016 May; 63(5): 1493–1505. doi:10.1002/hep.28446.

[71] Lawitz E, Poordad F, Gutierrez J, Kakuda T, Picchio G, De La Rosa G, et al. Simeprevir (SMV) plus daclatasvir (DCV) and sofosbuvir (SOF) in treatment-naïve and -experienced patients with chronic hepatitis C virus genotype 1 or 4 infection and decompensated liver disease: interim results from the Phase II IMPACT study. J Hepatol. 2015; 62(Suppl 2): S266–S267. doi:10.1016/S0168-8278(15)30161-6

[72] Derbala M, Amer A, Alkaabi S, Kamel Y, Sultan K, et al. Safety and efficacy of two IFN-free DAAs regimens in genotype 4 chronic HCV patients: first real clinical practice data in gulf from qatar HCV registry. Annual Meeting of the American Association for the Study of Liver Diseases, November 13–17, 2015. Hepatology, 62: 93A–207A. doi: 10.1002/hep.28162

[73] Hézode C, Asselah T, Reddy KR, Hassanein T, Berenguer M, et al. Ombitasvir plus paritaprevir plus ritonavir with or without ribavirin in treatment-naive and treatment-experienced patients with genotype 4 chronic hepatitis C virus infection (PEARL-I): a randomised, open-label trial. Lancet. 2015; 385(9986): 2502–2509. doi:10.1016/S0140-6736(15)60159-3

[74] Asselah T, Hassanein T, Qaqish R, Feld J, Hezode C, et al. Efficacy and safety of ombitasvir/paritaprevir/ritonavir co-administered with ribavirin in adults with genotype 4 chronic hepatitis C infection and cirrhosis (AGATE-I). Annual Meeting of the American Association for the Study of Liver Diseases, November 13–17, 2015. Hepatology, 62: 93A–207A. doi:10.1002/hep.28162

[75] Feld JJ, Moreno C, Trinh R, Tam E, Bourgeois S, Horsmans Y, et al. Sustained virologic response of 100% in HCV genotype 1b patients with cirrhosis receiving ombitasvir/paritaprevir/r and dasabuvir for 12 weeks. J Hepatol. 2016; 64(2): 301–307. doi:10.1016/j.jhep.2015.10.005

[76] Waked I, Shiha G, Qaqish R, et al. Ombitasvir, paritaprevir, and ritonavir plus ribavirin for chronic hepatitis C virus genotype 4 infection in Egyptian patients with or without compensated cirrhosis (AGATE-II): a multicentre, phase 3, partly randomised open-label trial. Lancet Gastroenterol Hepatol. 2016 (In press).

[77] Asselah T, Reesink HW, Gerstoft J, et al. High efficacy of grazoprevir and elbasvir with or without ribavirin in 103 treatment-naive and experienced patients with HCV genotype 4 infection: a pooled analysis. Presented at the American Association for the Study of Liver Diseases Liver Meeting, San Francisco CA, November 13–17, 2015. Hepatology, 62: 337A–341A. doi:10.1002/hep.28207

[78] Feld JJ, Jacobson IM, Hézode C, Asselah T, Ruane PJ, et al. Sofosbuvir and velpatasvir for HCV genotype 1, 2, 4, 5, and 6 infection. N Engl J Med. 2015; 373(27): 2599–2607. doi:10.1056/NEJMoa1512610

[79] Curry MP, O'Leary JG, Bzowej N, Muir AJ, Korenblat KM, Fenkel JM, et al. Sofosbuvir and Velpatasvir for HCV in Patients with Decompensated Cirrhosis. N Engl J Med. 2015; 373(27): 2618–2628. doi:10.1056/NEJMoa1512614

[80] Bzowej N, Nelson DR, Terrault NA, Everson GT, Teng LL, Prabhakar A, et al. PHOENIX Study Group. PHOENIX: a randomized controlled trial of peginterferon alfa-2a plus ribavirin as a prophylactic treatment after liver transplantation for hepatitis C virus. Liver Transpl. 2011; 17: 528–538. doi: 10.1002/lt.22271

[81] Chalasani N, Manzarbeitia C, Ferenci P, Vogel W, Fontana RJ, Voigt M, et al. Peginterferon alfa-2a for hepatitis C after liver transplantation: two randomized, controlled trials. Hepatology. 2005; 41: 289–298. doi:10.1002/hep.20560

[82] Dabbous HM, Elmeteini MS, Sakr MA, Montasser IF, Bahaa M, Abdelaal A, et al. Optimizing outcome of recurrent hepatitis C virus genotype 4 after living donor liver transplantation: moving forward by looking back. Transplant Proc. 2014; 46: 822–827. doi:10.1016/j.transproceed.2013.11.152

[83] Ponziani FR, Milani A, Gasbarrini A, Zaccaria R, Viganò R, Donato MF, et al. Treatment of recurrent genotype 4 hepatitis C after liver transplantation: early virological response

is predictive of sustained virological response. An AISF RECOLT-C group study. Ann Hepatol. 2012; 11: 338–342.

[84] Al-Hamoudi W, Mohamed H, Abaalkhail F, Kamel Y, Al-Masri N, Allam N, et al. Treatment of genotype 4 hepatitis C recurring after liver transplantation using a combination of pegylated interferon alfa-2a and ribavirin. Dig Dis Sci. 2011; 56: 1848–1852. doi:10.1007/s10620-010-1526-5

[85] Zeuzem S, Andreone P, Pol S, Lawitz E, Diago M, Roberts S, et al. REALIZE Study Team. Telaprevir for retreatment of HCV infection. N Engl J Med. 2011; 364: 2417–2428. doi: 10.1056/NEJMoa1013086

[86] Manns MP, Markova AA, Calle Serrano B, Cornberg M. Phase III results of Boceprevir in treatment naïve patients with chronic hepatitis C genotype 1. Liver Int. 2012; 32(Suppl 1): 27–31. doi:10.1111/j.1478-3231.2011.02725.x

[87] Armignacco O, Andreoni M, Sagnelli E, Puoti M, Bruno R, Gaeta GB, et al. Recommendations for the use of hepatitis C virus protease inhibitors for the treatment of chronic hepatitis C in HIV-infected persons. A position paper of the Italian Association for the Study of Infectious and Tropical Disease. New Microbiol. 2014; 37: 423–438.

[88] Burton JR, O'Leary JG, Verna EC, Saxena V, Dodge JL, Stravitz RT, et al. A US multicenter study of hepatitis C treatment of liver transplant recipients with protease-inhibitor triple therapy. J Hepatol. 2014; 61(3): 508–514. doi:10.1016/j.jhep.2014.04.037

[89] Ajlan A, Al-Jedai A, Elsiesy H, Alkortas D, Al-Hamoudi W, Alarieh R, et al. Clinical study sofosbuvir-based therapy for genotype 4 HCV recurrence post-liver transplant treatment-experienced patients. Can J Gastroenterol Hepatol. 2016; 2016: 2872371. doi: 10.1155/2016/2872371

[90] Dabbous HM, Montasser IF, Sakr MA, Refai R, Sayam M, Abdelmonem A, et al. Safety, efficacy, and tolerability of sofosbuvir and ribavirin in management of recurrent hepatitis C virus genotype 4 after living donor liver transplant in Egypt: what have we learned so far? Hepat Mon. 2016; 16(5): e35339. doi:10.5812/hepatmon.35339

[91] Charlton M, Gane E, Manns MP, Brown RS Jr, Curry MP, Kwo PY, et al. Sofosbuvir and ribavirin for treatment of compensated recurrent hepatitis C virus infection after liver transplantation. Gastroenterology. 2015; 148: 108–117. doi:10.1053/j.gastro.2014.10.001

[92] Forns X, Charlton M, Denning J, McHutchison JG, Symonds WT, Brainard D, et al. Sofosbuvir compassionate use program for patients with severe recurrent hepatitis C after liver transplantation. Hepatology. 2015; 61: 1485–1494. doi:10.1002/hep.27681

[93] Abergel A, Loustaud-Ratti V, Metivier S, Jiang D, Kersy K, Knox SJ, et al. Ledipasvir plus sofosbuvir for 12 weeks in patients with hepatitis C genotype 4 infection. Hepatology. 2016 Oct;64(4):1049–56. doi: 10.1002/hep.28706.

[94] Manns M, Forns X, Samuel D, Denning J, Arterburn S, Brandt-Sarif T, et al. Ledipasvir/sofosbuvir with ribavirin is safe and efficacious in decompensated and post-liver

transplantation patients with HCV infection: preliminary results of the SOLAR-2 trial. J Hepatol. 2015; 62: S187.

[95] Samuel D, Manns M, Forns X, Flamm SL, Reddy KR, Denning J, et al. Ledipasvir/sofosbuvir with ribavirin is safe in >600 decompensated and post-liver transplantation patients with HCV infection: an integrated safety analysis of the SOLAR-1 and SOLAR-2 trials. Lancet Infect Dis. 2016; 16(6): 685–697. doi:10.1016/S1473-3099(16)00052-9

[96] Dumortier J, Leroy V, Duvoux C, de Ledinghen V, Francoz C, Houssel-Debry P, et al. 5 Sofosbuvir-based treatment of hepatitis C with severe fibrosis (METAVIR F3/F4) after liver transplantation: Liver Transpl. 2016 Oct;22(10):1367–78. doi: 10.1002/lt. 24505.

[97] Coilly A, Fougerou-Leurent C, de Ledinghen V, Houssel-Debry P, Duvoux C, Di 9 Martino V, et al. Multicentre experience using daclatasvir and sofosbuvir to treat 10 hepatitis C recurrence after liver transplantation – The CO23 ANRS CUPILT study. J Hepatol. 2016 Oct;65(4):711–8. doi: 10.1016/j.jhep.2016.05.039.

[98] Fontana RJ, Brown RS Jr, Moreno-Zamora A, Prieto M, Joshi S, Londo-o MC, et al. Daclatasvir combined with sofosbuvir or simeprevir in liver transplant recipients with severe recurrent hepatitis C infection. Liver Transpl. 2016; 22(4): 446–458. doi:10.1002/lt.24416

[99] Leroy V, Dumortier J, Coilly A, Sebagh M, Fougerou-Leurent C, Radenne S, et al. Efficacy of sofosbuvir and daclatasvir in patients with fibrosing cholestatic hepatitis C after liver transplantation. Clin Gastroenterol Hepatol. 2015; 13(11): 1993–2001. doi: 10.1016/j.cgh.2015.05.030

[100] Ascha M, Ascha M, Zein NN, Alkhouri N, Eghtesad B, Abu-Elmagd K, et al. Treatment of recurrent hepatitis c genotype-4 post-liver transplantation with sofosbuvir plus simeprevir. Int J Organ Transplant Med. 2015; 6: 86–90.

[101] Obed A, Jarrad A, Bashir A, Moog G. Combination therapy of simeprevir and sofosbuvir in recurrent HCV genotype 4 after liver retransplantation: case report. Am J Case Rep. 2016; 17: 357–359. doi:10.12659/AJCR.896810

[102] Belli LS, Berenguer M, Cortesi PA, Strazzabosco M, Rockenschaub SR, Martini S, Morelli C, et al. Delisting of liver transplant candidates with chronic hepatitis C after viral eradication: A European study. J Hepatol. 2016 Sep;65(3):524–31. doi: 10.1016/j.jhep.2016.05.010.

[103] Afdhal N, Everson GT, Calleja JL, McCaughan G, Bosch J, Denning J, et al. Effect of long term viral suppression with sofosbuvir + ribavirin on hepatic venous pressure gradient in HCV-infected patients with cirrhosis and portal hypertension. J Hepatol. 2015; 62(Suppl 2): S269–S270. doi:10.1016/S0168-8278(15)30167-7

Chapter 6

HCV Treatment Failure in the Era of DAAs

Mohamed Hassany and Aisha Elsharkawy

Additional information is available at the end of the chapter

http://dx.doi.org/10.5772/67149

Abstract

Hepatitis C virus (HCV) has six well-known genotypes in worldwide and has a very high genetic diversity. Introduction of DAAs leads to improvement of treatment results with SVR rates exceeding 95%. Development of HCV treatment resistance is a problematic issue that needs sufficient solutions. Many hosts, viral, and drug factors are implemented in the process of treatment resistance. Lack of clinical trials on treatment failure leads to lag in development of certain consensuses for retreatment.

Keywords: HCV-DAAs, viral resistance, treatment failure

1. Introduction

Chronic hepatitis C virus (HCV) infection is a major health problem all over the world. The global prevalence of viremic HCV infection was reestimated between 64 and 103 million patients [1]. Chronic HCV patients suffered a long time from the complications of their disease until the first discovery of interferon treatment. However, its modest response rate and the development of many adverse events were the major problem. Soon the dream seems to become true with the introduction of HCV direct acting antivirals (DAAs) in 2014. Their higher rates of response and minimally observed adverse events encourage more patients to go for treatment. In addition, patients with advanced fibrosis and cirrhosis find a new hope to stop the progression of their disease. Three classes of DAAs (protease inhibitors, NS5A inhibitors, and polymerase inhibitors) targeting three HCV enzymatic nonstructural proteins were approved for treatment in many countries [2]. Variability of treatment efficacy among patients makes it difficult to control the infection; while for some patients, weak antivirals and short-term treatments are sufficient, others require combination therapies with several highly active antivirals for longer durations [3].

Despite the high rates of virological cure achieved with these treatments, the infection is not eliminated from a substantial number of patients (1–15%, depending on the patient status and regimen used) [4]. Patients and researchers started to face the new problem of drug resistance. In this review, HCV treatment failure in the era of DAAs will be discussed in the context of factors affecting development of resistance, diagnosis, and management.

2. Treatment from interferon to DAAs

Hepatitis C virus (HCV) has six well-known genotypes in worldwide [5–10] with multiple subtypes (a, b, c, etc.). RNA sequence may vary by 35% between different genotypes. HCV has a very high genetic diversity and very high rate of replication (>10 trillion virions/day), and due to this replication rate, significant genetic errors occur and a continuous process of correction is already running to optimize the replication and sequencing of the virus genes; failure of error correction leads to the formation of genetic drifts [5]; these drifts are represented either in the form of genotypes or quasispecies. **Table 1** shows the difference among genotypes, subtypes, and quasispecies.

The presence of different HCV genotypes does not exhibit a major clinical implication on the natural history of the disease and its progression, yet it has a great influence on treatment outcome. The best results for treatment in the past era of pegylated interferon (PegIFN) and ribavirin (RBV) were achieved in genotypes 2, 3 (80–90%) with less favorable results in genotypes 1, 4 (40–50%) and intermediate results in genotypes 5, 6 (60–70%). Failure of treatment during this era had no satisfactory solutions rather than retreatment using the same regimen or changing the pegylated interferon type (between alpha 2a and alpha 2b) or even extending the treatment duration.

Introduction of the direct acting antivirals (DAAs) in the playground of HCV treatment represents a major challenge with the rising number of approved molecules and its coming followers in the pipe of production and approval as shown in **Table 2**, although the very high response to these drugs, which sometimes exceeds 95% yet its limited failure, represents a problematic issue.

DAAs permit to treat different categories of patients who could not be treated easily in the past due to the low efficacy and safety of pegylated interferon such as those with advanced liver disease (CHILD-PUGH B, C), autoimmune diseases, polymedicated patients, renal impairment, postorgan transplantation, etc. Implementation of larger groups to the treatment pipe leads to expulsion of more numbers of treatment failures asking for better solutions for retreatment.

Genotypes, subtypes	Quasispecies
Difference in RNA sequence	Mutation during replication
Major genetic differences	Minor genetic differences
Does not change	Continue to evolve over time

Table 1. Differences between genotypes, subtypes, and quasispecies.

http://dx.doi.org/10.5772/67149

Agent class	Generation	Compound	Phase of clinical development
NS3-4A protease inhibitors	First-wave First-generation	Telaprevir Boceprevir	Approved
	Second-wave First-generation	Simeprevir Paritaprevir/ritonavir	Approved
		Asunaprevir Vaniprevir Sovaprevir	In clinical development
	Second-generation	Grazoprevir	Approved
		ACH-2684	In clinical development
Nucleoside/nucleotide analogues	Nucleotide analogues	Sofosbuvir	Approved
		MK-3682 ACH-3422 AL-335	In clinical development
Nonnucleoside inhibitors	Palm domain I inhibitors	Dasabuvir	Approved
	Thumb domain I inhibitors	Beclabuvir	In clinical development
	Thumb domain II inhibitors	GS-9669	In clinical development
NS5A inhibitors	First-generation	Daclatasvir Ledipasvir Ombitasvir	Approved
	Second-generation	Elbasvir Velpatasvir	Approved
		ACH-3102	In clinical development

Table 2. DAAa pipeline current situation (April 2016).

All the previously mentioned molecules have different characteristics regarding the potency, genotype coverage, and barrier to resistance. **Table 3** shows the characteristics of DAAs molecules [6].

Different continental guidelines for HCV management describe different treatment regimens:

1. *PegIFN-based regimens* (e.g., PegIFN + RBV + Sofosbuvir, PegIFN+RBV + Simeprevir, PegIFN + RBV + Daclatasvir)

2. *PegIFN-free sofosbuvir-based regimens ± ribavirin* (Sofosbuvir + Daclatasvir, Sofosbuvir + Simeprevir, Sofosbuvir + Ledipasvir, Sofosbuvir + Velpatasvir)

3. *PegIFN-free Sofosbuvir-free regimens ± ribavirin* (Paritaprevir/r + Ombitasvir ± Dasabuvir, Grazoprevir + Elbasvir)

Drug group	Potency	Genotype coverage	Resistance barrier
NS3-4A protease inhibitors	+++	+++	++
NS5A inhibitors	+++	+++	++
Nucleoside/nucleotide analogues	+++	+++	+++
Nonnucleoside inhibitors	++	+	+

Table 3. Characteristics of DAAs molecules.

3. Definitions

The terms RAVs, RASs, resistant variants, and sensitive variants were recently used in clinical practice to describe the susceptibility to an administered DAA. Using these definitions paved the way to understand more about HCV treatment failure when using DAAs. Pawlotsky has described well these terms as mentioned below [4]:

3.1. Viral resistance

Positive selection of viral variants with reduced susceptibility to an administered DAA.

3.2. Resistance-associated variant (RAV)

It is often used to indifferently describe the amino acid substitutions that reduce the susceptibility of a virus to a drug or drug class or, alternatively, the viral variants with reduced susceptibility that carry these substitutions.

3.3. Resistance-associated substitutions (RASs)

The amino acid substitutions that confer resistance.

3.4. Resistant variants

The viral variants carrying these RASs and thereby have reduced susceptibility to the DAA.

3.5. Sensitive variants

Viral variants that do not contain amino acids that confer reduced susceptibility to the antiviral action of an HCV DAA (contain only the original wild-type amino acids of the viral strains).

3.6. Fitness-associated substitution(s)

Single amino acid changes that do not alter DAA susceptibility but increase the power of replication (fitness of the resistant variants).

http://dx.doi.org/10.5772/67149

Prior to therapy, multiple baseline HCV resistant-associated variants (RAVs) are already present but usually at a very low undetectable limit. After treatment with DAAs, a sharp decline of HCV viremia occurs within the first treatment days and a competition between sensitive variants and resistant variants will determine which of the following scenarios will be encountered after stoppage of the administered drug:

(1) The drugs success to eliminate both sensitive and resistant variants and the patient succeed to achieve sustained virologic response (SVR).

(2) The drug eliminates the HCV sensitive variants and rendering the resistant variants and after stoppage of treatment both resistant and sensitive variants are restored to the same baseline picture and continue to replicate.

(3) The drug eliminates the HCV sensitive variants and rendering the resistant variants and after stoppage of treatment the resistant variants replicate as a dominant virus.

4. Factors affecting the outcome and HCV resistance

Failure of treatment and development of resistance are a multifactorial process depending on host-related factors, virus-related factors, and drug-related factors as shown in **Figure 1**.

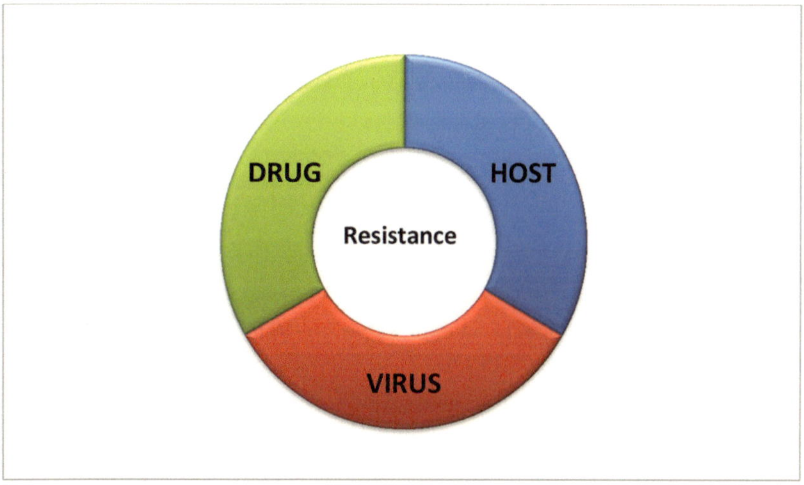

Figure 1. Factors affecting treatment outcome and development of resistance.

4.1. Host-related factors

Introduction of DAAs eliminates multiple host factors, which affect previous treatment with PegIFN and ribavirin, yet several host factors still persist:

(1) Adherence to therapy: achievement of the best drug response surely will be better in case of proper administration of the drug with its proper dose at regular times and respect of food relations as recommended by the manufacturer.

(2) HIV, post-organ transplantation and polymedicated patients: revision of the drug-drug interactions map is necessary in those patients to avoid the effect of other drugs in reducing the plasma level of anti-HCV drugs.

(3) Treatment status: most of clinical trials on DAAs showed mild better response in treatment naïve patients than those who previously failed treatment with PegIFN/RBV.

(4) Hepatic fibrosis stage: patients with advanced fibrosis stage remain the most difficult to treat group even under the umbrella of DAAs which showed a wide variable results in cirrhotics ranged between 33 and 100% [7]. Addition of ribavirin and prolonged treatment duration may offer the best chance for those patients in achieving sustained virological response.

4.2. Virus-related factors

(1) Genotype: treatment with PegIFN/RBV/Sofosbuvir represents the regimen that showed remarkable potency against all HCV genotypes. IFN-free regimens should be selected primarily based on genotype as we have pangenotypic regimens (Sofosbuvir + Velpatasvir ± RBV, Sofosbuvir + Daclatasvir ± RBV, Paritaprevir-ritonavir/Ombitasvir ± Dasabuvir ± RBV), regimens fit for all genotypes except genotype 3 (Sofosbuvir + Simeprevir ± RBV, Sofosbuvir + Ledipasvir ± RBV), and individualized regimens for genotypes 2-3-4 (Sofosbuvir + RBV).

(2) Baseline RAVs: The presence of baseline RAVs seems to be associated with variable degrees of treatment response. Zeuzem et al. [8], observed no significant difference in response in noncirrhotic genotype 1 patients treated with Sofosbuvir and ledipasvir between those with baseline RAVs and others without RAVs in different treatment status and durations (98% in RAVs group vs. 99% in no RAVs group in naïve patients treated for 8 weeks, 99% in RAVs group vs. 99% in no RAVs group in naïve patients treated for 12 weeks, 90% in RAVs group vs. 99% in no RAVs group in experienced patients treated for 12 weeks). However, a significant difference was observed in cirrhotic patients (88% in RAVs group vs. 100% in no RAVs group in naïve patients treated for 24 weeks, 87% in RAVs group vs. 100% in no RAVs group in experienced patients treated for 24 weeks) [4]. In C-EDGE study, Zeuzem et al. showed a great influence of baseline RAVs on treatment outcome in HCV GT1 patients treated with grazoprevir/elbasvir combined with very low SVR (22%) in GT1a patients with NS5A baseline RAVs > fivefolds potency loss [9]. No effect on SVR in genotype 1 HCV patients with or without cirrhosis with baseline RAVs treated with combination of ombitasvir, r-paritaprevir, and dasabuvir, with or without ribavirin, for 12 or 24 weeks in four phase three clinical trials [11]. When Sofosbuvir/Daclatasvir combination was used, the presence of NS5A baseline RAVs is associated with reduced rates of SVR in under-treated (too short duration, no ribavirin) patients with cirrhosis and genotype 3 infection

http://dx.doi.org/10.5772/67149

[12]. In addition, the presence of NS3 protease RAS Q80K was associated with a reduced rate of SVR in patients with HCV genotype 1a infection and cirrhosis, especially if they failed to respond to previous pegylated IFN–based treatment [13, 14].

4.3. Drugs-related factors

(1) Potency and genetic barrier: the ideal drug for HCV treatment is not only potent but also could keep this potency against all HCV strains until cure which is known as resistant barrier (**Table 3**).

(2) Drugs combinations: lessons learned from HIV and TB management of drug resistance, multiple drug resistance and extensive drug resistance, outlining the frame of HCV treatment. Using multiple potent drugs for ideal durations is the best way to achieve HCV cure.

(3) Posttreatment RAVs: emergence of posttreatment RAVs has a major impact on retreatment decision. NS3-4a RAVs appearing after treatment failure usually persists for short durations (12–18 months) posttreatment [10] while longer durations were observed in NS5A RAVs which sometimes persist for years [4, 15]. On the other hand, appearance of RAVs to Nucleoside/nucleotide analogues is extremely rare, and if happened, it is usually nonreplicative [16]. **Tables 4–6** show the different amino acid variants causing either resistance or cross-resistance in different DAAs classes.

Variant	Boceprevir	Telaprevir	Simeprevir	Paritaprevir
V36	R	R	-	S
T54	R	R	-	-
V55	R	-	-	S
V107	S	-	-	-
R155	R	R	R	S
A156	R	R	-	-
V158	S	-	-	-
D168	S	S	R	R
I/V 170	R	-	R	-
M175	S	-	-	-
I132	-	S	-	-
Q80	-	-	R	-
S122	-	-	R	-
Y56	-	-	-	R

Table 4. Resistance and cross-resistance in NS3-4A protease inhibitors.

Variant	Daclatasvir	Ledipasvir	Ombitasvir	Elbasvir	Velpatasvir
M/L/L28	R	-	-	-	-
P29	S	-	-	-	-
Q/R/L30	R	-	-	-	-
L31	R	R	-	R	-
P32	S	-	-	-	-
H/P58	R	-	-	-	-
E62	S	-	-	-	-
A92	S	-	-	-	-
Y93	R	R	R	R	R
M28	-	S	R	R	-
Q30	-	R	R	R	-
H58	-	S	S	-	-
M/L28	-	-	R	-	

Table 5. Resistance and cross-resistance in NS5A inhibitors.

Variant	Sofosbuvir	Dasabuvir
S282T	R	R
A421V	-	R
P495S/Q/L/A/T	-	R
C316Y/N	-	R
L419S	-	R
S368T	-	R
R422K	-	R
M414T/I/V/L	-	R
M423T/I/V/L	-	R
Y448C/H	-	R
I482L/V/T	-	R
G554D/S	-	R
A486/V/I/T/M	-	R
S556G	-	R
V494A	-	R
D559G	-	R

Table 6. Resistance in NS5B inhibitors.

http://dx.doi.org/10.5772/67149

5. Diagnosis of HCV RAVs

5.1. Diagnosis of resistance in clinical practice is conducted by two methods

(1) Phenotypic analysis: used to determine the optimum plasma concentration (effective concentration, EC_{50} EC_{90}) of the dug sufficient to inhibit the viral replication.

RAVs are typically associated with a change in the shape of the binding or interaction site of DAAs to HCV target proteins. RAVs harbor different levels of resistance due to different locations within the sites of interaction and different chemical structures of DAAs targeting the same site on the same HCV protein [3].

(2) Genotypic analysis (sequence analysis): used to detect the amino acids substitutes which cause drug resistance and treatment failure [17]. Clonal and deep sequencing technologies allow reliable detection of viral variants with a frequency down to 0.5–1% and commonly accepted level reached to 15% [18]. Generally, due to the high heterogeneity of HCV isolates and methodological restrictions all sequencing technologies may miss detection of RAVs due to nonamplification based on HCV RNA secondary structures, primer selection, and low frequencies within HCV quasispecies [3].

Resistance testing in clinical practice is not so easy, but it is actually very difficult. Limited number of well-equipped virological labs all over the world that can deal with these tests, experienced hands and the ability to interpret the results correctly, make testing for resistance a time and money consuming procedure and balancing the benefit versus the cost should be considered especially when dealing with large populations having different genotypes.

5.2. Timing of HCV resistance testing

Because of the above-mentioned limitations, resistance testing is not recommended before starting therapy with DAAs for the first time; especially in areas where HCV is highly endemic. Instead, trying to give patients the best chance of cure through using multiple drugs, adding ribavirin or prolongation of the treatment duration if needed may be a good decision; also testing at the time of treatment failure usually associated with high prevalence of quasispecies and RAVs.

On the other hand, testing of resistance before retreatment of patients who fail to achieve virological response with DAAs may have a benefit for the proper selection of the best DAA drug for retreatment [4].

6. Management of drug failure and drug resistance

Clear evidence is still not available about the best regimens, best duration, and best time for retreatment of patients with DAAs failures, yet European association for the study of the liver (EASL) [19] and American association for the study of the liver diseases (AASLD) [20] released their interim opinions for retreatment options.

EASL guidelines recommend that Sofosbuvir should be a cornerstone in any retreatment trial due to its high barrier to resistance, addition of 1 or 2 other DAAs preferably with no cross-resistance with the failed drug, addition of ribavirin if tolerable and prolongation of treatment duration to 24 weeks especially in cirrhotics.

AASLD guidelines using Sofosbuvir-based triple or quadruple DAAs with ribavirin if tolerable for 12–24 weeks in case of failure of Sofosbuvir-based dual regimen, RAVs testing prior to retreatment and the final treatment options is tailored based on its results.

Review of some recent published data in **Table 7** for retreatment of clinical trials appears to be insufficient to justify a competent guidelines, more data is needed to reach to the nearest figure to ideal. From these trials, we could choose one of the following models:

(1) The patients have no RAVs, so retreatment using the same failed regimen (or adding other drugs) could be allowed but add ribavirin if needed but not previously added and choose the ideal duration according to the patient status.

(2) The patient has RAVs to protease or polymerase inhibitors, which will disappear after few weeks or months, so we could choose either to wait until reset point or to use another family of DAAs like NS5A inhibitors plus sofosbuvir.

(3) The patient has RAVs to NS5A inhibitor drug without cross-resistance, so the failed drug could not be used but other drugs from the same family could be.

(4) The patient has RAVs to NS5A inhibitor at certain sites leading to resistance and cross-resistance, so the whole NS5A members from the same wave could not be used, shifting to different wave of the family or changing the whole group to protease inhibitors will be the best way.

	Description	**Retreatment regimen**	**Results**	**RAVs impact**
Wyles et al. [21]	51 GT1 patients with previous treatment failure 25 patients failed PegIFN/RBV/Sofosbuvir 20 patients failed Sofosbuvir/RBV 5 failed Sofosbuvir placebo/PegIFN/RBV 1 failed GS-0938 monotherapy	Sofosbuvir + Ledipasvir + Ribavirin for 12 weeks	50/51 (98%) SVR	NA
Forns et al. [22]	79 GT1 patients with previous treatment failure 66 patients failed PegIFN/RBV/protease inhibitor 12 patients intolerable to treatment with PegIFN/RBV/protease inhibitor	Grazoprevir + Elbasvir + Ribavirin for 12 weeks	76/79(96.2%) SVR	-100% in patients without baseline RAVs -91.2% with baseline NS3 RAVs -75% with baseline NS5A RAVs -66.7% in both NS3, NS5A RAVs

	Description	Retreatment regimen	Results	RAVs impact
Hézode et al. [23]	Real world data 16 GT1, 4 patients with previous treatment failure 13 patients failed PegIFN/ RBV/daclatsvir/asunaprevir 3 patients failed PegIFN/ RBV/daclatasvir	Sofosbuvir + Simeprevir for 12 weeks without ribavirin	14/16 (87.5%) SVR	Presence of Simeprevir RAVs (R155K and Q80K) had no effect on treatment outcome
Lawitz et al., C-SWIFT [24]	25 GT1 patients failed Grazoprevir + Elbasvir + Sofosbuvir for 4, 6, or 8 weeks	Grazoprevir + Elbasvir + Sofosbuvir + RBV for 12 weeks	100% SVR	No impact
Poordad et al. QUARTZ 1 [25]	22 GT1 patients with previous treatment failure to DAAs 14 patients to OBV/PTV/r + DSV 2 patients to OBV/PTV/r 2 patients to telaprevir 2 patients to SOF 1 patient to simeprevir/ samatasvir 1 patient to simeprevir + SOF	-OBV/PTV/r + DSV + SOF for 12 weeks in patients without cirrhosis -OBV/PTV/r + DSV + SOF + RBV for 12 weeks in GT1a patients without cirrhosis -OBV/PTV/r + DSV + SOF + RBV for 24 weeks in GT1a patients with cirrhosis	14/15 (93%) SVR 12 IN patients treated for 12 weeks, 7/7 (100 %) SVR 4 in patients received 24 weeks	No impact

Table 7. Review of recent data for retreatment.

7. Conclusion

HCV elimination is a worldwide goal; curing infection with oral drugs for short duration and minimal adverse events is going on. Appearance of resistance to DAAs is disappointing to the clinicians and the researchers yet choosing the proper treatment regimen initially leading to minimizing this problem. The ideal RAVs testing and interpretation lead to the best options to justify the retreatment regimen.

Author details

Mohamed Hassany[1] and Aisha Elsharkawy[2]*

*Address all correspondence to: a_m_sharkawy@yahoo.com

1 National Hepatology & Tropical Medicine Research Institute (NHTMRI), Cairo, Egypt

2 Endemic Medicine and hepatogastroentrology, Faculty of Medicine, Cairo University, Cairo, Egypt

References

[1] Gower E, Estes C, Blach S, Razavi-Shearer K, Razavi H. Global epidemiology and genotype distribution of the hepatitis C virus infection. J Hepatol. 2014;61:S45–S57

[2] Bartenschlager R, Lohmann V, Penin F. The molecular and structural basis of advanced antiviral therapy for hepatitis C virus infection. Nat Rev Microbiol. 2013;11:482–496.

[3] Sarrazin C. The importance of resistance to direct antiviral drugs in HCV infection in clinical practice. J Hepatol. 2016 Feb;64(2):486–504.

[4] Pawlotsky J-M. Hepatitis C virus resistance to direct-acting antiviral drugs in interferon-free regimens. Gastroenterology. 2016 Jul;151(1):70–86.

[5] Farci P, Purcell RH. Clinical significance of hepatitis C virus genotypes and quasispecies. Semin Liver Dis. 2000 Jan;20(1):103–126.

[6] Asselah T, Marcellin P. Interferon free therapy with direct acting antivirals for HCV. Liver Int. 2013 Mar;33(Suppl 1):93–104.

[7] Majumdar A, Kitson MT, Roberts SK. Systematic review: current concepts and challenges for the direct-acting antiviral era in hepatitis C cirrhosis. Aliment Pharmacol Ther. 2016 Jun;43(12):1276–1292.

[8] Zeuzem S, Mizokami M, Pianko S, Mangia A, Han K, Martin R.et al. Prevalence of pretreatment NS5A resistance associated variants in genotype 1 patients across different regions using deep sequencing and effect on treatment outcome with LDV/SOF. AASLD. 2015. p. Abstract 91.

[9] Zeuzem S, Ghalib R, Reddy KR, Pockros PJ, Ben Ari Z, Zhao Y, et al. Grazoprevir-elbasvir combination therapy for treatment-naive cirrhotic and noncirrhotic patients with chronic hcv genotype 1, 4, or 6 infection: a randomized trial. Ann Intern Med. 2015 Apr 24;163(1):1–13.

[10] Lenz O, Verbinnen T, Fevery B, Tambuyzer L, Vijgen L, Peeters M, et al. Virology analyses of HCV isolates from genotype 1-infected patients treated with simeprevir plus peginterferon/ribavirin in Phase IIb/III studies. J Hepatol. 2015 May;62(5):1008–1014.

[11] Krishnan P, Tripathi R, Schnell G, et al. Resistance analysis of baseline and treatment-emergent variants in hepatitis C virus genotype 1 in the AVIATOR study with paritaprevir-ritonavir, ombitasvir, and dasabuvir. Antimicrob Agents Chemother. 2015;59:5445–5454.

[12] Nelson DR, Cooper JN, Lalezari JP, et al. All-oral 12- week treatment with daclatasvir plus sofosbuvir in patients with hepatitis C virus genotype 3 infection: ALLY-3 phase III study. Hepatology. 2015;61:1127–1135

[13] Kwo P, Gitlin N, Nahass N, et al. Simeprevir plus sofosbuvir (12 and 8 weeks) in HCV genotype 1-infected patients without cirrhosis: OPTIMIST-1, a Phase 3, randomized study. Hepatology. 2016 Aug;64(2):370–380.

[14] Lawitz E, Matusow G, DeJesus E, et al. Simeprevir plus sofosbuvir in patients with chronic hepatitis C virus genotype 1 infection and cirrhosis: a phase 3 study (OPTIMIST-2). Hepatology. 2016 Aug;64(2):360–369.

[15] McPhee F, Hernandez D, Yu F, Ueland J, Monikowski A, Carifa A, et al. Resistance analysis of hepatitis C virus genotype 1 prior treatment null responders receiving daclatasvir and asunaprevir. Hepatology. 2013 Sep;58(3):902–911.

[16] Svarovskaia ES, Dvory-Sobol H, Parkin N, Hebner C, Gontcharova V, Martin R, et al. Infrequent development of resistance in genotype 1-6 hepatitis C virus-infected subjects treated with sofosbuvir in phase 2 and 3 clinical trials. Clin Infect Dis. 2014 Dec 15;59(12):1666–1674.

[17] Fourati S, Pawlotsky J-M. Virologic tools for HCV drug resistance testing. Viruses. 2015 Dec;7(12):6346–6359.

[18] Dietz J, Schelhorn SE, Fitting D, Mihm U, Susser S, Welker MW, et al. Deep sequencing reveals mutagenic effects of ribavirin during monotherapy of hepatitis C virus genotype 1-infected patients. J Virol. 2013;87:6172–6181

[19] EASL Recommendations on Treatment of Hepatitis C 2015. J Hepatol. 2015 Apr 21;63(1):199–236.

[20] Hepatitis C guidance: AASLD-IDSA recommendations for testing, managing, and treating adults infected with hepatitis C Virus. Hepatology. 2015 Jun 25.

[21] Wyles D, Pockros P, Morelli G, Younes Z, Svarovskaia E, Yang JC, et al. Ledipasvir-sofosbuvir plus ribavirin for patients with genotype 1 hepatitis C virus previously treated in clinical trials of sofosbuvir regimens. Hepatology. 2015 Jun;61(6):1793–1797.

[22] Forns X, Gordon SC, Zuckerman E, Lawitz E, Calleja JL, Hofer H, et al. Grazoprevir and elbasvir plus ribavirin for chronic HCV genotype-1 infection after failure of combination therapy containing a direct-acting antiviral agent. J Hepatol. 2015 Sep;63(3):564–572.

[23] Hézode C, Chevaliez S, Scoazec G, Soulier A, Varaut A, Bouvier-Alias M, et al. Retreatment with sofosbuvir and simeprevir of patients with HCV GT1 or 4 who previously failed a daclatasvir-containing regimen. Hepatology. 2016 Jun;63(6):1809–1816.

[24] Lawitz EJ, Poordad F, Gutierrez J, Wells J, Landaverde C, Reiling J, et al. C-SWIFT retreatment final results: highly successful retreatment of GT1-infected patients with 12 weeks of elbasvir/grazoprevir plus sofosbuvir and ribavirin after failure of short-duration all-oral therapy. EASL 2016. Abstract SAT 148.

[25] Poordad F, Bennett M, Sepe TE, Cohen E, Reindollar RW, Everson G, et al. ombitasvir/paritaprevir/r, dasabuvir, and sofosbuvir treatment of patients with hcv genotype 1-infection who failed a prior course of daa therapy: the QUARTZ-I study. EASL 2016. Abstract SAT 156.

Chapter 7

Treatment of Chronic Hepatitis B: An Update and Prospect for Cure

Andrew Dargan and Hie-Won Hann

Additional information is available at the end of the chapter

http://dx.doi.org/10.5772/66724

Abstract

Since the discovery of the hepatitis B virus (HBV) by Blumberg et al., nearly half a century ago, the subsequent development of a vaccine, understanding of the pathogenesis, and the advent of antiviral drugs, the prevalence of chronic hepatitis B has decreased from approximately 5% to 3.61% of the worldwide population. Despite this improvement, approximately 248 million individuals are still infected with the virus. Effective treatment of chronic hepatitis B is extremely important as a positive correlation has been observed between baseline viral load and the risk for the development of hepatocellular carcinoma (HCC). While there have been significant advancements in the management of hepatitis B virus with available nucleos(t)ide analogues, there remains much work to be done to prevent HCC. The molecular mechanism and the subsequent carcinogenesis and progression of chronic HBV carriers to HCC remain in large part poorly understood. While current treatment with nucleos(t)ide analogues has succeeded in maintaining undetectable viral levels in patients with chronic hepatitis B, eradication of the virus has not been possible, and there remains the risk of development of HCC. Therefore, more effective treatment regimens aiming for HBV cure are urgently needed. With multiple new therapies in the pipeline, the future of treating hepatitis B is an exciting and developing one, and hopefully, it will soon become a disease of the past.

Keywords: hepatitis B, hepatocellular carcinoma, anti-HBV drugs, nucleos(t)ide analogues, HBV cure, HBV therapy

1. Introduction

In the past 50 years, since the discovery of the hepatitis B virus [1], the development of a vaccine, understanding of the pathogenesis, and the advent of antiviral drugs, the prevalence of chronic hepatitis B has decreased from approximately 5% to 3.61% of the worldwide population [2]. Nevertheless, hepatitis B remains a common and frequently encountered condition, affecting approximately 248 million individuals in the world.

The vast majority of individuals with chronic hepatitis B are located in Africa and Eastern Asia. In the United States, over 2 million Americans are afflicted and the majority (1.5 million) are immigrants from foreign countries [3, 4]. Effective treatment of chronic hepatitis B remains of extremely high importance, as patients who have been found to have higher baseline viral loads have been shown to have increased rates of hepatocellular carcinoma (HCC) [5]. As the treatment landscape of hepatitis B has shifted from earlier regimens of interferon and lamivudine to newer agents, namely tenofovir and entecavir, there remains much work to be done to reduce viral loads in patients and prevent long-term sequelae of cirrhosis and HCC. This chapter will discuss the natural history and potential carcinogenesis of hepatitis B virus, and will discuss current and possible future treatments, and the hope for an eventual cure.

2. Natural history of hepatitis B virus

In contrast to many known pathogens, hepatitis B virus (HBV) is not directly cytopathic to hepatocytes. Although not completely understood, the injury to the liver cells is in part through a host immune mechanism. Replicating HBV in hepatocytes produces HBsAg particles and virions which are taken up by the antigen presenting cells. The viral proteins are degraded to peptides, which are presented on the cell surface bound to MHC class I or II molecules. MHC class I molecules are recognized by CD8 T cells and MHC II by CD4 T cells. Virus-specific CD8+ cytotoxic T cells, with help from CD4+ T cells, recognize viral antigens presented on MHC class I chains on infected hepatocytes. This recognition reaction can lead to either direct lysis of the infected hepatocyte or the release of interferon-γ and TNF-$\boldsymbol{a}$, which can down-regulate viral replication in surrounding hepatocytes without direct cell killing [6].

In order to further discuss advancements in the understanding and treatment of HBV, it is important first to review the natural history of the disease. The cycle of chronic HBV infection primarily consists of five phases as shown in **Figure 1** [7, 8].

In the initial infection phase, or so-called immune tolerant phase, patients have very minimal inflammation. The hallmark of this phase is that these patients are found to be positive for HBeAg with high viral loads, typically >20,000 IU/mL (> 10^5 copies/mL) [9]. Conversely, they have normal aminotransferase (ALT) levels, and near-normal liver parenchyma on biopsy [10]. This "immune tolerant" phase is relatively short when HBV is acquired in adulthood, but can be sustained for much longer periods of time with infections acquired at birth or in early childhood [11, 12]. The risk of progressing to the chronic carrier state is significantly higher in infections acquired at a younger age, including up to a 90% risk when infected perinatally, as compared to a less than 1% risk of progression when acquired as an adult [13, 14].

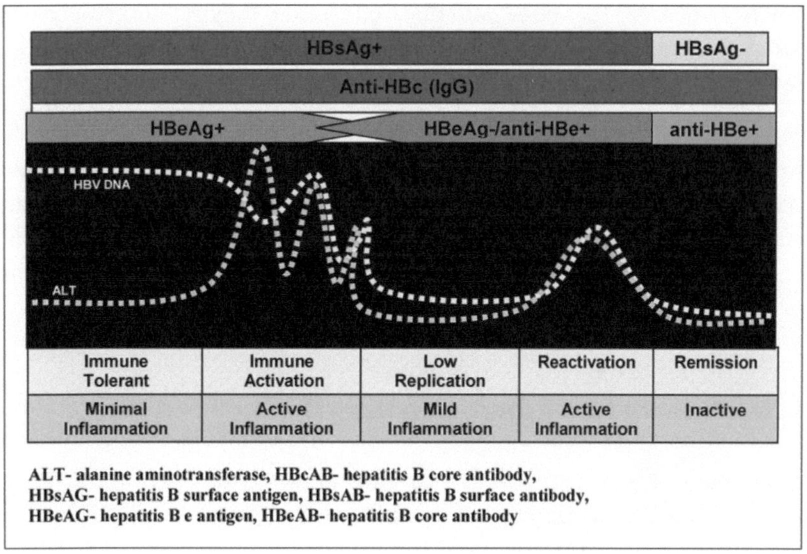

Figure 1. Five phases of chronic hepatitis B *. * *Adapted from Tong et al. (7) and modified by Halegoua-DeMarzio and Hann (8).*

Following the "immune tolerant" phase, patients progress into the "immune clearance" phase, which again consists of high viral loads and a persistently positive HBeAg. However, at this point patients begin experiencing increased inflammation, with elevated ALT levels, and potential hepatic decompensation [15, 16]. It is at this point when the viral DNA levels of HBV begin to decline, as does the presence of HBeAg. This is in large part due to the activated T-cell immune response, and subsequent destruction of infected hepatocytes [6]. An outcome of the immune clearance phase is HBeAg seroconversion, which has been found to be critical in predicting progression to cirrhosis and HCC.

Following HBeAg seroconversion, patients typically enter an "inactive carrier" phase, where HBeAg becomes undetectable, and HBe antibodies (anti-HBe) appear [17]. Typically the patient's viral load is low or undetectable and ALT returns to normal. Biopsy at this time will show minimal fibrosis and mild hepatitis. If the patient had experienced severe liver injury during the "immune clearance" phase, cirrhosis can also be present [17].

During the "reactivation phase", patients who were previously infected with HBV again have a detectable viral load, elevated ALT, and inflammation seen on biopsy [18]. In contrast to the "immune tolerant" phase, however, these patients do not have HBeAg positivity, but do have positive anti-HBe. As a result, this phase is known as the "HBeAg negative chronic hepatitis B" phase. As with the "immune clearance" phase, these patients can exhibit marked inflammation and hepatocyte destruction, and can experience hepatic decompensation during this phase.

The final phase of HBV infection is known as the "remission" or "inactive" phase, in which HBsAg may become negative, but anti-HBe and anti-HBc remain positive. Transaminases are normal at this time, and HBV viral loads are very low or undetectable.

It is important to remember that once patients are infected, they remain positive for anti-HBc IgG throughout even after they lose HBsAg and after they acquire anti-HBs. Also, anti-HBe may often remain detectable.

Furthermore, as part of the infection of HBV into human hepatocytes, HBV DNA converts itself into a covalently closed circular DNA, known as cccDNA, inside the hepatocyte nucleus [19]. This cccDNA serves as a template for transcription of HBV viral mRNAs, which translate and produce HBV proteins as well as provide a template for HBV DNA synthesis [20]. Thus, although a patient's viral load may be undetectable and HBsAg may become negative, the patient is not cured of HBV, as cccDNA will remain within hepatocytes.

3. Current treatments for chronic hepatitis B

Anti-HBV treatment drugs have made significant progress in improving the health and lifespan of patients with HBV. Beginning with interferon in 1991, therapies have become more targeted with lower resistance profiles and more tolerable side effects. The ultimate goal of hepatitis B treatment is to achieve remission, i.e., sustained suppression of viral replication. This, in turn, will lead to prevention of progression to cirrhosis and/or HCC. Several studies have demonstrated the reduction of HCC development with antiviral drugs [21–26].

Currently there are six approved treatments for HBV. The details of drugs and efficacy are shown in **Table 1**.

Pegylated interferon alpha-2a. The first treatment approved for HBV in 1991, pegylated interferon alpha-2a, or peg-IFN α-2a, is an immunomodulator, which also displays a weak effect against the virus itself [27]. It is administered as an injection, which patients receive weekly for a total treatment of 48 weeks. It has been shown to produce HBeAg seroconversion in 27% of patients, and 25% of patients develop an undetectable HBV DNA load [28]. It has been shown to have the best response for those individuals with genotype A with either ALT > 2x ULN or low HBV DNA, and for genotypes B and C with ALT > 2x ULN and low HBV DNA [29]. Although an effective treatment in the past, peg-IFN α-2a is a small percentage of current HBV treatments in the US [30]. Much of this is likely due to the requirement of an injection weekly, a large percentage of patients who fail to respond, and a significant side effect profile.

Lamivudine. The first nucleoside analogue approved for treatment of HBV, lamivudine (LMV) is a reverse transcriptase inhibitor. Functioning as a nucleoside analogue, it inhibits DNA synthesis of HBV. The treatment is extended across 1 year, and has been associated with a seroconversion rate of 16–18% at 1 year, and increases up to nearly 50% at 4 years [31, 32]. It is the least expensive of the nucleotide/nucleoside analogues, and is safe to use in pregnancy, which is one of its most common uses in current times. LMV has also been shown to reduce the rate of development of both fibrosis and HCC [33]. The most significant evidence of the effectiveness of LMV was shown in a randomized, controlled trial by Liaw et al., comparing LMV versus placebo in patients with chronic hepatitis B and high serum levels of HBV DNA

Name	Trade Name	Strong Points	Weak Points	Approved
Interferon alpha-2b and Pegylated Interferon 2a	Intron A Pegasys	-Finite duration of treatment -Durable response post-treatment -No known resistance	-Needle injection -High cost -65-70% fail to respond -Significant side effects	1991 2005
Lamivudine (LAM)	Epivir	-Oral -Safe with negligible side effects -Least expensive -Effective and safe in pregnancy	-Long term treatment is necessary -High incidence of resistance	1998
Adefovir Dipivoxil (ADV)	Hepsera	-Oral -Low resistance	-Long term treatment is necessary -Long term renal toxicity -Less potent than other treatments	2002
Entecavir (ETV)	Baraclude	-Oral -Potent viral suppression -Safe with negligible side effects -Low resistance	-Long term treatment is necessary -High cost	2005
Telbivudine (TLV)	Tyzeka	-Oral -Potent viral suppression -Effective and safe in pregnancy	-Long term treatment is necessary -High incidence of resistance	2006
Tenofovir (TDF)	Viread	-Oral -Most potent viral suppression -Safe with negligible side effects -No known resistance	-Associated with osteopenia -Long term treatment is necessary	2008

** Adapted from Halegoua-De Marzio and Hann (8).*

Table 1. Treatment options of chronic hepatitis B*.

[33]. The primary endpoint was progression of liver disease identified as either an increase in Child-Pugh score, bleeding from esophageal varices, or development of HCC. The study was discontinued early given that it demonstrated such a clear benefit of LMV compared to placebo [33]. Despite the success that has been shown with LMV, its use is limited, mainly due to the high incidence of resistance, especially compared with newer nucleotide/nucleoside analogues [34]. In one study, however, much lower resistance was observed if the baseline HBV DNA was < 10^6 copies/mL [35], and there has been an extensive review as to the discrepancies

of LMV resistance among the multiple studies regarding the incidence of LMV resistance [36]. LMV also reduced vertical HBV transmission from highly viremic mothers to their newborns [37]. Currently, the use of oral antiviral agents during the first and second trimesters of pregnancy is not recommended.

Adefovir dipivoxil. The first nucleotide analogue, adefovir dipivoxil (ADV), was approved by the FDA for use in 2002. Similar to LMV in its mechanism of action, ADV functions as a reverse transcriptase inhibitor. As compared with LMV, however, ADV had both an increased antiviral potency, and an intrinsic stereoscopic structure that prevents emergence of viral resistance. HBe seroconversion was achieved in 12% of patients after 1 year of therapy with ADV, and a 53% rate of histological improvements in patients who were positive for HBeAg [38]. Of the patients who did seroconvert, it was found to be sustained in 91% of these patients [39]. Like LMV, however, prolonged use is associated with an increase in resistance, progressing from 3% at 2 years to 29% at 5 years [40]. Due to this, in addition to associated renal toxicity, the use of ADV has become increasingly rare with the development of newer, more effective therapies.

Entecavir. The second nucleoside analogue approved for treatment of chronic HBV, entecavir (ETV), was approved by the FDA for treatment in 2005. It has been shown to be superior at reducing HBV DNA levels, as compared with LMV [41]. In a phase 3 study comparing ETV to LMV after 1 year of treatment, patients were found to have improved virological response with HBV DNA < 400 copies/mL (67% vs 36%), improvement on histologic examination (72% vs 62%), and improvement in aminotransferases, namely ALT (78% returned to normal as compared to 70%) [41]. In longer term studies, up to 96% of patients had improvement in histologic examination, and improvement in fibrosis score after 6 years [42]. Improvements were even found in patients with cirrhosis. Entecavir also was shown to keep HBeAg-positive patients with HBV DNA levels below 300 copies/mL in 94% of patients at 5 years [43]. It has been shown to cause viral suppression quicker than ADV, and has been shown to significantly decrease the incidence of HCC in chronic HBV patients, with a 3.7% incidence in the ETV group as compared with 13.7% in the untreated group [23]. One of the most important features of entecavir, and a reason why it remains one of the two recommended treatments for chronic HBV today, is that it has a high genetic barrier and a very low incidence of resistance. The cumulative incidence of resistance after 6 years has been found to be 1.2% in nucleoside-naïve patients [44].

Telbivudine. Another nucleoside analogue similar in structure to LMV, telbivudine (TLV) was approved by the FDA for treatment of chronic HBV in 2006. In HBeAg-positive patients, the seroconversion with TLV was found to be 22% at 1 year and 30% at 2 years [45, 46]. Viral suppression to less than 300 copies of DNA/mL was found to be 60% after 1 year of TLV therapy, and 56% after two years of therapy [45, 46]. Unfortunately, although TLV was shown to have promising effects and to have a higher barrier to resistance than LMV, resistance has been found to be as high as 21.6% in HBeAg-positive patients, and 8.6% in HBeAg-negative patients [47]. Because of this, TLV currently is not a recommended first-line treatment. However, TLV is shown to be highly effective for those with low baseline HBV DNA and achieves undetectable HBV DNA at week 24. Therefore, TLV is highly effective for patients with the above characteristics [48]. Furthermore, recent studies report the renoprotective effect of TLV, its role in preventing ADV-induced nephrotoxicity, and increased GFR improvement of renal function in liver transplant patients and in patients with compensated or decompensated HBV-related liver diseases [49–52]. The rate of vertical transmission was reduced when telbivudine was given to mothers with high viral loads during the third trimester of pregnancy [53]. Currently, the use of oral antiviral agents during the first and second trimesters of pregnancy is not recommended.

Tenofovir. The most recent nucleotide analogue, tenofovir disoproxil fumarate (TDF), was approved by the FDA for treatment of patients with chronic hepatitis B in 2008. Structurally similar but a more potent drug than ADV, TDF has been shown to produce more viral suppression in HBeAg-positive patients, with 76% of patients achieving viral loads < 400 copies/mL as compared with 13% of patients treated with ADV after 48 weeks of treatment [54]. ALT normalization, histologic improvement, and HBsAg loss were all also found to be significantly increased in patients treated with TDF as compared with ADV [54]. Data have shown an excellent continued response, with a 7-year viral suppression (HBV DNA levels < both 69 IU/mL and 29 IU/mL) of greater than 99% in both HBeAg-negative and HBeAg-positive patients [55]. In addition to its effectiveness, TDF has also been shown to have an extremely favorable resistance profile [56]. Due to the effectiveness and the virtual absence of resistance, TDF has been recommended as a first-line treatment in patients with chronic hepatitis B.

Several currently used guidelines are shown in **Table 2**.

Since the majority of chronic hepatitis B patients in the United States are immigrants form endemic countries, especially from Asia, where infection takes place commonly at birth or in early childhood, Asian-American algorithm is frequently used for treatment for this majority of HBV patients. These guidelines are as follows [7]:

1. For HBeAg (+) or (-) patient with chronic HBV with DNA > 10^4 copies/mL (> 2000 IU/mL) and ALT > ULN, treatment should be started with a first-line agent (ETV or TDF).

2. For cirrhotic patients with detectable HBV DNA, treatment should be started with ETV or TDF.

3. In HBeAg (-) patients with HBV DNA > 10^4 copies/mL (> 2000 IU/mL) and normal ALT, a liver biopsy is recommended. If not available, further stratification for risk factors (albumin ≤ 3.5 g/dL or platelets ≤ 130,000/μL, HCC first degree relative, age ≥ 40, male gender, ALT > 30 U/L for male and 19 U/L for female) should be conducted prior to treatment.

4. ***Monitoring treatment:*** Test for serum ALT every 3 months. Measure HBV DNA every 3 months until negative, then every 3–6 months. Measure HBeAg every 6 months until negative, then test for anti-HBe.

5. After seroconversion from HBeAg-positive to anti-HBe, test for HBsAg every 12 months. In HBeAg (-) patients, test for HBsAg every 12 months after sustained suppression of HBV DNA.

	Chronic Hepatitis			
	HBeAg (+)		HBeAg (-)	
Guidelines (last updated)	HBV DNA (IU/ml)	ALT (U/L)	HBV DNA (IU/ml)	ALT (U/L)
EASL (2012)	> 2,000	> ULN	> 2,000	> ULN
US Algorithm (2015)	> 20,000	> ULN* or (+) biopsy	> 2,000	> ULN
APASL (4) (2016)	> 20,000	> ULN	> 2,000	> 2x ULN
AASLD (5) (2016)	> 20,000	> 2x ULN* or (+) biopsy	> 2,000	> 2x ULN
Asian American Algorithm (2011)	> 2,000	> ULN	> 2,000	> ULN

**EASL (European Association for the Study for the Liver) (72),*
US Algorithm (73)
APASL (Asian Pacific Association of the Study of the Liver (74)
AASLD (American Association of the Study of Liver Diseases) (75)
Asian American Algorithm (7)
ULN = Upper limit of normal; NS = Not stated).
** UNL: 30 IU/mL for men, 19 IU/mL for women*
2000 IU/mL = 104copies/mL
20,000 IU/mL=105copies/mL

Table 2. Current treatments for hepatitis B in chronic hepatitis, as recommended by different guidelines (ref. 7, 69–72).

6. ***Monitoring of resistance:*** Viral breakthrough with confirmation of single drug resistance requires switching to another first-line oral antiviral agent.

7. Surveillance for HCC with Alpha-fetoprotein (AFP) and abdominal ultrasound should be performed every 6 months in HBsAg-positive patients with chronic hepatitis, cirrhosis, and for patients with a family history of HCC.

8. ***With regard to stopping treatment,*** for HBeAg (+) patients, following HBeAg seroconversion, continue consolidation for 1–2 years before stopping therapy. However, the relapse rate is high, and longer consolidation therapy may be needed. For HBeAg (-) patients, antiviral therapy should be indefinite therapy until HBsAg seroconversion.

Before the antiviral drugs became available, 25–40% of HBV-infected individuals used to progress from chronic hepatitis to cirrhosis and eventually to HCC as shown in **Table 3**

http://dx.doi.org/10.5772/66724

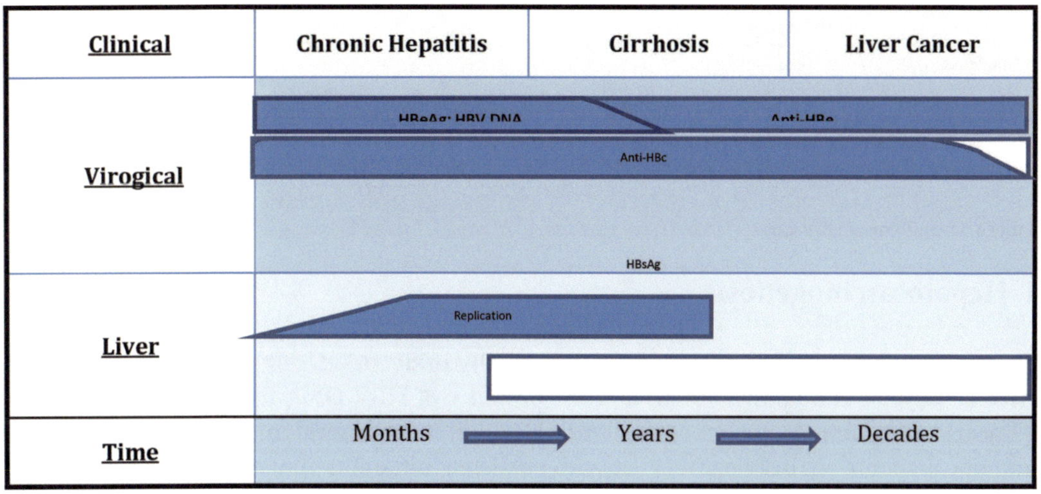

Table 3. Natural history of chronic hepatitis B infection.

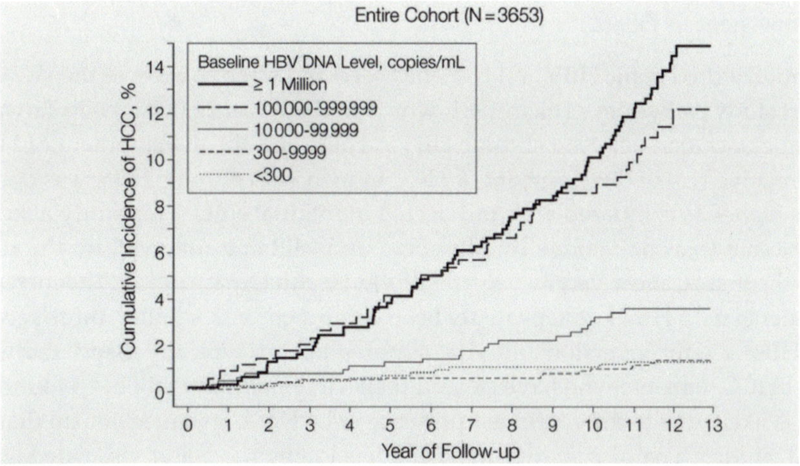

**From Chen, et. al. (5).*

Figure 2. Higher baseline viral loads are associated with increased rate of HCC. **From Chen, et al. (5).*

In their 13-year follow-up study of HBV-infected carriers, Chen et al. have noted that higher baseline viral loads were associated with an increased rate of HCC [5] (**Figure 2**).

During the last 10 years, several studies have demonstrated that antiviral treatment significantly reduced the incidence of HCC [21–26]. However, all these treatment modalities are to suppress HBV replication. They do not fully eradicate the virus. The inability to eradicate HBV still leaves infected individuals at the risk for HCC. Current anti-HBV treatment can achieve "functional cure" but not "complete cure", the terminology as coined by Zeisel et al. [19]. (**Table 4**).

	HBsAg	Anti-HBs	Viremia	cccDNA
Functional cure	-	+	-	+
Complete cure	-	+	-	-

**Ab, antibodies; cccDNA, covalently closed circular DNA*
Adapted and edited from Zeisel et al. (19)

Table 4. Definitions of HBV Cure.

4. Hepatocarcinogenesis

The pathogenesis for HBV-related HCC is not fully understood, but is likely multifactorial. HBV DNA level is a known factor, and the presence of HBV DNA has been shown to have a linear relationship to the development of HCC [5]. A high viral load leads to a persistent immune response against hepatocytes, with persistent inflammation, regeneration, and fibrosis. This up-regulated state of inflammation can in turn predispose to a malignant transformation [57]. Several studies have also suggested that the integration of HBV DNA into the host DNA can lead to chromosomal instability and eventual gene rearrangement. These rearrangements can, in effect, lead to deregulation and instability of gene expression, subsequently leading to oncogenesis [58–60].

The association with chronic HBV and HCC has been described as early as the 1970s. The landmark cohort study by Beasley et al. in 1981, which studied over 22,000 men in Taiwan, showed a significant association between chronic HBV carriers and the development of HCC. In this study, the relative risk of development of HCC in men with chronic HBV was determined to be 63 times higher as compared with uninfected individuals [61]. This study also designated the HBV vaccine (plasma vaccine by Blumberg and Millman followed by the recombinant vaccine) as the first "Cancer Vaccine" by the World Health Organization. The increased risk of HCC in patients with HBV has repeatedly been confirmed with smaller, more recent studies. Although HBsAg seroconversion and viral suppression are typically associated with protection against HCC, patients who have cleared their viral load have still been found to acquire HCC. This is likely due to the continued presence of cccDNA, in a mechanism that is not well understood. Studies have also shown that HCC development is better associated with patients who have had active HBV infection for longer time periods, including patients who were infected at younger ages. Thus, it is thought that HCC progression is likely a result of HBV replication itself and subsequent liver injuries that follow [62]. It also raises the point that in individuals infected earlier, carcinogenic processes may have already been in play prior to the halt of viral replication later in life, and the ability of HBV to integrate into the infected host's hepatocyte genome is one of the most important direct pro-oncogenic properties.

In addition to chronic HBV carrier status, other risk factors have been identified which predispose patients with hepatitis B to HCC. These factors include co-infection with hepatitis C (HCV), a family history of prior HCC, concurrent alcohol use, and a predominance of genotype C [63–66]. Additionally, the presence of core promoter mutations, the most common of which is the HBx protein, a potent activator of multiple genes, including oncogenes, has been discovered [67].

5. Future treatments

Most current guidelines recommend against HBV treatment of patients in the immune tolerant phase (**Table 2**). However, recent reports have indicated evidence that immune reactivity is in fact present in patients during this immune tolerant stage [68–70]. There is a growing opinion that to prevent HCC, we should consider earlier treatment of chronic hepatitis B as lucidly reasoned by Zoulim and Mason [71]. Given the emergence of HCC even in patients who had become seronegative, these guidelines should be readdressed in order to treat patients starting at a younger age, in order to prevent progression of disease and the development of HCC, as viral suppression alone has not proven effective for the absolute prevention of HCC. Additionally, the required long-term therapy imposes not only financial burden but may also put patients at risk for potential drug resistance and unknown toxicity.

Along with nucleoside/nucleotide analogues, treatment may need to include targeting the cccDNA and inhibiting viral entry into the newly formed hepatocytes. This may be accomplished via a T-cell vaccine which specifically targets HBV, enhancing innate immunity with toll-like receptor agonist. Several compounds have been identified which have the

	Targets	Compounds	Stage of development
DAAs	HBV capsid	Phenylproenamide derivatives Heteroaryldihydropyrimidines	Preclinical and early clinical phase Morphothiadine mesilate (GLS4) in phase II
	rcDNA-cccDNA conversion	Disubstituted sulfonamide	Preclinical
	cccDNA	DNA cleavage enzymes	Preclinical
	HBV RNA	siRNA antisense	ARC-520 in phase II ISIS-HBVRx in phase I
HTAs	NTCP	HBV preS1-derived lipopeptide Cyclosporine A, ezetimibe	Myrcludex-B in phase II FDA approved but not tested for HBV
	Host factors involved in HBV secretion and budding	Iminosugar derivatives of butyldeoxynojirimycin and related glycolipids α-glucosidase inhibitors triazol-o-pyrimidine derivatives benzimidazole derivative phosphorothioate oligonucleotides	Preclinical Preclinical Preclinical Preclinical REP 9 AC in phase II
	Innate immune responses	LTβR agonists TLR7 agonists Thymosin α1 Nitazoxanide Interleukin-7 IFN-λ	Preclinical Phase II Phase IV Phase I Phase I/II Phase II
	Adaptive immune responses	PD1 blockade X-S-Core proteins (antigen-based vaccine) HBV DNA (DNA-based vaccine)	Phase I/II for HCC GS-4774 in phase II DV-601 in phase I DNA vaccine pCMVS2.S in phase I/II

cccDNA, covalently closed circular DNA; DAA, direct-acting antiviral; FDA, US Food and Drug Administration; HCC, hepatocellular carcinoma; HTA, host-targeting agent; IFN, interferon; LTβR, lymphotoxin-β receptor; NTCP, sodium taurocholate co-transporting polypeptideAdapted and edited from Zeisel et al. (19)

Table 5. Emerging drugs against HBV.

potential for eradicating the virus. The clinical trials are in progress at different phases to further investigate these compounds [19]. Among these are direct-acting antagonists against the HBV capsid, against the HBV cccDNA, and against the HBV RNA. While the targets enhancing the innate immunity are mainly in the preclinical phase, they pose exciting possibilities for the future of HBV treatment. The potential drugs in the pipelines are shown below [19] (**Table 5**).

6. Conclusion

While there have been significant advancements in the understanding and management of hepatitis B virus, there remains much to be learned. The molecular mechanism and the subsequent carcinogenesis and progression of chronic HBV carriers to HCC remain in large part poorly understood. While significant improvements in treatment of HBV continue to be made, research toward HBV complete cure and the treatment landscape now is much different than it was at the end of the twentieth century. The development of nucleotide and nucleoside analogues, particularly entecavir and tenofovir, has significantly improved the ability of chronic HBV carriers to remain with undetectable viral levels. There remains, however, the possibility of development of HCC, in part likely in the early stages of infection, as well as the viral incorporation into hepatocyte DNA. Therefore, more effective treatment regimens need to be developed, and the prospect of treating individuals at earlier stages of HBV should be addressed. With multiple new therapies in the pipeline, the future of treating hepatitis B is an exciting and developing one, and hopefully, it will soon become a disease of the past.

Disclosures:

AD, no conflict, HWH, receives research grants from Bristol Myers-Squibb and Gilead Sciences.

Author details

Andrew Dargan[2] and Hie-Won Hann[1, 2*]

*Address all correspondence to: hie-won.hann@jefferson.edu

1 Liver Disease Prevention Center, Department of Medicine, Thomas Jefferson University Hospital, Philadelphia, PA, USA

2 Division of Gastroenterology and Hepatology, Department of Medicine, Thomas Jefferson University Hospital, Philadelphia, PA, USA

References

[1] Blumberg BS, Alter HJ, Visnich S. A "new" antigen in leukemia sera. JAMA. 1965; 191:541–546.

[2] Schweitzer A, Horn J, Mikolajczyk RT, Krause G, Ott JJ. Estimations of worldwide prevalence of chronic hepatitis B virus infection: a systematic review of data published between 1965 and 2013. Lancet. 2015; 386:1546–1555.

[3] Cohen C, Evans AA, London WT, Block J, Conti M, Block T. Underestimation of chronic hepatitis virus infection in the United States of America. J Viral Hepatitis. 2008; 15:12–13.

[4] Kim WR. Epidemiology of hepatitis B in the United States. Hepatology. 2009; 49:S28–S34.

[5] Chen C-J, Yang H-I, Su J, Jen C-L, You S-L, Lu S-N, Huang GT, Iloeje UH. Risk of hepatocellular carcinoma across a biological gradient of serum hepatitis B virus DNA level. JAMA. 2006; 295:65–73.

[6] Ganem D, Prince AM. Hepatitis B virus infection, natural history and clinical consequences. N Engl J Med. 2004; 350:1118–1129.

[7] Tong MJ, Pan CQ, Hann HW, Kowdley KV, Han SH, Min AD, Leduc TS. The management of chronic hepatitis B in Asian Americans. Dig Dis Sci. 2011; 56:3143–3162.

[8] Halegoua-DeMarzio D, Hann HW. Prevention of hepatocellular carcinoma and its recurrence with anti-hepatitis B viral therapy. Minerva Gastroenterol Dietol. 2014; 60:191–200.

[9] Croagh CMN, Lubel JS. Natural history of chronic hepatitis B: phases in a complex relationship. World J Gastroenterol. 2014; 20:10395–10404.

[10] Chu CM, Karayiannis P, Fowler MJ, Monjardino J, Liaw YF, Thomas HC. Natural history of chronic hepatitis B virus infection in Taiwan: studies of hepatitis B virus DNA in serum. Hepatology. 1985; 5:431–434.

[11] Fattovich G, Bortolotti F, Donato F. Natural history of chronic hepatitis B: special emphasis on disease progression and prognostic factors. J Hepatol. 2008; 48:335–352.

[12] Villa E, Fattovich G, Mauro A, Pasino M. Natural history of chronic HBV infection: special emphasis on the prognostic implications of the inactive carrier state versus chronic hepatitis. Dig Liver Dis [Internet]. 2011; 43(Suppl 1):S8–S14.

[13] Beasley RP, Hwang LY, Lin CC, Leu ML, Stevens CE, Szmuness W, Chen KP. Incidence of hepatitis B virus infections in preschool children in Taiwan. J Infect Dis. 1982; 146:198–204.

[14] Beasley RP, Trepo C, Stevens CE, Szmuness W. The e antigen and vertical transmission of hepatitis B surface antigen. Am J Epidemiol. 1977; 105:94–98.

[15] Liaw YF, Tai DI, Chu CM, Chen TJ. The development of cirrhosis in patients with chronic type B hepatitis: a prospective study. Hepatology. 1988; 8:493–496.

[16] McMahon BJ, Holck P, Bulkow L, Snowball M. Serologic and clinical outcomes of 1536 Alaska natives chronically infected with hepatitis B virus. Ann Intern Med. 2001; 135:759–768.

[17] Yim HJ, Lok AS-F. Natural history of chronic hepatitis B virus infection: what we knew in 1981 and what we know in 2005. Hepatology. 2006; 43(2 Suppl 1):S173–S181.

[18] Hadziyannis SJ, Vassilopoulos D. Hepatitis B e antigen-negative chronic hepatitis B. Hepatology. 2001; 34:617–624.

[19] Zeisel MB, Lucifora J, Mason WS, Sureau C, Beck J, Levrero M, Kann M, Knolle PA, Benkirane M, Durante D, Michel ML, Autran B, Cosset FL, Strick-Marchand H, Trepo C, Kao JH, Carrat F, Lacombe K, Schinazi RF, Barre-Sinoussei F, Delfraissy JF, Zoulim F. Towards an HBV cure: state-of-the-art and unresolved questions-report of the ANRS workshop on HBV cure. Gut. 2015; 64:1314–1326.

[20] Summers J, Mason WS. Replication of the genome of a hepatitis B-like virus by reverse transcription of an RNA intermediate. Cell. 1982; 29:403–415.

[21] Liaw YF, Sung JJ, Chow WC, Farrell G, Lee CZ, Yuen H, et al. Lamivudine for patients with chronic hepatitis B and advanced liver disease. N Engl J Med. 2004; 351:1521–1531.

[22] Eun JR, Lee HJ, Kim TN, Lee KS. Risk assessment for the development of hepatocellular carcinoma: according to on-treatment viral response during long-term lamivudine therapy in hepatitis B virus-related liver disease. J Hepatol. 2010; 53:118–125

[23] Hosaka T, Suzuki F, Kobayashi M, Seko Y, Kawamura Y, Sezaki H, Akuta N, Suzuki Y, Saitoh S, Arase Y, Ikeda K, Kobayashi M, Kumada H. Long-term entecavir treatment reduces hepatocellular carcinoma incidence in patients with hepatitis B virus infection. Hepatology. 2013; 58:98–107.

[24] Wong GL, Chan HL, Chan HY, Tse YK, Mark CW, Lee SK, Ip ZM, Lam AT, Iu JW, Leung JM, Wong VW. Accuracy of risk scores for patients with chronic hepatitis B receiving entecavir treatment. Gastroenterology. 2013; 144:933–944.

[25] Ahn J, Lim JK, Lee HM, Lok AS, Nguyen M, Pan CQ, Mannalithara A, Te H, Reddy KR, Trinh H, Chu D, Tran T, Lau D, Leduc T-S, Min A, Le LT, Bae H, Tran SV, Do S, Hann HW, Wong C, Han S, Pillai A, Park JS, Tong M, Scaglione S, Woog J, Kim WR. Lower observed hepatocellular carcinoma incidence in chronic hepatitis B patients treated with entecavir: results of the ENUMERATE study. Am J Gastroenterol. 2016; 111:1297–1304.

[26] Kim WR, Loomba R, Berg T, Schall REA, Yee LJ, Dinh PV, et al. Impact of long-term tenofovir disoproxil fumarate on incidence of hepatocellular carcinoma in patients with chronic hepatitis B. Cancer. 2015; 121:3631–3638

[27] Dianzani F. Biological basis for the clinical use of interferon. Gut. 1993; 34(2 Suppl):S74–S76.

[28] Lau GKK, Piratvisuth T, Luo KX, Marcellin P, Thongsawat S, Cooksley G, et al. Peginterferon Alfa-2a, lamivudine, and the combination for HBeAg-positive chronic hepatitis B. N Engl J Med. 2005; 352(26):2682–2695.

[29] Buster EHCJ, Hansen BE, Lau GKK, Piratvisuth T, Zeuzem S, Steyerberg EW, et al. Factors that predict response of patients with hepatitis B e antigen-positive chronic hepatitis B to peginterferon-alfa. Gastroenterology. 2009; 137:2002–2009.

[30] Zoulim F, Perrillo R. Hepatitis B: reflections on the current approach to antiviral therapy. J Hepatol. 2008; 48:S2–S19.

[31] Dienstag JL, Schiff ER, Wright TL, Perrillo RP, Hann HW, Goodman Z, et al. Lamivudine as initial treatment for chronic hepatitis B in the United States. N Engl J Med. 1999; 341:1256–1263.

[32] Chang TT, Lai CL, Chien RN, Guan R, Lim SG, Lee CM, et al. Four years of lamivudine treatment in Chinese patients with chronic hepatitis B. J Gastroenterol Hepatol. 2004; 19:1276–1282.

[33] Liaw Y-F, Sung JJY, Chow WC, Farrell G, Lee C-Z, Yuen H, Tanwandee T, Tao QM, Shue K, Keene ON, Dixon JS, Gray DE. Sabbat J. Lamivudine for patients with chronic hepatitis B and advanced liver disease. N Engl J Med. 2004; 351:1521–1531.

[34] Lok ASF, Lai CL, Leung N, Yao GB, Cui ZY, Schiff ER, Dienstag JL, Heathcote EJ, Little NR, Griffiths DA, Gardner SD, Castiglia M. Long-term safety of lamivudine treatment in patients with chronic hepatitis B. Gastroenterology. 2003; 125:1714–1722.

[35] Chae HB, Hann HW. Baseline HBV DNA level is the most important factor associated with virologic breakthrough in chronic hepatitis B treated with lamivudine. World J Gastroenterol. 2007; 13:4085–4090.

[36] Hann HW, Gregory VL. Dixon JS, Barker KF. A review of the one year incidence of resistance to lamivudine in the treatment of chronic hepatitis B. Hepatology Int. 2008; 2:440–456.

[37] Xu W-M, Cui Y-T, Wang L, Yang H, Liang ZQ, Li XM, Zhang SL, Qiao FY, Campbell F, Chang CN, Gardner S, Atkins M. Lamivudine in late pregnancy to prevent perinatal transmission of hepatitis B virus infection: a multicentre, randomized, double-blind, placebo-controlled study. J Viral Hepat. 2009; 16:94–103.

[38] Marcellin P, Chang T-T, Lim SG, Tong MJ, Sievert W, Shiffman ML, Jeffers L, Goodman Z, Wulfsohn MS, Xiong S, Fry J, Brosgart CL. Adefovir dipivoxil for the treatment of hepatitis B e antigen-positive chronic hepatitis B. N Engl J Med. 2003; 348:808–816.

[39] Hadziyannis SJ, Tassopoulos NC, Heathcote EJ, Chang T-T, Kitis G, Rizzetto M, Marcellin P, Lim SG, Goodman Z, Wulfsohn MS, Xiong S, Fry CL, Brosgart CL. Adefovir dipivoxil for the treatment of hepatitis B e antigen-negative chronic hepatitis B. N Engl J Med. 2003; 348:800–807.

[40] Hadziyannis SJ, Tassopoulos NC, Heathcote EJ, Chang TT, Kitis G, Rizzetto M, Marcellin P, Lim SG, Goodman Z, Ma J, Brosgart CL, Borroto-Esoda K, Arterburn S, Chuc S. Long-term therapy with adefovir dipivoxil for HBeAg-negative chronic hepatitis B for up to 5 years. Gastroenterology. 2006; 131:1743–1751.

[41] Chang TT, Gish RG, de Man R, Gadano A, Sollano J, Chao YC, Lok AS, Han KH, Goodman Z, Zhu ZJ, Cross A, DeHertogh D, Wilber R, Colonno R, Apelian D. A comparison of entecavir and lamivudine for HBeAg-positive chronic hepatitis B. N Engl J Med. 2006; 354:1001–1010.

[42] Chang TT, Liaw YF, Wu SS, Schiff E, Han KH, Lai CL, Safasi R, Lee SS, Halota W, Goodman Z, Chi YC, Zhang H, Hindes R, Iloeje S, Kreter B. Long-term entecavir therapy results in the reversal of fibrosis/cirrhosis and continued histological improvement in patients with chronic hepatitis B. Hepatology. 2010; 52:886–893.

[43] Chang T-T, Lai C-L, Kew Yoon S, Lee SS, Coelho HSM, Carrilho FJ, Poordad F, Halota W, Horsmans Y, Tsai N, Zhang H, Tenney DJ, Tamez R, Iloeje U. Entecavir treatment for up to 5 years in patients with hepatitis B e antigen-positive chronic hepatitis B. Hepatology. 2010; 51:422–430.

[44] Tenney DJ, Rose RE, Baldick CJ, Pokornowski KA, Eggers BJ, Fang J, Wichroski MJ, Xu D, Yang J, Wilber RB, Colonno RJ. Long-term monitoring shows hepatitis B virus resistance to entecavir in nucleoside-naive patients is rare through 5 years of therapy. Hepatology. 2009; 49:1503–1514.

[45] Liaw YF, Gane E, Leung N, Zeuzem S, Wang Y, Lai CL, Heathcote EJ, Manns M, Bzowej N, Niu J, Han SH, Hwang SG, Cakaloglu Y, Tong MJ, Papatheodoridis G, Chen Y, Brown NA, Albanis E, Galil K, Naoumov NY. 2-year GLOBE trial results: Telbivudine is superior to lamivudine in patients with chronic hepatitis B. Gastroenterology. 2009; 136:486–495.

[46] Lai CL, Gane E, Liaw YF, Hsu CW, Thongsawat S, Wang Y, Chen Y, Heathcote EJ, Rasenack J, Bzowej N, Naoumov NV, Di Bisceglie AM, Zeuzem S, Moon YM, Goodman Z, Chao G, Constance BF, Brown NA. Telbivudine versus lamivudine in patients with chronic hepatitis B. N Engl J Med. 2007; 357:2576–2588.

[47] Sonneveld MJ, Janssen HLA. Chronic hepatitis B: peginterferon or nucleos(t)ide analogues? Liver Int. 2011; 31(Suppl. 1):78–84.

[48] Hann HW. Telbivudine for the treatment of hepatitis B. Expert Opin Pharmacother. 2010; 11:2243–2249.

[49] Gane EJ, Deray G, Liaw Y-F, Lim SG, Lai CL, Rasenack J, Wang Y, Papatheodoridisl G, Di Bisceglie A, Bull M, Samuel D, Uddin A, Bosset S, Trylesinski A. Telbivudine improves renal function in patients with chronic hepatitis B. Gastroenterology. 2014; 146:138–135.

[50] Lee M, Oh S, Lee HJ, Yeum TS, Lee JH, Yu SJ, Kim HY, Yoon JH, Lee HS, Kim YJ. Telbivudine protects renal function in patients with chronic hepatitis B infection in conjunction with adefovir-based combination therapy. J Viral Hepatol. 2014; 21:873–881.

[51] Li W, Zhang D. Influence of monotherapy with telbivudine or entecavir on renal function in patients with chronic hepatitis B. Zhonghua Ganzangbing Zazhi Chin J Hepatol. 2015; 23:407–411.

[52] Perrella A, Lanza A, Pisaniello D, DiCostanzo G, Calise F, Cuomo O. Telbivudine prophylaxis for hepatitis B virus recurrence after liver transplantation improves renal function. Transplant Proc. 2014. 2319–2321.

[53] Han G-R, Cao M-K, Zhao W, Jiang H-X, Wang C-M, Bai S-F, et al. A prospective and open-label study for the efficacy and safety of telbivudine in pregnancy for the

http://dx.doi.org/10.5772/66724

prevention of perinatal transmission of hepatitis B virus infection. J Hepatol. 2011; 55:1215–1221.

[54] Marcellin P, Heathcote EJ, Buti M, Gane E, de Man R A, Krastev Z, Germanidis G, Lee SS, Flisiak R, Kaita K, Manns M, Kotzev I, Tchernev K, Buggisch P, Weilert F, Kurdas OO, Shiffman ML, Trinh H, Washington MK, Sorbek K, Anderson J, Snow-Lampart A, Mondou E, Quinn J, Rousseau F. Tenofovir disoproxil fumarate versus adefovir dipivoxil for chronic hepatitis B. N Engl J Med. 2008; 359:2442–2455.

[55] Buti M, Tsai N, Petersen J, Flisiak R, Gurel S, Krastev Z, Schall RA, Flaherty JF, Martins EB, Charuworn P, Kitrinos KM. Seven-year efficacy and safety of treatment with tenofovir disoproxil fumarate for chronic hepatitis B virus infection. Dig Dis Sci. 2015; 60:1457–1464.

[56] Tsai N, Gane E, Weilert F, Buti M, Jacobson I, Washington MK, et al. Five years of treatment with tenofovir disoproxil fumarate (TDF) for chronic hepatitis B (CHB) infection in lamivudine-experienced patients is associated with sustained viral suppression and histological improvement. Hepatol Int. 2012; 6:106.

[57] Chisari FV, Isogawa M, Wieland SF. Pathogenesis of hepatitis B virus infection. Pathol Biol (Paris). 2010; 58:258–266.

[58] Bréchot C. Pathogenesis of hepatitis B virus-related hepatocellular carcinoma: old and new paradigms. Gastroenterology. 2004; 127(5 Suppl. 1):S56–S61.

[59] Fourel G, Trepo C, Bougueleret L, Henglein B, Ponzetto A, Tiollais P, et al. Frequent activation of N-myc genes by hepadnavirus insertion in woodchuck liver tumours. Nature. 1990; 347:294–298.

[60] Matsubara K, Tokino T. Integration of hepatitis B virus DNA and its implications for hepatocarcinogenesis. Mol Biol Med. 1990; 7:243–260.

[61] Beasley RP, Lin C-C, Hwang L-Y, Chien C-S. Hepatocellular carcinoma and hepatitis B virus. Lancet. 1981; 318:1129–1133.

[62] Kremsdorf D, Soussan P, Paterlini-Brechot P, Brechot C. Hepatitis B virus-related hepatocellular carcinoma: paradigms for viral-related human carcinogenesis. Oncogene. 2006; 25:3823–3833.

[63] Benvegnu L. Natural history of compensated viral cirrhosis: a prospective study on the incidence and hierarchy of major complications. Gut. 2004; 53:744–749.

[64] Yu MW, Chang HC, Liaw YF, Lin SM, Lee SD, Liu CJ, et al. Familial risk of hepatocellular carcinoma among chronic hepatitis B carriers and their relatives. J Natl Cancer Inst. 2000; 92:1159–1164.

[65] Ohnishi K, Ilda SH, Iwama S, Goto N, Nomura F, Takahashi M, Mishima A, Kono K, Kimura K, Musha H, Kotota K. The effect of chronic habitual alcohol intake on the development of liver cirrhosis and hepatocellular carcinoma: relation to hepatitis B surface antigen carriage. Cancer. 1982; 49:672–677

[66] Tsubota A, Arase Y, Ren F, Tanaka H, Ikeda K, Kumada H. Genotype may correlate with liver carcinogenesis and tumor characteristics in cirrhotic patients infected with hepatitis B virus subtype adw. J Med Virol. 2001; 65:257–265.

[67] Zheng Y, Li J, Ou J. Regulation of hepatitis B virus core promoter by transcription factors HNF1 and HNF4 and the viral X protein. J Virol. 2004; 78:6908–6914.

[68] Bertoletti A, Kennedy PT. The immune tolerant phase of chronic HBV infection: new perspectives on an old concept. Cell Mol Immunol. 2015; 12:258–263.

[69] Kennedy PT, Sandalova E, Jo J, et al. Preserved T-cell function in children and young adults with immune-tolerant chronic hepatitis B. Gastroenterology. 2012; 143:637–645.

[70] Levy O. Innate immunity of the newborn: basic mechanisms and clinical correlates. Nat Rev Immunol. 2007; 7:379–390.

[71] Zoulim F, Mason WS. Reasons to consider earlier treatment of chronic HBV infections. Gut. 2012; 61:333–336.

[72] European Association for the Study of the Liver. EASL clinical practice guidelines: management of chronic hepatitis B virus infection. J Hepatol. 2012; 57:167–185.

[73] Martin P, Lau DT-Y. Nguyen MH, Janssen HLA, Dietrich DT, Peters MG, Jacobson IM. Treatment algorithm for the management of chronic hepatitis B virus infection in the United States: 2015 update. Clin Gastroenterol Hepatol. 2015; 13:2071–2087.

[74] Sarin SK, Kumar M, LauGK. Abbas Z, Chan HLY, Chen CJ, Chen DS, Chen HL, Chen PJ, Chien RN, Dokmec AK, Gane E, Hou JL, Jafri W, Jia J, Kim JH, Lai CL, Lee HC, Lim SG, Liu CJ, Locarnini S, Mahtab MAI, Mohamed R, Omata M, Park J, Piratvisuth T, Sharma BC, Sollano J, Wang FS, Wei L, Yuen MF, Zheng SS, Kao JH. Asian-Pacific clinical practice guidelines on the management of hepatitis B: a 2015 update. Hepatol Int. 2016; 10:1–98.

[75] Terrault NA, Bzowej NH, Chang KM, Hwang JP, Jonas MM, Murad MH. AASLD guidelines for treatment of chronic hepatitis B. Hepatology. 2016; 63(1):261–283.

Chapter 8

Recent Advancement in Hepatitis B Virus, Epigenetics Alterations and Related Complications

Mankgopo Magdeline Kgatle

Additional information is available at the end of the chapter

http://dx.doi.org/10.5772/66879

Abstract

Worldwide, it is estimated that more than 400 million people are currently living with chronic hepatitis B virus (HBV) infection, contributing to more than one million deaths annually as a result of liver cirrhosis and hepatocellular carcinoma (HCC). HBV DNA integrates into the cellular DNA in liver tissue of patients with chronic HBV infection and HCC. Following HBV infection, DNA methyltransferases (DNMTs) methylate any HBV DNA integrated into the human genome. This novel epigenetic mechanism enables the suppression of HBV antigens, leading to reduced viral replication. HBV is thought to induce DNA methylation via hepatitis B x (HBx) protein, which modulates cellular signalling pathways by activating DNMT 1 and 3 to benefit the virus. Activation of DNMT 1 and 3 inappropriately methylates host cellular genes including tumour suppressor genes whose disruption causes transformation of hepatocytes and hepatic malignancy. By being localised in the cytoplasm, nucleus and mitochondria of HBV-infected hepatocytes, it appears that HBx protein manages to exploit the entire body of cellular signalling pathways for viral survival and propagation. HBx protein may achieve its transcriptional transactivation action by either interacting with key genes or altering their related cellular signalling pathways or by hijacking their binding partners and taking over their roles. Although the underlying mechanisms are still unclear, processes such as cell cycle progression, calcium homeostasis, hepatic metabolism, protein ubiquitination, RNA splicing and vitamin D receptor regulation are key mechanisms that HBx protein alters to favour viral replication and cell survival. These detrimental effects would connect HBV infection to malignant transformation by inducing uncontrolled cell growth, proliferation and disrupting apoptosis.

Keywords: epigenetics alterations, viral integration, hepatitis B virus, hepatocellular carcinoma, hepatitis X antigen

1. Hepatitis B virus

Hepatitis B virus (HBV) is one of the most prevalent infections in humans and important cause of acute and chronic hepatitis. Chronic infection is defined as the presence of hepatitis B surface antigen (HBsAg) in the blood more than 6 months following initial infection. Without treatment, chronic HBV infection may result in the development of liver cirrhosis and hepatocellular carcinoma (HCC) [1–3].

HBV was first identified in the 1960s and was the first human hepatitis virus to be well characterised at a molecular level [3, 4]. Long-term inflammatory changes due to chronic hepatitis cause hepatocyte injury and the release of reactive oxygen species (ROS) and Kupffer cells activation. These produce proinflammatory and fibrogenic cytokines resulting in the recruitment of immune cells. The Kupffer cells also activate hepatic stellate cells which produce extracellular matrix proteins and cytokines. Repeating cycles of this activation and inflammation lead to cirrhosis characterised by regenerative nodules and irreversible fibrosis [2, 3, 5].

The ability of the virus to cause liver injury is associated with genetic changes that affect both viral and host DNA leading to mutations that predispose to liver injury and possible cancer. These events link chronic HBV infection with HCC. More than 80% of HCC cases arise in chronic HBV infection, strongly suggesting that HBV is an important contributor to the development of tumour [2, 3].

Possible mechanisms by which HBV infection causes HCC have been described, and these include HBV DNA integration, epigenetic alterations (change in gene expression) and aberrant transcriptional activities of HBx protein [3, 6, 7]. Nearly 90% of HBV-related HCC cases show evidence of HBV integration into the host genome [3, 8]. This is associated with genetic changes such as genomic instability, deletions and chromosomal translocations in the host cells, which may lead to accumulation of mutations and epigenetic changes with a malignant phenotype. Several contributing environmental and viral factors such as chronic tobacco smoking, alcohol consumption, aflatoxins, HBV e antigen positive status, high viral load and HBV genotype have been identified in HBV-related HCC cases and are associated with many epigenetic changes [3, 8–10].

1.1. Transmission Routes of HBV

HBV can be stable for 7 days or more on dry environmental surfaces. The two major routes of HBV transmission are horizontal and perinatal or vertical transmission. The efficient modes of transmission are blood and sexual contact with an infected person. The virus is horizontally transmissible during child to child physical contact or through contact with blood or infected toys. Horizontal transmission can also occur through body fluids such as semen and vaginal secretions. Perinatal or vertical transmission of HBV occurs through blood or secretions from an infected mother to the newborn baby during delivery. Perinatal transmission is high in mothers who are positive for hepatitis B e antigen (HBeAg) at 85–90% and lower in those who are negative for HBeAg where the rate is 5–20% [1, 3, 11–13].

1.2. Global epidemic of HBV infection

Worldwide, it is estimated that more than 400 million people are currently living with chronic HBV infection, contributing to more than one million deaths annually [1]. The prevalence of HBV infection is determined by the seroprevalence of HBsAg. HBV is highly endemic in Asia and sub-Saharan Africa with HBsAg seroprevalence rates exceeding 8% (**Figure 1**) [3, 14]. In these regions, the infection is typically acquired at birth or in early childhood. Progression to chronic HBV infection is common in these regions and is associated with prevalence rates of 30% for hepatic cirrhosis and 53% for HCC [16].

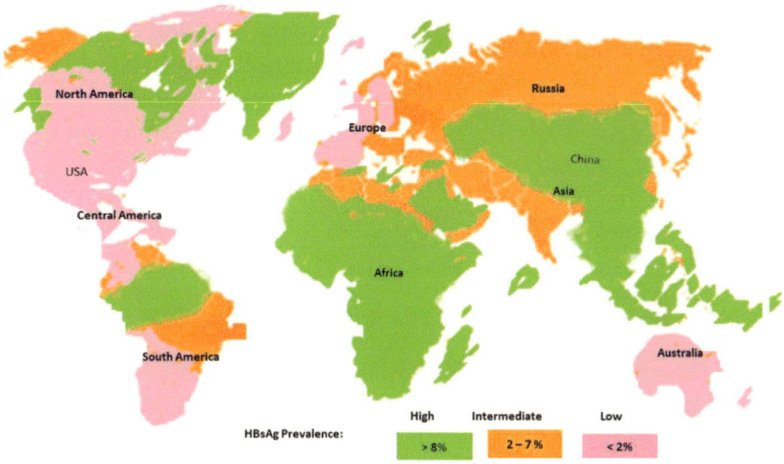

Figure 1. Global geographical distribution of chronic hepatitis B infection (Adapted from Lavanchy D **[13]**).

Annually, approximately one million people are diagnosed with HCC worldwide, and more than half of these people die within a year of diagnosis. Studies show that the highest HCC incidence rates of 70–80% occur in South-East Asia and sub-Saharan Africa, the regions with a high prevalence of chronic HBV infection [16]. This is due to various factors that include the late presentation of patients with large tumours, failure to recognise those at risk, high prevalence of risk factors in the population, lack of medical facilities for early diagnosis and limited access to effective treatment after diagnosis [3, 16].

An intermediate HBsAg seroprevalence of 2–7% is seen in some parts of Asia, Europe, America and Russia. The prevalence of HBV infection is low in Western Europe, Australia and United States where HBsAg seroprevalence is <2% [3, 17].

1.3. Epidemic of HBV infection in Africa

There are 65 million individuals infected with chronic HBV in Africa and 250,000 of these people die annually due to HBV-related diseases. The prevalence of chronic HBV infection in Africa varies by geographic region. It is high in sub-Saharan Africa, with HBsAg seroprevalence rates of more than 8%. In Kenya, Sierra Leone, Zambia, Senegal and Liberia, the prevalence of HBV infection is intermediate with HBsAg seroprevalence rates ranging from 2 to 8%. North African countries including Morocco, Egypt, Algeria and Tunisia have low prevalence rates of <2%.

In South Africa and other African countries, the prevalence of HBV infection is much higher in rural compared to urban areas [18]. Low socio-economic status, infected household contact, unsafe sexual intercourse, sharing of partially eaten sweets or chewing gum, dental work and bathing towels may be some of the contributing factors for the high prevalence of HBV infection in rural areas [3, 12, 18].

1.4. HBV genotypes and genomic alterations

HBV is classified into eight genotypes (A–J) with four major serotypes (adw, adr, ayw and ayr) [3, 19, 20]. HBV genotypes are differentiated by more than 8% sequence divergence in the entire genome and more than 4% at the level of S gene. They have distinct geographical distribution as illustrated in **Table 1**. Genotype A is predominant in sub-Saharan Africa, North-West Europe and North America.

Genotype	Geographic distribution	Mutation	Host CpG promoter methylation
A	North America, Sub-Saharan Africa, North-West Europe	G1888A 1762T1764A G1862T	Induces hypomethylation and down-regulation of the *DLEC1* gene
B	Indonesia, China, Vietnam	Unknown	Unknown
C	East Asia, Korea, China, Japan, Polynesia, Vietnam	Unknown	Unknown
D	Mediterranean area, Middle East	G1896A	Induces hypermethylation and down-regulation of *GSTP1* gene
E	Africa	Unknown	Unknown
F	Central and South America, Polynesia	Unknown	Unknown
G	France, America	Unknown	Unknown
H	Mediterranean area, Middle East	Unknown	Unknown
I	South-East Asia	Unknown	Unknown
J	Japan	Unknown	Unknown

Abbreviations: A, adenine; CpG, cytosine-phosphate-guanine; DLEC1, deleted in lung and esophageal cancer 1; G, guanine; GSTP1, glutathione S transferase pi 1; HBV, hepatitis B virus; T, thymine.

Table 1. The global geographic distribution of HBV genotypes, mutations and associated CpG promoter DNA methylation.

Genotype A has four subgenotypes. Subgenotype 1A is common in South Africa, Malawi, Tanzania, Uganda, Somalia, Yemen, India, Nepal, Brazil and the Philippines [3, 20]. There are three CpG islands within HBV genotype A, which are associated with methylation of the promoter of *Deleted in Lung and Esophageal Cancer 1* (*DLEC*) gene and down-regulation of its expression in HBV-induced HCC. *DLEC* is a tumour suppressor gene and has been reported to be down-regulated in ovarian, liver, lung and EBV-related cancers [3, 21].

Genotypes B and C are more prevalent in Asia, Indonesia and Vietnam [20]. Based on the phylogenetic analysis, it was demonstrated that HBV genotype C is subdivided into 5 subgenotypes (C1–C5). Geographical clustering of these subgenotypes was clear. The subgenotype C1 was found to be prevalent in East Asia, subgenotype C2 in South-East Asia, subgenotypes C3 and C4 in Southern Pacific Ocean and subgenotype C5 in Philippines [3, 22–34]. Genotype D is commonly found in the Mediterranean region and Middle East. The hepatitis B x (HBx) protein is associated with hypermethylation and down-regulation of the *GSTP1* gene which plays an important role in the development of cancer. Genotype E is found mainly in Africa. Genotype F is found in Europe and the United States, and genotype G, in France and America. Genotype H is predominant in Central America, California and Mexico. Genotype I and J are prevalent in South-East Asia and Japan, respectively [3, 20].

HBV has a mutation rate of 10%, which is relatively high compared to other viruses. It replicates via reverse transcription of RNA intermediates that result in random mismatched base errors during genomic replication. HBV DNA polymerase lacks the ability to proofread these errors, and this predisposes HBV to mutations [3, 25]. HBV develops four major mutations which are the precore, basic core promoter, tyrosine-methionine-aspartate-aspartate (YMDD) and asparagines-to-threonine (rtN236T) mutations. The precore mutants were the first to be identified and are characterised by a nonsense G1896A mutation [3, 26]. The G1896A mutation is responsible for HBeAg negativity in chronic HBV carriers and induces the down-regulation of HLA class II molecules in hepatocytes. This mutation is common in individuals infected with HBV genotype D [3, 27]. The basic core promoter mutations include A1762T and G1764A and were identified after the precore mutations. Similar to the precore mutations, the basic core promoter mutations are found in HBeAg-negative individuals where they prevent HBeAg expression [3, 28].

1.5. Prevention and treatment

HBV infection can be prevented by avoiding direct contact with any HBV-contaminated fluids and materials. Immunisation with recombinant hepatitis B vaccines is recommended for all infants at birth and in individuals who are at high risk of acquiring the infection. Passive immunoprophylaxis with hepatitis B immunoglobulin derived from sera of positive HBV individuals is used to prevent mother-to-child HBV transmission at birth, after liver transplantation for HBV infection, needle-stick injuries and sexual intercourse [3, 20, 29].

Acute HBV infection does not require treatment as it usually resolves spontaneously. Two major classes of drugs available for treating chronic HBV infection include the injectable standard interferon-α and pegylated interferon-α2, and the oral nucleos(t)ide analogues. Nucleoside analogues are lamivudine, entecavir, telbivudine, whilst nucleotide analoques are adefovirdipivoxil and tenofovir. The main aims of treatment are to improve long-term survival by reducing the risk of developing cirrhosis and HCC [3, 30, 31].

Treatment with oral nucleos(t)ide analogues is associated with the development of mutations. Lamivudine induces point mutations in the YMDD motif of the HBV polymerase, and these include rtM204V and rtM204I mutations. The viral replication rate increases in the presence of lamivudine resistance, and when lamivudine treatment is stopped, the wild-type virus reestablishes itself. Lamuvidine resistance mutations are responsible for the development of resistance in entecavir that is also associated with similar mutations and more including rtI169T, rtT184G, rtS202I and rtM250V [3, 32, 33]. Telbivudine has a high antiviral potency and relatively low resistance than lamuvidine and entecavir. It is associated with mutations at rtL80I/V, rtL180M, rtA181T/V, rtM204I and rtL229W/V. Telbivudine results in myoparthy and neuropathy when used simultaneously with pegylated interferon-α2, and therefore, combination of these two agents is avoided [3, 32, 34].

Adevovir treatment causes mutations that are associated with the emergence of resistant strains such as the rtN236T mutation which is downstream to the YMDD motif [35]. The use of adevovir treatment is now rare as it is associated with severe kidney injury, which may be a consequence of mitochondrial DNA depletion and activity of multidrug resistance-associated protein 4 [3, 36].

Despite the availability of treatment for chronic HBV infection, many patients will develop cancer, and this remains a major medical problem worldwide. This may be attributed to HCC-associated risk factors such as the HBV genotype, alanine aminotransferase (ALT), HBV load and HBV surface antigen level, which may influence the response to chronic HBV treatment. The response to interferon is significantly higher in patients infected with HBV genotype A compared to D and in patients with lower levels of HBV DNA and higher levels of ALT [3, 37, 38].

Aberrant methylation of promoter CpG islands is the primary epigenetic change seen during the course of HBV infection as it progresses to cirrhosis and HCC. Such methylation is detected at higher rates in HCC tissues compared to liver cirrhosis without cancer [10]. In a recent large cohort study report by Tseng et al., high HBV surface antigen levels are associated with a risk of developing HCC even in the presence of low HBV DNA levels. This finding may be due to a higher degree of viral HBV surface antigen integration into the host genome that would result in mutations and epigenetic alteration particularly DNA methylation, causing chronic liver damage, malignant transformation and HCC [3, 38–40].

The association of DNA methylation with chronic HBV treatment was first observed during telbivudine treatment. Telbivudine is a thymidine agent that interacts with protein kinases to form telbivudine 5′–triphosphate via phosphorylation. Telbivudine 5′–triphosphate competes with thymidine 5′–triphosphate, leading to the suppression of HBV DNA polymerase and reduced viral replication. Interestingly, telbivudine was recently reported to correct HBV-induced histone methylation in HBV-infected hepatocytes [3, 41].

http://dx.doi.org/10.5772/66879

1.6. Virological characteristics of HBV

HBV virions are infectious double-shelled particles of approximately 40–42 nanometre (nm) in diameter. They consist of a nucleocapsid core of 27 nm in diameter, which forms the inner part of enveloped virions known as Dane particles. The nucleocapsid core is surrounded by an outer surface antigen coat of ~4 nm thickness. It contains HBsAg and hepatitis B core antigen (HBcAg), which are detected in the sera of HBV-infected individuals in the form of spherical and filamentous particles [1, 3, 19, 42].

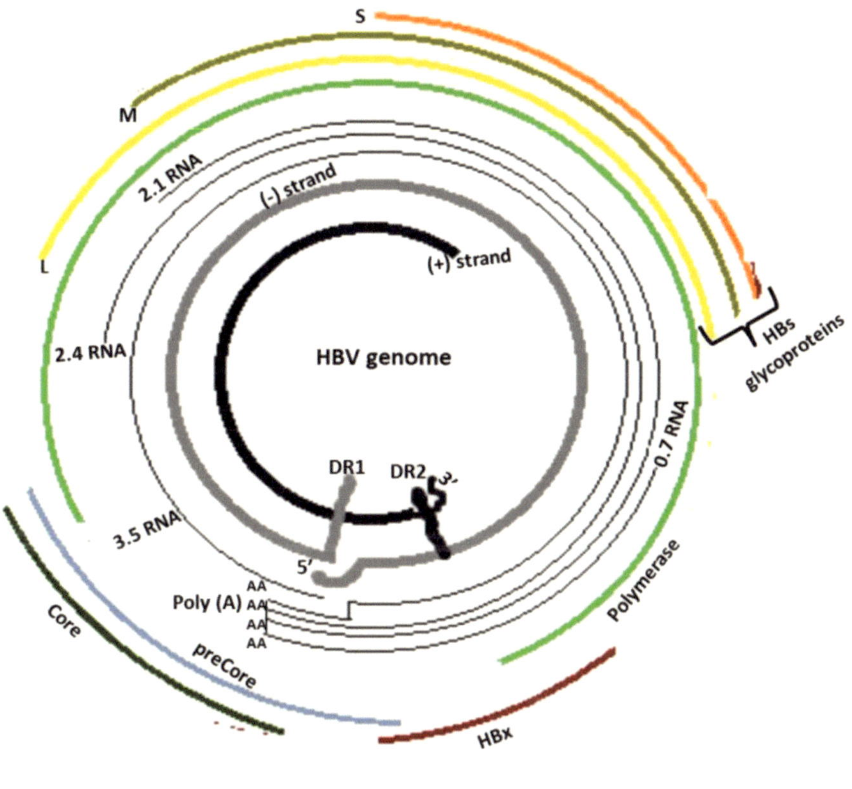

Figure 2. The structure of the HBV genome.

HBV is classified as an *Orthohepadnavirus* which belongs to the family *Hepadnaeviridae*. Contained in this family are other viruses such as the hepatic viruses of woodchucks, ducks, herons, ground and tree squirrels. These viruses replicate via reverse transcription of RNA intermediates, the step in which the DNA is packaged into hepadnaviral infectious particles. They are classified as *Hepadnaeviridae*due to their structure and genomic organisation being similar to that of HBV. HBV genome is a small and relaxed circular molecule of 3.2 kb in size. It contains two strands of different length, a long minus strand and a short plus strand as illustrated in **Figure 2**. The minus strand is terminally redundant and contains a second copy of direct repeat 1 (DR1), ε signal and poly A tail. It serves as a template for reverse transcription of a plus strand and also as a transcript for the translation of viral proteins including polymerase, HBcAg and HBeAg. The 5′ end of a minus strand is covalently linked to the viral reverse transcriptase and polymerase through a phosphor-tyrosine bond. The plus strand overlaps part of the minus strand whilst its 5′ end bears the oligoribonucleotides [3, 42, 43].

The HBV genome contains four ORFs, which have the same orientation and partially overlap. These ORFs encode the viral envelope pre-S/S, a pre-core/core, a polymerase and X proteins. The viral envelope also encodes three surface glycoproteins, which are the large (L), middle (M) and small (S) glycoproteins (**Figure 2**). These surface glycoproteins are synthesised by the initial transcription of pre-S/S. The L surface glycoprotein is important for viral assembly and infectivity, whilst the function of M surface glycoprotein is unknown. The longest open reading frame encodes the viral polymerase which serves as a reverse transcriptase and DNA polymerase. The pre-S/S envelope open reading frame overlaps the precore/core and X open reading frames and encodes HBsAg. The precore/core open reading frame produces HBeAg and HBcAg through cleavage by cellular proteases. HBcAg is the nucleocapsid and encloses the viral DNA [3, 11, 42, 43].

HBx protein is a transactivating protein that alters the expression of some genes via DNA methylation leading to tumourigenesis. It consists of 154 amino acid residues with a molecular weight of 27 kDa and is encoded by the smallest ORF. It stimulates viral replication either by activating viral transcription or by enhancing the reverse transcription of the viral polymerase [44, 45]. In hepatoma cell lines, HBx protein enhances viral replication by interacting with DNA binding protein 1 which interferes with cell growth and viability. In mice infected with wild-type HBV, viral replication is stimulated by HBx protein, suggesting that HBx protein is required for viral replication in normal hepatocyte cells [3, 44, 46, 47].

1.7. Life cycle of HBV

Due to the lack of efficient in vitro infection systems and animal models in which to study the life cycle of HBV infection, a lot of data are from the duck model infected with duck hepatitis B virus (DHBV) [3, 48]. HBV life cycle begins through the interaction of HBsAg with cellular receptor/s at the surface of hepatocytes. A number of potential cellular receptors that interact with HBsAg during HBV infection have been previously identified, but the mechanisms of action still remain controversial as none of them has been proved to be functional to HBV. These receptors include retinoid X receptor (RXR), peroxisome proliferator-activated receptor (PPAR) and farnesoid X receptor (FXR) [3, 49, 50].

Sodium taurocholate cotransporting polypeptide (NTCP) was discovered as the potential receptor for HBV infection (**Figure 2**). NTCP is abundantly expressed in the liver and is involved in the transportation and clearance of bile acids from portal blood into hepatocytes. Yan et al. [51] have shown by using near-zero-distance photo-cross-linking, tandem affinity purification and mass spectrophotometry that the pre-S/S envelope domain, a key determinant for receptor/s binding, selectively interacts with NTCP to facilitate HBV infection. Knockdown of the NTCP

http://dx.doi.org/10.5772/66879

expression in duck primary hepatocytes infected with DHBV significantly decreased HBV infection, suggesting that NTCP is actually required for HBV infection [3, 51, 52].

HBV requires DNA polymerase and reverse transcriptase to replicate through RNA intermediates known as pregenomic RNA. Following the interaction of surface antigen with NTCP, the viral nucleocapsid enters the host cell's nucleus to deliver dsDNA (**Figure 3**) [3, 51, 52]. In the nucleus, the dsDNA gets repaired and converted to covalently closed circular super-coiled DNA (cccDNA) by DNA polymerase. The cccDNA molecule serves as a template for the transcription of four viral RNA transcripts 3.5, 2.4, 2.1 and 0.4 kb in size, pregenomic RNA and RNA intermediate for viral replication before moving to the cytoplasm. The mRNA transcripts are then translated to produce the envelope (pre-S/S), precore/core, viral polymerase and X proteins. The 3.5 RNA transcript is reverse-transcribed into viral dsDNA [3, 8, 11, 40, 48, 53]. Some of the resulting viral DNA and polymerase-containing capsids are enveloped via budding into the endoplasmic reticulum (ER). The rest of the viral DNA is recycled or is migrated back to the nucleus where it produces new generations of cccDNA which maintains persistent HBV infection [1, 3, 11, 36, 40].

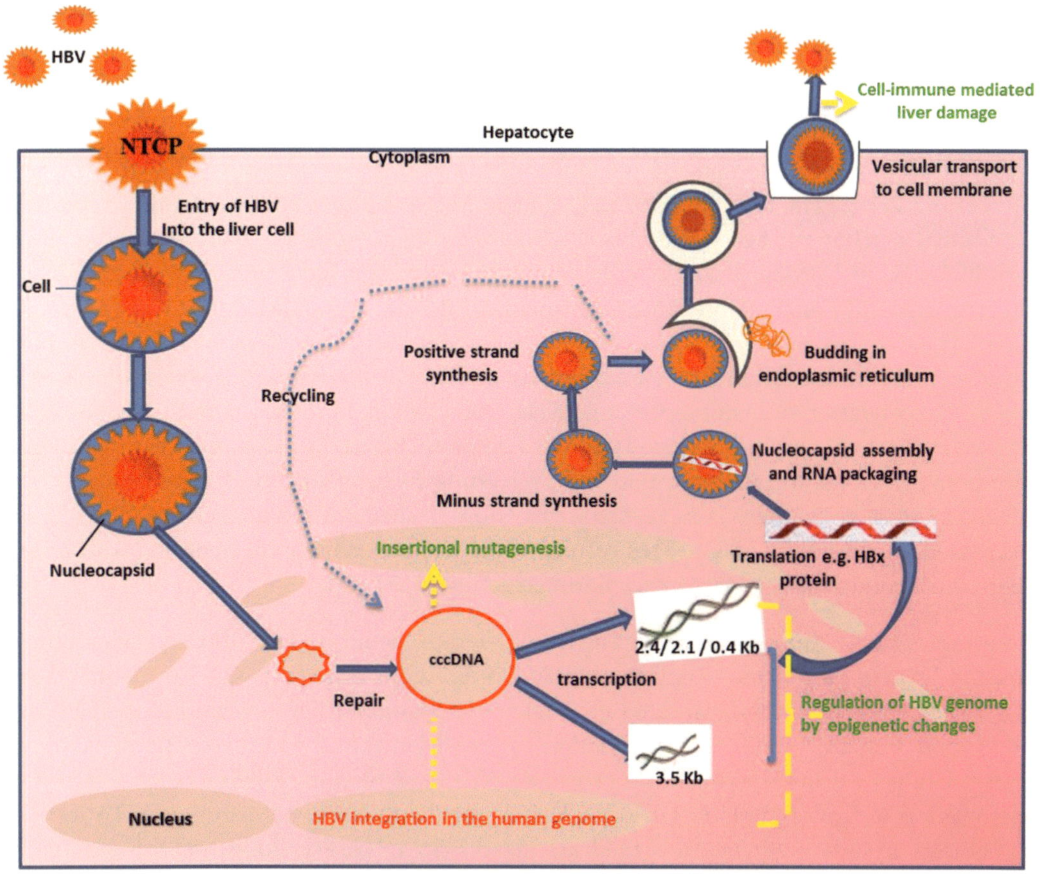

Figure 3. The life cycle of HBV infection and underlying mechanisms.

2. Epigenetics and HBV-induced hepatocarcinogenesis

Epigenetics involves attachment of chemical compounds and proteins on the DNA sequence leading to altered gene expression and normal function. There are two major ways through which gene transcription can be regulated through epigenetic changes. One way of regulating gene transcription is directly through DNA methylation. This involves the addition of a methyl group into DNA sequence. Methyl groups are carbon and hydrogen molecules which bind to the genome through the action of methyl cytosine-phosphate-guanine (CpG)-binding proteins (MeCPs), DNA methyltransferases (DNMTs), histone acetyltransferases (HATs) and histone deacetylases (HDACs), which inactivate gene transcription. Other transcription repressors including nuclear factor kappa B (NF-κB), c-myc/c-myn, activator protein (AP)-2, E2 promoter binding factor (E2F) and cyclic adenosine monophosphate (cAMP) response element binding protein (CREB) may also be activated by methyl groups to inhibit gene transcription [3, 53, 54].

In addition to DNA methylation, epigenetics can also be regulated by histone protein modifications. Histone protein modifications may be caused by over-expression or aberrant recruitment of HDACs that remodel the chromatin shape and structure. The two basic mechanisms responsible for chromatin remodelling are histone acetylation and deacetylation [3, 53, 55]. These mechanisms are controlled by the enzyme activity of HATs and HDACs, respectively [3, 54].

Acetylation of histone proteins is generally acknowledged as playing a key role in gene regulation. For a gene to be transcribed, it must become physically accessible to the transcriptional machinery. Acetylation by HATs substitutes the positive charges on the amino terminal tails of histone proteins with an acetyl group derived from acetyl coenzyme A, causing uncoiling of the DNA and euchromatin into an open-relaxed form of chromatin. Consequently, this makes genes accessible to several binding factors such as RNA polymerase II and transcriptional factors, allowing gene expression to occur and proteins to be made. Deacetylation of histone proteins by HDACs results in the tight coiling of the DNA and closed form of chromatin regions known as heterochromatin. This prevents the interaction between DNA and transcription factors leading to suppression of gene transcription. In some cancer cells, there is increased expression or aberrant recruitment of HDACs and decreased expression of HATs. This results in the hypoacetylation of histone proteins and therefore a condensed or closed chromatin structure [3, 54–56].

Epigenetics plays important roles in oncogenic viruses including HBV, human papillomavirus and Epstein Barr virus. In episomal HBV DNA, 3 CpG islands have been identified and described. These are island 1 located on nucleotide positions 55–286, island 2 on 1224–1667 and island 3 on 2257–2443 [57]. Methylation of CpG islands in the human genome is known to regulate gene transcription. These prompted Vivekanandan et al. [58] to hypothesise that methylation of CpG islands in HBV DNA may regulate viral gene expression. To test this hypothesis, in vitro methylation of the transfected HBV DNA was done, and this resulted in decreased expression of HBV mRNA and proteins in the cells. In addition, the effect of viral cccDNA methylation in the liver tissue of patients with chronic HBV infection was investigated and found to be associated with reduced HBV replication [58]. These findings support the work of Pollicino et al. [3, 58] who showed that HBV replication is regulated by the acetylation of HBV cccDNA bound H3 and H4 histone proteins. Although these data suggest that HBV DNA methylation is a novel mechanism that influences the regulation of viral gene expression, the mechanisms of action are still not known.

Previous human studies have shown that DNA viruses integrate into the host genome and that the expression levels of DNMTs increase in response to active viral replication [59]. Vivekanandan et al. [58] hypothesised that the up-regulation of DNMTs gives infected cells the ability to methylate viral DNA and therefore control viral replication. To investigate this, the expression of DNMTs was measured in cell lines exposed to HBV DNA using two experimental systems, one of temporary transfection of cells and another that mimicked natural chronic infection. High-level expressions of DNMT 1, 2 and 3 were observed in response to persistent HBV infection. This correlated with suppressed viral replication associated with methylation of HBV DNA and increased methylation of host CpG islands [3, 58].

The seminal work of Vivekanandan et al. [58] allows for the development of a model that explains the development of liver injury and HCC in chronic HBV infection (**Figure 4**). In this model, infected host cells respond to HBV infection by up-regulating the expression of DNMTs. Up-regulation of DNMTs can also result from interaction with HBx transcriptional

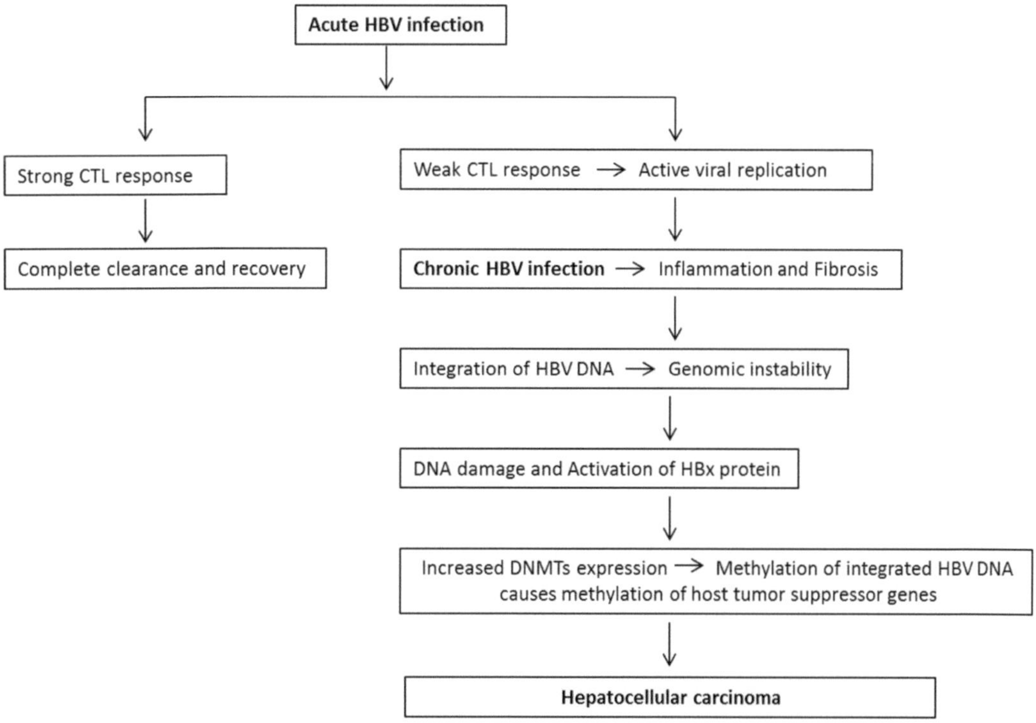

Figure 4. Model of chronic HBV infection and DNA methylation.

activator protein. Once activated, DNMTs methylate HBV DNA and switch off the expression of viral mRNA and proteins, thereby reducing viral replication. The methylation of integrated HBV DNA may be detrimental to the host genome through the inappropriate methylation of the neighbouring host genome, particularly if the promoter CpG islands regions of the gene are affected. A consequence of this effect would be the transcriptional repression of host immunoregulatory and tumour suppressor genes that prevent the development of cancer [3, 58].

Chromosomal fragile sites	Target gene	Role in tumour development
FRA1A (1p36)	TCEA; RAR; CHML	Alters gene expression and promote cell survival
FRA2C (1q)	EMX2-like gene	Modulates β-catenin signalling pathway and cell survival
FRA4E (4p)	Cyclin A	Stimulate cell cycle and anti-apoptotic effect
FRA3D (3q25.3)	IRAK2	Promotes apoptosis and tumour progression
FRA5C (5p31.1)	PDGFRβ	Regulates DNA synthesis and fibrotic genes
FRA7 (7p)	SERCA 1; NCF1	β-Catenin activation
FRA9 (9q)	KLF1; CASPR3	Promote cell growth; regulates DNA methylation
FRA10A (10q)	PTEN; PI3K	Promotes metastasis; promotes cell cycle progression
FRA11A (11q13)	EMS1, FGF4; BIRC3	Modulates β-catenin signaling pathway; alters cell fate
FRA12A (12q24)	ErbB3; Mill2	Promotes tumour progression
FRA13A (13q32)	CTGF; CCNL; IMP-2	Tumour suppression
FRA18 (18q)	DCC; DPC4	Regulates methyl-CpG-binding proteins
FRA19A (19q13)	Cyclin E	Delays DNA synthesis and promotes immortalisation
FRA20 (20P12.3)	hTERT	Alters gene expression and promotes cell survival

Abbreviations: BIRC3, baculoviral IAP repeat containing 3; CASPR3, contactin-associated protein-like 3;CCNL, cyclin L1;CHML, choroideremia-like gene; CTGF, connective tissue growth factor; DCC, deleted in colorectal cancer; DPC4, deleted in pancreatic cancer 4; EMSL, EMSL; EMX2, empty spiracle homeobox 2; ErbB3, V-erb-b2 erythroblasticleukemia viral oncogene homolog 3; FGF4, fibroblast growth factor 4; FRA, fragile site; hTERT, human telomerase reverse transcriptase; IMP-2, insulin-like growth factor II mRNA binding protein 2; IRAK2, interleukin-1 receptor-associated kinase 2; KLF1, Krueppel-like factor 1; Mill2, major histocompatibility complex I like leukocyte 2; NCF1, neutrophil cytosolic factor 1; PDGFRβ, platelet-derived growth factor receptor beta; PI3K, phosphatidylinositol 3 kinase; PTEN, phosphatise and tension homolog; RAR, retinoic acid receptor; SERCA, sarco/endoplasmic reticulum calcium transport ATPase; TCEA, transcription elongation factor A.

Table 2. Examples of chromosomal fragile sites associated with HBV insertions and their roles in tumour development.

HBV integrates into the host genome and promotes viral persistence. Infected cells increase the expression of DNMTs in response to viral replication. This causes methylation of HBV cccDNA and reduces viral replication. The same methylation system methylates the adjacent host tumour suppressor and immunoregulatory genes leading to hepatocarcinogenesis.

2.1. Integration of HBV DNA into the human genome

HBV integration was first discovered in 1980 using Southern blot hybridisation. It was associated with genomic instability such as loss of heterozygocity (LOH), resulting in the rearrangements, deletions, duplications and inversions of the host and viral genomic sequences. Viral integration results in the insertion of HBV DNA sequences such as HBx gene in the host genome and enables viral persistence [3, 7, 8].

Integration of HBV in the host genome also occurs in woodchucks and other animal models. In woodchucks and California ground squirrels (Spermophilusbeecheyi), HBV genome integrates close to *ras* and *myc* family oncogenes including *c-myc, N-myc1* and *N-myc2*. Modulation of *myc* and *ras* family oncogenes through *cis*-activation enhances cell proliferation and transformation. These events occur via transactivation action of HBx protein and favour the development of cancer [3, 60, 61].

The occurrence of integrated HBV DNA at preferential sites in the human chromosomes has been identified using Alu-PCR-based technique. The preferential sites are known as chromosomal fragile sites (CFS) and are non-random [3, 8]. HBV DNA integrates into the human genome soon after the repair and conversion of HBV DNA to cccDNA [3, 57, 58, 62]. The HBV genome integrates within the coding sequence or close to an array of key regulatory cellular genes that can deregulate proto-oncogenes and tumour suppressor genes. Activation or inactivation of such genes promotes genomic chromosomal instability by altering various cellular signalling pathways, triggering genetic mutations and epigenetic alteration. Mutagenesis and epigenetic alteration result in the abnormal regulation of the targeted genes. This promotes malignant transformation by altering the control of cell growth, differentiation, proliferation and apoptosis [3, 57, 58, 63]. The integration of HBV at or within *cyclin A* and *RARβ* genes is associated with increased protein activities and hepatocellular growth in HBV-induced HCC, suggesting that HBV integration contributes to hepatocytes transformation [60]. Examples of known active CFS targeted by HBV integration are outlined in **Table 2**. The 60s ribosomal protein, *hTERT, major histocompatibility complex I like leukocyte* (*Mill*), *platelet-derived growth factor receptor* (*PDGFR*) and *calcium signalling-related* genes are also common sites or targets of HBV integration. These genes are important in cellular signalling pathways that control DNA damage, oxidation stress and cell growth, and their alteration is associated with the development and progression of cancer [3, 9, 64].

2.2. HBx protein and its carcinogenic effects

HBx protein is a transcriptional transactivator that HBV uses to integrate into the host cellular DNA and is associated with malignant transformation in hepatocytes. It interacts with nuclear transcription factors such as NF-κB, AP1, CREB, TATA-binding protein (TBP), peroxisome proliferator-activated receptor γ (PPARγ) and transcription factor II H (TFIIH) [44]. Interaction of HBx protein with these transcription factors disrupts multiple cellular signalling pathways that include janus kinase 1 (JAK1)-signal transducer activator of transcription (STAT), mitogen-activated protein kinase (MAPK), phosphatidylinositol 3-kinase (PI3K) and p53 signalling pathways. Cellular signalling pathways are important in regulating DNA repair, cell growth, differentiation, adhesion, proliferation and apoptosis. Although the precise mechanisms of action are still being elucidated, HBx protein has also been shown to induce methylation of important tumour suppressor genes critical in HBV-induced hepatocarcinogenesis by modulating DNMTs [3, 44, 45, 47, 63, 65, 66].

The transcriptional transactivation role of HBx protein on the transforming growth factor beta 1 (TGF-β1) protein may be important in explaining liver inflammation and fibrosis. TGF-β1, encoded by *TGF-β1* gene, is a cytokine that is produced in response to liver injury by activated hepatocytes, platelets and Kupffer cells. It triggers apoptosis, cell growth and differentiation in human hepatocytes, hepatoma cell lines and transgenic mice [3, 67, 68]. It promotes the development of fibrosis and cirrhosis in chronic HBV infection and other liver-related diseases. HBx protein induces the expression of TGF-β1 through the transactivation of *TGF-β1* gene, the down-regulation of α_2-macroglobulin and the induction of TGF-β1 mediator Smad4. High levels of TGF-β1 protein are observed in the sera of chronic HBV-induced HCC patients and correlate with the mutation and loss of mannose-6-phosphate/IGF-II receptor that mediates TGF-β1 signalling [3, 67, 69, 70]. In addition, HBx protein alters the signalling pathway of TGF-β1 from being tumour suppressive to oncogenic in early chronic HBV infection. This occurs via the activation of c-Jun N-terminal kinase (JNK) which shifts epithelial tumour suppressive pSmad3C signal to mesenchymal oncogenic pSmadL signal pathway [3, 70].

Studies show that in HBx transgenic mice and hepatoma cell lines, HBx protein can transactivate the NF-κB, MAPK/ERK, STAT3 and PI3K/Akt cellular signalling pathways by inducing the production of ROS. Accumulation of ROS in human cancers is associated with anti-apoptotic activity, DNA damage and mutations which promote malignant transformation. HBx-induced ROS and 8-oxoguanine alter the expression of PTEN protein by oxidising cysteine residues within the promoter region encoding *PTEN* gene, which activates Akt pathway and contributes to hepatocarcinogenesis [3, 65, 70–72].

2.3. HBx protein and DNA methylation

HBx protein has been labelled an epigenetic deregulating agent. It uses its oncogenic ability to induce promoter methylation of some cellular tumour suppressor genes that contribute to the development of liver cancer [3, 73]. Cancer-associated DNA methylation may be global hypomethylation (less methylation) or hypermethylation (increased methylation). Abnormal hypermethylation of various cellular genes including host tumour suppressors has been described in liver cancer, and it is associated with silencing of genes critical for preventing malignant transformation [3, 56]. Altered gene expression has been reported in HBV infection where the DNA methylation machinery is induced as a host defence mechanism to suppress viral genes [3, 53, 57, 58]. This correlates with loss of normal activity in genes important for wound healing and immune processes. Disruption of these processes will interfere with normal cell proliferation and apoptosis and potentiates the ability to metastasize in abnormal cells as seen in chronic liver disease and malignant transformation [3, 58, 63]. By modulating the transcriptional activation of DNMTs, HBx protein induces the hypermethylation of tumour suppressor gene promoters and silences their expression [3, 74–77].

HBx protein induces the hypermethylation of *RARβ2* gene by up-regulating DNMT1 and 3A activities and down-regulating the expression of RARβ2 protein [3, 73, 77]. *RARβ2* binds to and inactivates the E2F1 transcription factor, which is essential for cell cycle progression [3, 64, 73, 77]. Down-regulation of RARβ2 protein expression is associated with activation of E2F1 transcription factor, which abolishes the ability of retinoic acid to regulate the expression of G_1 checkpoint regulators, leading to up-regulation of p16, p21 and p27 proteins. The activation of E2F1 transcription factor is associated with uncontrolled cell proliferation which contributes to carcinogenesis [3, 77].

Insulin-like growth factor binding 3 (*IGJBP-3*) is another potential tumour suppressor gene which is both hyper- and hypomethylated in HBV-induced HCC. Hypermethylation of *IGJBP-3* gene is mediated by DNMT 1 and 3A which are upregulated via the transcriptional activities of HBx protein, and this is associated with loss of *IGJBP-3* gene expression. In contrast, HBx protein reduces the transcriptional activities of DNMT 3B, leading to hypomethylation and up-regulation of the *IGJBP-3* gene [3, 45].

DLEC1 is a functional tumour suppressor gene silenced by promoter methylation in lung, gastric, colon and nasopharyngeal cancers. Similar methylation has also been observed in HCC where it is associated with induction of G1 cell cycle arrest and loss of gene expression. Silencing of *DLEC 1* gene expression is mediated by both DNA hypermethylation and histone acetylation [3, 21, 78]. HBx protein encoded by HBV genotype A enhances the transcription of *DLEC 1* gene by increasing the level of histone acetylation through the activation of HATs, leading to suppression of tumour progression. Through the activation of DNMT1 expression mediated by the pRB-E2F pathway, HBx protein induces DNA hypermethylation of *DLEC1* gene and suppresses its transcriptional activities [3, 78].

Caveolin-1, encoded by *caveolin-1* gene, is an integral membrane protein abundantly expressed in adipose, fibrous and endothelial tissue. High-level expression of caveolin-1 protein disrupts growth factor signalling pathways, which in turn alters cell growth, proliferation and differentiation. HCC cells expressing high levels of caveolin-1 are associated with uncontrolled cell growth, motility, in vivo tumour aggressiveness and metastasis. Conversely, HBx-induced methylation of *Caveolin-1* gene promoter region suppresses its transcriptional activities, and this correlates with reduced tumour aggressiveness and metastasis, indicating a role of DNA methylation in HBV-related HCC [3, 80, 81].

Hypermethylation of $p16^{ink4a}$gene is a frequent event in several malignancies including HBV-induced HCC. HBx protein silences the expression of $p16^{ink4a}$gene through the activation of DNA methyltransferase 1 and the cyclin D1-CDK 4/6-pRb-E2F1 pathway. Methylation of $p16^{ink4a}$gene is associated with increased viral replication, integration and loss of protein expression [3, 80, 81].

HBx-protein-induced DNA hypermethylation has also been connected with loss of expression and normal function of *LINE-1, pRB, ASPP, E-cadherin, GSTP1* and *hTERT* tumour suppressor genes [3, 76, 78, 82, 83]. This methylation is associated with increased up-regulation of DNMTs with DNMT1 being the most active one. Aberrant methylation of these genes is associated with perturbed cellular signalling pathways such as ubiquitination, DNA repair, transcription, proliferation and apoptosis, which may lead to the development of HBV-related HCC [3, 21, 45, 78].

Genome-wide studies aided in identifying DNA methylation, histone modifications and miRNA expression profiling across the entire samples with CHB and HBV-related HCC [3, 84–86]. Preliminary data conducted by Kgatle et al. [84] demonstrate that HBV-induced methylation may affect cellular processes such as cell cycle progression, calcium homeostasis, hepatic metabolism, protein ubiquitination, RNA splicing and vitamin D receptor regulation, which are key mechanisms that HBx protein alters to favour viral replication and cell survival. Disruption in these cellular processes could cause genetic instability, hepatocyte transformation and tumour development. However, amongst most conducted genome-wide studies, there are some discrepancies and data variations due to lack of proper normal control, heterogeneity of disease, variations of samples source, use of different technologies for analysis and validation with gene expression analysis, suggesting need for further validations [3, 84].

3. Summary

Substantial data show that there is an association between the methylation of CpG islands and transcriptional changes in gene promoter regions. Transcriptional alterations within gene promoter regions interfere with the normal function of a wide spectrum of cellular genes including tumour suppressor genes which are potential inducers of malignancies. Oncogenic viruses integrate themselves into the human genome and alter gene transcription through DNA methylation. During HBV infection, the expression levels of DNMTs are elevated in response to viral replication as viral genes are methylated to suppress viral replication. This may result in inappropriate random methylation of neighbouring host cellular genes, including tumour suppressor genes. This would cause malignant transformation and ultimately liver cancer. In addition, other genes affected by methylation may contribute to the development of liver inflammation, fibrosis and cirrhosis. As a multifunctional viral transactivator, the HBx protein may be the driving force behind the activation of DNMTs, causing gene promoter hypermethylation and gene silencing. The epigenetic alteration of genes may affect cellular signalling pathways and favour uncontrolled hepatocyte proliferation and HBV-induced inflammation, fibrosis and cancer.

Author details

Mankgopo Magdeline Kgatle

Address all correspondence to: mankgopo.kgatle@gmail.com

Department of Medicine, Faculty of Health Sciences, University of Cape Town, Groote Schuur Hospital, Cape Town, South Africa

References

[1] Liaw Y, Chu C: Hepatitis B virus infection. Lancet 2009, 373: 582–592.

[2] Beasley RP: Rocks along the road to the control of HBV and HCC. Ann. Epidemiol. 2009, 19: 231–234.

[3] Kgatle MM: An investigation of genome-wide promoter region cytosine-phosphate-guanine (CpG) Island methylation profiles in patients with chronic hepatitis B virus infection. University of Cape Town Thesis; 2014: 19–43.

[4] Blumberg BS, Gerstley BJS, Hungerford DA, London WT, Sutnick AI: A serum antigen (Australia antigen) in Down's syndrome, leukemia, and hepatitis. Ann. Intern. Med. 1967, 66: 924–931.

[5] Fausto N, Campbell JS, Riehle KJ: Liver regeneration. Hepatology 2006, 43.

[6] Brechot C, Pourcel C, Louise A, Rain B, Tiollais P: Presence of integrated hepatitis B virus DNA sequences in cellular DNA of human hepatocellular carcinoma 1980.

[7] Sung W, Zheng H, Li S, Chen R, Liu X, Li Y, Lee NP, Lee WH, Ariyaratne PN, Tennakoon C: Genome-wide survey of recurrent HBV integration in hepatocellular carcinoma. Nat. Genet. 2012, 44: 765–769.

[8] Murakami Y, Saigo K, Takashima H, Minami M, Okanoue T, Brechot C, Paterlini-Brechot P: Large scaled analysis of hepatitis B virus (HBV) DNA integration in HBV related hepatocellular carcinomas. Gut 2005, 54: 1162–1168.

[9] Popescu NC, Zimonjic D, DiPaolo JA: Viral integration, fragile sites, and proto-oncogenes in human neoplasia. Hum. Genet. 1990, 84: 383–386.

[10] Yang H, Lu S, Liaw Y, You S, Sun C, Wang L, Hsiao CK, Chen P, Chen D, Chen C: Hepatitis B e antigen and the risk of hepatocellular carcinoma. N. Engl. J. Med. 2002, 347: 168–174.

[11] Shepard CW, Simard EP, Finelli L, Fiore AE, Bell BP: Hepatitis B virus infection: epidemiology and vaccination. Epidemiol. Rev. 2006, 28: 112–125.

[12] Karayiannis P, Novick DM, Lok AS, Fowler MJ, Monjardino J, Thomas HC: Hepatitis B virus DNA in saliva, urine, and seminal fluid of carriers of hepatitis B e antigen. Br. Med. J. (Clin. Res. Ed) 1985, 290: 1853–1855.

[13] Zonneveld M, Nunen A, Niesters H, Man R, Schalm S, Janssen H: Lamivudine treatment during pregnancy to prevent perinatal transmission of hepatitis B virus infection. J. Viral Hepat. 2003, 10: 294–297.

[14] Lavanchy D: Hepatitis B virus epidemiology, disease burden, treatment, and current and emerging prevention and control measures. J. Viral Hepat. 2004, 11: 97–107.

[15] Fattovich G, Stroffolini T, Zagni I, Donato F: Hepatocellular carcinoma in cirrhosis: incidence and risk factors. Gastroenterology 2004, 127: S35–S50.

[16] Bréchot C: Pathogenesis of hepatitis B virus—related hepatocellular carcinoma: old and new paradigms. Gastroenterology 2004, 127: S56–S61.

[17] Wasley A, Kruszon-Moran D, Kuhnert W, Simard EP, Finelli L, McQuillan G, Bell B: The prevalence of hepatitis B virus infection in the United States in the era of vaccination. J. Infect. Dis. 2010, 202: 192–201.

[18] Kramvis A, Kew MC: Epidemiology of hepatitis B virus in Africa, its genotypes and clinical associations of genotypes. Hepatol. Res. 2007, 37.

[19] Glebe D: Hepatitis B virus taxonomy and hepatitis B virus genotypes. World J. Gastroentrol. 2007, 13: 14–21.

[20] Lin C, Kao J: The clinical implications of hepatitis B virus genotype: recent advances. J. Gastroenterol. Hepatol. 2011, 26: 123–130.

[21] Qiu G, Salto-Tellez M, Ross JA, Yeo W, Cui Y, Wheelhouse N, Chen GG, Harrison D, Lai P, Tao Q: The tumor suppressor gene DLEC1 is frequently silenced by DNA methylation in hepatocellular carcinoma and induces G1 arrest in cell cycle. J. Hepatol. 2008, 48: 433–441.

[22] Kramvis A, Arakawa K, Yu MC, Nogueira R, Stram DO, Kew MC: Relationship of serological subtype, basic core promoter and precore mutations to genotypes/subgenotypes of hepatitis B virus. J. Med. Virol. 2008, 80: 27–46.

[23] Norder H, Courouce AM, Coursaget P, Echevarria JM, Lee SD, Mushahwar IK, Robertson BH, Locarnini S, Magnius LO: Genetic diversity of hepatitis B virus strains derived worldwide: genotypes, subgenotypes, and HBsAg subtypes. Intervirology 2004, 47: 289–309.

[24] Sakamoto T, Tanaka Y, Orito E, Clavio J, Sugauchi F, Ito K, Ozasa A, Quino A, Ueda R, Sollano J: Novel subtypes (subgenotypes) of hepatitis B virus genotypes B and C among chronic liver disease patients in the Philippines. J. Gen. Virol. 2006, 87: 1873–1882.

[25] Echevarría JM, Avellón A: Hepatitis B virus genetic diversity. J. Med. Virol. 2006, 78: S36–S42.

[26] Min XC, Miao XH, Zhao SM, Zhao KK, Yang DG: The spontaneous YMDD mutation rate in chronic hepatitis B patients. Zhonghua Gan Zang Bing Za Zhi 2009, 17: 887–890.

[27] Yang HI, Yeh SH, Chen PJ, Iloeje UH, Jen CL, Su J, Wang LY, Lu SN, You SL, Chen DS, et al.: Associations between hepatitis B virus genotype and mutants and the risk of hepatocellular carcinoma. J. Natl. Cancer Inst. 2008, 100: 1134–1143.

[28] Fang Z, Sabin CA, Dong B, Wei S, Chen Q, Fang K, Yang J, Wang X, Harrison TJ: The association of HBV core promoter double mutations (A1762T and G1764A) with viral load differs between HBeAg positive and anti-HBe positive individuals: a longitudinal analysis. J. Hepatol. 2009, 50: 273–280.

[29] Kao JH, Chen PJ, Lai MY, Chen DS: Genotypes and clinical phenotypes of hepatitis B virus in patients with chronic hepatitis B virus infection. J. Clin. Microbiol. 2002, 40: 1207–1209.

[30] Shaw T, Locarnini S: Entecavir for the treatment of chronic hepatitis B. Expert review of anti-infective therapy 2014.

[31] Trépo C, Chan HL, Lok A: Hepatitis B virus infection. Lancet 2014, 384: 2053–2063.

[32] Perrillo R, Hann H, Mutimer D, Willems B, Leung N, Lee WM, Moorat A, Gardner S, Woessner M, Bourne E: Adefovir dipivoxil added to ongoing lamivudine in chronic hepatitis B with YMDD mutant hepatitis B virus. Gastroenterology 2004, 126: 81–90.

[33] Chon CY, Han K, Ahn SH: Long-term adefovir dipivoxil monotherapy for up to 5 years in lamivudine-resistant chronic hepatitis B. Antivir. Ther. (Lond.) 2010, 15: 235–241.

[34] Han G, Cao M, Zhao W, Jiang H, Wang C, Bai S, Yue X, Wang G, Tang X, Fang Z: A prospective and open-label study for the efficacy and safety of telbivudine in pregnancy for the prevention of perinatal transmission of hepatitis B virus infection. J. Hepatol. 2011, 55: 1215–1221.

[35] Yeon JE, Yoo W, Hong SP, Chang YJ, Yu SK, Kim JH, Seo YS, Chung HJ, Moon MS, Kim SO, et al.: Resistance to adefovir dipivoxil in lamivudine resistant chronic hepatitis B patients treated with adefovir dipivoxil. Gut 2006, 55: 1488–1495.

[36] Tan J, Degertekin B, Wong SN, Husain M, Oberhelman K, Lok AS: Tenofovir monotherapy is effective in hepatitis B patients with antiviral treatment failure to adefovir in the absence of adefovir-resistant mutations. J. Hepatol. 2008, 48: 391–398.

[37] Kao J, Chen P, Chen D: Recent advances in the research of hepatitis B virus-related hepatocellular carcinoma: epidemiologic and molecular biological aspects. Adv. Cancer Res. 2010, 108.

[38] Tseng T, Liu C, Yang H, Su T, Wang C, Chen C, Kuo SF, Liu C, Chen P, Chen D: High levels of hepatitis B surface antigen increase risk of hepatocellular carcinoma in patients with low HBV load. Gastroenterology 2012, 142: 1140–1149. e3.

[39] Zeng L, Lian J, Chen J, Jia H, Zhang Y, Xiang D, Yu L, Hu J, Lu Y, Zheng L: Hepatitis B surface antigen levels during natural history of chronic hepatitis B: a Chinese perspective study. World J. Gastroenterol. 2014, 20: 9178–9184.

[40] Nguyen T, Thompson AJ, Bowden S, Croagh C, Bell S, Desmond PV, Levy M, Locarnini SA: Hepatitis B surface antigen levels during the natural history of chronic hepatitis B: a perspective on Asia. J. Hepatol. 2010, 52: 508–513.

[41] Tian Y, Ni D, Yang W, Zhang Y, Zhao K, Song J, Mao Q, Tian Z, van Velkinburgh JC, Yang D: Telbivudine treatment corrects HBV-induced epigenetic alterations in liver cells of patients with chronic hepatitis B. Carcinogenesis 2014, 35: 53–61.

[42] Ganem D, Prince AM: Hepatitis B virus infection—natural history and clinical consequences. N. Engl. J. Med. 2004, 350: 1118–1129.

[43] Scaglioni PP, Melegari M, Wands JR: Recent advances in the molecular biology of hepatitis B virus. Baillière's Clin. Gastroenterol. 1996, 10: 207–225.

[44] Murakami S: Hepatitis B virus X protein: a multifunctional viral regulator. J. Gastroenterol. 2001, 36: 651–660.

[45] Park IY, Sohn BH, Yu E, Suh DJ, Chung Y, Lee J, Surzycki SJ, Lee YI: Aberrant epigenetic modifications in hepatocarcinogenesis induced by hepatitis B virus X protein. Gastroenterology 2007, 132: 1476–1494.

[46] Chung TW, Lee YC, Kim CH: Hepatitis B viral HBx induces matrix metalloproteinase-9 gene expression through activation of ERK and PI-3K/AKT pathways: involvement of invasive potential. FASEB J. 2004, 18: 1123–1125.

[47] Shih WL, Kuo ML, Chuang SE, Cheng AL, Doong SL: Hepatitis B virus X protein inhibits transforming growth factor-beta -induced apoptosis through the activation of phosphatidylinositol 3-kinase pathway. J.Biol.Chem. 2000, 275: 25858–25864.

[48] Weiner AJ, Choo QL, Wang KS, Govindarajan S, Redeker AG, Gerin JL, Houghton M: A single antigenomic open reading frame of the hepatitis delta virus encodes the epitope(s) of both hepatitis delta antigen polypeptides p24 delta and p27 delta. J. Virol. 1988, 62: 594–599.

[49] Dandri M, Lutgehetmann M, Volz T, Petersen J: Small animal model systems for studying hepatitis B virus replication and pathogenesis 2006, 26: 181–191.

[50] Mangelsdorf DJ, Evans RM: The RXR heterodimers and orphan receptors. Cell 1995, 83: 841–850.

[51] Yan H, Zhong G, Xu G, He W, Jing Z, Gao Z, Huang Y, Qi Y, Peng B, Wang H, et al.: Sodium taurocholate cotransporting polypeptide is a functional receptor for human hepatitis B and D virus. Elife 2012, 1: e00049.

[52] Yan H, Peng B, Liu Y, Xu G, He W, Ren B, Jing Z, Sui J, Li W: Viral entry of hepatitis B and D viruses and bile salts transportation share common molecular determinants on sodium taurocholate cotransporting polypeptide. J.Virol. 2014, 88: 3273–3284.

[53] Esteller M: Epigenetics in cancer. N.Engl.J.Med. 2008, 358: 1148–1159.

[54] Holliday R: Epigenetics: a historical overview. Epigenetics 2006, 1: 76–80.

[55] Grunstein M: Histone acetylation in chromatin structure and transcription. Nature 1997, 389: 349–352.

[56] Bestor TH, Chandler VL, Feinberg AP: Epigenetic effects in eukaryotic gene expression. Dev. Genet. 1994, 15: 458–462.

[57] Vivekanandan P, Thomas D, Torbenson M: Hepatitis B viral DNA is methylated in liver tissues. J. Viral Hepat. 2008, 15: 103–107.

[58] Vivekanandan P, Thomas D, Torbenson M: Methylation regulates hepatitis B viral protein expression. J. Infect. Dis. 2009, 199: 1286–1291.

[59] Pollicino T, Belloni L, Raffa G, Pediconi N, Squadrito G, Raimondo G, Levrero M: Hepatitis B virus replication is regulated by the acetylation status of hepatitis B virus cccDNA-bound H3 and H4 histones. Gastroenterology 2006, 130: 823–837.

[60] Wang Y, Lau SH, Sham JS, Wu M, Wang T, Guan X: Characterization of HBV integrants in 14 hepatocellular carcinomas: association of truncated X gene and hepatocellular carcinogenesis. Oncogene 2004, 23: 142–148.

[61] Jacob JR, Sterczer A, Toshkov IA, Yeager AE, Korba BE, Cote PJ, Buendia M, Gerin JL, Tennant BC: Integration of woodchuck hepatitis and N-myc rearrangement determine size and histologic grade of hepatic tumors. Hepatology 2004, 39: 1008–1016.

[62] Shafritz DA, Shouval D, Sherman HI, Hadziyannis SJ, Kew MC: Integration of hepatitis B virus DNA into the genome of liver cells in chronic liver disease and hepatocellular carcinoma: studies in percutaneous liver biopsies and post-mortem tissue specimens. N. Engl. J. Med. 1981, 305: 1067–1073.

[63] Lupberger J, Hildt E: Hepatitis B virus-induced oncogenesis. World J. Gastroenterol. 2007, 13: 74.

[64] Edamoto Y, Hara A, Biernat W, Terracciano L, Cathomas G, Riehle H, Matsuda M, Fujii H, Scoazec J, Ohgaki H: Alterations of RB1, p53 and Wnt pathways in hepatocellular carcinomas associated with hepatitis C, hepatitis B and alcoholic liver cirrhosis. Int. J. Cancer 2003, 106: 334–341.

[65] Lee Y, Yun Y: HBx protein of hepatitis B virus activates Jak1-STAT signaling. J. Biol. Chem. 1998, 273: 25510–25515.

[66] Zhang X, Zhang H, Ye L: Effects of hepatitis B virus X protein on the development of liver cancer. J. Lab. Clin. Med. 2006, 147: 58–66.

[67] Gressner A, Weiskirchen R: Modern pathogenetic concepts of liver fibrosis suggest stellate cells and TGF-β as major players and therapeutic targets. J. Cell. Mol. Med. 2006, 10: 76–99.

[68] Yoo YD, Ueda H, Park K, Flanders KC, Lee YI, Jay G, Kim SJ: Regulation of transforming growth factor-beta 1 expression by the hepatitis B virus (HBV) X transactivator. Role in HBV pathogenesis. J. Clin. Invest. 1996, 97: 388–395.

[69] Lee DK, Park SH, Yi Y, Choi SG, Lee C, Parks WT, Cho H, de Caestecker MP, Shaul Y, Roberts AB, Kim SJ: The hepatitis B virus encoded oncoprotein pX amplifies TGF-beta family signaling through direct interaction with Smad4: potential mechanism of hepatitis B virus-induced liver fibrosis. Genes Dev. 2001, 15: 455–466.

[70] Murata M, Matsuzaki K, Yoshida K, Sekimoto G, Tahashi Y, Mori S, Uemura Y, Sakaida N, Fujisawa J, Seki T: Hepatitis B virus X protein shifts human hepatic transforming growth factor (TGF)-β signaling from tumor suppression to oncogenesis in early chronic hepatitis B. Hepatology 2009, 49: 1203–1217.

[71] Murata M, Thanan R, Ma N, Kawanishi S: Role of nitrative and oxidative DNA damage in inflammation-related carcinogenesis. J. Biomed. Biotechnol. 2012, 2012: 623019.

[72] Lim W, Kwon S, Cho H, Kim S, Lee S, Ryu W, Cho H: HBx targeting to mitochondria and ROS generation are necessary but insufficient for HBV-induced cyclooxygenase-2 expression. J. Mol. Med. 2010, 88: 359–369.

[73] Zheng D, Zhang L, Cheng N, Xu X, Deng Q, Teng X, Wang K, Zhang X, Huang J, Han Z: Epigenetic modification induced by hepatitis B virus X protein via interaction with de novo DNA methyltransferase DNMT3A. J. Hepatol. 2009, 50: 377–387.

[74] Lee J, Kwun HJ, Jung JK, Choi KH, Jang KL: Hepatitis B virus X protein represses E-cadherin expression via activation of DNA methyltransferase 1. Oncogene 2005, 24: 6617–6625.

[75] Liu J, Lian Z, Han S, Waye M, Wang H, Wu M, Wu K, Ding J, Arbuthnot P, Kew M: Downregulation of E-cadherin by hepatitis B virus X antigen in hepatocellullar carcinoma. Oncogene 2006, 25: 1008–1017.

[76] Zhao J, Wu G, Bu F, Lu B, Liang A, Cao L: Epigenetic silence of ankyrin-repeat-containing, and proline-rich region-containing protein 1 (ASPP1) and ASPP2 genes promote tumour growth in hepatitis B virus-positive hepatocellular carcinoma. Hepatology 2010, 51: 142–153.

[77] Jung JK, Arora P, Pagano JS, Jang KL: Expression of DNA methyltransferase 1 is activated by hepatitis B virus X protein via a regulatory circuit involving the p16INK4a-cyclin D1-CDK 4/6-pRb-E2F1 pathway. Cancer Res. 2007, 67: 5771–5778.

[78] Niu D, Feng H, Chen WN: DLEC1 Expression is modulated by epigenetic modifications in hepatocelluar carcinoma cells: role of HBx genotypes. Cancers 2010, 2: 1689–1704.

[79] Tse T, Yuk E, Ko F, Chi F, Tung K, Kwok E, Chan LK, Lee W, Kin T, Ngan W: Caveolin-1 overexpression is associated with hepatocellular carcinoma tumourigenesis and metastasis. J. Pathol. 2012, 226: 645–653.

[80] Yan J, Lu Q, Dong J, Li X, Ma K, Cai L: Hepatitis B virus X protein suppresses caveolin-1 expression in hepatocellular carcinoma by regulating DNA methylation. BMC Cancer 2012, 12: 353.

[81] Zhu Y, Zhu R, Fan J, Pan Q, Li H, Chen Q, Zhu H: Hepatitis B virus X protein induces hypermethylation of p16INK4A promoter via DNA methyltransferases in the early stage of HBV-associated hepatocarcinogenesis. J.Viral Hepat. 2010, 17: 98–107.

[82] Ferber MJ, Montoya D, Yu C, Aderca I, McGee A, Thorland EC, Nagorney D, Gostout B, Burgart L, Boix L: Integrations of the hepatitis B virus (HBV) and human papillomavirus (HPV) into the human telomerase reverse transcriptase (hTERT) gene in liver and cervical cancers. Oncogene 2003, 22: 3813–3820.

[83] Takai D, Yagi Y, Habib N, Sugimura T, Ushijima T: Hypomethylation of LINE1 retrotransposon in human hepatocellular carcinomas, but not in surrounding liver cirrhosis. Jpn. J. Clin. Oncol. 2000, 30: 306–309.

[84] Kgatle MM, Spearman CW, Wayne M, Ramesar R, Kalla AA, Kandpal M, Vivekanandan P, Hairwadzi HN: Genome-wide analysis of core promoter region cytosine-phosphate-guanine islands hypermethylation profiles in chronic hepatitis B virus patients in South Africa. J. Med. Health Sci. 2016, 6.

[85] Tao R, Li J, Xin J, Wu J, Guo J, Zhang L, Jiang L, Zhang W, Yang Z, Li L: Methylation profile of single hepatocytes derived from hepatitis B virus-related hepatocellular carcinoma. PLoS One 2011, 6: e19862.

[86] Zhao Y, Xue F, Sun J, Guo S, Zhang H, Qiu B, Geng J, Gu J, Zhou X, Wang W: Genome-wide methylation profiling of the different stages of hepatitis B virus-related hepatocellular carcinoma development in plasma cell-free DNA reveals potential biomarkers for early detection and high-risk monitoring of hepatocellular carcinoma. Clin. Epigenet. 2014, 6: 1.

Chapter 9

Response-Guided Therapy Based on the Combination of Quantitative HBsAg and HBV DNA Kinetics in Chronic Hepatitis B Patients

Valeriu Gheorghiță and Florin Alexandru Căruntu

Additional information is available at the end of the chapter

http://dx.doi.org/10.5772/67128

Abstract

Chronic hepatitis B (CHB) remains a difficult-to-treat disease because no current treatments provide an optimal virological and immunological control, there is a high rate of relapse following any antiviral therapy, and there are no identified clinical useful treatment stopping rules, especially in hepatitis B e antigen (HBeAg)-negative patients treated with nucleoside or nucleotide analogues (NUCs). Taking into account the limited options of antiviral drugs, the response-guided therapy seems to be the best approach for optimization of treatment response. Hepatitis B surface antigen (HBsAg) can be considered a surrogate marker of HBV immune control during antiviral therapy, regardless of virological response reflected by serum HBV DNA. Thus, the decrease of HBV DNA level represents a reduction of viral replication, while serum HBsAg decline signifies a reduction of messenger RNA translation. The most important on-treatment predictors of the antiviral treatment response, especially Peg-IFN α-2a, are the quantitative HBsAg and HBV DNA evolution during therapy. A combination of no HBsAg decline and <2 log10 IU/mL decrease of HBV DNA seems to be a predictor of nonresponse in European HBeAg-negative patients with genotype D. The reduction of HBsAg levels during NUCs treatment in HBeAg-positive patients may identify cases with subsequent HBeAg or HBsAg loss.

Keywords: chronic hepatitis B, antiviral treatment strategy, quantitative HBsAg, algorithm of chronic hepatitis B treatment

1. Introduction

Worldwide, hepatitis B virus (HBV) infection has a high prevalence (350–400 million people are chronic HBV surface antigen carriers) and an increased morbidity and mortality (0.5–1 million deaths annually) [1]. To date, chronic hepatitis B (CHB) remains a difficult-to-treat disease due to the inability to achieve an optimal viral and immunological control with the available treatments, the high rate of relapse following any antiviral therapy and the absence of clinically useful predictors of sustained serological and viral responses.

Although existing potent nucleoside and nucleotide analogues (NUCs) with high genetic barriers have improved patient prognosis via suppression of viral load, there are still concerns that need to be addressed such as the need for long-term therapy, reactivation of the disease after cessation of therapy, hepatocellular carcinoma (HCC) risk persistence and the low rate of hepatitis B surface antigen (HBsAg) seroconversion.

In the last years, many published studies assessed the role of serum HBsAg quantification as predictor of treatment response in CHB patients treated mainly with pegylated interferon (Peg-IFN)-based regimens [2]. Some authors have proposed an early stopping rule using the combination between serum HBsAg and HBV DNA levels for hepatitis B e antigen (HBeAg)-negative CHB patients treated with Peg-IFN α-2a [2, 3].

2. Natural history of chronic hepatitis B

CHB is distinguished in five different phases according to HBeAg status, HBV DNA level, HBsAg status, alanine aminotransferase (ALT) level and histologic damages [1, 4]. Thus, the five evolutionary phases are as follow: the "immune-tolerant" phase, the "immune-active" HBeAg-positive phase, the "inactive HBV carrier" state, the "immune-escape" HBeAg-negative phase and the HBsAg-negative phase or "occult" HBV infection phase [1, 4]. In the evolution of chronic HBV infection, a patient may pass through each phase consecutively, especially after vertical transmission of the virus. Also, some phases are not identifiable in every patients, either because it may not be an obligatory step in the overall natural course of the infection or because it is of very short duration [5]. This feature seems to be dependent on age at the time of infection and the host immune reactivity against the virus.

The "immune-tolerant" phase is recognized usually in perinatally HBV-infected patients, which may last for about one to four decades in different populations and individuals [4, 5]. There is a highly replicative phase of the virus denoted by the presence of the HBeAg and high levels of HBV DNA ($>2 \times 10^7$ IU/mL) in the serum despite a low inflammatory reaction reflected by normal ALT levels (<19 U/L for females and <30 U/L for males) and mild or no liver inflammation and no or slow progression of fibrosis [1, 2, 4, 5].

The "immune-active" phase, in which the immune system is trying to eliminate the virus, is defined by the HBeAg positivity in conjunction with high or fluctuating serum HBV DNA levels, persistent or intermittent elevation of ALT levels and active inflammation with accelerated progression of fibrosis compared to the previous phase [1, 2, 5]. The hallmark of transition to the inactive phase of chronic HBV infection is the HBeAg seroconversion achieved in the natural course of the disease or therapeutically induced.

The "inactive HBV carrier" state represents the most desirable phase of the disease for HBsAg-positive patients. It is characterized by absence of HBeAg, positive anti-HBe, persistently normal ALT values, low or undetectable HBV DNA (usually <2000 IU/mL) and mild or no inflammatory reaction on liver histology [1, 2, 5]. In clinical practice, one of the main issues is to distinguish between truly inactive HBV carriers and HBeAg-negative active CHB phase. It is well known that HBeAg-negative CHB patients could have intermittent normal transaminases and relatively low level of viral replication. However, these patients often have a long-term chronic HBV infection with advanced fibrosis score and a high probability of progression in the absence of treatment intervention. Considering that, we reinforced the recommendation to regularly check these patients based on individual clinical and biological characteristics.

The "immune-escape" phase may follow either by a spontaneous HBeAg seroconversion to anti-HBe (10–30%) or by reactivation of HBV replication and exacerbations of hepatitis following years of persistent inactive carrier state (10–20%) [1, 2, 5]. Moreover, this phase is defined by a fluctuating evolution of the disease activity with intermittent increase in ALT and HBV DNA serum levels [2]. Most of the patients harbor a pre-core or core promoter HBV variants which are unable to express or express low levels of HBeAg [1, 2].

The "occult" HBV infection phase follows after HBsAg disappearance and represents the persistence of minimum viral replication with detectable HBV DNA into the liver and no or low levels of HBV DNA in serum (<200 IU/mL) [1]. The clinical relevance of this phase is explained by the increasing number of patients who need immunosuppressive or cytotoxic therapy. Thus, to avoid the reactivation of the HBV replication, all guidelines recommend checking for HBsAg, immune globulins G (IgG) anti-HBc, anti-HBs, ALT and HBV DNA serum levels in conjunction with preemptive antiviral therapy depending on the blood test results and type of immunosuppressive agent [1, 2, 5, 9].

3. Treatment objective

As HBV cannot be truly eliminated with available treatment due to the persistence of covalently closed circular (ccc) DNA into the nuclei of the hepatocytes, the current goal of therapy in patients with CHB is improving the quality of life and prolonging their life expectancy by preventing the progression of the disease to the cirrhosis, decompensated cirrhosis, end-stage liver disease, hepatocellular carcinoma (HCC) and deaths [1, 2]. One of the efficient strategies to reach this goal is achieving and maintaining indefinitely the complete inhibition of viral replication. HBsAg loss and anti-HBs seroconversion, events rarely achieved nowadays, represent the ultimate aim of any antiviral treatment strategy and reflect especially the immune control of the virus without need for further medication, except decompensated cirrhosis or necessity of cytotoxic/immunosuppressive prolonged treatment [4].

Virtually, all patients diagnosed with chronic HBV infection are potential candidates for antiviral therapy. However, considering that current antiviral cannot completely eradicate the virus, all international guidelines agree that treatment is not required in the immune-tolerant phase and inactive carrier state of chronic HBV infection [1, 2, 5, 6]. In addition, it has been proved that patients with CHB who persist for years in immune-tolerant phase or inactive carrier state do not register a significant disease progression and the likelihood of response, in particular HBeAg seroconversion, is very low (<5%) [6, 7]. Nevertheless, even in these populations some controversy still remains about the risk of developing HCC and the risk of virus transmission into the population, respectively. The REVEAL (Risk Evaluation of Viral Load Elevation and Associated Liver Disease/Cancer) study has been concluded that persistently high serum HBV DNA levels are associated with increased risk of cirrhosis, HCC and liver-related death. On the other hand, 67% of populations in this study were older than age 39 [8]. For all these reasons some experts have proposed that immune-tolerant patients older than age of 40 should receive antiviral treatment, especially if they have elevated HBV DNA (>10^6 IU/mL) and significant necroinflammation or fibrosis [2, 6]. Given that HBV infection is a chronic and dynamic condition, having the possibility of crossing a stage to the other and vice versa, regular monitoring is critical in patients without indication for antiviral therapy at a single-point assessment, in order to identify the best timing for treatment intervention [6].

From the clinical perspective, usually the decision to initiate the antiviral treatment in patients diagnosed with HBV infections is made by taking into consideration several important parameters: clinical status, ALT and HBV DNA levels, HBeAg status and the severity of liver inflammation and fibrosis [1, 2, 5, 6]. Indications for treatment may also depend on age, familial history of HCC, coinfection with other viruses, immunosuppression conditions, planning to become pregnant within the next 2–3 years in female patients [1, 6]. There are some absolute indications for antiviral treatment necessity such as HBV infection–associated life-threatening liver disease: acute liver failure or severe acute hepatitis (prolonged jaundice and coagulation abnormality), decompensated cirrhosis, severe exacerbation of CHB as well as for preventing reactivation in patients receiving immunosuppressive therapy, regardless of HBV DNA and ALT levels [1, 2, 5, 6]. In patients with compensated cirrhosis, we follow the European Association for the Study of the Liver (EASL) guideline which recommends antiviral treatment when the serum HBV DNA is detectable, irrespective of ALT levels [1]. In supporting of this approach, we mention the availability of potent NUCs with high genetic barrier to resistance along with slowing the progression of the disease to decompensated cirrhosis, end-stage liver disease and death. In noncirrhotic CHB patients, the treatment is generally recommended when they have a serum HBV DNA levels above 2000 IU/mL, persistently increased ALT levels above upper limit of normal (ULN) and/or histologic assessment showing moderate/severe inflammation or fibrosis [1, 6]. However, there are slight differences between the guidelines regarding the cutoff for HBV DNA and ALT values and the need for liver biopsy in order to establish the indication for antiviral treatment.

The EASL guideline recommends an HBV DNA cutoff value of 2000 IU/mL for initiating treatment, irrespective of HBeAg status [1]. The American Association for the Study of Liver Disease (AASLD) and Asian Pacific Association for the Study of the Liver (APASL) guidelines suggest an HBV DNA level of 20,000 IU/mL for HBeAg-positive patients and 2000 IU/mL for

HBeAg-negative patients [2]. All international guidelines agree that, for patients who fulfill the criteria for HBV DNA, treatment should be recommended whenever the ALT levels are above 2×ULN or less than 2×ULN, even in normal range, whether are evidences for moderate/severe inflammation or fibrosis [1, 2, 5].

4. Antiviral treatment strategy with available options: Peg-IFN and NUCs

To date, there are currently available two different classes of antiviral agents for treatment of CHB patients: IFN-α (conventional or pegylated) and oral drugs (NUCs) [4]. Despite the availability of seven approved drugs, only three of them are preferred as first-line options in the international American and European guidelines, as follow: Peg-IFN α-2a, entecavir (ETV) and tenofovir (TDF). Obviously, each of these agents is selected based on patient characteristics, considering that neither IFN nor NUCs are the best treatment options in any clinical condition. Thus, baseline as well as on-treatment predictive markers are needed to identify which patients benefit most from a finite course of IFN treatment or indefinite treatment with oral NUCs.

Both IFN-alfa and NUCs have different mechanisms of action in order to achieve the predefined goals of treatment in CHB patients: ALT normalization, suppression of viral replication, HBeAg and HBsAg seroconversion [9]. In addition, the reduction of the risk of progression to cirrhosis and HCC are among the desired therapeutic objectives [9].

IFN is a pro-inflammatory cytokine with dual mechanism of action, both antiviral and immunomodulatory activities, enhancing host immunity defense against HBV, which may lead to a sustained off-therapy response known as immune control [5, 6, 9]. Although the antiviral potency of IFN (Peg-IFN, respectively) is modest, the international guidelines have positioned it in the first-line treatment option, considering the major advantages associated with usage of this drug: finite duration of therapy, immunomodulatory effect with the potential to increase the chance of HBeAg and HBsAg seroconversion as well as a long-term immune control of the disease at least in a well-selected population [1, 2, 5, 10]. In addition, the National Institute for Health and Care Excellence (NICE) guideline for CHB recommend that a 48-week course of Peg-IFN α-2a should be offered as first-line treatment in adults with HBeAg-positive and-negative CHB and compensated liver disease [10].

It has been identified pretreatment predictors of IFN/Peg-IFN α-2a response in HBeAg-positive CHB patients: young age, high serum ALT levels (>2×ULN), low viral load, HBV genotype A and B, high histologic activity index and wild-type pre-core and basal-core promoter sequence [6, 9]. In HBeAg-negative patients, there were no such well-defined baseline predictors of IFN treatment [6]. From the clinical point of view, the presence of these baseline predictors in an individual patient with CHB does not assure the response to a 48-week course of Peg-IFN treatment. For this reason, of great significance are early predictive factors, such as ALT flares and quantitative HBsAg decline at 12 and 24 weeks during treatment [11–13].

On the other hand, there are some limitations of IFN-based treatment in CHB due to the parenteral weekly administration, the broad spectrum of side effects and the restriction of administration in several circumstances of the disease according to licensed indications (e.g., decompensated cirrhosis, uncontrolled psychiatric illness, pregnancy, hematologic neoplasia with need for cytotoxic or immunosuppressive treatment) [14].

NUCs, known as drugs with direct antiviral mechanism of action, targeting the HBV polymerase, represent another major class available in the therapeutic armamentarium of CHB. These antiviral drugs have become the mainstay therapy in CHB given the oral administration, the easy management, the absence of contraindications to start treatment, the high antiviral potency and a narrow spectrum of side effects [6, 9]. Among the available NUCs, lamivudine (LAM), telbivudine (LdT) and adefovir (ADV) are no longer recommended as first-line monotherapy because of the resistance concerns, while ETV and TDF are ranked by all international guidelines in the pole position of antiviral treatment [1, 2, 5].

Mitochondrial toxicity is a potential side effect of any NUCs, but fortunately is very rare event. There are reported specific side effects for each NUC, such as myopathy and neuropathy related to LdT, lactic acidosis related with administration of ETV in patients with severely impaired liver function and renal dysfunction and bone mineral density impairment in patients treated with ADV and TDF [6].

ETV and TDF suppress viral replication in over 90% of CHB patients within a defined period of time (months to years), although undetectable HBV DNA is much faster achieved when the baseline viral load is lower [9]. Furthermore, HBeAg seroconversion rate increase over time with around 40% in Asian studies and 20% of HBeAg-positive, genotype A, patients from Europe, respectively, while HBsAg seroconversion occurs in approximately 3–10% of all CHB patients over 5 years of follow-up [6, 9]. Despite the inability of NUCs to act directly on the cccDNA, the level of the intrahepatic cccDNA seems to decrease over prolonged treatment with NUCs, as the nuclear replenishment with new chains of viral DNA is interfered by blocking the transcription of pregenomic viral RNA. It is estimated that with current NUCs treatment, the median number of years needed to clear HBsAg is 52.2 years [15]. The similar study predicted a median time for HBsAg loss of 36 years in HBeAg-positive and 39 years in HBeAg-negative HBV infection, respectively [16]. High baseline ALT level seems to be the most important pretreatment predictor of response to NUC treatment in HBeAg-positive patients [6]. In the HBeAg-negative CHB patients, there have not been defined baseline predictors of treatment with NUCs [6]. Unlike Peg-IFN treatment, it has not been demonstrated that HBV genotype could influence the NUCs treatment response [6].

The long-term completely viral suppression is associated with liver histology improvement and in some patients even with reversion of cirrhosis over a treatment period of 5 years [17, 18]. The impact of long-term treatment with NUCs on HCC risk is questionable. At least from the theoretically point of view, the inhibition of viral replication could decrease the cumulative incidence of HCC, considering that HBV DNA levels have been identified as an independent risk factor for HCC occurrence [8]. Thus, there have been published some studies which established that long-term treatment with potent NUCs have been linked to the reduction of the incidence of HCC [19, 20]. On the opposite, the risk of HCC could not be eliminated with any available treatments because of the truncated sequences of HBs genes integrated in the DNA of the infected hepatocytes, which is believed to be associated with carcinogenesis.

However, it is still unresolved issue related to the NUCs treatment in CHB, such as the safety of long-term usage of these antivirals, the extent of the optimal duration of treatment and when the treatment discontinuation is suitable [21]. Despite the highest antiviral efficacy, NUCs do not have immunomodulatory effects and induce only a transient increase of immune activity, being unlikely to provide a sustained off-treatment control of viral replication [21]. Thus, treatment with NUCs is indefinite in most cases. It has been proposed that the best and safest endpoint for NUCs discontinuation in any CHB patient is HBsAg seroconversion, defined as HBsAg loss and anti-HBs appearance at a level over 100–200 IU/mL [9]. However, around 30% of patients who achieve HBsAg loss during NUCs treatment do not develop anti-HBs even with prolongation of antiviral treatment [9]. According to the guidelines, the NUCs treatment endpoints in CHB patients are different depending on the HBeAg status. In HBeAg-positive CHB, it seems reasonable to discontinue the NUCs treatment in noncirrhotic patients who undergone HBeAg seroconversion and who have maintained the undetectable HBV DNA at least 1 year thereafter, although approximately 50% relapse [1, 9]. On the other hand, indefinite treatment with NUCs is necessary for HBeAg-negative patients and HBeAg-positive patients who do not develop anti-HBe seroconversion [1]. The same approach is recommended in patients with cirrhosis irrespective of HBeAg status or anti-HBe seroconversion on treatment [1]. In some instances, discontinuations could be attempted in HBeAg-negative patients after treatment for at least 2 years (preferably 4–5 years) with undetectable HBV DNA documented on three separate occasions, 6 months apart [5, 9]. Once it has been decided to stop the NUC-based treatment, regular monitoring of virological and biochemical parameters is mandatory, considering that there are potential life-threatening clinical consequences associated with NUCs discontinuation such as hepatitis flare and hepatic decompensation [9].

5. Response-guided therapy based on serum HBsAg and HBV DNA kinetics

One of the modern and cost-efficient concepts in the management of CHB in terms of antiviral treatment is "response guided therapy" depending on the kinetics of the serum HBsAg and HBV DNA levels during treatment. In the current international guidelines, there are some validated rules that support either continuation of antiviral regimen, based on a positive prediction of response, or contrary, cessation/switching therapy to another regimen, depending on a high negative prediction of sustained response.

The clinical relevance of quantitative serum HBsAg arises from the correlation with the intrahepatic amount and transcriptional activity of cccDNA, the main replicative template of HBV [22–24]. It is assumed that quantitative HBsAg could be used as a surrogate marker for immune control of the virus, regardless of the HBV DNA response during treatment and thereafter [23]. A HBV DNA decline directly reflects a reduction of viral replication, while serum HBsAg decline signifies a reduction of transcriptional activity of intranuclear cccDNA and integrated DNA sequences [24, 25].

Several studies have been published to identify the useful surrogate markers for selecting the initial antiviral regimen, for guiding the treatment as well as for early prediction of the favorable or unfavorable outcome [4]. These markers have been stratified as pretreatment and on-treatment predictors. The majority of the studies have investigated the significance of HBsAg and HBV DNA levels as the most powerful predictive factors for antiviral treatment response. It is well known that the most important decrease of HBsAg levels occurred during the Peg-IFN treatment because of the dual mechanism of action, including the modulation of the immune activity. On the other hand, the long-term treatment with NUCs induces only a minimal reduction of serum HBsAg, especially in HBeAg-positive patients. Thus, the HBsAg quantification has various benefits in the management of CHB patients depending on the HBeAg status and the antiviral treatment.

Quantification of HBsAg levels can be used to guide the treatment with Peg-IFN α-2a. In addition, different studies proposed the role of HBsAg level as a "stopping rule" at week 12 of Peg-IFN treatment in both HBeAg-positive and HBeAg-negative patients [5].

In HBeAg-positive CHB patients with genotype A and D, an absence of any HBsAg decline at 12 weeks of Peg-IFN treatment has been associated with a negative predictive value (NPV) of 97% for sustained response [26]. Moreover, in HBeAg-positive, genotype B and C chronic HBV infections, it has been observed that a level of HBsAg over 20,000 IU/mL at 12 weeks of treatment with Peg-IFN could predict a low chance of HBeAg seroconversion [1, 5]. Thus, the European and Asian guidelines have proposed an early stopping rule in CHB, HBeAg-positive patients, who do not achieve any HBsAg decline or who have an HBsAg levels over 20,000 IU/mL after 12 weeks of Peg-IFN-based treatment [1, 5]. Also, a level of HBsAg over 20,000 IU/mL at 24 weeks could be applied as another stopping rule, irrespective of HBV genotype [27]. Overall, around 20–30% of the HBeAg-positive patients would be eligible for an early stopping of treatment with Peg-IFN, at 12/24 weeks, due to the high negative prediction of the sustained response after 48 weeks course of standard of care [9]. On the other hand, it has been proved that HBeAg seroconversion rates 6 months posttreatment were significantly higher in patients with HBsAg <1500 IU/mL at weeks 12 and 24 (56.7 and 54.4%, respectively) versus patients with HBsAg <20,000 IU/mL (16.3 and 15.4%, respectively) [28]. Another on-treatment positive predictor is based on HBV DNA decline at 12 weeks. An HBV DNA level less than 20,000 IU/mL has been associated with 50% chance of anti-HBe seroconversion [29].

In HBeAg-negative genotype D patients treated with Peg-IFN α-2a, it has been validated a stopping rule depending on a combination of HBsAg and HBV DNA assessment at 12 weeks. According to this rule, we can identify early, with a NPV of 100%, all CHB, HBeAg-negative, genotype D patients who will not achieve sustained response at 48 or 96 weeks of treatment with Peg-IFN α-2a [30]. A less than 10% decline of HBsAg levels at 12 weeks for patients with nongenotype D infections and at 24 weeks for genotype D has been shown to be associated with 16% probability of treatment response at 1 year posttherapy [31]. Similar to HBeAg-positive patients, approximately 50% of HBeAg-negative CHB patients with an HBV DNA decrease <20,000 IU/mL at 12 weeks during Peg-IFN treatment would achieve a sustained off-treatment response [1].

In 2013, we published a Romanian real-life small cohort study which included 57 patients with CHB treated 48 weeks with Peg-IFN α-2a and followed for another 24 weeks. The majority of patients had HBeAg-negative CHB (68%, $n = 39$) and genotype D (approximately 80%). During treatment, patients who achieved sustained response showed a marked decrease in serum HBsAg in comparison with non-responders (mean decrease of 1.06 ± 1.3 $\log_{10}$ IU/mL versus 0.04 ± 0.5 $\log_{10}$ IU/mL at 48 weeks, $p = 0.005$). On therapy, HBV DNA reduction >2 $\log_{10}$ IU/mL with any decrease of HBsAg level at week 12 had a positive predictive value (PPV) of 80% (95% CI: 51.91–95.43%) for sustained response, while HBV DNA decline <2 $\log_{10}$ IU/mL without any decline of HBsAg had a NPV of 85.71% (95% CI: 42.23–97.63%) for sustained response. One interesting findings of our study showed that relapsers had the same HBsAg declining profile as non-responder patients [3].

Considering that the rate of virological relapse after cessation of NUCs treatment is estimated to be 50%, the decline of HBsAg may help identify patients in whom treatment can be safely stopped without a high risk of relapse. Together with serum ALT and HBV DNA assessment, HBsAg quantification has been proposed as a clinically useful tool to monitor treatment responses during NUCs treatment, especially the prediction of future HBsAg loss [4].

The magnitude of HBsAg reduction during NUCs treatment could also predict the later HBsAg loss [4]. An HBsAg decline more than 1 $\log_{10}$ IU/mL after 1 year of oral antiviral treatment in HBeAg-positive CHB patients have been shown to predict the HBsAg loss [32].

Lower HBsAg levels at the end of treatment were predictive for later HBsAg loss, as well as for maintenance of HBV suppression after discontinuation of long-term NUCs treatment [4].

In HBeAg-positive CHB patients, an HBsAg levels <100 IU/mL was highly predictive of sustained response at 2 years off treatment [33]. In a recent Asian study, it has been showed that post-treatment virological relapse rate was significantly higher in patients over 50 years old and in patients with an HBsAg level >2 $\log_{10}$ IU/mL at the ETV cessation [34]. In the same study, an HBsAg level of 2.5 $\log_{10}$ IU/mL at HBeAg seroconversion has been established as an optimal cutoff for prediction of post-treatment virological relapse [34]. Thus, patients aged <50 years who achieved an HBsAg level <2.5 $\log_{10}$ IU/mL at HBeAg seroconversion had the lowest rate of relapse, 5% respectively [34]. In HBeAg-positive CHB patients treated with ETV, a serum HBsAg level below 2.5 $\log_{10}$ IU/mL at HBeAg seroconversion could be a useful predictor of post-treatment virological relapse [34].

Although previous studies have shown that quantitative HBsAg levels could be a useful predictor of relapse after cessation of treatment with NUCs in HBeAg-negative patients, in other recent prospective studies, neither HBsAg level at the end of treatment nor the kinetics of HBsAg were not able to predict the off-treatment relapse [35]. However, at the end of treatment, both HBsAg ≤2 $\log_{10}$ IU/mL and reduction by >1 $\log_{10}$ IU/mL from baseline were associated with a sustained virological response, defined as HBV DNA <200 IU/mL 12 month posttreatment [36].

6. Other clinical benefits of serum HBsAg quantifications in management of chronic hepatitis B

Since its discovery, besides the using of qualitative HBsAg as a diagnostic marker, there have been identified several roles of HBsAg in the management of chronic HBV infections, as follows.

6.1. Defining different phases of CHB

It is well known that HBsAg levels vary during the natural history of chronic HBV infections [3]. The highest values of HBsAg are reported in immune-tolerant phase (5.0 $\log_{10}$ IU/mL for HBsAg) and progressively decrease in "immune-active" phase (medium level of 3.0–4.0 $\log_{10}$ IU/mL) [24, 37, 38]. The lowest values of HBsAg levels have been reported in the "inactive carrier state" [24, 38]. Moreover, there is a variability of the quantitative HBsAg across different viral genotypes [3]. Patients with genotype A and D have the highest mean value of serum HBsAg (4.5 $\log_{10}$ IU/mL) compared to genotypes B and C (4.3 $\log_{10}$ IU/mL and 3.8 $\log_{10}$ IU/mL, respectively) [32, 39].

From the clinical point of view, combining a single-point determination of HBsAg <1500 IU/mL and HBV DNA <2000 IU/mL may identify "true inactive carriers" with a NPV of 96.7% for genotype D CHB patients [40]. This strategy could be useful especially in HBeAg-negative CHB patients with an HBV DNA level around 2000 IU/mL and normal transaminases, considering that in some patients is difficult to distinguish between active HBeAg-negative hepatitis and inactive carriers.

6.2. Predictor of liver fibrosis

Both HBV DNA and HBsAg levels have a declining evolution as long as liver disease progress from the immune-tolerant status to the active hepatitis and cirrhosis in HBeAg-positive patients [41]. Although previous studies showed that HBV DNA level could predict the risk of cirrhosis and HCC, it has been proved a poor correlation between HBsAg level and HBV DNA across different phases of the chronic HBV infection [8, 41]. Given that ALT measurement is a suboptimal marker for prediction of significant liver disease, it is recommended to have, as accurate as possible, an estimation of fibrosis and inflammation based on a reliable tool in order to decide antiviral treatment indication [42]. Nowadays, liver biopsy became rarely used in evaluation of patients with chronic hepatitis viral diseases due to the risk of the procedure, inter- and intraobservers variability, costs, as well as the availability of several noninvasive tests. All international guidelines agree that any HBV carriers who fulfill the criteria of HBV DNA have indication of antiviral treatment, whether there are evidences of significant necroinflammation and/or moderate/severe fibrosis [1, 2, 5]. Transient elastography, an imaging noninvasive test for assessing liver fibrosis, has a low accuracy in distinguished between intermediate stages of fibrosis (F1–F3). Also, the results are influenced by some confounding factors such as steatosis, ALT elevation [43].

There is emerging evidence suggesting association between HBsAg level and liver fibrosis stage in HBeAg-positive CHB patients. It has been proposed different cutoff levels of HBsAg for prediction of liver fibrosis among HBeAg-positive patients. Thus, serum HBsAg over 100,000 IU/mL was 100% predictive of insignificant fibrosis in patients with ALT below 2×ULN [42]. In HBeAg-positive patients with ALT ≤2×ULN, an HBsAg level over 25,000 IU/mL has been proved to be the best independent predictor of insignificant liver fibrosis (PPV of 92.7%, odds ratio 9.042) [42]. Based on these results, it has been suggested that HBeAg-positive patients with ALT ≤2×ULN and HBsAg ≥ 25,000 IU/mL could be followed without the need of liver biopsy [42]. On the other hand, there are evidences which support that lower serum levels of HBsAg are associated with more severe liver fibrosis in HBeAg-positive CHB patients [41]. A cutoff of 4.7 $\log_{10}$ IU/mL predicted moderate to advanced fibrosis (F2-F4) in HBeAg-positive patients, with an accuracy of 89% and a NPV of 91% [41]. Thus, a single-point baseline assessment of HBsAg level in HBeAg-positive chronic HBV-infected patients could become an accurate surrogate marker for distinguish moderate to advanced fibrosis from no or mild fibrosis [41]. However, in HBeAg-negative patients, there were no reported significant differences in serum HBsAg levels between patients with moderate to severe fibrosis and those with no or mild fibrosis [41].

6.3. Predictor of HCC

One of the remaining concerns in the management of CHB patients is the individual prediction of the HCC risk. There is very well known that the risk of HCC cannot be eliminated with any available therapy because of integrated sequences of viral DNA into the host genome. Even in cases of acute HBV naturally resolved infections the risk of HCC is estimated to be very low but higher compared to the general populations. The REVEAL study showed that viral replication is the major driver of disease progression and is an individual risk factor for HCC occurrence in patients with baseline HBV DNA ≥2000 IU/mL [8]. From the clinical practice point of view, it is very important to identify risk factors for HCC in an individual with CHB in order to adjust our HCC screening strategy. There are preliminary data which suggest an existing correlation between higher HBsAg level and an increased risk of HCC appearance [44]. From the clinical point of view, a particular interest would be in noncirrhotic patients with low level of HBV DNA (<2000 IU/mL) in whom the risk of HCC is difficult to be estimated. Thus, in HBeAg-negative patients with HBV DNA <2000 IU/mL an HBsAg level ≥1000 IU/mL has been has been identified as a new independent risk factor of HCC with a hazard ratio of 13.7 (95% CI: 4.8–39.3) compared to patients with HBsAg level <1000 IU/mL [44]. Moreover, HBV DNA has not been associated with HCC risk in these patients. Contrary, in HBeAg-negative patients with HBV DNA level above 2000 IU/mL, the HCC risk has not been proved to be linked to serum HBsAg levels [44]. These data support the role of HBsAg as a complementary tool by the side of HBV DNA in predicting the risk of HCC occurrence. According to the existing evidences, high risk factors for HCC related to HBV chronic infection include male gender, age over 50 years, HBV genotype B and C, pre-core and basal-core promoter HBV variants, pre-S deletion mutants, high serum of ALT, HBV DNA ≥ 2000 IU/mL and last but not least HBsAg ≥1000 IU/mL in low viremic HBeAg-negative patients [45].

7. Conclusions

In summary, there have been identified several clinical benefits of using quantitative HBsAg in the management of CHB. In case of IFN-based treatment, the most important role of HBsAg measurement is attributed to the highest NPV for sustained post-treatment response. Thus, in routinely clinical practice, different early stopping rules after 12 weeks of treatment can be used, depending on the HBeAg status. In HBeAg-positive CHB patients, Peg-IFN should be stopped after 12 weeks whether HBsAg does not decline more than standard error or HBsAg level is above 20,000 IU/mL. In HBeAg-negative CHB patients, an absence of HBsAg reduction combined with a less than 2 $\log_{10}$ IU/mL decline of HBV DNA at week 12 of treatment should be used as another stopping rule. On the other hand, in NUCs treatment, the exact roles of the HBsAg have not been defined yet. However, one of the proposed roles of HBsAg quantification during long-term NUCs therapy is identifying those patients in whom treatment discontinuation can be safely decided. Moreover, there are robust evidences that support the role of HBsAg quantification as a useful tool for identification of true inactive HBV carriers, for distinguishing between HBeAg-positive patients with moderate to advanced fibrosis and no or mild fibrosis, as well as for predicting the risk of HCC occurrence especially in HBeAg-negative low viremic patients.

Author details

Valeriu Gheorghiță[1,2]* and Florin Alexandru Căruntu[1,3]

*Address all correspondence to: gvaleriu21@yahoo.com

1 "Carol Davila" University of Medicine and Pharmacy, Bucharest, Romania

2 "Carol Davila" Central Military Emergency University Hospital, Bucharest, Romania

3 National Institute for Infectious Diseases "Prof Dr Matei Balș," Bucharest, Romania

References

[1] European Association for the Study of the Liver. EASL clinical practice guidelines: management of chronic hepatitis B virus infection. Journal of Hepatology 2012; 57:167–185.

[2] Terrault NA, Bzowej NH, Chang K-M, Hwang JP, Jonas MM, Murad MH. American Association for the Study of Liver Diseases. AASLD guidelines for treatment of chronic hepatitis B. Hepatology 2015; 1–23.

[3] Gheorghita V, Caruntu FA, Curescu M et al. Use of quantitative serum HBsAg for optimization of therapy in chronic hepatitis B patients treated with pegylated interferon alfa-2a: a Romanian cohort study. J Gastrointestin Liver Dis 2013; 22 (1):27–32.

[4] Siederdissen CH, Cornberg M. The role of HBs Ag levels in the current management of chronic HBV infection. Annals of Gastroenterology 2014;27:105–112.

[5] Sarin S K, Kumar M, Lau GK et al. Asian-Pacific clinical practice guidelines on the management of hepatitis B: a 2015 update. Hepatol Int 2016;10:1–98.

[6] Yapali S, Talaat N, Lok AS. Management of hepatitis B: our practice and how it relates to the guidelines. Clinical Gastroenterology and Hepatology 2014;12:16–26.

[7] Chu CM, Hung SJ, Lin J, Tai DI, Liaw YF. Natural history of hepatitis B e antigen to antibody seroconversion in patients with normal serum aminotransferase levels. Am J Med 2004;116:829–834.

[8] Chen C, Yang HI, Su J, et al. Risk of hepatocellular carcinoma across a biological gradient of serum hepatitis b virus DNA level. JAMA. 2006;295(1):65–73.

[9] Lampertico P, Maini M, Papatheodoridis G. Optimal management of hepatitis B virus infection—EASL Special Conference. Journal of Hepatology 2015;63:1238–1253.

[10] Hepatitis B (chronic): Diagnosis and management of chronic hepatitis B in children, young people and adults. National Institute for Health and Care Excellence. National Clinical Guideline Centre, 2013 (https://www.nice.org.uk/guidance) 2 September 2016.

[11] Marcellin P, Lau GK, Bonino F, et al. Peginterferon alfa-2a alone, lamivudine alone, and the two in combination in patients with HBeAg-negative chronic hepatitis B. N Engl J Med 2004;351:1206–1217.

[12] Brunetto MR, Moriconi F, Bonino F, et al. Hepatitis B virus surface antigen levels: a guide to sustained response to peginterferon alfa-2a in HBeAg-negative chronic hepatitis B. Hepatology 2009;49:1141–1150.

[13] Moucari R, Mackiewicz V, Lada O, et al. Early serum HBsAg drop: a strong predictor of sustained virological response to pegylated interferon alfa-2a in HBeAg-negative patients. Hepatology 2009;49:1151–1157.

[14] Package Insert. PEGASYS® (peginterferon alfa-2a). Hoffmann-La Roche Inc. http://www.accessdata.fda.gov/drugsatfda_docs/label/2002/pegihof101602LB.htm. 2 September 2016.

[15] Chevaliez S, Hézode C, Bahrami S, Grare M, Pawlotsky J-M. Long-term hepatitis B surface antigen (HBsAg) kinetics during nucleoside/nucleotide analogue therapy: finite treatment duration unlikely. J Hepatol 2012;58:683–676.

[16] Zoutendijk R, Hansen BE, van Vuuren AJ, Boucher CAB, Janssen HLA. Serum HBsAg decline during long-term potent nucleos(t)ide analogue therapy for chronic hepatitis B and prediction of HBsAg loss. J Infect Dis 2011;204:415–418.

[17] Marcellin P, Gane E, Buti M, et al. Regression of cirrhosis during treatment with tenofovir disoproxil fumarate for chronic hepatitis B: a 5-year open-label follow-up study. Lancet 2013;381:468–475.

[18] Chang T-T, Liaw Y-F, Wu S-S, et al. Long-term entecavir therapy results in the reversal of fibrosis/cirrhosis and continued histological improvement in patients with chronic hepatitis B. Hepatology 2010;52:886–893.

[19] Papatheodoridis GV, Lampertico P, Manolakopoulos S, Lok A. Incidence of hepatocellular carcinoma in chronic hepatitis B patients receiving nucleos(t)ide therapy: a systematic review. J Hepatol 2010;53:348–356.

[20] Hosaka T, Suzuki F, Kobayashi M, et al. Long-term entecavir treatment reduces hepatocellular carcinoma incidence in patients with hepatitis B virus infection. Hepatology 2013;58:98–107.

[21] Lee CH. Oral antiviral therapy for chronic hepatitis b virus infection: is continuous treatment needed? Gastroenterol Hepatol Open Access 2014;1(1):00005. DOI: 10.15406/ghoa.2014.01.00005.

[22] Chan HL, Thompson A, Martinot-Peignoux M, et al. Hepatitis B surface antigen quantification: why and how to use it in 2011—a core group report. J Hepatol 2011;55:1121–1131.

[23] Sonneveld MJ, Zoutendijk R, Janssen HL. Hepatitis B surface antigen monitoring and management of chronic hepatitis B. J Viral Hepat 2011;18:449–457.

[24] Liaw YF. Clinical utility of hepatitis B surface antigen quantitation in patients with chronic hepatitis B: a review. Hepatology 2011; 53:2121–2129.

[25] Brunetto MR. A new role for an old marker, HBsAg. J Hepatol 2010;52:475–477.

[26] Sonneveld MJ, Rijckborst V, Boucher CA, Hansen BE, Janssen HL. Prediction of sustained response to peginterferon alfa-2b for hepatitis B e antigen-positive chronic hepatitis B using on treatment hepatitis B surface antigen decline. Hepatology 2010;52:1251–1257.

[27] Sonneveld MJ, Hansen BE, Piratvisuth T, et al. Response-guided peginterferon therapy in hepatitis B e antigen-positive chronic hepatitis B using serum hepatitis B surface antigen levels. Hepatology 2013;58:872–880.

[28] Piratvisuth T, Marcellin P, Popescu M, Kapprell HP, Rothe V, Lu ZM. Hepatitis B surface antigen: association with sustained response to peginterferon alfa-2a in hepatitis B e antigen-positive patients. Hepatol Int 2011;7(2):429–436.

[29] Fried MW, Piratvisuth T, Lau GK, et al. HBeAg and hepatitis B virus DNA as outcome predictors during therapy with peginterferon alfa-2a for HBeAg-positive chronic hepatitis B. Hepatology 2008;47:428–434.

[30] Rijckborst V, Hansen BE, Ferenci P, et al. Validation of a stopping rule at week 12 using HBsAg and HBV DNA for HBeAg-negative patients treated with peginterferon alfa-2a. J Hepatol 2012;56:1006–1011.

[31] Marcellin P, Bonino F, Yurdaydin C, et al. Hepatitis B surface antigen levels: association with 5-year response to peginterferon alfa-2a in hepatitis B e-antigen-negative patients. Hepatol Int 2013;7:88–97.

[32] Wursthorn K, Jung M, Riva A, et al. Kinetics of hepatitis B surface antigen decline during 3 years of telbivudine treatment in hepatitis B e antigen-positive patients. Hepatology 2010;52:1611–1120.

[33] Cai W, Xie Q, An B, et al. On-treatment serum HBsAg level is predictive of sustained off-treatment virologic response to telbivudine in HBeAg-positive chronic hepatitis B patients. J Clin Virol 2010;48:22–26.

[34] Qiu Y-w, Huang L-h, Yang W-l, et al. Hepatitis B surface antigen quantification at hepatitis B e antigen seroconversion predicts virological relapse after the cessation of entecavir treatment in hepatitis B e antigen-positive patients. Int J Infect Dis 2016;43:43–48.

[35] Jung KS, Park JY, Chon YE, et al. Clinical outcomes and predictors for relapse after cessation of oral antiviral treatment in chronic hepatitis B patients. J Gastroenterol 2016;51:830–839.

[36] Chan HL-Y, Wong GL-H, Chim AM-L, et al. Prediction of off treatment response to lamivudine by serum hepatitis B surface antigen quantification in hepatitis B e antigen-negative patients. Antivir Ther 2011;16:1249–1257.

[37] Chan HL, Wong VW, Wong GL, Tse CH, Chan HY, Sung JJ. A longitudinal study on the natural history of serum hepatitis B surface antigen changes in chronic hepatitis B. Hepatology 2010; 52:1232–1241.

[38] Jaroszewicz J, Calle Serrano B, Wursthorn K, et al. Hepatitis B surface antigen (HBsAg) levels in the natural history of hepatitis B virus (HBV)-infection: a European perspective. J Hepatol 2010; 52:514–522.

[39] Sonneveld MJ, Rijckborst V, Senturk H, et al. HBsAg decline during peginterferon alfa-2b therapy for HBeAg-positive chronic hepatitis B depends on HBV genotype: relation to sustained response. Hepatology 2010; 52: 441 (Abstract).

[40] Brunetto MR, Oliveri F, Colombatto P, et al. Hepatitis B surface antigen serum levels help to distinguish active from inactive hepatitis B virus genotype D carriers. Gastroenterology 2010; 139:483–490.

[41] Goyal SK, Jain AK, Dixit VK, et al. HBsAg level as predictor of liver fibrosis in HBeAg positive patients with chronic hepatitis B virus infection. J Clin Exp Hepatol 2015;5:213–220.

[42] Seto W-K, Wong DK-H, Fung J, et al. High hepatitis B surface antigen levels predict insignificant fibrosis in hepatitis B e antigen positive chronic hepatitis B. PLoS One. 2012;7(8):e43087/www.plosone.org.

[43] Fung J, Lai CL, Seto WK, Yuen MF. The use of transient elastography in the management of chronic hepatitis B. Hepatol Int 2011;5: 868–875.

[44] Tseng T-C, Liu C–J, Yang H–C, et al. High levels of hepatitis B surface antigen increase risk of hepatocellular carcinoma in patients with low HBV load. Gastroenterology 2012;142:1140–1149.

[45] Lin C-L, Kao J-H. Risk stratification for hepatitis B virus related hepatocellular carcinoma. J Gastroenterol Hepatol 2013;28:10–17.

Chapter 10

Current Management Strategies in Hepatitis B During Pregnancy

Letiția Adela Maria Streba, Anca Pătrașcu,
Aurelia Enescu and Costin Teodor Streba

Additional information is available at the end of the chapter

http://dx.doi.org/10.5772/66068

Abstract

Hepatitis B virus (HBV) infection remains a major health problem worldwide and a major risk factor for end-stage liver disease and hepatocellular carcinoma. Notable differences of chronic hepatitis B prevalence were observed in geographic area. In highly endemic areas, at least 50 % of HBV infections are most commonly acquired either perinatally or in early childhood, during the first 5 years of life. The prevalence of chronic HBV infection in pregnant women is expected to mirror those in the general populations of each geographic area. Chronic hepatitis B during pregnancy is associated with high risk of maternal complications and an increased risk of mother-to-child transmission (MTCT). Thus, chronic hepatitis B during pregnancy can now be considered an important contributor to new HBV infections and to the global burden of disease. As a result, HBV infection during pregnancy requires management strategies for both the mother and the fetus/neonate, including prevention/elimination of MTCT and lessening the HBV effects on maternal and fetal health. This chapter will review current management strategies for hepatitis B in the pregnancy and the postpartum period, including special considerations on the effects of pregnancy on the course of HBV infection, MTCT, and antiviral therapy during the pregnancy.

Keywords: hepatitis B virus, pregnancy, mother-to-child transmission, disease burden, antiviral treatment, HBV vaccination, hepatitis B immune globulin (HBIG)

1. Introduction

Hepatitis B is caused by hepatitis B virus (HBV), a partially double-stranded DNA virus, member of the Hepadnaviridae family. The hepatitis B virion is a 42-nm particle composed of a 27-nm nucleocapsid consisting of the hepatitis B core antigen (HBcAg) surrounded by an outer lipoprotein coat envelope containing the hepatitis B surface antigen (HBsAg) [1, 2].

To date, 10 HBV genotypes (A–J) have been defined based on intergroup divergence of above 8 % in the complete nucleotide sequence and over 30 subgenotypes. The genotypes show heterogeneity in their global geographic distribution and have also been associated with different clinical features and different responses to antiviral therapy [3–6].

HBV infection remains a major health problem worldwide and a major risk factor for end-stage liver disease and hepatocellular carcinoma. Two billion people worldwide have been infected with HBV, and more than 240 million people have chronic hepatitis B infection defined as HBsAg positive for more than 6 months. Despite the fact that in many countries HBV infections have declined substantially because of effective prevention strategies, more than 780,000 people die every year worldwide due to HBV complications, including cirrhosis and liver cancer [2].

HBV infection is transmitted by percutaneous and mucous membrane *via* blood or infected body fluids [7]. HBV mother-to-child transmission (MTCT), defined as HBsAg positivity at 6–12 months of life in an infant born to an infected mother, has been recognized as a major mode of transmission and at the same time the most important phase for the chronic hepatitis B prevention. In Asia, up to 50 % of new cases of HBV infection are due to MTCT [8–10]. In Europe, MTCT is the most important and frequent transmission route of HVB infection, which accounted for 41.1 % of all cases, according to the results of the first enhanced surveillance data collection of HVB infections across 30 countries of the European Union and the European Economic Area [11].

Infants born to HBsAg-positive mothers who do not become infected perinatally remain at risk of HBV infection during early childhood [12]. More than one third of patients with HBV acquired the infection during the perinatal period or in early childhood, even in low-endemic areas [13]. In highly endemic areas, at least 50 % of HBV infections are most commonly acquired either perinatally or in early childhood, during the first 5 years of life [2]. Moreover, the rate of chronicity is about 90 % for perinatally acquired HVB infection or during the first year of life, 30–50 % in infected children between ages 1 and 6 years, and 5–10 % in children over the age of 6 years and in adults [2, 14].

Thus, chronic hepatitis B during pregnancy is now an important contributor to the new HBV infections and to the global burden of disease.

2. Epidemiologic aspects of HBV infection in pregnant women

Notable differences of chronic hepatitis B prevalence were observed by geographic area, with the highest endemicity levels in the sub-Saharan Africa and East Asia (5–10 %) and low prevalence (<1 %) in the United States (USA), Canada, and Western Europe. High rates of prevalence have also been found in the southern regions of Eastern and Central Europe [2, 15].

According to the technical report of the European Centre for Disease Prevention and Control (ECDC), based on literature review, the prevalence of HBsAg in the general population ranged from 0.1 to more than 7 % by country. Countries in the central or southern part of the Europe (EU) have a higher prevalence of HBV infection than countries in the northern or western part of the EU. Thus, Romania, Greece, and Turkey have a high HBV prevalence (>2 %); Italy has medium HBV prevalence (>1 and ≤2 %), while Belgium, France, Spain, Germany, the Netherlands, Slovakia, Sweden, Switzerland, and the United Kingdom have a low HBV prevalence (≤1 %). Among countries with available data, Turkey has the largest number of HBV-infected individuals (national and regional estimates ranged from 2.5 to 9.0 % in adults and 1.7 to 2.7 % in children only), followed by Romania (5.6 %) [16].

The prevalence of chronic HBV infection in pregnant women is expected to mirror those in the general populations of each geographic area. Thus, in higher endemicity areas, rates are proportionately higher [9].

In the United States, a country of low endemicity, estimated chronic HBV infection prevalence in pregnant women is 0.7–0.9 % [17]. In Europe, the chronic HBV infection prevalence in pregnant women is generally higher than in the general population (0.1–4.4 %) in countries where both estimates were available (e.g., Germany, Greece, Ireland, Italy, the Netherlands, and Slovakia), according to the ECDC study. This difference in prevalence can be attributed to the fact that migrant women, whom have a relatively high HBV infection prevalence, are better represented in pregnancy studies than in general population studies. Conversely, Spain reported in Catalonia in 2004 a lower prevalence of chronic hepatitis B in pregnant women than the prevalence in the general population in the same region in 2002 (0.7 %), attributing these aspects to the higher vaccination rate [16]. In France, the prevalence of chronic HBV infection is about 1 % in pregnant women [18]. In Denmark, country where all pregnant women have been screened for HBV since November 2005, the overall prevalence of HBV infection among pregnant women has increased from 0.11 % in 1971 to 0.26 % in 2007. In the same period, the prevalence among pregnant native Danes decreased from 0.11 to 0.01 % [19].

Available data suggest a wide variation in prevalence of chronic HBV infection among pregnant women globally. However, there are insufficient epidemiological data and limitations to estimate the epidemiology of HVB infection among pregnant women globally.

3. Serological markers of HBV infection

Measurement of several HBV antigens and/or antibodies plays an important role in diagnosis, assessment, and monitoring the disease progression and its response to treatment.

There are three clinical useful antigen-antibody groups used in the serological diagnosis of HVB:

1. Hepatitis B surface antigen and antibody: antigen (HBsAg) and antibody to HBsAg (anti-HBs)

2. Core antigen and antibodies: antigen (HBcAg does not appear in the blood) and antibody to HBcAg (anti-HBc), IgM antibody subclass of anti-HBc (IgM anti-HBc), and IgG antibody subclass of anti-HBc (IgG anti-HBc)

3. Hepatitis B e antigen (HBeAg) and antibody to HBeAg (anti-HBe)

Additionally, the presence and concentration of circulating HBV DNA can also be tested [20–22].

HBsAg is the serological hallmark of both acute and chronic forms of HBV infection and the most commonly used diagnostic and blood screening marker for HBV infection. It usually appears in serum 1–10 weeks (average, 4 weeks) after acute exposure to the virus, and its persistence for six months or more implies progression to chronic HBV infection. The presence of HBsAg indicates that the person is infected with HBV and is therefore potentially infectious. More than 95–99 % of adults with acute HBV infection will recover spontaneously, without antiviral therapy [23, 24].

In patients that recover completely from their HBV infection, HBsAg usually becomes undetectable after four to six months, and its disappearance is followed several weeks later by the appearance of anti-HBs. Therefore, there is a gap ("window period") of several weeks to months between the disappearance of HBsAg and the appearance of anti-HBs, and during this period, the detectable marker of HBV infection is anti-HBc. The persistence of anti-HBs for a lifetime provides long-term immunity against HBV. Therefore, the presence of anti-HBs in serum attests to previous HBV exposure and acquired immunity. In some patients, anti-HBs may not become detectable after disappearance of HBsAg. These patients do not appear to be susceptible to recurrent infection [20, 23, 24].

Total anti-HBc (IgM and IgG) appears before anti-HBs, and its presence in serum attests both past exposure and current HBV infection. Its presence during the "window period" makes it a reliable indicator of HBV infection, in the absence of other HBV markers [25].

IgM anti-HBc develops in acute HBV infection and may usually persist for four to six months if the infection resolves [20, 22]. Although it is considered a reliable serologic marker for acute infection, IgM anti-HBc can also become positive during a chronic hepatitis B flare in patients who have long-standing hepatitis B [26, 27].

A negative IgM anti-HBc in conjunction with a positive HBsAg likely suggests a chronic HBV infection. As a result, routine testing for IgM anti-HBc is not generally recommended to screen for acutely infected patients [28, 29].

IgG anti-HBc develops in the late acute phase of infection and generally remains detectable for lifetime [20]. IgG anti-HBc may be the only serologic marker remaining in patient serum who recover from acute HBV infection. The presence of IgG anti-HBc can indicate progression to chronic disease [22].

HBeAg is a viral soluble protein that develops in the serum of persons with acute or chronic HBV infection. HBeAg appears in serum early during acute HBV infection and usually disappears about three weeks before HBsAg disappears. Persistence of HBeAg three or more months after the onset of illness indicates a carrier state and the risk of developing chronic

HVB. The HBeAg presence in the serum of HBV carriers and chronic hepatitis B patients indicates greater infectivity and a high level of viral replication [20, 30].

The small-size soluble HBeAg can cross the placental barrier from the mother to the fetus especially through villous capillary endothelial cells. The maternal HBeAg-positive serological status and high serum HBV DNA levels increase the risk of MTCT. By contrast, the absence of the HBeAg in serum is associated with lower levels of viral replication and with a significantly lower risk of intrauterine HBV transmission. The infants born to HBeAg-positive mothers have up to 90 % chance of acquiring perinatal HBV without prophylaxis [13, 14, 31, 32].

Anti-HBe appears in the resolution phase of the disease, when HBeAg disappears. Its presence correlates to a decreased infectivity. A seroconversion of HBeAg to anti-HBe marks a transition to the inactive carrier state in the majority of cases [20].

Spontaneous or treatment-induced HBeAg seroconversion is associated with lower rates of disease progression [33].

In addition to viral antigens and antibodies detected or measured, serum HBV DNA can also be measured both qualitatively and quantitatively (HBV viral load). HBV DNA is the most sensitive and specific marker of viral replication [29].

Serologic pattern of acute HBV infection is characterized by the transient presence of HBsAg (<6 months) and IgM anti-HBc. HBeAg and HBV DNA are also present during the initial phase of infection. The disappearance of HBV DNA, HBeAg to anti-HBe seroconversion, and loss of HBsAg or HBsAg to anti-HBs seroconversion designate recovery. The presence of IgG anti-HBc in the absence of HBsAg usually indicates a past HBV infection, while the presence of anti-HBs only reveals immunity to HBV infection after vaccination [20, 22, 25].

Three standard tests (HBsAg, anti-HBs, and anti-HBc) are usually indicated to determine if a person is currently infected with HBV, has recovered from HBV infection, or is susceptible to HBV infection [20].

Combinations of serologic HBV markers are used to identify different phases of HBV infection (**Table 1**).

Serological markers	Results	Interpretation
HBsAg	Negative	Never infected. Susceptible
Total anti-HBc	Negative	Vaccination should be recommended
Anti-HBsAg	Negative	
HBsAg	Negative	Recovered from past infection and immune
Total anti-HBc	Positive	
IgM anti-HBc	Negative	
Anti-HBsAg	Positive	
HBsAg	Negative	Immune due to hepatitis B vaccination
Total anti-HBc	Negative	

Serological markers	Results	Interpretation
Anti-HBsAg	Positive	
HBsAg	Positive	Acute HBV infection
Total anti-HBc	Positive	
IgM anti-HBc	Positive	
Anti-HBsAg	Negative	
HBsAg	Positive	Chronic HBV infection
Total anti-HBc	Positive	
IgM anti-HBc	Negative	
Anti-HBsAg	Negative	
HBsAg	Negative	Interpretation of isolated detection of anti-HBc
Total anti-HBc	Positive	Resolved infection
Anti-HBsAg	Negative	Window period of acute HBV (anti-HBc-predominantly IgM)
		False-positive test results
		"Low level" chronic infection

Table 1. Most common serological profiles of HBV infection [20, 22, 28].

4. Mechanisms and predictors for MTCT of HBV infection

Perinatal transmission of hepatitis B is highest in mothers with acute hepatitis, especially in HBe-positive mothers in the third trimester (50–80 %), lower in mothers with anti-HBe (25 %), and lowest in carriers (5 %) [34].

The World Health Organization (WHO) defines "perinatal" as the time period starting at 22 completed weeks (154 days) gestation and ending seven complete days after birth [35]. However, the perinatal period is defined in various ways, and depending on the definition, it starts at the 20th–28th week of gestation and ends 1–4 weeks after birth [36]. The term MTCT is entitled and covers the transmission of all HBV infections from mother to her child during pregnancy (intrauterine transmission), childbirth, or after birth. As a result, there are three main possible routes for MTCT of HBV infection: transplacental transmission of HBV, transmission during delivery, and postnatal transmission during child care and breastfeeding [37].

Intrauterine transmission of HBV is considered the most important cause for the failure of passive-active immunoprophylaxis in preventing MTCT, although it is presumed to cause a minority of HBV infections [38]. The main risk factors for intrauterine HBV infection are maternal serum HBeAg positivity, high HBV DNA level, history of threatened preterm labor, and HBV presence in the villous capillary endothelial cells of the placenta. One of the proposed mechanisms involved in the HBV intrauterine transmission is the transplacental leakage of

HBeAg-positive maternal blood induced by uterine contractions during pregnancy and by the disruption of placental barriers. In addition, HBeAg can pass through the placenta via the "cellular route." Although the risk of fetal hepatitis B infection through amniocentesis is considered to be low, the maternal HBeAg status would be valuable in the counseling regarding risks associated with amniocentesis. Another possible route of HBV intrauterine transmission could be via germ cells, maternally or paternally dependent [14, 37, 39].

HBV transmission during delivery is recognized as the most important route of MTCT in endemic areas for HBV infection, as a result of exposure to maternal cervical secretions and maternal blood that contain HBV. There is no consensus regarding the effect of delivery mode on MTCT (vaginal delivery vs. cesarean section). While some studies suggest that cesarean section might reduce the risk of MTCT, other studies assert that the mode of delivery does not influence the rate of HBV transmission as long as all infants received both hepatitis B vaccine and hepatitis B immune globulin (HBIG) at birth [37].

There is little evidence that cesarean delivery prevents HBV transmission, and current guidelines do not recommend cesarean section to decrease the risk of MTCT. As for elective cesarean section (ECS), there are studies that show alike an absolute risk reduction of MTCT of HBV compared with immunoprophylaxis alone and studies that report no benefit to ECS. According to recent clinical guidelines of American College of Gastroenterology (ACG) concerning liver disease and pregnancy, validation studies are needed to determine the relative safety and efficacy of ECS and immunoprophylaxis versus immunoprophylaxis alone in reducing MTCT of HVB [40].

Although markers of HBV are detectable in breast milk from HBsAg-positive women, there is no evidence that breastfeeding is a risk factor for HBV infection if the infant received hepatitis B vaccine and HBIG. According to the WHO and the American Academy of Pediatrics recommendations, in infants who receive full immunoprophylaxis, breastfeeding in HBs-positive mothers is not a contraindication [9, 41, 42].

5. Clinical and laboratory features of HBV infection in pregnancy

The clinical manifestations of HBV infection may be variable in both acute and chronic diseases. In acute HBV infection, clinical manifestations usually range from anicteric hepatitis to icteric hepatitis, while in the chronic phase, manifestations range from an asymptomatic carrier state to chronic hepatitis, cirrhosis, and hepatocellular carcinoma. Fulminant hepatic failure, most probably due to massive immune-mediated lysis of infected hepatocytes, is unusual but can occur in some cases. Extrahepatic manifestations may be present in both acute and chronic infections [25, 40, 42].

Testing for HBsAg should be performed in all women at the first prenatal visit, even if they have been previously vaccinated or tested, and repeated later in pregnancy if appropriate [25, 43].

The first step in assessing a woman presenting at any stage of pregnancy with acute or chronic HBV infection should be the same as with any nonpregnant patient: complete history, physical

Phase	ALT	HBV DNA	HBeAg	Notes
"Immune tolerant"	Normal	Elevated	Positive	Perinatal or early childhood-acquired HBV infection Patients are highly contagious Low spontaneous HBeAg loss Minimal liver inflammation and fibrosis
HBeAg-positive immune-active phase "Immune active"	Elevated	Elevated	Positive	Moderate-to-severe liver inflammation or fibrosis HBeAg to anti-HBe seroconversion possible, leading to "immune-control" phase
Inactive chronic hepatitis "Immune control"	Normal	Low or undetectable	Negative	Low risk for cirrhosis Minimal liver necroinflammation, variable fibrosis
HBeAg-negative chronic hepatitis "Immune escape mutant"	Elevated persistent or intermittently	Moderate to elevated	Negative	Generally in older persons Liver necroinflammation Risk for fibrosis or cirrhosis
"Reactivation" or "acute-on-chronic hepatitis" or HBeAg-negative immune reactivation phase	Elevated	Elevated	Negative	Spontaneously or precipitated by immunosuppressive therapy, transplantation, antiviral resistance, HIV infection, withdrawal of antiviral therapy Moderate-to-severe liver necroinflammation and fibrosis

Table 2. Phases of chronic hepatitis B [44–46].

exam, standard serological workup, laboratory test which should include assessment of liver disease activity and function, markers of HBV replication, and tests for coinfection with hepatitis C virus [8, 16, 40, 43, 44].

The clinical spectrum of acute HBV infection in pregnant women usually is not different from that of nonpregnant women; however, the risk of preterm delivery and low birth weight is higher than in the general population [9, 14, 42]. It seems that acute HBV infection does not increase mortality or have teratogenic effects [9].

Common symptoms of acute HBV infection in pregnant women are indistinguishable from those of nonpregnant, including upper quadrant discomfort, fatigue, nausea, vomiting, diarrhea, headaches, myalgia, anorexia, low-grade fever, and jaundice. The icteric phase of acute viral hepatitis usually begins within 10 days of the initial symptoms and disappears about 4–12 weeks afterwards. Diagnosis is based on the detection of HBsAg and the presence of IgM anti-HBc. Recovery is accompanied by HBsAg clearance with seroconversion to anti-HBs, usually within 3 months. Concentrations of alanine and aspartate aminotransferase (ALT and AST) levels usually increase, with ALT typically higher than AST. In patients who recover, normalization of serum aminotransferases usually occurs within one to four months [20, 25, 42, 45].

Acute exacerbation or flare of hepatitis in chronic HBV infections can be present during pregnancy, and it may be difficult to differentiate from acute HBV infection. HBV testing with HBsAg and IgM anti-HBc is recommended in pregnant women presenting with acute hepatitis [40].

Most chronic HBV infections are asymptomatic and pregnancy is well tolerated. Some patients may complain of fatigue, anorexia, and nonspecific malaise. Significant symptoms will develop only if the liver disease progresses. Cirrhosis, condition usually associated with amenorrhea and infertility, is relatively uncommon in the younger age group of pregnant women, and severe cases are fortunately rare [9, 42, 45]. The chronic hepatitis B is usually mild in pregnant women but may flare at the end of pregnancy or shortly after delivery [9].

The natural history of chronic HBV infection consists of several phases of variable duration, which are not necessarily sequential (**Table 2**) [44–46]. Pregnancy is a hormone-induced immune-tolerant state, and there is limited understanding of the natural history of chronic HBV infection during pregnancy [47]. Increased levels of adrenal corticosteroids and estrogen hormones during pregnancy may be responsible for an increase in HBV viral load and a decrease in ALT levels. A postpartum decline in HBV DNA level, associated with increased ALT levels and active hepatitis, requires close monitoring of the mother [9, 42].

6. Current management strategies for chronic hepatitis B in pregnancy

HBV infection during pregnancy requires management strategies for both mother and fetus/neonate, including prevention/elimination of MTCT and lessening the HBV effects on maternal and fetal health [48, 49].

Current management strategies for hepatitis B during pregnancy include antenatal maternal screening for HBV infection, initial assessment of mother with HBV infection (severity of liver disease, level of viral replication, presence of comorbidities), prophylactic HBV vaccination and HBIG administration to all infants born to HBV-infected mothers as soon as possible after birth, the use of antiviral medications for pregnant women with chronic hepatitis B, safe delivery practices, and strengthened maternal and child health services [8, 40, 45, 50].

Few countries have national hepatitis strategies, plans, and budgets, and as a consequence, the WHO recently published a 5-year global health sector strategy on viral hepatitis. This includes testing algorithms, strategies for hepatitis B, diagnosis and management of acute hepatitis B, as well as management of advanced liver disease [8, 45].

Antenatal screening for HBV infection in all pregnant women is a well-established, evidence-based standard of practice to prevent MTCT. Therefore, the first step is to identify all HBsAg-positive pregnant women in the first trimester by universal screening [45].

All pregnant women who are HBsAg positive should be assessed the same way as any non-pregnant individual: a complete history with special emphasis on risk factors for coinfection, physical exam and laboratory tests for assessment of liver disease activity and function, markers of HBV replication, and tests for coinfection (hepatitis C virus, hepatitis delta virus, or human immunodeficiency virus in those at risk) [24, 44, 48, 50].

Assessment of the severity of liver disease should include measurement of ALT, AST, alkaline phosphatase (ALP), gamma-glutamyl transpeptidase, total bilirubin, full blood count, serum albumin and globulins, prothrombin time, and an ultrasound examination. Assessment of the level of viral replication in chronic hepatitis B using quantification of serum HBV DNA and HBeAg and anti-HBe is an important step in determining the risk of MTCT and therefore in guiding antiviral therapy decisions and the need for surveillance [24, 44, 48, 50]. Elevated serum ALT and HBV DNA levels are strongly predictive of risk of liver complications [44].

According to the WHO Strategic Advisory Group of Experts, the currently recommended practice to reduce perinatal MTCT of HBV relies on the administration of HBV vaccine and, in some countries, concurrent administration of HBIG. The infants of all HBsAg-positive women should receive immunoprophylaxis with HBV vaccination ± HBIG. Hepatitis B vaccine and HBIG should be administered at different injection sites [45].

The timing of administration of the first dose of hepatitis B vaccine to infants in relation to birth is the most important factor in determining the efficacy of vaccination [41, 51]. As a result, the recommended timing of administration of the first dose of hepatitis B vaccine in newborns has evolved in the last decades, in order to optimize prevention of MTCT hepatitis B infections. The WHO recommends that all infants receive the hepatitis B vaccine as soon as possible after birth, within 24 h of the birth [2].

Passive immunization against hepatitis B with HBIG in conjunction with HBV vaccination may be of additional benefit for newborn whose mothers are HBsAg positive, particularly if they are also HBeAg positive [45]. According to the Centers for Disease Control, all preterm infants born to HBsAg-positive mothers and mothers with unknown HBsAg status must receive HBIG and hepatitis B vaccine within 12 h of birth [52].

Unfortunately, despite postnatal active-passive immunization of the newborns, MTCT of HBV still occurs, especially if the mother has very a high maternal concentration of HBV DNA, typically observed in HBeAg-positive women [45].

There are emerging data based on open-label nonrandomized studies which suggest that short-term maternal antiviral therapy used in pregnant women with stable liver disease during the third trimester may reduce the risk of MTCT occurring during the perinatal period, by lowering maternal viral load prior to delivery [24, 47].

Current guidelines of the American Association for the Study of Liver Diseases (AASLD), ACG, European Association for the Study of the Liver (EASL), and Asian Pacific Association for the Study of the Liver (APASL) suggest or recommend antiviral therapy to reduce the risk of perinatal transmission of hepatitis B in HBsAg-positive pregnant women with a HBV DNA above 200,000 IU/mL [24, 44, 48, 50]. As for the WHO current position, the Guidelines Development Group did not make a formal recommendation on the use of antiviral therapy to prevent MTCT, due to the fact that key trials are still ongoing and there is a lack of consensus regarding the programmatic implications of a policy of more widespread antiviral use in pregnancy [45].

There are only three therapeutic antiviral agents studied and used for the treatment of chronic hepatitis B in pregnant women: lamivudine, telbivudine (nucleoside analogues (NAs)), and tenofovir disoproxil fumarate (nucleotide analogue). According to the US Food and Drug Administration classification of oral antiviral, based on the risk of teratogenicity in preclinical evaluation, only two drugs from the nucleoside/nucleotide analogues (NAs) class—tenofovir and telbivudine—are classified in risk category B (no risk in animal studies, but unknown in humans), while lamivudine, entecavir, and adefovir dipivoxil are classified as category C drugs (teratogenic in animals, but unknown in humans) [24, 44]. Additionally, tenofovir received category B classification based on data collected from human exposure [53].

Lamivudine, the first and the most studied NAs in pregnant women with chronic hepatitis B, is not considered an optimal choice for prevention of MTCT due to its poor antiviral activity and low barrier to resistance. Its administration, even for short periods, is associated with the selection of resistant mutants. Lamivudine reaches higher concentrations in amniotic fluid than in serum and has been found to be excreted in breast milk [49, 54, 55].

The results of small human pregnancy trials show that telbivudine reduces MTCT in highly viremic pregnant women and its use appears to be safe in late pregnancy [47].

Tenofovir is considered a preferred choice in pregnant women with chronic hepatitis B, due to its antiviral potency, the available safety data of use during pregnancy, and its better resistance profile [44, 45].

As for other antiviral drugs, the safety of entecavir in pregnancy is not known, and interferon (IFN) therapy is contraindicated during pregnancy [44, 45].

Antiviral therapy was started at 28–32 weeks of gestation in most studies, and therefore NAs starting from 28 to 32 weeks of gestation are recommended [24, 45]. A careful examination to exclude maternal systemic disorder and fetal anomalies is required prior to the administration of NAs [44, 50]. For pregnant women with immune-active chronic hepatitis B, monitoring therapeutic response to NAs, both serological and virological, as well as for potential side effects, should be based on recommendations for nonpregnant women [24, 44, 45]. Tenofovir therapy requires monitoring serum creatinine and serum phosphate levels every three months, due to potential nephrotoxicity. The risks of maternal liver disease, fetal development, HBV MTCT, and long-term plan for treatment should be discussed with pregnant women [24, 50].

Although there are no studies on the duration of NA therapy (cessation at delivery vs. after delivery), cessation of NA therapy (at delivery or 4–12 weeks after delivery) is recommended in females without ALT flares [24, 44, 45]. According to EASL guidelines, if NA therapy is given only for prevention of MTCT, it may be discontinued within the first 3 months after delivery [50]. If the anti-HBV therapy is discontinued during pregnancy or early after delivery, women need to be closely monitored for the risk of hepatic flares, especially after delivery [44, 50].

In certain situations, such as ALT flares detected during the treatment period, continuation of antiviral treatment after delivery is needed. As a result, this raises the issue of safety of NA therapy during breastfeeding. Due to limited data on the effect of these medications on infants, the safety of NA therapy during breastfeeding is considered uncertain [24, 50].

The safety of lamivudine and tenofovir during breastfeeding in HBV infection has not been well studied. Additionally, tenofovir and lamivudine concentrations in breast milk have been reported. However, due to its poor oral bioavailability, the breastfeeding infants are exposed to only small tenofovir concentrations [50].

According to drug labels, tenofovir disoproxil fumarate and lamivudine should not be used during breastfeeding. Breastfeeding is discouraged during maternal NA treatment according to APASL current guidelines, but in the case of ALT flares, continuation of antiviral may be indicated, depending on the liver disease status of mother [24]. A recent review of available data concluded that tenofovir and lamivudine should not be contraindicated during breast-feeding. However, there are insufficient data based on long-term studies to establish the safety of infant exposure to different antiviral therapies during breastfeeding [56].

7. Conclusions

Despite advancements in the prevention, diagnosis, and treatment of HBV infection, it remains a serious global health issue and one of major risk factors for end-stage liver disease and hepatocellular carcinoma. Given that chronic hepatitis B in pregnant women is an important contributor worldwide to the new HBV infections, most effective and sustainable measures are required for prevention of MTCT. Universal screening of pregnant women for HBsAg and passive and active immunoprophylaxis are important tools in MTCT of HBV. The causes of immunoprophylaxis failure in some infants are not yet not fully understood, and, therefore, studies are needed in order to clarify this issue. Longitudinal cohort studies are also required to determine the safety of infant exposure to different NA therapies during breastfeeding.

Author details

Letiția Adela Maria Streba, Anca Pătrașcu, Aurelia Enescu and Costin Teodor Streba*

*Address all correspondence to:costinstreba@gmail.com

University of Medicine and Pharmacy of Craiova, Romania

References

[1] Zuckerman AJ. Hepatitis viruses. In: Baron S, eds. Medical Microbiology, 4th ed. The University of Texas Medical Branch at Galveston, Galveston, Texas, 1996, ISBN: 10: 0-9631172-1-1 Chapter 70:849–863.

[2] World Health Organization. Media Centre. Hepatitis B. 2013. Available from: http://www.who.int/mediacentre/factsheets/fs204/en/ [Accessed April 19, 2016].

[3] Okamoto H, Tsuda F, Sakugawa H et al. Typing hepatitis B virus by homology in nucleotide sequence: comparison of surface antigen subtypes. J Gen Virol 1988;69:2575–2583.

[4] Norder H, Courouce AM, Magnius LO. Complete genomes, phylogenetic relatedness, and structural proteins of six strains of the hepatitis B virus, four of which represent two new genotypes. Virology 1994;198:489–503.

[5] Arauz-Ruiz P, Norder H, Robertson BH, Magnius LO. Genotype H: a new Amerindian genotype of hepatitis B virus revealed in Central America. J Gen Virol 2002;83:2059–2073.

[6] Sunbul M. Hepatitis B virus genotypes: global distribution and clinical importance. World J Gastroenterol 2014; 20(18):5427–5434.

[7] Alter MJ. Epidemiology and prevention of hepatitis B. Semin Liver Dis 2003;23:39–46.

[8] WHO. Global health sector strategy on viral hepatitis, 2016–2021. Geneva: World Health Organization; 2016 for submission to WHO Executive Board. Available from: http://apps.who.int/iris/bitstream/10665/246177/1/WHO-HIV-2016.06-eng.pdf?ua=1 [Accessed 24 July 22, 2016]

[9] Jonas MM. Hepatitis B and pregnancy: an underestimated issue. Liver Int 2009;29 Suppl 1:133–139.

[10] Gambarin-Gelwan M. Hepatitis B in pregnancy. Clin Liver Dis. 2007;11:945–963.

[11] Duffell EF, van de Laar MJW, Amato-Gauci AJ. Enhanced surveillance of hepatitis B in the EU, 2006–2012. J Viral Hepat. 2015;22(7):581–589.

[12] Kim WR. Epidemiology of hepatitis B in the United States. Hepatology 2009;49(5 Suppl):S28–S34.

[13] Panpan Yi, Ruochan Chen, Yan Huang, Rong-Rong Zhou, Xue-Gong Fan. Management of mother-to-child transmission of hepatitis B virus: propositions and challenges. J Clin Virol 2016;77:32–39.

[14] Borgia G, Carleo MA, Gaeta GB, Gentile I. Hepatitis B in pregnancy. World J Gastroenterol 2012;18(34):4677–4683.

[15] Ott JJ, Stevens GA, Groeger J, Wiersma ST. Global epidemiology of hepatitis B virus infection: new estimates of age-specific HBsAg seroprevalence and endemicity. Vaccine 2012;30:2212–2219.

[16] European Centre for Disease Prevention and Control. Technical Report: Hepatitis B and C in the EU neighbourhood: prevalence, burden of disease and screening policies. 2010. Available from: http://ecdc.europa.eu/en/publications/Publications/TER_100914_Hep_B_C%20_EU_neighbourhood.pdf [Accessed April 23, 2016]

[17] Dionne-Odom J, Tita AT, Silverman NS. #38: Hepatitis B in pregnancy screening, treatment, and prevention of vertical transmission. Am J Obstet Gynecol 2016;214(1):6–14. doi: 10.1016/j.ajog.2015.09.100.

[18] Fouquet A, Jambon AC, Canva V, Bocket-Mouton L, Gottrand F, Subtil D. Hepatitis B and pregnancy. Part 1. Thirteen practical issues in antenatal period. J Gynecol Obstet Biol Reprod (Paris). 2016, Mar 7. pii: S0368-2315(16)00029-6.

[19] Hansen N, Hay G, Cowan S, Jepsen P, Bygum Krarup H, Obel N, Weis N, Brehm Christensen P. Hepatitis B prevalence in Denmark – an estimate based on nationwide registers and a national screening programme, as on 31 December 2007. Euro Surveill 2013;18(47):pii=20637. DOI: http://dx.doi.org/10.2807/1560-7917.ES2013.18.47.20637

[20] World Health Organization. Hepatitis B. 2016. Available from: http://www.who.int/csr/disease/hepatitis/HepatitisB_whocdscsrlyo2002_2.pdf?ua=1 [Accessed June 17]

[21] Bessone F. Re-appraisal of old and new diagnostic tools in the current management of chronic hepatitis B. Liver Int 2014;34:991–1000.

[22] Centers for Disease Control and Prevention. Recommendations for Identification and Public Health Management of Persons with Chronic Hepatitis B Virus Infection. MMWR 2008;57(RR-8):3. Available at: http://www.cdc.gov/mmwr/PDF/rr/rr5708.pdf [Accessed on July 13, 2016].

[23] Chen Y-P, Qiao Y-Y, Zhao X-H, Chen H-S, Wang Y, Wang Z. Rapid detection of hepatitis B virus surface antigen by an agglutination assay mediated by a bispecific diabody against both human erythrocytes and hepatitis B virus surface antigen. Clin Vaccine Immunol 2007;14(6):720–725. doi:10.1128/CVI.00310-06.

[24] Sarin SK, Kumar M, Lau GK, et al. Asian-Pacific clinical practice guidelines on the management of hepatitis B: a 2015 update. Hepatol Int 2016;10:1–98.

[25] Petersen J. Hepatitis B. In Mauss S, Berg T, Rockstroh J, Sarrazin C, Wedemeyer H. Hepatology: A clinical textbook. 7th ed., Fokus Verlag, Hamburg, 2016, pp. 145–155.

[26] Maruyama T, Schodel F, Iino S, Koike K, Yasuda K, Peterson D, Milich DR. Distinguishing between acute and symptomatic chronic hepatitis B virus infection. Gastroenterology 1994;106:1006–1015

[27] Craxí A, Marino L, Aragona E, Patti C. IgM anti-HBc in acute and chronic hepatitis B virus (HBV) infection: diagnostic value and correlation with viral replication and disease activity. Boll Ist Sieroter Milan 1988;67:275–282.

[28] Petersen J. Hepatitis B. In: Mauss S, Berg T, Rockstroh J, Sarrazin C, Wedemeyer H: Hepatology: A clinical textbook. 7th ed. Fokus Verlag, Hamburg, 2016, pp. 145–155.

[29] Krajden M, McNabb G, Petric M. The laboratory diagnosis of hepatitis B virus. Can J Infect Dis Med Microbiol 2005;16(2):65–72

[30] Perrillo R. Hepatitis B and D. In: Feldman M, Friedman LS, Brandt LJ, eds. Sleisenger and Fordtran's Gastrointestinal and Liver Disease. 9th ed. Philadelphia, PA: Elsevier Saunders; 2010: 78, pp. 1287–1312.

[31] Singh AE, Plitt SS, Osiowy C, Surynicz K, Kouadjo E, Preiksaitis J, et al. Factors associated with vaccine failure and vertical transmission of hepatitis B among a cohort of Canadian mothers and infants. J Viral Hepat 2011;18:468–473.

[32] Apuzzio, J., Block, J.M., Cullison, S., et al. Chronic hepatitis B in pregnancy: a workshop consensus statement on screening, evaluation, and management part 1. Female Patient 2012;37:22–27.

[33] Liaw Y-F. HBeAg seroconversion as an important end point in the treatment of chronic hepatitis B. Hepatol Int. 2009;3(3):425–433. doi:10.1007/s12072-009-9140-3.

[34] Hay JE. Liver disease in pregnancy. Hepatology 2008;47:1067–1076. doi:10.1002/hep.22130.

[35] World Health Organization. Maternal and perinatal health 2016. Available from: http://www.who.int/maternal_child_adolescent/topics/maternal/maternal_perinatal/en/ [Accessed July 18].

[36] European Comission. Infant and Perinatal health 2016. Available from: http://ec.europa.eu/health/population_groups/gender/perinatal/index_en.htm [Accessed on July 18].

[37] Navabakhsh B, Mehrabi N, Estakhri A, Mohamadnejad M, Poustchi H. Hepatitis B virus infection during pregnancy: transmission and prevention. Middle East J Digest Dis 2011;3(2):92–102.

[38] Zhang SL, Han XB, Yue YF. Relationship between HBV viremia level of pregnant women and intrauterine infection: nested PCR for detection of HBV DNA. World J Gastroenterol 1998;4:61–63.

[39] Davies G, Wilson RD, Desilets V et al. Society of Obstetricians and Gynaecologists of Canada: amniocentesis and women with hepatitis B, hepatitis C or human immunodeficiency virus. J Obstet Gynaecol Can 2003;25(2):145–148, 149–152

[40] Tran TT, Ahn J, Reau NS. ACG clinical guideline: liver disease and pregnancy. Am J Gastroenterol 111:176–194.

[41] Umar M, Hamama-Tul-Bushra, Umar S, Khan HA. HBV perinatal transmission. Int J Hepatol 2013;2013:875791.

[42] Nelson NP, Jamieson DJ, Murphy TV. Prevention of perinatal hepatitis B virus transmission. J Pediatric Infect Dis Soc. 2014;3 Suppl 1:S7–S12.

[43] US Preventive Services Task Force. Screening for hepatitis B Virus infection in pregnancy: US Preventive Services Task Force Reaffirmation recommendation statement. Ann Intern Med 2009;150:869–873.

[44] Terrault NA, Bzowej NH, Chang KM, Hwang JP, Jonas MM, Murad MH. AASLD guidelines for treatment of chronic hepatitis B. Hepatology 2016;63(1):261–283.

[45] World Health Organization, Guidelines for the Prevention, Care and Treatment of Persons with Chronic Hepatitis B Infection, WHO, 2015, http://apps.who.int/iris/bitstream/10665/154590/1/9789241549059_eng.pdf [Accessed on April 24].

[46] World Gastroenterology Organisation Global Guideline. Hepatitis B 2015. Available from: http://www.spg.pt/wp-content/uploads/2015/11/2015-hepatitis-b.pdf [Accessed on July 25].

[47] Pan CQ, Lee HM. Antiviral therapy for chronic hepatitis B in pregnancy. Semin Liver Dis 2013;33:138–146.

[48] Visvanathan K, Dusheiko G, Giles M, et al. Managing HBV in pregnancy. Prevention, prophylaxis, treatment and follow-up: position paper produced by Australian, UK and New Zealand key opinion leaders. Gut 2016;65(2):340–350

[49] Degli Esposti S, Shah D. Hepatitis B in pregnancy: challenges and treatment. Gastroenterol Clin North Am 2011;40(2):355–372.

[50] European Association for the Study of the Liver. EASL clinical practice guidelines: Management of chronic hepatitis B virus infection. J Hepatol 2012;57(1):167–185.

[51] André FE, Zuckerman AJ. Review: protective efficacy of hepatitis B vaccines in neonates. J Med Virol 1994;44:144–151.

[52] Centers for Disease Control and Prevention. Hepatitis B in the Pink Book: Course Textbook. 13th ed. 2015. Available from: http://www.cdc.gov/vaccines/pubs/pinkbook/downloads/hepb.pdf

[53] Guclu E, Karabay O. Choice of drugs in the treatment of chronic hepatitis B in pregnancy. World J Gastroenterol 2013;19(10):1671–1672. DOI: 10.3748/wjg.v19.i10.1671.

[54] Han L, Zhang H-W, Xie J-X, Zhang Q, Wang H-Y, Cao G-W. A meta-analysis of lamivudine for interruption of mother-to-child transmission of hepatitis B virus. World J Gastroenterol 2011;17(38):4321–4333.

[55] Ayres A, Yuen L, Jackson KM, et al. Short duration of lamivudine for the prevention of hepatitis B virus transmission in pregnancy: lack of potency and selection of resistance mutations. J Viral Hepat 2014;21:809–817.

[56] Ehrhardt S, Xie C, Guo N, Nelson K, Thio CL. Breastfeeding while taking lamivudine or tenofovir disoproxil fumarate: a review of the evidence. Clin Infect Dis 2015;60:275–278.

Chapter 11

Treatment and Prognosis of Hepatitis B Virus Concomitant with Alcoholism

Chih-Wen Lin, Chih-Che Lin and Sien-Sing Yang

Additional information is available at the end of the chapter

http://dx.doi.org/10.5772/66981

Abstract

Hepatitis B virus (HBV) infection is a global disease worldwide. The Asia-Pacific region has a high prevalence of viral hepatitis, and Taiwan is a region of high prevalence of chronic hepatitis B (CHB) with increasing alcoholic liver disease. We have investigated the prognosis and treatment of patients with concomitant hepatitis B virus (HBV) infection and alcoholism. The 10-year cumulative incidence of hepatocellular carcinoma (HCC) is much higher in patients with concomitant alcoholism and HBV infection than in those with alcoholism or HBV infection alone. Treatment with antiviral therapy and abstinence may be started in patients with decompensated cirrhosis and compensated cirrhosis with high HBV DNA. In pre-cirrhotic cases, treatment with antiviral therapy and abstinence may be started in patients with persistently elevated ALT levels and high HBV DNA, and significant fibrosis with minimal elevated or normal ALT levels and mild high HBV DNA. Treatment with antiviral therapy and abstinence reduces the incidence of HCC in patients with concomitant HBV infection and alcoholism. In conclusion, patients with concomitant HBV infection and alcoholism have high incidence of cirrhosis, HCC, and mortality. Treatment with antiviral therapy and abstinence may be started to reduce the incidence of cirrhosis, HCC, and mortality in these patients.

Keywords: chronic hepatitis B, hepatitis B virus DNA, nucleos(t)ides analogues, alcoholism, hepatocellular carcinoma, treatment, prognosis

1. Introduction

Hepatitis B virus (HBV) infection is a global disease, affecting approximately 350 million people worldwide [1]. The Asia-Pacific region has a high prevalence of viral hepatitis, and Taiwan is a region with high prevalence of chronic hepatitis B (CHB) [2]. It is particularly endemic in Taiwan, where the infection is usually acquired perinatally or in early childhood [2]. The morbidity and mortality associated with CHB are substantial in that 15% to approximately 40% of infected patients will develop serious sequels including persistent hepatitis, hepatic failure, liver cirrhosis and hepatocellular carcinoma (HCC) during their lifetime [2].

Alcohol-related morbidity and mortality represent a major public health issue worldwide [3, 4]. The United States National Institute on Alcohol Abuse and Alcoholism defines "heavy drinking" as consuming more than fourteen drinks per week for males and seven drinks per week for females. The risk threshold for developing alcohol-related liver disease is consuming 20–30 g of alcohol per day, and the development of cirrhosis occurs in 10–20% of those consuming more than 80 g of alcohol daily [3]. The Asia-Pacific region has a high prevalence of viral hepatitis, and Taiwan is a region of high prevalence of chronic hepatitis B (CHB) with increasing alcoholic liver disease [5–7]. The affordability of alcohol and changes in life style and drinking behavior have the causes for the increase in cases of hospitalization for alcoholic liver disease [6].

In the animal model system, mice fed with ethanol have an increased serum hepatitis B surface antigen (HBsAg) by up to seven folds accompanied by an increased in viral DNA load [8]. In addition, these ethanol-fed mice have elevated expression of HBV surface, core, and X antigens in the liver, accompanied by an increase in HBV RNA levels. Chronic ethanol consumption is found to stimulate hepatitis B virus replication and gene expression in HBV transgenic mice [8]. Our recent study also reveals that patients with concomitant alcoholism and HBV infection have high percentages of hepatitis B viral load in clinics [9]. Moreover, the lipid composition of cellular membranes in lipid rafts is altered by alcohol exposure, and alcohol exposure may thereby influences HBV infectivity [10]. Furthermore, alcohol can influence anti-HBV immunity, an effect involving the cellular membrane as well as the lipid rafts. HBV is known to interfere with the T-cell receptor (TCR) responsible for interacting and recognizing foreign antigens, thereby preventing the initiation of an immune response. This results in a defective adaptive immune response during chronic HBV infection [8, 11]. Thus, alcohol can acts synergistically with HBV to limit antiviral immunity. Since the adaptive immunity plays a key role in viral clearance, the consequences of alcohol's effects on the TCR of HBV infection are of high interest in the field of hepatology [12].

2. Epidemiology

HBV infection is a serious global health problem, with 2 billion people infected worldwide and 350 million suffering from chronic HBV infection. HBV infections result in 0.5–1.2 million deaths per year caused by chronic hepatitis, cirrhosis, and HCC. HBV-related end-stage liver disease or HCC is responsible for over 0.5–1 million deaths per year and currently represents 5–10% of cases of liver transplantation. Morbidity and mortality in CHB are linked to persistence of viral replication and evolution to cirrhosis and/or HCC [1, 2].

In Taiwan, the introduction of universal vaccination of neonates in 1983–1985 has drastically decreased the prevalence of HBsAg in children below the age of 15 from 9.8 % in 1984 to 0.5 % in 2004 [13]. This is accompanied by a significant decrease in the incidence of infant fulminant hepatitis associated with chronic liver disease, mortality, and HCC [14, 15].

Alcohol is abused by more than 18 million adults in the United States. A daily consumption of alcohol exceeding 80 g for more than 10 years increases the risk for HCC by fivefold, while daily consumption of alcohol below 80 g is not significantly associated with an increased risk for HCC [3, 4]. The risk for HCC in decompensated alcoholic cirrhosis is close to 1% per year [3, 4]. Alcohol consumption is one of the top five causes of disease and disability in almost all European countries [16]. In the United States, about 50% of liver-related death is attributed by alcohol consumption, accounting for $3 billion annually loss, and is the third leading cause of preventable deaths in the U.S. [17]. It is estimated that alcohol is responsible for 5.9% of global mortality worldwide [18] and 2.5 million deaths per annual [19, 20].

3. Prognosis

Based on a large nationwide Risk Evaluation of Viral Load Elevation and Associated Liver Disease/Cancer-Hepatitis B Virus (REVEAL-HBV) study performed in Taiwan for CHB without alcoholism, detectable serum HBV DNA at study entry is demonstrated to be a significant risk predictor of HCC in HBV patients [21–23]. Those with detectable HBsAg are at 5- to 98-fold higher risk of developing HCC [24]. The seropositivity for HBeAg is also found associated with an increase in risk for HCC [25]. Compared to those who are seronegative for HBsAg and HBeAg, the hazard ratio (HR) of developing HCC is about 10 and 60, respectively, for individuals with seropositivity for HBsAg and both HBsAg and HBeAg [25, 26]. The serum level of HBV DNA is therefore a strong risk predictor of HCC [21], and it is also an important and independent risk factor for disease progression prognosis (including cirrhosis, risk of death, metastasis, and recurrence following surgery) in chronic hepatitis B [22]. Alcohol has a synergistic effect in increasing the risk of HCC incidence in HBsAg-positive men [27].

In one of our study, 966 cirrhotic patients in Taiwan, consisting of 632 patients with HBV infection, 132 patients with HBV infection and alcoholism, and 202 patients with alcoholism, are evaluated for HCC development [6]. We show that 15.8, 28.8 and 10.4% of the patients with HBV infection alone, concomitant HBV infection and alcoholism, and alcoholism alone, respectively, are found to have newly developed HCC after a period of 10 years of follow-up. The 1-, 3-, 5-, and 10-year cumulative incidence of HCC is 1.2, 9.4, 18.4, and 39.8%, respectively, for patients with HBV infection alone; 3.1, 28.7, 36.8, and 52.8%, respectively, for patients with concomitant HBV infection and alcoholism; and 1.1, 6.1, 10.7, and 25.6%, respectively, for patients with alcoholism alone (**Figure 1**). The 10-year cumulative incidence of HCC is much higher in patients with concomitant alcoholism and HBV infection than in those with alcoholism alone or HBV infection alone (52.8% vs. 25.6% vs. 39.8%, $p < 0.001$). The mean

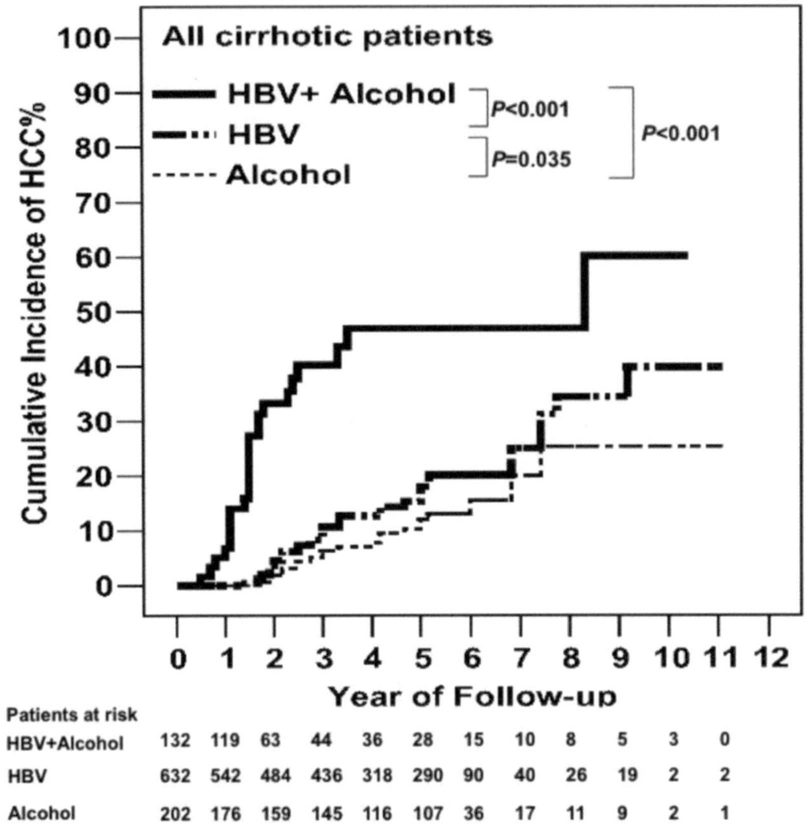

Figure 1. Cirrhotic patients with concomitant HBV infection and alcoholism have higher cumulative incidence of HCC than those with alcoholism alone or HVB infection alone.

follow-up period is 2.9, 5.2, and 3.9 years for patients with concomitant HBV infection and alcoholism, alcoholism alone, and HBV infection alone, respectively. The annual incidence of HCC is 9.9, 2.1, and 4.1%, respectively, for patients with concomitant HBV infection and alcoholism, alcoholism alone, and HBV infection alone. Our findings reveal that heavy alcohol consumption significantly increases the risk of developing HCC in HBV-related cirrhotic patients [6].

The baseline serum HBV DNA level, antiviral nucleos(t)ide analogues [NA(s)] therapy, serum α-fetoprotein, daily amount of alcohol intake, and years of alcohol intake are also found to be significantly associated with the incidence of HCC by univariate analyses. In multivariate logistic regression analyses, antiviral NUCs therapy (OR = 0.01) and baseline high serum HBV DNA levels (OR = 16.8) are significantly linked to a reduction in the incidence of HCC. In addition, the cumulative incidence of HCC during the follow-up period is significantly higher in patients with higher baseline serum HBV DNA levels than those with lower baseline serum HBV DNA levels. Alcoholic cirrhotic patients with higher serum HBV DNA levels have higher incidence of HCC than those with lower serum HBV DNA levels, and increasing HBV DNA levels precipitates the progression of liver cirrhosis to HCC [6].

In another case-control and hospital-based study conducted in Italy, the relative risks of HCC for HBsAg and heavy alcohol intake are 11.4 and 4.6, respectively [28]. Positive synergisms between HBsAg positivity and heavy alcohol intake are reported, suggesting a stronger additive effect of viral infections and alcohol drinking on the risk of HCC. On the basis of population attributable risks (AR), heavy alcohol intake seems to be the single most relevant cause of HCC in this area (AR: 45%) followed by HBV (AR: 22%) infection [28]. Similarly, another study by Sagnelli and colleagues has demonstrates that alcohol abuse can increase the risk of hepatitis B infection progressing to liver cirrhosis by threefold [29].

Furthermore, in another hospital-based, case-control study carried out in USA, the ORs for HCC based on multivariate analysis are 12.6, 4.5, and 4.3, respectively, for patients with HBsAg, heavy alcohol consumption (daily consumption of more than 80 mL of alcohol), and diabetes mellitus. Based on the additive model, synergistic interactions are observed between heavy alcohol consumption and diabetes mellitus (OR, 9.9) and chronic hepatitis virus infection (OR, 53.9). The significant synergy observed between heavy alcohol consumption, hepatitis virus infection, and diabetes mellitus may suggest the presence of a common pathway for hepatocarcinogenesis [30].

In another Taiwanese men prospective and community-based study carried out in the REVEAL-HBV study cohort over a period of 14 years, 20% of the patients are reported to be alcohol users [27]. Based on analyses adjusted for multivariable, alcohol abuse and extreme obesity (BMI ≥30 kg/m^2) have synergistic effects on the risk of incident HCC (HR, 3.40). Obesity and alcohol are also reported to have synergistic effects in increasing risk of incident HCC in HBsAg-positive men [27]. It is therefore concluded that lifestyle interventions might significantly reduce the incidence of HCC [27].

4. Treatment in patients with concomitant HBV infection and alcoholism

Antiviral therapies including lamivudine, adefovir dipivoxil, entecavir, telbivudine, tenofovir, and Peg-interferon have been widely prescribed for the treatment of HBV-related liver diseases worldwide [14, 31, 32]. Several large population-based and international studies have reveal that antiviral therapy could reduce the incidence of hepatic failure, cirrhosis, HCC, and mortality in CHB patients without alcoholism [33–40].

In patients with concomitant HBV infection and alcoholism, the prescription of both antiviral therapy and abstinence is important for the treatment of disease progression. Oral NA(s) can reduce the disease progression for HBV infection-induced liver diseases. Abstinence is one of the most important therapies for patients with alcohol-induced liver diseases [41]. In addition, abstinence has been shown to improve the histological features of hepatic injury and reduce the outcome of disease progression to cirrhosis, HCC, and mortality in patients with alcoholic liver diseases [5, 6, 41–45].

The indications of treatment for patients with concomitant HBV infection and alcoholism are based on three criteria: severity of liver disease, serum HBV DNA levels, and serum ALT

Alcoholic patients with HBsAg positive	HBV DNA (IU/mL)	ALT	Treatment
Decompensated cirrhosis	Detectable	Any	Treat with NA(s) and abstinence
Compensated cirrhosis	>2000	Any	Treat NA(s) and abstinence
Severe reactivation of chronic HBV	Detectable	Elevated	Treat with NA(s) or Peg-interferon and abstinence immediately
Non-cirrhotic HBeAg-positive chronic hepatitis B	>20,000	>2× ULN	Observation for 3 months. Treat with NA(s) or Peg-interferon and abstinence
		1–2× ULN	Monitor every 3 months Treat with NA(s) or Peg-interferon and abstinence if noninvasive tests suggest significant fibrosis
		Persistently normal	Monitor every 3 months Treat with NA(s) or Peg-interferon and abstinence if noninvasive tests suggest significant fibrosis
	2000–20,000	Any ALT	Monitor every 3 months. Assess fibrosis noninvasively. Monitor every 3 months Treat with NA(s) and abstinence if noninvasive tests suggest evidence of significant fibrosis.
	<2000	<ULN	Monitor every 3 months Treat with NA(s) or Peg-interferon and abstinence if noninvasive tests suggest significant fibrosis
		>ULN	Monitor every 3 months Treat with NA(s) or Peg-interferon and abstinence if noninvasive tests suggest significant fibrosis
	Undetectable	Any ALT	Treat with abstinence
Non-cirrhotic HBeAg-negative chronic hepatitis B	>2000	>2× ULN	Observation for 3 months. Treat with NA(s) or Peg-interferon and abstinence
		1–2× ULN	Monitor every 3 months Treat with NA(s) or Peg-interferon and abstinence if noninvasive tests suggest significant fibrosis

Alcoholic patients with HBsAg positive	HBV DNA (IU/mL)	ALT	Treatment
		Persistently normal	Monitor every 3 months Treat with NA(s) or Peg-interferon and abstinence if noninvasive tests suggest significant fibrosis
	<2000	>ULN	Monitor every 3 months Treat with NA(s) or Peg-interferon and abstinence if noninvasive tests suggest significant fibrosis
	Undetectable	Any	Treat with abstinence

Table 1. Treatment indications for patients with concomitant HBV infection and alcoholism.

levels [14]. The treatment in patients with concomitant HBV infection and alcoholism is summarized in **Table 1**.

4.1. In cirrhotic patients or patient with severe HBV reactivation with concomitant HBV infection and alcoholism

1. Alcoholic cirrhotic patients with decompensated cirrhosis and detectable HBV DNA require urgent antiviral treatment with NA(s) and abstinence [46, 47].
2. Alcoholic cirrhotic patients with compensated cirrhosis and HBV DNA >2000 IU/mL should be treated with NA(s) and abstinence.
3. Alcoholic patients with severe reactivation of HBV infection (the presence of high ALT, high bilirubin, INR more than 1.5 with impending or overt hepatic decompensation, and detectable HBV DNA) should be treated immediately with NA(s) and abstinence to prevent the development or deterioration of hepatic decompensation.

4.2. In pre-cirrhotic patients with concomitant HBV infection and alcoholism

1. Patient have persistently elevated ALT levels >2 times the upper limit of normal (ULN) (at least 3 months between observations) and HBV DNA >20,000 IU/mL if HBeAg positive and >2000 IU/mL if HBeAg negative. Treatment with antiviral therapy [NA(s) or Peg-interferon] and abstinence may be started. A noninvasive method for the estimation of the extent fibrosis is useful in such patients. Antiviral therapy and abstinence prevent further progression of fibrosis and other complications of liver disease.
2. Patients have minimally elevated or normal ALT levels (at least 3 months between observations) and HBV DNA >20,000 IU/mL if HBeAg positive and >2000 IU/mL if HBeAg negative, and a noninvasive method shows the presence of a significant fibrosis.

Treatment with antiviral therapy [NA(s) or Peg-interferon] and abstinence may be started. Antiviral therapy and abstinence prevent further progression of fibrosis and other complications of liver disease.

3. Patients have persistently elevated, minimally elevated, or normal ALT levels or HBV DNA <20,000 IU/mL if HBeAg positive and <2000 IU/mL if HBeAg negative, and a noninvasive method shows the presence of a significant fibrosis. Treatment with antiviral therapy [NA(s) or Peg-interferon] and abstinence may be started. NA(s) and abstinence prevent further progression of fibrosis and other complications of liver disease.

4. Patients have normal or elevated ALT levels and undetectable HBV DNA. Treatment with abstinence may be started. Abstinence prevents further progression of fibrosis and other complications of liver disease.

Our previous study shows that oral antiviral therapy significantly reduces the incidence of HCC in alcoholic cirrhotic patients with concomitant HBV infection (**Figure 2**) [6]. Therefore, aggressive NA(s) therapy should be considered in patients with alcoholic cirrhosis and detectable serum HBV DNA, in order to reduce the incidence of HCC [6].

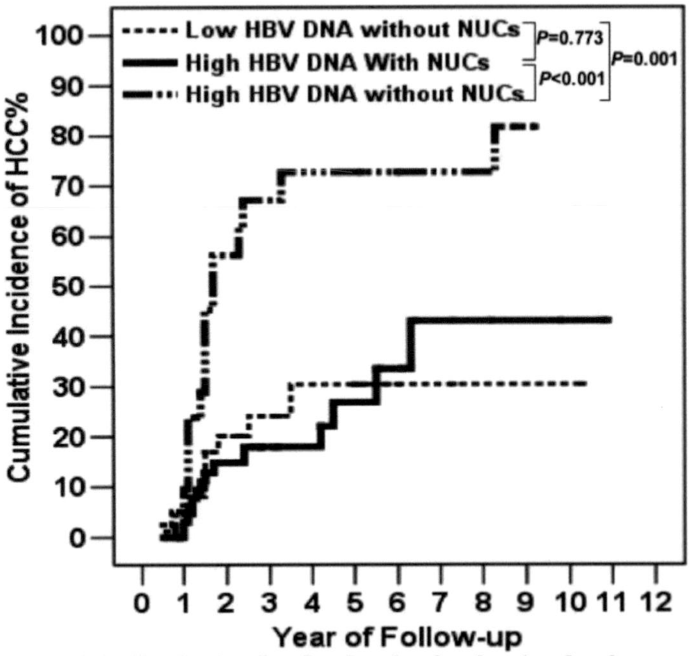

Patients at ris												
High HBV DNA without NUCs	21	20	8	6	5	5	4	3	3	1	0	0
High HBV DNA with NUCs	71	65	32	22	20	12	8	5	4	3	2	0
High HBV DNA Without NUCs	40	34	23	16	11	11	3	2	1	1	1	0

Figure 2. The cumulative incidence of HCC in cirrhotic patients with concomitant alcoholism and HBV infection is significantly reduced in patients receiving oral antiviral therapy.

5. Conclusion

Patients with concomitant HBV infection and alcoholism have high incidence of cirrhosis, HCC, and mortality. Treatment with antiviral therapy and abstinence may be started with the aim to reduce the incidence of cirrhosis, HCC, and mortality in patients with concomitant HBV infection and alcoholism.

Acknowledgements

We thank Jen-Chien Chen, Chia-Chang Hsu, and Kah Wee Koh for collection of the data.

Author details

Chih-Wen Lin[1,2,3,*], Chih-Che Lin[4] and Sien-Sing Yang[5]

*Address all correspondence to: lincw66@gmail.com

1 School of Medicine, College of Medicine, I-Shou University, Kaohsiung, Taiwan

2 Division of Gastroenterology and Hepatology, Department of Medicine, E-DA Dachang Hospital, I-Shou University, Kaohsiung, Taiwan

3 Department of Health Examination, E-Da Hospital, I-Shou University, Kaohsiung, Taiwan

4 Department of Surgery, Kaohsiung Chang Gung Memorial Hospital and Chang Gung University College of Medicine, Kaohsiung, Taiwan

5 Liver Unit, Cathay General Hospital and Fu-Jen Catholic University, Taipei, Taiwan

References

[1] Lee, W.M., *Hepatitis B virus infection*. N Engl J Med, 1997. **337**(24): p. 1733–45.

[2] Chen, C.J., L.Y. Wang, and M.W. Yu, *Epidemiology of hepatitis B virus infection in the Asia-Pacific region*. J Gastroenterol Hepatol, 2000. **15 Suppl**: p. E3–6.

[3] Voigt, M.D., *Alcohol in hepatocellular cancer*. Clin Liver Dis, 2005. **9**(1): p. 151–69.

[4] Morgan, T.R., S. Mandayam, and M.M. Jamal, *Alcohol and hepatocellular carcinoma*. Gastroenterology, 2004. **127**(5 Suppl 1): p. S87–96.

[5] Lin, C.W., et al., *Esophagogastric varices predict mortality in hospitalized patients with alcoholic liver disease in Taiwan*. Hepatogastroenterology, 2010. **57**(98): p. 305–8.

[6] Lin, C.W., et al., *Heavy alcohol consumption increases the incidence of hepatocellular carcinoma in hepatitis B virus-related cirrhosis*. J Hepatol, 2013. **58**(4): p. 730–5.

[7] Yang, S.-S., *Alcoholic liver disease: clinical and sonographic features*. J Med Ultrasound, 2008. **16**(2): p. 140–9.

[8] Larkin, J., et al., *Chronic ethanol consumption stimulates hepatitis B virus gene expression and replication in transgenic mice*. Hepatology, 2001. **34**(4 Pt 1): p. 792–7.

[9] Lin, C.W., et al C.-C.H., *The histological assessment of hepatitis B viral activity in patients with heavy alcohol consumption*. J Liver, 2016. 3(5): p. 1–4.

[10] Dolganiuc, A., et al., *Acute ethanol treatment modulates Toll-like receptor-4 association with lipid rafts*. Alcohol Clin Exp Res, 2006. **30**(1): p. 76–85.

[11] Barboza, L., et al., *A deficient translocation of CD3zeta, ZAP-70 and Grb2 to lipid raft, as a hallmark of defective adaptive immune response during chronic hepatitis B infection*. Cell Immunol, 2013. **284**(1–2): p. 9–19.

[12] Barve, S.S., et al., *Mechanisms of alcohol-mediated CD4+ T lymphocyte death: relevance to HIV and HCV pathogenesis*. Front Biosci, 2002. **7**: p. d1689–96.

[13] Ni, Y.H., et al., *Two decades of universal hepatitis B vaccination in taiwan: impact and implication for future strategies*. Gastroenterology, 2007. **132**(4): p. 1287–93.

[14] Sarin, S.K., et al., *Asian-Pacific clinical practice guidelines on the management of hepatitis B: a 2015 update*. Hepatol Int, 2016. **10**(1): p. 1–98.

[15] Chiang, C.J., et al., *Thirty-year outcomes of the national hepatitis B immunization program in Taiwan*. JAMA, 2013. **310**(9): p. 974–6.

[16] Addolorato, G., et al., *Treatment of alcohol use disorders in patients with alcoholic liver disease*. J Hepatol, 2016. **65**(3): p. 618–30.

[17] Mokdad, A.H., et al., *Actual causes of death in the United States, 2000*. JAMA, 2004. **291**(10): p. 1238–45.

[18] *Global status report on alcohol and health* 2014. World Health Organization.

[19] European Association for the Study of, L., *EASL clinical practical guidelines: management of alcoholic liver disease*. J Hepatol, 2012. **57**(2): p. 399–420.

[20] Mackenbach, J.P., et al., *Inequalities in alcohol-related mortality in 17 European countries: a retrospective analysis of mortality registers*. PLoS Med, 2015. **12**(12): p. e1001909.

[21] Chen, C.J., et al., *Risk of hepatocellular carcinoma across a biological gradient of serum hepatitis B virus DNA level*. JAMA, 2006. **295**(1): p. 65–73.

[22] Chen, C.J., et al., *Hepatitis B virus DNA levels and outcomes in chronic hepatitis B*. Hepatology, 2009. **49**(5 Suppl): p. S72–84.

[23] Chen, C.F., et al., *Changes in serum levels of HBV DNA and alanine aminotransferase determine risk for hepatocellular carcinoma*. Gastroenterology, 2011. **141**(4): p. 1240–8, 1248 e1–2.

[24] Chen, C.J., M.W. Yu, and Y.F. Liaw, *Epidemiological characteristics and risk factors of hepatocellular carcinoma*. J Gastroenterol Hepatol, 1997. **12**(9–10): p. S294–308.

[25] Yang, H.I., et al., *Hepatitis B e antigen and the risk of hepatocellular carcinoma*. N Engl J Med, 2002. **347**(3): p. 168–74.

[26] You, S.L., H.I. Yang, and C.J. Chen, *Seropositivity of hepatitis B e antigen and hepatocellular carcinoma*. Ann Med, 2004. **36**(3): p. 215–24.

[27] Loomba, R., et al., *Obesity and alcohol synergize to increase the risk of incident hepatocellular carcinoma in men*. Clin Gastroenterol Hepatol, 2010. **8**(10): p. 891–8, 898 e1–2.

[28] Donato, F., et al., *Hepatitis B and C virus infection, alcohol drinking, and hepatocellular carcinoma: a case-control study in Italy. Brescia HCC Study*. Hepatology, 1997. **26**(3): p. 579–84.

[29] Sagnelli, E., et al., *Impact of comorbidities on the severity of chronic hepatitis B at presentation*. World J Gastroenterol, 2012. **18**(14): p. 1616–21.

[30] Hassan, M.M., et al., *Risk factors for hepatocellular carcinoma: synergism of alcohol with viral hepatitis and diabetes mellitus*. Hepatology, 2002. **36**(5): p. 1206–13.

[31] Terrault, N.A., et al., *AASLD guidelines for treatment of chronic hepatitis B*. Hepatology, 2016. **63**(1): p. 261–83.

[32] European Association For The Study Of The, L., *EASL clinical practice guidelines: management of chronic hepatitis B virus infection*. J Hepatol, 2012. **57**(1): p. 167–85.

[33] Liaw, Y.F., et al., *Lamivudine for patients with chronic hepatitis B and advanced liver disease*. N Engl J Med, 2004. **351**(15): p. 1521–31.

[34] Eun, J.R., et al., *Risk assessment for the development of hepatocellular carcinoma: according to on-treatment viral response during long-term lamivudine therapy in hepatitis B virus-related liver disease*. J Hepatol, 2010. **53**(1): p. 118–25.

[35] Papatheodoridis, G.V., et al., *Incidence of hepatocellular carcinoma in chronic hepatitis B patients receiving nucleos(t)ide therapy: a systematic review*. J Hepatol, 2010. **53**(2): p. 348–56.

[36] Liaw, Y.F., *Impact of hepatitis B therapy on the long-term outcome of liver disease*. Liver Int, 2011. **31 Suppl 1**: p. 117–21.

[37] Peng, C.Y., R.N. Chien, and Y.F. Liaw, *Hepatitis B virus-related decompensated liver cirrhosis: benefits of antiviral therapy*. J Hepatol, 2012. **57**(2): p. 442–50.

[38] Hsu, Y.C., et al., *Entecavir versus lamivudine in the treatment of chronic hepatitis B patients with hepatic decompensation*. Antivir Ther, 2012. **17**(4): p. 605–12.

[39] Su, T.H., et al., *Four-year entecavir therapy reduces hepatocellular carcinoma, cirrhotic events and mortality in chronic hepatitis B patients*. Liver Int, 2016. 36(12): p. 1755–1764.

[40] Lim, Y.S., et al., *Mortality, liver transplantation, and hepatocellular carcinoma among patients with chronic hepatitis B treated with entecavir vs lamivudine*. Gastroenterology, 2014. **147**(1): p. 152–61.

[41] Pessione, F., et al., *Five-year survival predictive factors in patients with excessive alcohol intake and cirrhosis. Effect of alcoholic hepatitis, smoking and abstinence*. Liver Int, 2003. **23**(1): p. 45–53.

[42] O'Shea, R.S., et al., *Alcoholic liver disease*. Hepatology, 2010. **51**(1): p. 307–28.

[43] Borowsky, S.A., S. Strome, and E. Lott, *Continued heavy drinking and survival in alcoholic cirrhotics*. Gastroenterology, 1981. **80**(6): p. 1405–9.

[44] Brunt, P.W., et al., *Studies in alcoholic liver disease in Britain. I. Clinical and pathological patterns related to natural history*. Gut, 1974. **15**(1): p. 52–8.

[45] Luca, A., et al., *Effects of ethanol consumption on hepatic hemodynamics in patients with alcoholic cirrhosis*. Gastroenterology, 1997. **112**(4): p. 1284–9.

[46] Shim, J.H., et al., *Efficacy of entecavir in treatment-naive patients with hepatitis B virus-related decompensated cirrhosis*. J Hepatol, 2010. **52**(2): p. 176–82.

[47] Liaw, Y.F., et al., *Tenofovir disoproxil fumarate (TDF), emtricitabine/TDF, and entecavir in patients with decompensated chronic hepatitis B liver disease*. Hepatology, 2011. **53**(1): p. 62–72.

Chapter 12

Hepatitis B and C in Kidney Transplantation

Smaragdi Marinaki, Konstantinos Drouzas,

Chrysanthi Skalioti and John N. Boletis

Additional information is available at the end of the chapter

http://dx.doi.org/10.5772/65381

Abstract

The prevalence of chronic hepatitis B and C virus infection has declined among the dialysis population during the past decades. However, it still comprises a major health problem with high morbidity and mortality. Renal transplantation is the optimal treatment for patients with end-stage renal disease and hepatitis B or C, although it is associated to lower patient and allograft survival compared to seronegative kidney recipients. Novel therapeutic strategies with the use of new antiviral agents, especially direct-acting antiviral agents in hepatitis C, have significantly changed the natural history of both hepatitis B and C not only in the general population but also in renal-transplant recipients. We believe that future research should focus on the impact of new antiviral medications in this specific subset of patients.

Keywords: hepatitis B, hepatitis C, transplantation, direct-acting antiviral agents

1. Introduction

Though the prevalence of both hepatitis B and C is decreasing at least in developed countries, it still ranges from 0.1 to 20% for hepatitis B and from 2.5 to 13% for hepatitis C. General hygiene measures as well as specific measures in dialysis units and vaccination programs contributed to the reduction of hepatitis B and C prevalence in the dialysis population. However, hepatitis B and C seropositivity still remain an important clinical problem in this patient population associated with a high risk of morbidity and mortality. Although kidney transplantation is the treatment of choice for hepatitis B- and C-infected dialysis patients, morbidity and mortality are worse compared to seronegative patients. Major causes of death are liver cirrhosis and hepatocellular carcinoma.

This review focuses on pretransplant and posttransplant evaluation of prospective donors and recipients emphasizing the optimal use of grafts from hepatitis B- or C-seropositive donors and the impact of hepatitis B or C infection in patient and allograft survival. Additionally, it focuses on the role of novel antiviral agents.

2. Kidney transplantation and hepatitis B virus infection

2.1. Epidemiology

The human hepatitis B virus (HBV) is a small enveloped DNA virus causing acute and chronic hepatitis. Although a safe and effective vaccine has been developed and it has been available for the last two decades, HBV infection still represents a major global health problem. It is estimated that approximately 30% of the world's population has had contact with or are carriers of the HBV. An estimated 350 million of them are HBV carriers [1]. Around one million persons die of HBV-related causes annually. HBV prevalence varies from 0.1% in Western Europe, United States, Canada, Australia, and New Zealand, up to 20% in southern Asia, China, and sub-Saharan Africa. Intermediate prevalence (3–5%) is the Mediterranean countries, Japan, Central Asia, the Middle East, and South America. Acute infection occasionally results in fulminant hepatitis, but more importantly can progress to a chronic state, with decompensation, cirrhosis, and hepatocellular carcinoma being the most serious complications. The progression rate is approximately 90% for an infection acquired perinatally, and decreases to 5% for infections acquired during adulthood [2].

Hemodialysis (HD) patients are at an increased risk of acquiring HBV. Reasons include increased exposure to blood products, shared hemodialysis (HD) equipment, breaching of skin, and immunodeficiency. Hemodialysis, which requires access to the bloodstream, also may favor transmission of HBV between patients, and between patients and staff.

The prevalence of hepatitis B virus infection in hemodialysis patients has significantly decreased over the past few years. This is due to the implementation of effective prevention measures, such as general hygiene rules, separation during hemodialysis, and hepatitis B vaccination. The most important measure to prevent HBV infection is immunization against the virus. Chronic dialysis patients should receive vaccination against hepatitis B. Ideally, patients with chronic kidney disease (CKD) should receive vaccination against hepatitis B at earlier stages of the disease, before starting dialysis, since vaccine immunogenicity is low in dialysis patients (70%) compared to 90% in the general population. Intensified vaccination protocols have been used in hemodialysis patients with good responses. The presence of an adequate hepatitis B antibody (anti-HBs) titer should be checked annually. If the antibody titer is lower than 10 IU/ml, a booster dose of the vaccine should be administrated [3].

Although rates of new infection are decreasing [4], hepatitis B still remains a problem in dialysis populations. According to data from the United States Renal Data System (USRDS) in 2002, 1% of dialysis patients were seropositive for HBsAg [3]. A registry study of Asia-Pacific countries found the prevalence of hepatitis B surface antigen (HBsAg) positivity ranging from

1.3 to 14.6% [5]. Despite the decrease of HBsAg prevalence in dialysis patients, 350 million people worldwide are chronic HBV carriers and a large number of them will need transplantation in the future [6].

Hepatitis B virus–infected patients are at risk of exacerbation of the infection, progressive liver disease, and development of hepatocellular carcinoma after kidney transplantation. Renal transplantation offers higher survival and better quality of life compared to hemodialysis, which also applies to HBV patients, providing that they are receiving antiviral prophylaxis, since it is easier to prevent than treat HBV reactivation [7].

2.2. Evaluation of HBV-infected dialysis patients before transplantation

All dialysis patients should be checked routinely for HBsAg and when indicated with HBV DNA. HBV infected kidney transplant candidates should be tested for hepatitis B e antigen (HBeAg) and serum HBV DNA prior to transplantation. Patients who are HBeAg positive or have high levels of HBV DNA should receive antiviral treatment before transplantation with one of the available agents (lamivudine (LAM), entecavir (ETV), adefovir, tenofovir, and telbivudine (LdT)) until HBeAg becomes negative and viral replication is suppressed.

According to the Kidney Disease Improving Global Outcomes (KDIGO) guidelines, it is recommended that a liver biopsy is performed in HBsAg-positive hemodialysis patients on the waiting list for transplantation in order to evaluate liver disease status. If there is ongoing viral activity, candidates should repeat liver biopsy every 3–5 years [8]. Noninvasive testing for liver stiffness as fibroscan (elastography), which tends to replace liver biopsy in the general population, has not yet been validated neither in HBV-positive patients nor in patients on hemodialysis or after transplantation [9]. So, liver biopsy while on the waiting list still remains the "gold standard" for kidney transplant candidates.

Liver cirrhosis has for long been considered as an absolute contraindication for kidney transplantation alone; combined liver kidney transplantation is the treatment of choice in these patients. However, with the use of new nucleos(t)ide analogs, some dialysis patients with compensated cirrhosis achieve sustained viral response (SVR). If a follow-up biopsy after 12 months reveals partial reversibility of cirrhosis, those patients can be after that included in the waiting list and undergo kidney transplantation alone. This has been reported for HBV- and hepatitis C virus (HCV)-positive patients after SVR with the new antivirals [10].

HBsAg-positive renal transplant candidates should start antiviral treatment immediately after transplantation, regardless of the HBV DNA status or the findings of liver histology, due to the risk of severe reactivation, fibrosing cholestatic hepatitis, and rapid histological deterioration after the induction of immunosuppression.

2.3. Transmission of HBV infection from the donor

Besides HBV reactivation, HBV may be transmitted from the donor to the recipient. Renal transplantation from HBsAg-positive donors to HBV-naïve recipients is not recommended because it carries a significant risk of de novo infection, most often with an aggressive course

[11]. On the other hand, as shown by Jiang et al., allografts from HBsAg-positive donors can safely be transplanted into HBsAg-negative recipients with natural or acquired immunity (anti-HBs positive, titer above 10 IU/ml), with concurrent administration of hepatitis B hyperimmune globulin (HBIG) with or without booster vaccination [12]. In such cases, although the risk of transmission is relatively low, it is mandatory to inform patients and to obtain written consent in order to proceed with kidney transplantation. In a study by Singh et al., the successful procedure was described in 104 anti-HBs–positive recipients [13]. Prevention strategies included booster vaccination and concomitant administration of HBIG in combination with antiviral agents while vaccination alone was used in 27 patients.

In our center, we perform kidney transplantations from HBsAg-positive donors to HBsAg negative/HBsAb positive, that is, immunized either from past infection or from vaccination recipients. Those transplantations are performed only if the antibody titer of the recipient, measured immediately before transplantation, is at least 10 IU/ml and with concomitant administration of one dose of booster vaccination in combination with hepatitis B hyperimmune globulin(HBIG) while most of the recipients are started on antiviral prophylaxis postoperatively. The need and the duration of antiviral treatment in this patient population have not been investigated; moreover, data about monitoring long term are lacking. It seems logical to assume that antibody titer should be checked and booster vaccination should be administered when the titer falls below 10 IU/ml, since transplant recipients receiving immunosuppression are at risk for viral reactivation—if it has been transmitted from the donor —for long. However, to the best of our knowledge, current evidence is so sparse that only suggestions can be made.

Another issue regarding donor to recipient HBV transmission is that there is a very low but substantial risk of HBV transmission from HBsAg-negative, anti-HBc-positive, anti-HBs–negative donors to HBV-naïve recipients. In a recent review of 1385 HBsAg-negative kidney recipients from anti-HBc–positive donors, seroconversion to HbsAg positivity occurred in 0.28% (4/1385) and to anti-HBc positivity in 2.3% (32/1385) [14–16]. Ideally, those donors should be checked for anti-HBc IgM presence, indicating a more recent infection rather than ineffective immune response. Unfortunately, in the case of transplantation from deceased donors, this is impossible, due to the shortness of time. Given the organ shortage and the survival advantage of transplantation over remaining on hemodialysis, kidney transplantation could be considered in these cases too, since the risk for transmission is even lower than from HBsAg-positive donors. Again without data supporting the evidence, one may suggest that, in this case too, transplant candidates should be immunized and receive prophylaxis with booster vaccination and HBIG administration, while antiviral prophylaxis may not be indicated in this setting.

2.4. Outcome of HBV-infected patients after kidney transplantation

HBV-infected renal allograft recipients have worse survival compared to their seronegative counterparts. A meta-analysis of six observational studies, which included 6050 HBsAg-positive patients after kidney transplantation, showed that the relative risk of death and graft loss were 2.49 and 1.44, respectively [17].

The widespread use of antiviral agents since 1986 has significantly improved survival of HBV-infected kidney transplant recipients. In a small study from Italy, 42 HbsAg-positive patients who have been transplanted between 1976 and 1982 had a 12-year survival rate of 67% [18]. In a more recent study from Hong Kong, a 10-year survival of 63 HbsAg-positive renal transplant recipients who were treated with nucleoside/nucleotide analogs reached 81% [19]. However, liver failure remains the leading cause of death in this patient population. HBsAg-seropositive recipients who are HBeAg-negative have undetectable viral load, and for mild changes in liver biopsy they should receive preventive antiviral therapy immediately posttransplantation, in order to avoid viral reactivation due to immunosuppressive therapy. The only study that evaluated serial biopsies after kidney transplantation found histological deterioration in 85% of HBsAg-positive patients. No patient had cirrhosis before kidney transplantation while 28% of them had biopsy-proven liver cirrhosis after transplantation. Among those with cirrhosis, hepatocellular carcinoma was found in 23% [20].

2.5. Antiviral agents

The goal of treatment is suppression of viral replication and prevention of hepatic fibrosis, while minimizing resistance to the drugs. HBV DNA levels need to be measured systematically to assess response to therapy, because of the poor likelihood of seroconversion to anti-HBs and because of low reliability of alanine aminotransferase (ALT) as a marker of liver disease activity.

Treatment must be initiated before or immediately after transplantation. In a study of 15 patients, seven were started on lamivudine at the time of kidney transplantation. All patients had normal transaminase levels preoperatively. Half of those who were not treated initially showed transaminase elevations in the first year of follow-up requiring lamivudine therapy at that time. By contrast, all seven individuals who had received lamivudine at the time of transplantation remained negative for HBV DNA throughout the follow-up [21].

Currently, there are several medications available for the treatment of hepatitis B: interferon alfa-2b, pegylated interferon (PEG-INF) alfa 2a, and the nucleos(t)ide analogs lamivudine, adefovir, tenofovir, telbivudine, and entecavir.

2.5.1. Interferon and PEG-INF

In the current era of potent antiviral drugs as nucleoside analogs, the use of interferon-α (IFN) and PEG-IFN after transplantation is not recommended anymore. IFN-α has known immunomodulatory effects and its use in case series of kidney transplant recipients in the past has been associated with increased rates of graft loss due to rejection and with relapse rates approaching 80% after therapy discontinuation [22].

2.5.2. Lamivudine (LAM)

Lamivudine is a cytosine analog that inhibits HBV reverse transcriptase. The prophylactic use of lamivudine posttransplantation has proven efficacy long term. Since LAM was the first nucleoside analog approved for clinical use, most of the available data on the management of HBsAg-positive renal transplant recipients are with this agent. A meta-analysis of 14 clinical studies, which included 184 patients, showed that LAM administration results in undetectable viral load in 91% and a normalization of alanine aminotransferase (ALT) in 81% of patients, for a prolonged period of time [23]. Lamivudine has for long been the cornerstone of therapy in HBV-infected kidney transplant recipients and has increased survival rates. HBsAg-positive kidney recipients treated with lamivudine reached 10-year survival rates of 81%, comparable to HBsAg-negative patients [24].

Since it is eliminated by the kidney, its dose should be adapted to renal function: recommended dose is 100 mg/day in patients with estimated glomerular filtration rate (eGFR) >50 ml/min and 100 mg every other day in patients with less-preserved renal function.

The major problem with prolonged lamivudine treatment is the development of resistance. The presentation of the resistance varies. Some patients show only reappearance of serum HBA DNA, while others present with elevated liver enzymes. In most cases, resistance occurs due to a mutation in the tyrosine-methionine-aspartate-aspartate (YMDD) locus of the HBV DNA polymerase [25].

In a series of studies, the rates of lamivudine resistance vary from 20 up to 60% [26, 27]. In a study of 29 renal transplant recipients, after a mean follow-up of 69 months, 14 patients (48%) developed lamivudine resistance. Among them, 79% presented with a hepatitis flare. The YMDD mutation was found in all cases of resistance [25]. A meta-analysis of 2004 showed that increased duration of lamivudine therapy was positively associated with lamivudine resistance [22].

Patients with lamivudine resistance should be treated with adefovir, tenofovir, entecavir, or telbivudine.

2.5.3. *Tenofovir disoproxil fumarate (TDF)*

Tenofovir disoproxil fumarate (TDF) is a nucleotide analog and a potent inhibitor of human immunodeficiency virus type 1 reverse transcriptase and hepatitis B virus polymerase. Tenofovir is a potent antiviral agent for treatment-naïve patients and for patients with lamivudine resistance [28, 29]. Data for patients who have undergone kidney transplantation are limited and there are concerns for the development of kidney injury. Daude et al. conducted a study, which showed effective suppression of viral replication after 12 months of follow-up and preservation of stable kidney function in seven hepatitis B virus-positive solid-organ transplant recipients, with three renal-transplant recipients among them [30]. In a study of patients from the general population with HBV infection, tenofovir was effective in lamivudine-resistant cases, and did not induce resistance after up to 48 months of treatment [31].

2.5.4. *Telbivudine (LdT)*

Telbivudine is not effective in kidney transplant recipients with lamivudine-resistant HBV, because it shows cross-resistance to lamivudine and entecavir, since the virus develops the same mutations for both medications. Data about the use of telbivudine in renal transplantation are lacking.

2.5.5. Entecavir (ETV)

Entecavir, a guanosine analog, is 30 times more potent than lamivudine in suppressing viral replication and nowadays it is used as first-line prophylactic treatment in renal transplant recipients. This drug has a high antiviral potency, a high genetic barrier for resistance, and a good safety profile. There is sufficient evidence that it can effectively clear the viral load for a prolonged period. A recent prospective study included 27 renal transplant recipients, 18 (67%) were treatment naïve and 9 (33%) had been previously treated with LAM but had no resistant mutations. Entecavir cleared HBV DNA in 70, 74, 96, and 100% of patients after 12, 24, 52, and 104 weeks, respectively. Furthermore, entecavir reached higher rates of undetectable HBV DNA compared to lamivudine (32, 37, 63, and 63% at 12, 24, 52, and 104 weeks, respectively; $P < 0.005$) [32]. However, in patients with lamivudine-resistant HBV, complete response to entecavir can be delayed for more than 6 weeks, or not be achieved at all. The use of entecavir in renal transplant recipients who had developed lamivudine—or adefovir—resistance has been examined in a small study of 10 solid-organ-transplant recipients, with 8 kidney-allograft recipients among them, who were treated with entecavir for 16.5 months. There was a significant decrease in HBV DNA viral load (50%) without any significant adverse events [33]. Resistance to entecavir has not been documented in renal transplant recipients. In the general population, the rate of entecavir resistance is minimal (1.2%) in treatment-naïve patient after 5 years of therapy. However, in lamivudine-resistant patients, the probability of entecavir resistance at years 1–5 rises from 6 to 15, 36, 46, and 51%, respectively [34].

2.5.6. Adefovir dipivoxil (ADV)

Adefovir is an acyclic nucleotide adenosine analog. Adefovir is effective as monotherapy or in combination with entecavir in the general population with HBV infection and lamivudine resistance [35–38]. The problem with this agent is that it is potentially nephrotoxic. Studies in human immunodeficiency virus (HIV) patients show that high daily doses of adefovir (60–120 mg) may cause renal tubular injury. The drug is mainly used in lamivudine-resistant HBV cases [39]. Fontaine et al. studied the efficacy of adefovir as monotherapy at 11 renal-transplant recipients with lamivudine resistance. After 12 months, a satisfactory decline in serum HBV DNA and an absence of hepatitis flares were observed. Importantly, there were no significant clinical and laboratory adverse events [35]. In another study of 11 renal-transplant recipients with lamivudine resistance, adefovir was given at very low doses (10–2.5 mg/day) and it showed good efficacy, without nephrotoxicity [38]. In another study, evidence of nephrotoxicity implementing treatment discontinuation despite dosage adjustment was observed in 29% of patients [39].

2.6. Treatment duration

In the general population, the duration of treatment depends on the HBeAg status. HBeAg-positive patients should be treated until HBV DNA and HBeAg are cleared and anti-HBe seroconversion occurs. Additional treatment is needed for at least 6–12 months after anti-HBe seroconversion to prevent virological reactivation. Patients without HbeAg should be treated until HBsAg clearance. The duration of antiviral therapy for renal transplant recipients remains unclear, because outcomes after nucleos(t)ide analogs withdrawal in immunosuppressed patients allograft recipients are unknown.

One small retrospective study [40] evaluated the course of 6 out of 14 HBsAg(+) kidney-transplant recipients, in whom antiviral treatment had been discontinued after a median of 14 months. All of the six patients in whom antiviral agents had been discontinued were on stable, low-dose maintenance immunosuppression with undetectable HBV DNA and serological negativity for HBeAg. In four out of the six patients (67%), antiviral withdrawal was successful, without any sign of reactivation after a median follow-up of 60 months. In the remaining two patients, who had reactivated HBV, antiviral therapy was reintroduced immediately, with subsequent HBV clearance. Though the number of patients is indeed small, the study provides promising results for future investigation.

In the absence of robust data, we can suggest that antiviral treatment after kidney transplantation may be discontinued only in a subset of carefully selected patients who meet the following criteria: stable renal function and low immunological risk for rejection, low-dose maintenance immunosuppression for at least 6–9 months, no serological or biochemical evidence for HBV activity and previous antiviral treatment without resistance to any antiviral agent for at least 12 months. Close monitoring of HBV DNA every 3–6 months is essential, while antivirals should be reintroduced whenever immunosuppression must be intensified, that is, in the case of anti-rejection treatment.

2.7. Reactivation of HBV after renal transplantation: the role of immunosuppression

Immunosuppression is associated with hepatitis B virus reactivation not only in HBsAg-positive recipients but also in patients seropositive for anti-HBc/anti-HBs, usually in low titers, that is, past infection (reverse seroconversion) [41].

The majority of data come from studies in HBV patients treated for solid-organ or hematological malignancies [41, 42].

The main factors associated with HBV reactivation posttransplantation are the immunocompetence of the recipient, the total amount of immunosuppression, and finally the characteristics of the virus.

The status of immunosuppression changes the interaction between the HBV virus and the host, leading to potentially severe liver injury. Liver damage in the setting of immunosuppression may occur through two different mechanisms. The first mechanism is direct hepatotoxicity after the introduction of immunosuppression due to uncontrolled viral replication as a consequence of reduced immunosurveillance of the host. The second mechanism involves indirect, immune-mediated liver damage occurring after cessation of immunosuppression, during immune reconstitution. The second mechanism has been described in patients with solid-organ or hematologic malignancies even up to 6–12 months after completion of chemotherapy [43].

Since renal transplant recipients receive lifelong immunosuppression, hepatotoxicity in this setting may mostly be attributable to the first mechanism with the highest risk for viral reactivation being during the induction period, when the total amount of immunosuppression is high or whenever immunosuppression is intensified after that, as, for example, during anti-rejection treatment.

2.8. Immunosuppressive agents

Corticosteroids (CSs), calcineurin inhibitors (CNIs) (cyclosporine and tacrolimus), antimetabolites (mycophenolate mofetil (MMF) or mycophenolic sodium and azathioprine), and mammalian target of rapamycin (mTOR) inhibitors (sirolimus and everolimus) are the main immunosuppressants used in various combinations in kidney transplantation. Monoclonal antibodies (Rituximab, anti-IL2 Basiliximab) and polyclonal antibodies as antithymocyte globulin (ATG) are also part of the immunosuppressive regimen used for the induction or for the treatment of rejection. All of them are implicated in alterations of viral replication, mostly by inducing increased viral replication and enhance the risk of HBV reactivation. The risk of HBV reactivation according to specific immunosuppressive drug classes has been estimated by the American Gastroenterological Association (AGA) [44].

2.8.1. Rituximab

According to the AGA guidelines, Rituximab has the highest risk estimate of HBV reactivation (high >10%) from all immunosuppressants used in kidney transplantation. Moreover, the risk of HBV reactivation may persist up to 12 months, since the antibody has a prolonged phase of immune reconstitution.

Rituximab administration has been associated with HBV reactivation not only in HBsAg-positive but also in anti-HBc–positive and anti-HBs–positive patients (reverse seroconversion). In a prospective study of 314 HBsAg-negative patients with B-cell lymphoma treated with Rituximab, 16.2% were HBV carriers. All of them were anti-HBc positive, whereas half of them were also anti-HBs positive. Virus reactivation occurred in 12% of patients. HBV DNA clearance with the use of entecavir permitted readministration of Rituximab [45].

2.8.2. Polyclonal antibodies (antithymocyte globulin, ATG)

Increased viral replication following ATG administration has been described for herpes viruses, Epstein-Barr virus (EBV), and, to a lesser degree, cytomegalovirus (CMV). In those cases, ATG has been administered to patients with severe aplastic anemia concomitantly with cyclosporine [46]. Data about HBV reactivation after treatment with ATG are lacking.

2.8.3. Corticosteroids (CS)

Corticosteroids are the oldest and commonest immunosuppressants worldwide. Its use is undoubtedly associated with increased viral replication. Since they are used in many dosages, the risk of HBV reactivation depends on the dose and duration of CS administration. High corticosteroid doses increase viral replication, while ALT may be decreased. The opposite is observed during steroid tapering with elevated aminotransferases 4–6 weeks after steroid discontinuation [40]. According to the AGA guidelines, high CS doses (up to 20 mg/d of prednisone) and/or prolonged (>3 months) administration are considered as high risk for HBV reactivation while rapid tapering may also increase the risk for viral reactivation due to immune reconstitution.

In kidney transplantation, high CS doses are administered during the first weeks post transplantation; thereafter, they are tapered during a period of 3–6 months to a maintenance dose of 5 mg of prednisone daily or every other day. In stable, low-immunological risk patients they may be avoided completely (steroid-avoidance protocols) or they may be withdrawn after 4–6 weeks or even later (steroid-withdrawal protocols) with excellent outcomes. High CS doses, including intravenous pulses of methylprednisolone up to 500 mg/d, are used for the treatment of acute rejection.

In HBV kidney transplant recipients, steroids must be used at the lowest possible doses and preferably be discontinued or even completely avoided in patients with low immunological risk.

2.8.4. Calcineurin inhibitors

Calcineurin inhibitors are still the cornerstone of immunosuppression in kidney transplantation. It has been shown that cyclosporine reduces viral replication in vitro. Nowadays, most immunosuppressive regimens are tacrolimus based. Although there are no definite conclusions or guidelines, some suggest that cyclosporine may be preferable to Tacrolimus in HBV kidney transplant recipients. Nevertheless, since there are no definite conclusions, the choice of one of the two calcineurin inhibitors depends on the center's practice. Some others may argue that it is easier to withdraw steroids from a Tacrolimus-based regimen and would prefer this choice [47, 48].

2.8.5. Antimetabolites

Azathioprine, though hepatotoxic per se, has not been associated with an increased risk of HBV reactivation when given as monotherapy. Nevertheless, after the introduction of the more selective and more potent antimetabolites as the mycophenolic acids (MPAs), the use of azathioprine in kidney transplantation has been restricted to patients with special indications [49].

2.8.5.1. Mycophenolate acid derivates

Mycophenolate mofetil and the newer mycophenolate sodium have nowadays replaced azathioprine in most immunosuppressive regimens. Data about MPAs and HBV reactivation are lacking, but in general they are considered safe for HBV kidney-transplant recipients.

2.8.6. Mammalian target of rapamycin (mTOR) inhibitors

The reactivation of HBV with the use of mTOR inhibitors has not been studied in renal-transplant recipients and generally they are considered safe. Some case reports of HBV reactivation related to everolimus when used as a chemotherapeutic agent have been reported but everolimus dosage in this setting is much higher than the usual doses given as maintenance immunosuppression in kidney transplantation [50].

In conclusion, all immunosuppressants given in kidney transplantation can be used in HBV-positive recipients. The most important issue is the total amount of immunosuppression long term. It is crucial to maintain the lowest level of immunosuppression that is necessary to prevent rejection and to closely monitor the HBV status. Prophylactic antiviral treatment should be initiated immediately after transplantation and continued at least for 1 year after stable and low maintenance immunosuppression. In the carefully preselected patients in whom antivirals may be discontinued, close monitoring for HBV reactivation is mandatory.

2.9. In summarizing the existing evidence about kidney transplantation and HBV

- Though decreasing, HBV still remains a considerable problem in dialysis patients and kidney transplant recipients.
- Chronic kidney disease patients should be vaccinated before the initiation of dialysis.
- Intensified vaccination protocols should be applied to hemodialysis patients and antibody titer checked regularly.
- HBV-positive dialysis patients need monitoring with HBV DNA, viral serology (including HBeAg), and liver enzymes.
- HBsAg-positive candidates for kidney transplantation should be evaluated thoroughly with HBV DNA, liver enzymes, and liver biopsy.
- Antiviral treatment with tenofovir or entecavir (preferably to lamivudine) should be introduced to HBsAg-positive patients with viral activity on the waiting list.
- Patients with decompensated cirrhosis are candidates for combined liver-kidney transplantation, while compensated cirrhosis is no more an absolute contraindication for kidney transplantation alone.
- Kidney transplants from HBsAg-positive and from HBsAg-negative/anti-HBc–positive donors can be safely transplanted into immunized, HBsAg-negative recipients with concomitant prophylaxis.
- HBsAg-positive kidney transplant recipients should receive antiviral prophylaxis immediately after transplantation.
- In the current era of new antivirals, outcomes after transplantation are improving and long-term patient and graft-survival rates are approaching those of HBsAg-negative-matched recipients.
- The duration of antiviral prophylaxis after transplantation is unknown.
- Antivirals can be withdrawn in subsets of patients after transplantation.
- All immunosuppressants can be used in HBsAg-positive recipients.

- The total amount of immunosuppression must be kept at the lowest possible levels for the given donor/recipient.

In conclusion, with growing knowledge and evolving evidence in both fields, hepatitis B and transplantation, in the era of potent antivirals as nucleoside analogs, HBsAg-positive kidney-transplant candidates and recipients can be successfully treated and monitored and reach survival rates comparable to their HBsAg-negative counterparts.

3. Kidney transplantation and hepatitis C virus infection

3.1. Epidemiology of hepatitis C virus (HCV) infection

The prevalence of hepatitis C virus (HCV) infection worldwide is 3% and infected people are estimated to be approximately 170 millions. Prevalence rates in Africa, America, Europe, and South-East Asia are less than 2.5%. In the Western Pacific regions, the prevalence ranges between 2.5 and 4.9% while in some parts of the Middle East, it reaches 13% [51–53].

The prevalence of hepatitis C in patients with end-stage renal disease (ESRD) presents great variation worldwide. In northern Europe, it is below 5%, whereas in the US and southern Europe, it stands at 10%. In several North African, Asian, and Latin American countries, the relative disease prevalence varies between 10 and 70% [54]. In Greece, a 2003 collaborative study of the Hellenic Center for Infectious Diseases Control and the Hellenic Society of Nephrology showed that the percentage of patients with hepatitis C was 7.5% in a total of 7016 patients on dialysis [55].

Prior to 1990, the main routes of HCV transmission were blood-product transfusions, intravenous drug use, and unsafe medical procedures. Since the systematic screening of blood products, the risk of HCV infection related to transfusions is extremely low (1/20000000) [56]. Currently, the main routes of HCV infection are intravenous drug use, unsafe medical procedures, mother-to-child transmission, and the use of unsterilized materials in activities such as acupuncture and tattooing. Household and sexual transmission is extremely low. The dialysis-related risk is estimated at 2% per year. With the screening of blood products and the use of erythropoiesis-stimulating agents, the risk of transfusion-related HCV infection in dialysis patients has dramatically declined; however, they continue to comprise a "high-risk" group. In several studies, the prevalence of HCV infection correlated strongly with the time on dialysis, independently of the burden of transfusions and it was higher in HD than in home HD or peritoneal dialysis patients. These data strongly suggest that nosocomial transmission is of major importance [57].

Therefore, the KDIGO workgroup for the prevention of HCV transmission in dialysis patients focused on the implementation of hygienic precautions regarding the staff of HD units and the sterilization of the dialysis machines. Of major importance is the fact that the isolation of HCV-infected patients does not seem to protect against HCV transmission in HD units and therefore it is not recommended [53].

4. Kidney transplantation versus dialysis for HCV-infected dialysis patients

A meta-analysis of observational studies tried to establish the impact of hepatitis C virus infection on survival in dialysis patients. It showed that HCV-positive patients on dialysis have an increased risk of mortality compared with their HCV-negative counterparts, which is mainly attributed to liver-associated disease and its complications (relative risk, 5.89) [58].

Kidney transplantation is the treatment of choice for HCV-positive patients with ESRD. Three retrospective studies showed that transplantation offered a survival advantage in HCV-seropositive patients compared to those who remained on the waiting list [59–61]. A recent systematic review that included 9 studies with a total number of 2274 HCV-infected renal-transplant candidates and recipients showed that 5 years posttransplantation, anti-HCV–positive patients who had undergone kidney transplantation had approximately 55% lower risk of death compared to wait-listed patients [62].

5. Diagnosis and assessment of liver disease in HCV-positive kidney-transplant candidates

The clinical tools that are used for the assessment of liver damage for patients with ESRD do not differ from those used for the general population. Several studies have shown that aminotransferase (AST, ALT) levels are low in patients on dialysis and this reduction appears to occur in patients with advanced chronic kidney disease even before the initiation of renal-replacement treatment [63, 64].

All patients on the waiting list for a kidney allograft should be tested for hepatitis C, initially with an anti-HCV enzyme-linked immunosorbent assay (ELISA) and after a positive result by polymerase chain reaction assay (PCR) for the quantification of HCV RNA. Identification and classification of HCV genotype should follow. Screening for HCV must be a clinical routine and it must be performed once a year in all dialysis patients, since they are at constant risk of acquiring HCV infection. Dialysis units with a high prevalence of HCV should adopt a more strict protocol by examining their patient population for the presence of viremic activity, regardless of the result of the ELISA test [53].

Liver biopsy is recommended by the KDIGO guidelines as the "gold standard" for assessing the severity of hepatic damage and the prognosis of the disease. Furthermore, it can provide valuable assistance in planning the future treatment strategy [65]. A study on percutaneous liver biopsy in chronic hepatitis C patients found the procedure to be safe without increased risk in patients with ESRD [66]. The necessity of a liver biopsy is underlined by the following factors:

- There is no reliable correlation between the fluctuation of aminotransferases levels or the measurements of HCV RNA and the severity of liver injury as shown by histological findings in this group of patients [67].

- The percentage of HCV-positive renal transplant recipients that develop liver disease in the course of transplantation varies in different studies between 19 and 64% [59, 60].
- Studies have shown that up to 25% of ESRD patients with chronic hepatitis C infection have subclinical pre-cirrhotic disease in liver biopsy [68].
- The finding of advanced fibrosis in liver biopsy is a contraindication for renal transplantation, because 10-year survival is lower than 26% [52]. Patients with adequately compensated hepatic disease should be referred for simultaneous liver-kidney transplantation.

Novel, noninvasive, simple radiographic and serologic tests are used to validate hepatic fibrosis. Transient elastography (TE) evaluates the severity of fibrosis by liver-stiffness measurement. It has been used in non-uremic patients for the staging of fibrosis with satisfactory results [69]. In the dialysis population with chronic HCV infection, TE, performed with a Fibroscan machine, seemed to be efficient in estimating fibrosis in one study available [70]. Aspartate aminotransferase-to-platelet ratio index (APRI) is a serologic marker of fibrosis, easy to calculate. APRI is useful in diagnosing the degree of fibrosis [71], although it has a lower diagnostic accuracy than TE especially in cases of cirrhosis, in HD as well as in non-uremic patients with HCV [70]. Larger cohort studies are needed before noninvasive techniques can replace liver biopsy. Nevertheless, they can be useful when the biopsy cannot be performed because of contraindications or patient refusal.

6. Kidney donation from HCV-positive donors

All prospective donors should be evaluated for the risk of HCV infection based on blood tests, medical history, and lifestyle habits. Prior to transplantation, deceased and living donors should be screened for anti-HCV antibodies, preferably using ELISA third generation. However, the presence of antibodies against HCV in the donor may indicate a previous cleared infection and nontransmissibility. Thus, conducting PCR for HCV RNA is the next step for anti-HCV–positive donors. In the setting of cadaveric kidney transplantation, the results of HCV RNA will be available after transplantation. Therefore, the KDIGO guidelines advise against transplantation from HCV-positive donors to HCV-negative recipients [53], since it is well established that hepatitis C can be transmitted by solid-organ transplantation with a high frequency that approaches 100% in some studies [72, 73]. Viral transmission results in the occurrence of liver disease in the immunocompromised recipient, leading eventually to poor clinical outcomes due to infectious complications, development of cholestatic syndrome, and progression to hepatic failure [74].

Allocation of HCV-positive kidneys is controversial. The strategy of many transplant centers, including ours nowadays, is to accept kidneys from HCV-positive-deceased donors for HCV-positive-transplant candidates. According to the latest KDIGO guidelines [53], seropositive recipients should be tested by PCR for HCV RNA and must have an active viremia. This practice is based on the fact that kidney transplantation of HCV-infected dialysis patients from HCV-positive donors reduces the time in the transplant waiting list and is associated with superior survival compared to those who remain on the list waiting for a seronegative donor [75]. Additionally, a retrospective study by Morales et al. examined the differences between HCV-positive recipients who were transplanted either from HCV-positive donors or from HCV-negative donors. In terms of decompensated liver disease, no differences were observed between the two groups (10.3 vs. 6.2%). Moreover, 5- and 10-year patient survival were similar in the two groups, namely 84.8 and 72.7% in the subset of recipients from HCV-positive donors versus 86.6 and 76.5%, respectively, in those who received an HCV-negative renal allograft. Five- and ten-year graft survivals were decreased in the HCV-positive donor group (58.9% at 5 years and 34.4% at 10 years) compared to the HCV-negative donor group (65.5% at 5 years and 47.6% at 10 years, *p*: 0.006). However, this difference was not associated to HCV seropositivity in the multivariate regression analysis [76]. Ideally, donors and recipients should be matched for HCV genotype to minimize the risk of super-infection, even if this procedure is rarely performed during a deceased donor evaluation. However, two retrospective studies showed that the number of HCV genotypes has no significant effect on patient survival [77, 78]. In the new era of HCV treatment with the direct-acting antiviral agents (DAAs), the knowledge of the donors' genotype will be useful for the assessment of future treatment strategies.

Living donors with HCV infection and viremia should preferably receive appropriate treatment prior to donation, since the duration of therapy is short and it leads to sustained SVR [79]. On the other hand, prior to donation the transplant team should carefully consider and explain to the donor the risk for developing HCV-associated renal disease or diabetes mellitus in the future.

Based on the aforementioned data, the policy of transplanting a kidney from an anti-HCV–positive donor to an anti-HCV–positive recipient is considered to be a safe approach with good clinical outcomes in the long term. In any case prior to receiving an allograft, the HCV-infected-transplant candidate should be informed in detail about the HCV status of the donor, the risk of super-infection or other complications, the data regarding patient and graft survival, as well as the new treatment options.

7. Impact of HCV infection on posttransplant outcomes

Hepatitis C adversely affects the survival of both patients and grafts. Numerous, predominantly retrospective cohort studies report inferior 10-year survival rate of HCV-positive patients in comparison to uninfected kidney recipients [80–82]. Age at transplantation and the presence of anti-HCV antibodies were independently associated with patient survival [81]. However, a serious limitation of these studies is that histological data regarding the severity of hepatic disease pretransplantation were not available in the majority of them.

A recent meta-analysis of 18 observational trials that included 133,530 renal allograft recipients revealed an increased rate of all-cause mortality in HCV-positive patients after transplantation, regardless of the year of transplantation and thus the immunosuppressive regimen that was used, the country of origin or the number of patients. The main causes of death were cirrhosis and hepatocellular cancer. It is worth noting that hepatic disease developed late after transplantation. Cardiovascular mortality and cardiovascular disease were also more prevalent in this study group [83]. Additional extrahepatic causes of morbidity and mortality were new onset diabetes after transplantation (NODAT), de novo and recurrent glomerular diseases (mainly de novo type I membranoproliferative GN), and sepsis [84–86].

The abovementioned studies demonstrated also that graft survival is decreased in seropositive patients posttransplantation. More specifically, the meta-analysis by Fabrizi et al. showed that the adjusted relative risk of graft loss in these patients compared to those who are not infected was 1.76 [83]. Allograft failure has been attributed to the aforestated morbidity factors, namely diabetes and glomerulonephritides, as well as to the occurrence of transplant glomerulopathy and chronic allograft injury [83–87].

8. Therapy

Treatment of patients infected with HCV comprises the traditional approach with interferon and ribavirin, as well as novel regimens, interferon-a-free that consist of the direct-acting antiviral agents. Therapeutic regimens aim at the elimination of the virus. The viral load, based on HCV RNA quantification in serum, must be undetectable (10–15 IU/ml) 12 weeks after the end of treatment (SVR).

8.1. Traditional therapy

In the past decade, interferon and ribavirin were considered to be the cornerstone of HCV antiviral treatment. Nonetheless, these drugs were associated with considerable toxicity. More specifically, the use of interferon after kidney transplantation induced acute kidney injury, episodes of rejection resistant to steroid therapy, and graft loss [88, 89]. Therefore, before 2013 transplant candidates could only be treated prior to transplantation as the KDIGO guidelines recommended, with the exception of patients with fibrosing cholestatic hepatitis [53]. However, the Dialysis Outcomes Practice Patterns Study demonstrated that only a minority of ESRD patients on dialysis were treated for HCV [90]. Among 4589 HCV-positive HD patients who were observed from 1996 to 2011, only 48 (1%) were treated for HCV, whereas among the subset of patients waiting on the list for transplantation, only 3.7% were treated for HCV. The reasons for this approach were as follows:

- The use of ribavirin in this patient population aggravated anemia that was already present due to chronic kidney disease.
- Pegylated interferon-α (PegIFN-α) as monotherapy resulted in poor outcomes, with SVR 30–35% [91].
- Addition of ribavirin in low doses increased the SVR to 55% after 6 months, but also increased side effects [92].
- A substantial percentage of patients (18–30%) dropped out of therapy.

Nevertheless, HCV clearance when achieved was maintained posttransplantation in the vast majority of patients despite the use of immunosuppression [93].

8.2. Novel therapeutic agents

Thorough understanding of the HCV structure, replication mechanism, and cell cycle has led to the development of the DAAs. These drugs are small molecules that target nonstructural (NS) viral proteins and inhibit HCV replication. Four classes of DAAs exist, namely NS3/4A protease inhibitors (PIs) simeprevir, paritaprevir, and grazoprevir, NS5B nucleoside polymerase inhibitors (NPIs) and non-nucleoside polymerase inhibitors (NNPIs) sofosbuvir and dasabuvir, respectively, and NS5A inhibitors ledipasvir, daclatasvir, ombitasvir, and elbasvir [94].

The introduction of these new agents has modernized the therapeutic ammunition and has radically changed the treatment of patients with HCV infection; ongoing trials are expected to prove the safety and efficacy of DAAs in patients with impaired renal function and ESRD and establish proper dosing regimens. Besides the spectacular effectiveness of these drugs (SVR over 95%) in patients who had not received prior therapy [95], another important issue is the improved tolerance to treatment, due to reduced treatment duration and fewer side effects.

Different combinations of DAAs are administered based on the different HCV genotypes (**Table 1**).

Genotype 1α και 1b	***Genotype 4***
PegIFN-α, RBV, and Sofosbuvir	PegIFN-α, RBV, and Sofosbuvir
PegIFN-α, RBV, and Simeprevir	PegIFN-α, RBV, and Simeprevir
Sofosbuvir and Ledipasvir	Sofosbuvir and Ledipasvir
Ritonavir, Paritaprevir	Ritonavir, Paritaprevir, Ombitasvir
Ombitasvir and Dasabuvir	Sofosbuvir and Simeprevir or Daclatasvir
Sofosbuvir and Simeprevir or Daclatasvir	Grazoprevir, Elbasvir ± Ribavirin
Grazoprevir, Elbasvir ± Ribavirin	
Genotype 2	***Genotype 5***
PegIFN-α, RBV, and Sofosbuvir	PegIFN-α, RBV, and Sofosbuvir
Sofosbuvir and RBV	Sofosbuvir and Ledipasvir
Sofosbuvir and Daclatasvir	
Genotype 3	***Genotype 6***
PegIFN-α, RBV, and Sofosbuvir	PegIFN-α, RBV, and Sofosbuvir
Sofosbuvir and Daclatasvir	Sofosbuvir and Ledipasvir

Table 1. Treatment recommendation (EASL 2015) for chronic hepatitis C patients without liver cirrhosis.

The first studies that evaluated the effectiveness of DAAs excluded patients with estimated glomerular filtration rate (eGFR) less than 30 ml/min/1.73m^2, patients on dialysis, and renal-transplant recipients. It is worth noting that sofosbuvir is contraindicated for patients with eGFR <30 ml/min/1.73m^2 and for dialysis patients [94, 95]. Therefore, treatment options for this study group with HCV infection from genotypes 2, 3, 5, and 6 of HCV are limited, because all regimens include sofosbuvir. Severe, urgent cases should receive treatment after careful expert consultation. On the other hand, results are very promising for patients with genotypes 1 and 4 in comparison with the general population. Ruby-I is a single-arm multicenter study, in which 20 patients with HCV genotype 1 and CKD stage 4,5 or in dialysis were given ombitasvir co-formulated with paritaprevir and ritonavir, administered with dasabuvir for 12 weeks. Patients with HCV genotype 1a infection also received ribavirin (n:13), whereas those with genotype1b infection did not (n:7). The majority of patients, 90%, achieved the primary end point which was SVR 12 weeks after the end of treatment (SVR12). One patient did not achieve an SVR12 because of a relapse and another one died from causes not related to treatment. The most common adverse event was anemia (69%) due to ribavirin treatment, which led to drug discontinuation in nine cases [96]. C-Surfer is a multicenter, phase 3, randomized study of safety and observational study of efficacy regarding the combination of grazoprevir and elbasvir (both approved by the Food and Drug Administration (FDA) and wait to be approved by the European Medicines Agency (EMA) in 2016) for patients with genotype 1 infection and stage 4–5 CKD. The treatment group consisted of 111 patients, who received grazoprevir and elbasvir for 12 weeks. The results were remarkable. The SVR12 was 99%, with only one patient relapsing, whereas the drugs were well tolerated with minor adverse events that did not lead to drug discontinuation [97].

The use of interferon-free treatment regimens is of major importance in renal transplantation because it eliminates the risk of acute allograft rejection and subsequent graft loss. An important question that arises is when is the proper timing of treatment, pre- or post transplantation? The introduction of DAAs permits us to exceed the narrow timeframes before transplantation and treat our patients after transplantation. Thus, we have the advantage of using allografts from HCV-positive donors for recipients willing to accept them. This practice minimizes the time on the waiting list and subsequently the time on dialysis and all its deleterious effects as we have already mentioned, but it cannot be applied in small countries such as Greece with extremely long waiting time on the list. On the other hand, treatment with DAAs prior to transplantation may offer the advantage of increasing the overall survival of patients by diminishing the risk of hepatic and extrahepatic complications especially severe, evolving liver disease, glomerulonephritis and NODAT. Another important issue to consider when deciding the timing of treatment is the virus genotype. Eradication of the virus in patients infected with genotype 1 or 4 is plausible before transplantation, since sofosbuvir-free regimens are available.

In renal transplantation, the DAAs are used according to the guidelines applied to the general population and the liver-transplant recipients. Until 2016, there were no data to guide the use of these agents in kidney transplant patients and to demonstrate their efficacy and safety to this subpopulation of patients. The policy of many transplant centers, including ours, is that all kidney-transplant patients with chronic HCV infection and eGFR >30 ml/min/1.73m^2 receive appropriate therapy with a new, interferon-free antiviral regimen based on the detected genotype (**Table 1**). The dose of DAAs is not adjusted when eGFR is greater than 30 ml/min/

1.73m^2. Ribavirin is not recommended with eGFR <30 ml/min/1.73m^2 although it has been used in patients after renal transplantation with a close monitoring of hemoglobin levels [98].

Of great importance are the drug-drug interactions between the DAAs and the immunosuppressive agents and the mandatory dose adjustments (**Table 2**).

	Daclatasvir	Sofosbuvirκαι Ledipasvir	Ritonavir, Paritaprevir, Ombitasvirκαι Dasabuvir	Simeprevir	Sofosbuvir
Everolimus	[Orange]	[Orange]	[Orange]	[Orange]	[Green]
Azathioprine	[Green]	[Green]	[Green]	[Green]	[Green]
Ciclosporin	[Green]	[Orange]	[Orange]	[Red]	[Green]
Mycophenolate	[Green]	[Green]	[Orange]	[Green]	[Green]
Sirolimus	[Green]	[Orange]	[Orange]	[Orange]	[Green]
Tacrolimus	[Green]	[Orange]	[Orange]	[Orange]	[Green]

Green: No significant interaction is expected.

Orange: Possible interaction which requires close monitoring, changing the dosage, and/or drug-delivery time.

Red: Avoid concomitant use of drugs.

This table is based on data by the University of Liverpool on the site http://www.hep-druginteractions.org (University of Liverpool). For additional drug-drug interactions and for a more extensive range of drugs, detailed pharmacokinetic interaction data, and dosage adjustments, refer to the abovementioned website.

Table 2. Interactions between immunosuppressive drugs and DAA agents.

Since 2016, several studies have emerged. Kamar et al. tried to assess the efficacy and safety of an interferon-free regiment based on sofosbuvir. Twenty-five renal-transplant recipients with HCV infection (19/25 Genotype 1, 2/25 Genotype 2, 1/25 Genotype 3, 3/25 Genotype 4) received various combinations of sofosbuvir with other agents; ribavirin (n:3), daclatasvir (n:4), simeprevir (n:6), simeprevir and ribavirin (n:1), ledipasvir (n:9), ledipasvir and ribavirin (n:1), pegylated interferon and ribavirin (n:1). At week 12, an impressive SVR of 100% was recorded. During therapy, no significant adjustments in the dose of immunosuppressive drugs were required and kidney function remained stable [109]. However, after virus clearance, trough levels of tacrolimus decreased without any dose change. It is already known that HCV infection alters the pharmacokinetics of CNIs and results in increased drug exposure [99]. Therefore, we must be cautious after HCV clearance and adjust the dose of CNIs accordingly. A case series study of 20 HCV-infected kidney recipients (85% Genotype 1, 15% Genotype 2) who were treated off-label with sofosbuvir in combination with simeprevir (n:9), ribavirin (n:3), ledipasvir (n:7), and daclatasvir (n:1) demonstrated a sustained virological response of 100% at week 12 and it was maintained for a short median follow-up period of 8.6 months [100].

These impressive results show that the efficacy and safety of DAAs in renal transplant recipients is comparable with the general population. It remains to be determined if viral clearance after transplantation will improve long-term patient and kidney-allograft outcomes. The optimal timing of HCV therapy (posttransplantation or pretransplantation) has not clearly been determined. Taking into account that based on clinical trials the DAAs will be available for patients with eGFR <30/ml/min/1.73m^2 in the near future, treating these patients before transplantation may prevent posttransplantation complications and improve the overall outcomes. For the time being, ESRD patients infected with HCV Genotypes 2, 3, 5, 6 can be treated with DAAs only after transplantation or when it is absolutely obligatory in life-threatening conditions.

9. Immunosuppression in HCV-positive kidney transplant recipients

Immunosuppression may increase hepatitis C viral proliferation after transplantation and thus accelerate the evolution of hepatic damage [101]. Information regarding the use of immunosuppressive drugs in seropositive allograft recipients comes mostly from liver transplantation, as well as from the experience in the field of oncology-hematology. Large, prospective studies examining the effect of immunosuppressive drugs in HCV-seropositive recipients are lacking. However, the total amount of induction and maintenance immunosuppression may play an important role in the reactivation of the virus post transplantation.

10. Immunosuppressive agents

10.1. Rituximab

The use of anti-CD20 monoclonal antibody rituximab has been reported in a small number of seven HCV-positive patients after kidney transplantation. It was not related to the recurrence of the infection in a follow-up period of 19 months [102]. Larger studies in the field of hematology have shown a high incidence of hepatic flares in HCV-seropositive patients following treatment with Rituximab for lymphoma [103].

10.2. Induction therapy

Data from the Scientific Registry of Transplant Recipients (SRTRs) demonstrated that induction therapy, with polyclonal or monoclonal antibodies, has been associated with a lower risk of death. This finding could probably be attributed to lower rejection rates in patients receiving induction treatment [104]. Anti-CD3 monoclonal antibody OKT3, however, has been associated with recurrence of HCV in liver transplantation [105]. It is therefore avoided in HCV-infected patients after transplantation. On the other hand, the administration of the polyclonal antibody antithymocyte globulin (ATG) as induction therapy in 104 HCV-infected kidney-transplant patients did not induce viral replication [106], a finding that was confirmed by subsequent studies [107]. Contradictory data exist regarding monoclonal anti-IL2 antibodies, such as daclizumab. A single-center study in a small number of patients showed that therapy with daclizumab is followed by faster progression of liver fibrosis compared to ATG [108]. Large studies based on data from the United Network for Organ-Sharing UNOS base indicate that liver-transplant recipients with chronic HCV infection exhibit satisfactory graft and patient survival after receiving induction with daclizumab [109, 110].

10.3. Corticosteroids (CS)

High pulses of corticosteroids can cause up to 100 times increase of the viral load, but this has only been demonstrated in liver transplantation [107]. Although rapid steroid discontinuation leads to lower rates of diabetes and HCV recurrence, it has been associated with worst outcomes in liver transplantation [111, 112]. In the aforementioned study by Luan et al., in a total of 3708 HCV-positive kidney transplant patients, mortality rates were similar between those who received CS and those who did not [104].

10.4. Calcineurin inhibitors (CNIs)

In vitro studies have shown that cyclosporine may have an antiviral effect by suppressing HCV replication and the expression of proteins [113]. Moreover, cyclosporine is less diabetogenic in comparison with tacrolimus. However, in a cohort of 71 patients with HCV infection posttransplantation, liver fibrosis and viral replication were similar regardless of the CNI used [114]. Additionally, data from the Scientific Registry of Transplant Recipients (SRTR) [104] did not confer a survival advantage of cyclosporine over tacrolimus in renal allograft recipients.

10.5. Antimetabolites

MPAs appear to be safe in HCV-seropositive individuals after kidney transplantation. Notably, MMF administration was related to a reduced risk of death (hazard ratio (HR): 0.77, p: 0.005) in the study by Luan et al., implying a possible advantageous effect of the drug in renal recipients with chronic HCV infection [104].

10.6. Mammalian target of rapamycin (mTOR) inhibitors

Data regarding the use of mTOR inhibitors in transplant patients with HCV infection are limited. Sirolimus was associated with decreased evolution of hepatic fibrosis and cell proliferation in vitro, in an animal model of hepatic fibrosis [115]. This finding was not confirmed in a small cohort study of HCV-infected kidney recipients, where switch from CNI to sirolimus was not followed by lower viral load [116].

In conclusion, almost all immunosuppressive agents can be used in HCV-positive renal recipients. As in the case of HBV, the most important issue is the total level of immunosuppression, which should be kept as low as possible based on the specific conditions of transplantation and the immunological profile of the recipient. Close monitoring of HCV RNA is mandatory.

11. In summarizing the existing evidence about kidney transplantation and HCV

- The prevalence of hepatitis C in patients with ESRD presents great variation worldwide and is correlated with the time on dialysis.
- Kidney transplantation is the choice of therapy for HCV-infected patients with ESRD.
- Mortality is lower among patients who undergo kidney transplantation compared to those remaining on the waiting list.
- Liver biopsy should be performed in all HCV-infected renal transplant candidates.
- Systematic screening for HCV should be routinely done in all ESRD patients. Dialysis units with a high prevalence of HCV should preferably test all patients for HCV RNA, regardless of the presence of anti-HCV antibodies.
- Well-compensated cirrhosis is not a contraindication to kidney transplantation.
- Renal transplant recipients with chronic HCV infection have lower patient and allograft survival post transplantation compared with noninfected renal transplant recipients.
- Major causes of mortality in HCV-infected renal transplant recipients are cirrhosis and hepatocellular cancer. Additional causes of morbidity following kidney transplantation are de novo and recurrent and glomerular diseases and NODAT.
- Transplantation of a renal allograft from an HCV-infected donor may cause HCV infection to the recipient.
- All potential kidney donors, deceased and living, should be evaluated for the risk of HCV infection based on blood tests, medical history, and lifestyle habits.
- Kidneys from HCV-positive donors are donated to anti-HCV–positive recipients.
- Interferon should not be administered in renal transplant recipients with chronic HCV infection because it is associated with rejection episodes and graft loss.
- We suggest the following approach regarding antiviral treatment in HCV-infected renal allograft recipients:
  - All patients with eGFR >30 ml/min/1.73 m^2 should receive a new, interferon-free antiviral regimen based on the virus genotype.
  - Patients with eGFR <30 ml/min/1.73 m^2 should not be treated with sofosbuvir. Treatment options for genotypes 2, 3, 5, and 6 of HCV are limited. In severe conditions, treatment should be discussed with experts.
  - In the case of HCV genotype 1 or 4, the combination grazoprevir-elbasvir can be administered.

- Potential drug-drug interactions of antivirals with immunosuppressive agents present an important issue in selecting the appropriate immunosuppressive regimen after kidney transplantation.

- Immunosuppressive agents can safely be used in HCV-positive renal recipients with close monitoring of HCV RNA and minimization of immunosuppression.

In conclusion, the development of direct-acting antiviral agents (DAAs) may change the natural history of HCV infection in renal allograft recipients. Randomized, prospective trials are expected to prove the safety and efficacy, as well as the optimal dose of DAAs in patients with impaired renal function, ESRD, and kidney transplantation.

Author details

Smaragdi Marinaki, Konstantinos Drouzas, Chrysanthi Skalioti* and John N. Boletis

*Address all correspondence to: c_skalioti@yahoo.com

National and Kapodistrian University of Athens, Medical School, Nephrology Department and Renal Transplantation Unit, Laiko Hospital, Athens, Greece

References

[1] Goldstein ST, Zhou F, Hadler SC et al. A mathematical model to estimate global hepatitis B disease burden and vaccination impact. *Int J Epidemiol 2005*; 34: 1329–1339.

[2] Wasley A, Grytdal S, Gallagher K. Surveillance for acute viral hepatitis-United States, 2006. *MMWR Surveill Summ 2008*; 57: 1–24.

[3] Rangel MC, Coronado VG, Euler GL et al. Vaccine recommendations for patients on chronic dialysis. The Advisory Committee on Immunization Practices and the American Academy of Pediatrics. *Semin Dial 2000*; 13: 101–107.

[4] Finelli L, Miller JT, Tokars JI et al. National surveillance of dialysis-associated diseases in the United States, 2002. *Semin Dial 2005*; 18: 52–61.

[5] Johnson DW, Dent H, Yao Q et al. Frequencies of hepatitis B and C infections among haemodialysis and peritoneal dialysis patients in Asia–Pacific countries: Analysis of registry data. *Nephrol Dial Transplant 2009*; 24: 1598–1603.

[6] Hatzakis A, Wait S, Bruix J et al. The state of hepatitis B and C in Europe: report from the hepatitis B and C summit conference. *J Viral Hepat 2011*; 18: 1–16.

[7] Lu K, Wang HP, Chen HS. Outcomes of kidney transplantation recipients with hepatitis in the antiviral therapy era: a single-center experience. *Transplant Proc 2014*; 46: 460–463.

[8] KDIGO clinical practice guideline for the care of kidney transplant recipients. *Am J Transplant 2009*; 9 (3): S1–155.

[9] Foucher J, Chanteloup E, Vergniol J et al. Diagnosis of cirrhosis by transient elastography (FibroScan): a prospective study. *Gut 2006*; 55: 403–408.

[10] Poll S, Carnot F, Nalpas B et al. Reversibility of hepatitis C virus-related cirrhosis. *Hum Pathol 2004*; 35: 107–112.

[11] Wolf JL, Perkins HA, Schreeder MT et al. The transplanted kidney as a source of hepatitis B infection. *Ann Intern Med1979*; 91: 412–413.

[12] Jiang H, Wu J, Zhang X et al. Kidney transplantation from hepatitis B surface antigen positive donors into hepatitis B surface antibody positive recipients: a prospective nonrandomized controlled study from a single center. *Am J Transplant. 2009*; 9: 1853–1858.

[13] Singh G, Hsia-Lin A, Skiest D et al. Successful kidney transplantation from a hepatitis B surface antigen-positive donor to an antigen-negative recipient using a novel vaccination regimen. *Am J Kidney Dis 2013*; 61: 608–611.

[14] Mahboobi N, Tabatabaei SV, Blum HE et al. Renal grafts from anti-hepatitis B core-positive donors: A quantitative review of the literature. *Transplant Infect Dis 2012*; 14: 445–451.

[15] Wachs ME, Amend WJ, Ascher NL et al. The risk of transmission of hepatitis B from HBsAg(-), HBcAb(+), HBIgM(-) organ donors. *Transplantation 1995*; 59: 230–234.

[16] Madayag RM, Johnson LB, Bartlett ST et al. Use of renal allografts from donors positive for hepatitis B core antibody confers minimal risk for subsequent development of clinical hepatitis B virus disease. *Transplantation 1997*; 64: 1781–1786.

[17] Fabrizi F, Martin P, Dixit V et al. HBsAg seropositive status and survival after renal transplantation: meta- analysis of observational studies. *Am J Transpl 2005*; 5: 2913–2921.

[18] Aroldi A, Lampertico P, Montagnino G et al. Natural history of hepatitis B and C in renal allograft recipients. *Transplantation 2005*; 79: 1132–1136.

[19] Yap DY, Tanq CS, Yung S et al. Long term outcome of renal transplant recipients with chronic hepatitis B infection. Impact of antiviral treatments. *Transplantation 2010*; 90: 325–330.

[20] Fornairon S, Pol S, Legendre S et al. The long-term virologic and pathologic impact of renal transplantation on chronic hepatitis B virus infection. *Transplantation 1996*; 62: 297–299.

[21] Filik L, Karakayali H, Moray G et al. Lamivudine therapy in kidney allograft recipients who are seropositive for hepatitis B surface antigen. *Transplant Proc 2006*; 38: 496–498.

[22] Magnone M, Holley Jl, Shapiro R et al. Interferon-alpha-induced acute renal allograft rejection. *Transplantation 1995*; 59: 1068–1070.

[23] Fabrizi F, Dulai G, Dixit V et al. Lamivudine for the treatment of hepatitis B virus-related liver disease after renal transplantation: meta-analysis of clinical trials. *Transplantation 2004*; 77: 859–864.

[24] Fontaine H, Tiers V, Chretien Y et al. HBV genotypic resistance to lamivudine in kidney recipients and hemodialyzed patients. *Transplantation 2000*; 69(10): 2090–2094.

[25] Fabrizi F, Martin P. Management of Hepatitis B and C virus infection before and after transplantation. *Curr Opin Organ Transpl 2006*; 11: 583–588.

[26] Chan TM, Che KC, Tang CS. Prospective study on lamivudine-resistant hepatitis B in renal allograft recipients. *Am J Transpl 2004*; 4: 1103–1109.

[27] Lok AS, McMahon BJ. Chronic hepatitis B. *Hepatology 2007*; 45: 507–539.

[28] Jenh AM, Thio CL, Pham PA. Tenofovir for the treatment of hepatitis B virus. *Pharmacotherapy 2009*; 29: 1212–1227.

[29] Krummel T, Parvez-Braun L, Frantzen L et al. Tenofovir-induced acute renal failure in an HIV patient with normal renal function. *Nephrol Dial Transplant 2005*; 20: 473–474.

[30] Daudé M, Rostaing L, Sauné K et al. Tenofovir therapy in hepatitis B virus-positive solid-organ transplant recipients. *Transplantation 2011*; 91: 916–920.

[31] Marcellin P, Heathcote EJ, Buti M et al. Tenofovirdisoproxil fumarate versus adefovir-dipivoxil for chronic hepatitis B. *N Engl J Med 2008*; 359(23): 2442–2455.

[32] Hu TH, Tsai MC, Chien YS et al. A novel experience of antiviral therapy for chronic hepatitis B in renal transplant recipients. *Antivir Ther 2012*; 17(4): 745–753.

[33] Kamar N, Milioto O, Alric L et al. Entecavir therapy for adefovir-resistant hepatitis B infection in kidney and liver transplant recipients *Transplantation 2008*; 86: 611–614.

[34] Tenny DJ, Pokornowsky KA, Rose RE et al. Entecavir at five years shows long-term maintenance of high genetic barrier to hepatitis B virus resistance. *Hepatol Int 2008*; 2: A88–A89.

[35] Fontaine H, Vallet-Pichard A, Chaix ML et al. Efficacy and safety of adefovirdipivoxil in kidney recipients, hemodialysis patients, and patients with renal insufficiency. *Transplantation 2005*; 80: 1086–1092.

[36] de Silva HJ, Dassanayake AS, Manamperi A et al. Treatment of lamivudine-resistant hepatitis B infection in post-renal transplant patients with adefovirdipivoxil: preliminary results. *Transplant Proc 2006*; 38: 3118–3120.

[37] Lampertico P, Vigano M, Facchetti F et al. Long-term add-on therapy with adefovir in lamivudine-resistant kidney graft recipients with chronic hepatitis B. *Nephrol Dial Transplant 2011*; 26: 2037–2041.

[38] Kamar N, Huart A, Tack I et al. Renal side effects of adefovir in hepatitis B virus-(HBV) positive kidney allograft recipients. *Clin Nephrol 2009*; 71: 36–42.

[39] Lai HW, Chang CC, Chen TH et al. Safety and efficacy of adefovir therapy for lamivudine-resistant hepatitis B virus infection in renal transplant recipients. *J Formos Med Assoc 2012*; 111: 439–444.

[40] ChO JH, Lim JH, Park GY et al. Successful withdrawal of antiviral treatment in kidney transplant recipients with chronic hepatitis B viral infection. *Transpl Infect Dis 2014*; 16(2): 295–303.

[41] Cheng JC, Liu MC, Tsai SY et al. Unexpectedly frequent hepatitis B reactivation by chemoradiation and postgastrectomy patients. *Cancer 2004*; 101: 2126–2133.

[42] Nakamura Y, Motokura T, Fujita A et al. Severe hepatitis related to chemotherapy in hepatitis B virus carriers with haematologic malignancies. Survey in Japan 1987-1991. *Cancer 1996*; 78: 2210–2215.

[43] Patullo V. Prevention of hepatitis B reactivation in the setting of immunosuppression. *Clin Mol Hepatol 2016*; 22(2): 219–237.

[44] Reddy KR, Beavers KL, Hammond SP et al. American Gastroenterological Association Institute guidelines on the prevention and treatment of hepatitis B virus reactivation after immunosuppressive drug therapy. *Gastroenterology 2015*; 148: 215–237.

[45] Niitsu N, Hagiwara Y, Tanae K et al. Prospective analysis of hepatitis B virus reactivation in patients with diffuse Large B-cell lymphoma after Rituximab combination Chemotherapy. *J Clin Oncol 2010*; 28: 5097–5101.

[46] Scheinberg P, Fischer SH, Li L et al. Distinct EBV and CMV reactivation patterns following antibody-based immunosuppressive regimens in patients with severe aplastic anemia. *Blood 2007*; 109(8): 3219–3224.

[47] Watashi K, Sluder A, Daito T et al. Cyclosporine A and its analogs inhibit hepatitis B virus entry into cultured hepatocytes *through targeting* a membrane transporter, sodium taurocholate cotransporting polypeptide (NTCP). *Hepatology 2014*; 59(5):1726–1737.

[48] Xia WL, Shen Y, Zheng SS et al. Inhibitory effect of cyclosporine A on hepatitis B virus replication in vitro and its *possible mechan*isms. *Hepatobiliary Pancreat Dis Int 2005*; 4(1): 18–22.

[49] Wagner M, Early AK, Webster AC et al. Mycophenolic acid versus azathioprine as primary immunosuppression for kidney transplant recipients. *Cochrane Database Syst Rev 2015; (12): CD007746.*

[50] SezginGöksu S, Bilal S, Coskun HS. Hepatitis B reactivation related to everolimus. *World J Hepatol 2013*; 5(1): 43–45.

[51] Shepard CW, Finelli L, Alter MJ. Global epidemiology of hepatitis C virus infection. *Lancet Infect Dis. 2005*; 5: 558–567.

[52] Kidney Disease: Improving Global Outcomes (KDIGO) KDIGO clinical practice guidelines for the prevention, diagnosis, evaluation, and treatment of hepatitis C in chronic kidney disease. *Kidney Int Suppl 2008*; (109): S1–S99.

[53] Global surveillance and control of hepatitis C. Report of a WHO Consultation organized in collaboration with the Viral Hepatitis Prevention Board, Antwerp, Belgium. J *Viral Hepat 1999*; 6: 35–47.

[54] Chou CK, Wang LH, Lin HM et al. Glucocorticoid stimulates hepatitis B viral gene expression in cultured human hepatoma cells. *Hepatology 1992*; 16: 13–8.

[55] Marinaki S, Boletis JN, Sakellariou S, J Delladetsima. Hepatitis C in hemodialysis patients. *World J Hepatol 2015*; 7(3): 548–558.

[56] Jadoul M, Cornu C, Van Ypersele de Strihou C. Non-A, Non-B hepatitis in dialysis patients: diagnosis, prevention and treatment. In: *International Year Book of Nephrology, editor. London: Springer-Verlag; 1992*. pp. 253–270.

[57] Pereira BJ, Levey AS et al. Hepatitis C virus infection in dialysis and renal transplantation. *Kidney Int. 1997*; 51: 981–999.

[58] Fabrizi F, Takkouche B, Lunghi G et al. The impact of hepatitis C virus infection on survival in dialysis patients: meta-analysis of observational studies. *J Viral Hepat 2007*; 14: 697–703.

[59] Pereira BJ, Natov SN, Bouthot BA et al. Effects of hepatitis C infection and renal transplantation on survival in end- stage renal disease. The New England Organ Bank Hepatitis C Study Group. *Kidney Int 1998*; 53: 1374–1381.

[60] Bloom RD, Sayer G, Fa K et al. Outcome of hepatitis C virus-infected kidney transplant candidates who remain on the waiting list. *Am J Transplant 2005*; 5: 139–144.

[61] Kalantar-Zaden K, Kilpatrick RD, McAllist*er SJ et al. Hepatit*is C virus and death risk in hemodialysis patients. *J Am Soc Nephrol 2007*; 18: 1584–1593.

[62] Ingsathit A, Kamanamool N, Thankistian A, Sumethkul V. Survival advantage of kidney transplantation over dialysis in patients with hepatitis C: a systematic review and meta-analysis. *Transplantation 2013*; 95 (7): 943–948.

[63] Fabrizi F, Lunghi G, Finazzi S et al. Decreased serum aminotransferase activity in patients with chronic renal failure: impact on the detection of viral hepatitis. *Am J Kidney Dis 2001*; 38: 1009–1015.

[64] Yasuda K, Okuda K, Endo N et al. Hypoaminotransferasemia in patients undergoing long-term hemodialysis: clinical and biochemical appraisal. *Gastroenterology. 1995*; 109: 1295–1300.

[65] KDIGO Guideline 4: Management of HCV-infected patients before and after kidney transplantation. *Kidney Int* 2008; 73: S53–S68.

[66] Pawa S, Ehrinpreis M, Mutchnik M et al. Percutaneous liver biopsy is safe in chronic hepatitis C patients with end-stage renal disease. *Clin Gastroenterol Hepatol 2007*; 5(11): 1316–1320.

[67] Fabrizi F, Martin P, Dixit V et al. Acquisition of hepatitis C virus in hemodialysis patients: a prospective study by branched DNA signal amplification assay. *Am J Kidney Dis 1998*; 31: 647–654.

[68] Sterling RK, Sanyal AJ, Luketic VA et al. Chronic hepatitis C infection in patients with end stage renal disease: characterization of liver histology and viral load in patients awaiting renal transplantation. *Am J Gastroenterol 1999*; 94: 3576–3582.

[69] Friedrich-Rust M, Ong Mf, Martens S et al. Performance of transient elastography for the staging of liver fibrosis: a meta-analysis. *Gastroenterology 2008*; 134: 960–974.

[70] Liu CH, Liang CC, Huang KW et al. Transient elastography to assess hepatic fibrosis in hemodialysis chronic hepatitis C patients. *Clin J Am Soc Nephrol* 2011; 6: 1057–1065.

[71] Liu CH, Liang CC, Liu CJ et al. The ratio of aminotransferase to platelets is a useful index for predicting hepatic fibrosis in hemodialysis patients with chronic hepatitis C. *Kidney Int 2010*; 78: 103–109.

[72] Pereira BJ, Wright TL, Schmid CH et al. Screening and confirmatory testing of cadaver organ donors for hepatitis C virus infection: a U.S. National Collaborative Study. *Kidney Int 1994*; 46: 886–892.

[73] Pfau PR, Rho R, DeNofrio D et al. Hepatitis C transmission and infection by orthotopic heart transplantation. *J Heart Lung Transplant 2000*; 19: 350–354.

[74] Delladetsima I, Psichogiou M, Sypsa V et al. The course of hepatitis C virus infection in pretransplantation anti-hepatitis C virus-negative renal transplant recipients: a retrospective follow-up study. *Am J Kidney Dis 2006*; 47: 309–316.

[75] Abbott KC, Lentine KL, Bucci JR et al, The impact of transplantation with deceased donor hepatitis c-positive kidneys on survival in wait-listed long-term dialysis patients. *Am J Transplant 2004*; 4: 2032–2037.

[76] Morales JM, Campistol JM, Dominguez-Gil B et al. Long-term experience with kidney transplantation from hepatitis C-positive donors into hepatitis C-positive recipients. *Am J Transplant 2010*; 10: 2453–2462.

[77] Widell A, Mannson S, Persson NH et al. Hepatitis C superinfection in hepatitis C virus (HCV)-infected patients transplanted with an HCV-infected kidney. *Transplantation 1995*; 60: 642–647.

[78] Natov SN, Lau JY, Ruthazer R et al. Hepatitis C virus genotype does not affect patient survival among renal transplant candidates. *Kidney Int 1999*; 56: 700–706.

[79] Cruzado JM, Gil-Vernet S, Castellote J et al. Successful treatment of chronic HCV infection should not preclude kidney donation to an HCV negative recipient, *Am J Transplant 2013*; 13(10): 2773–2774.

[80] Bruchfeld A, Wilczek H, Elinder CJ et al. Hepatitis C infection, time in renal-replacement therapy, and outcome after kidney transplantation. *Transplantation 2004*; 78:745–750.

[81] Mathurin P, Mouquet C, Poynard T et al. Impact of hepatitis B and C virus on kidney transplantation outcome. *Hepatology 1999*; 29: 257–263.

[82] Fabrizi F, Martin P, Dixit V et al. Hepatitis C virus antibody status and survival after renal transplantation: meta-analysis of observational studies. *Am J Transplant 2005*; 5(6): 1452–1461.

[83] Fabrizi F, Martin P, Dixit V, Messa P. Meta-analysis of observational studies: hepatitis C and survival after renal transplant. *J Viral Hepat 2014*; 21 (5): 314–324.

[84] Abbott KC et al. Impact of diabetes and hepatitis after kidney transplantation on patients who are affected by hepatitis C virus. *Am Soc Nephrol 2004*; 15: 3166–3174.

[85] Scott Dr, Wong JK, Spicer TS et al. Adverse impact of hepatitis C virus infection on renal replacement therapy and renal transplant patients in Australia and New Zealand. *Transplantation 2010*; 90: 1165–1170.

[86] Baid-Agrawal S, Farris AB 3rd, Pascual M et al. Overlapping pathways to transplant glomerulopathy: chronic humoral rejection, hepatitis C infection, and thrombotic microangiopathy. *Kidney Int 2011*; 80: 879–885.

[87] Cruzado JM, Bestard O, Grinyo JM. Impact of extrahepatic complications (diabetes and glomerulonephritis) associated with hepatitis C virus infection after renal transplantation. *Contrib Nephrol 2012*; 176: 108–116.

[88] Ozgur O, Boyacioglu S, Telatur H et al. Recombinant alpha interferon in renal allograft recipients with chronic hepatitis C. *Nephrol Dial Transplant 1995*; 10: 2104–2106.

[89] Rostaing L, Izopet J, Baron E et al. Treatment of chronic hepatitis C with recombinant interferon alpha in kidney transplant recipients. *Transplantation 1995*; 59: 1426–1431.

[90] Goodkin DA, Bieber B, Gillepsie B et al. Hepatitis C infection is very rarely treated among hemodialysis patients. *Am J Nephrol 2013*; 38(5): 405–412.

[91] Liu CH, Huang CF, Liu CJ et al. Pegylated interferon-α2a with or without low-dose ribavirin for treatment-naive patients with hepatitis C virus genotype 1 receiving hemodialysis: a randomized trial. *Ann Intern Med 2013*; 159(11): 729–738.

[92] Rosen H. Chronic hepatitis C infection. *N Engl J Med 2011*; 364: 2429–2438.

[93] Kamar N, Toupance O, Buchler M et al. Evidence that clearance of hepatitis C virus RNA after alpha-interferon therapy in dialysis patients is sustained after renal transplantation. *J Am Soc Nephrol 2003*; 14: 2092–2098.

[94] Liang TJ, Ghany MG. Current and future therapies for hepatitis C virus infection. *N Engl J Med 2013*; 369(7): 679–680.

[95] Muir AJ. The rapid evolution of treatment strategies for hepatitis C. *Am J Gastroenterol 2014*; 100: 628–635.

[96] Pockros P, Reddy KR, Mantry PS et al. Efficacy of direct-acting antiviral combination for patients with HCV genotype 1 infection and severe renal impairment or end-stage renal disease. AASLD 2015; *Gastroenterology 2016* [Epub ahead of print].

[97] Roth D, Nelson DR, Bruchfeld A et al. Grazoprevir plus elbasvir in treatment-naive and treatment-experienced patients with hepatitis C virus genotype 1 infection and stage 4–5 chronic kidney disease (the C-SURFER study): a combination phase 3 study. *Lancet 2015*; 386: 1537–1545.

[98] American Association of the Study of Liver Disease (AASLD) guidelines. Available at: http://www.hcvguidelines.org.

[99] Kamar N, Marion O, Rostaing I et al. Efficacy and safety of sofosbuvir-based antiviral therapy to treat hepatitis C virus infection after kidney transplantation. *Am J Transplant 2016*; 16(5): 1474–1479.

[100] Sawinski D, Kaur N, Ajeti A et al. Successful treatment of hepatitis C in renal transplant recipients with direct-acting antiviral agents. *Am J Transplant 2016*; 16: 1588–1595.

[101] Somsouk M, Lauer GM, Casson D, et al. Spontaneous resolution of chronic hepatitis C virus disease after withdrawal of immunosuppression. *Gastroenterology 2003*; 124: 1946–1949.

[102] Kamar N, Sandres-Saune K, Rostai*ng L. Influence of ri*tuximab therapy on hepatitis C virus RNA concentration in kidney- transplant patients. *Am J Transplant 2007*; 7: 2440.

[103] Ennishi D, Maeda Y, Niitsu N et al. Hepatic toxicity and prognosis in hepatitis C virus-infected patients with diffuse large B- cell lymphoma treated with rituximab-containing chemotherapy regimens: a Japanese multicenter analysis. *Blood 2010*; 116: 5119–5125.

[104] Luan FL, Schaubel DE, Zhang H et al. Impact of immunosuppressive regimen on survival of kidney transplant recipients with hepatitis C. *Transplantation 2008;* 85: 1601–1606.

[105] Rosen HR, Shackleton CR, Higa L et al. Use of OKT3 is associated with early and severe recurrence of hepatitis C after liver transplantation. *Am J Gastroenterol 1997*; 92: 1453–1457.

[106] Rodrigues A, Pinho L, Lobato L et al. Hepatitis C virus genotypes and the influence of the induction of immunosuppression with anti- thymocyte globulin (ATG) on chronic hepatitis in renal graft recipients. *Transpl Int 1998*; 11(1): S115–S118.

[107] Lake JR. The role of immunosuppression in recurrence of hepatitis C. *Transplantation 2003*; 9: S63–S66.

[108] Roth D, Gaynor JJ, Reddy KR et al. Effect of kidney transplantation on outcomes among patients with hepatitis C. *J Am Soc Nephrol 2011*; 22: 1152–1160

[109] Uemura T, Schaefer E, Hollenbeak CS, Khan A, Kadry Z. Outcome of induction immunosuppression for liver transplantation comparing anti- thymocyte globulin, daclizumab, and corticosteroid. *Transpl Int 2011*; 24: 640–650.

[110] Moonka DK, Kim D, Kapke A, Brown KA, Yoshida A. The influence of induction therapy on graft and patient survival in patients with and without hepatitis C after liver transplantation. *Am J Transplant 2010*; 10: 590–601

[111] Humar A, Crotteau S, Gruessner A et al. Steroid minimization in liver transplant recipients: impact on hepatitis C recurrence and post- transplant diabetes. *Clin Transplant 2007*; 21: 526–531.

[112] Berenguer M, Aguilera V, Prieto M et al. Significant improvement in the outcome of HCV- infected transplant recipients by avoiding rapid steroid tapering and potent induction immunosuppression. *J Hepatol 2006*; 44: 717–722.

[113] Watashi K, Hijikata M, Hosaka M, Yamaji M, Shimotohno K. Cyclosporine A suppresses replication of hepatitis C virus genome in cultured hepatocytes. *Hepatology 2003*; 38: 1282–1288.

[114] Kahraman A, Witzke O, Scherag A et al. Impact of immunosuppressive therapy on hepatitis C infection after renal transplantation. *Clin Nephrol 2011*; 75: 16–25.

[115] Zhu J, Wu J, Frizell E et al. Rapamycin inhibits hepatic stellate cell proliferation in vitro and limits fibrogenesis in an in vivo model of liver fibrosis. *Gastroenterology 1999*; 117: 1198–1204.

[116] Gallego R, Henriquez F, Oliva E et al. Switching to sirolimus in renal transplant recipients with hepatitis C virus: a safe option. *Transplant Proc 2009*; 41: 2334–2336.

Section 3

Investigational Treatment Strategies

Chapter 13

Strategies to Preclude Hepatitis C Virus Entry

Thierry Burnouf, Ching-Hsuan Liu and
Liang-Tzung Lin

Additional information is available at the end of the chapter

http://dx.doi.org/10.5772/65470

Abstract

Without a preventive vaccine, hepatitis C virus (HCV) remains an important pathogen worldwide with millions of carriers at risk of end-stage liver diseases. Despite the introduction of novel direct-acting antivirals (DAAs), resistance problems, challenges with the difficult-to-treat populations and high costs limit the widespread application of these drugs. Antivirals with alternative mechanism(s) of action, such as by restricting viral entry or cell-to-cell spread, could help expand the scope of antiviral strategies for the management of hepatitis C. Transfusion-associated HCV infection remains another issue in endemic and resource-limited areas around the world. This chapter describes some of the latest developments in antiviral strategies to preclude HCV entry, such as through monoclonal antibodies and small molecules, as well as measures to enhance the safety of therapeutic plasma products in blood transfusion.

Keywords: hepatitis C virus, viral entry, antivirals, entry inhibitors, monoclonal antibodies, small molecules, therapeutic plasma products

1. Introduction

Hepatitis C virus (HCV) is a major pathogen that predisposes about 170–300 million people worldwide to risks of end-stage liver diseases (ESLD), including cirrhosis and hepatocellular carcinoma (HCC). The hepatotropic virus remains one of the top indications for liver transplantation in treating ESLD [1]. While a preventive vaccine remains unavailable, the recent introduction of direct-acting antivirals (DAAs) has revolutionized the treatment for hepatitis C, phasing out the decade-old interferon (IFN)-based regimens. The majority of DAAs, however, focus on targeting viral replication such as via inhibition of the HCV NS3/4A protease, the NS5A cofactor, and the NS5B polymerase [2]. Although the DAAs have significantly improved the rate of sustained virological response (SVR) in the most prevalent genotype 1 patients, several challenges persist in real-world setting including high cost, drug-drug interactions, emergence of drug resistance, hard-to-treat populations (e.g., human immunodeficiency virus [HIV] coinfection, ESLD, and transplant patients), and management of DAA failures [3–5]. With the advent of hepatitis C treatment in larger populations and borrowing from the experience with HIV cocktail therapy, it is becoming clear that developing therapeutic strategies with different modes of action would be necessary to address the various limitations of current DAAs. In addition, HCV transmission due to transfusion of contaminated blood products remains an issue in endemic areas around the world. This is particularly the case in resource-limited countries that face inadequate supply of safe blood products or have poorly controlled blood screening practices, leading to significant risk of transfusion-associated HCV infection [6]. Measures to enhance the safety of therapeutic plasma products such as through the implementation of viral inactivation treatments are therefore a necessity to reduce such risk.

The multistep process of HCV entry makes it an attractive target since it is the foremost fundamental prerequisite in establishing an infection. Following successful entry, the viral life cycle initiates to produce more virions, and with this development the underlying disease begins its progression. Blocking HCV infection by targeting its entry therefore has important implications for both prophylactic and therapeutic purposes since it abolishes the viral life cycle. As a prophylactic treatment, it can be used to prevent infection or reinfection. This is particularly useful in liver transplant setting of hepatitis C wherein the liver allograft is inevitably reinfected [7, 8]. As a therapeutic treatment, precluding HCV entry via de novo infection or cell-to-cell transmission helps to restrict viral spread in an infected person which could slow the progression of the disease. In addition, incorporation of strategies to block HCV entry into existing DAA treatments is expected to maximize the treatment response rate, even producing a synergistic effect [9], as with the experience of using multiple inhibitors in HIV cocktail therapy to concomitantly target various stages of the viral life cycle. Since more steps are being targeted in such a multipronged approach, the inclusion of entry inhibitors to existing DAAs could impose a higher genetic barrier to drug-resistance development. Such tactic not only aids in disrupting persistent HCV infection but could also help to ultimately achieve viral clearance. These aspects therefore make the development of HCV entry blocking strategies highly advantageous in both expanding the scope of antiviral treatments against hepatitis C and providing new insights into antiviral management. This chapter describes some of the latest development of strategies in precluding HCV entry for the management of hepatitis C.

2. Overview of HCV entry

Owing to the development of infectious HCV culture systems (e.g., cell-culture-derived HCV, HCVcc) and viral pseudoparticles bearing HCV glycoproteins (e.g., HCV pseudoparticles, HCVpp), a scenario of how HCV entry occurs has slowly emerged over the last decade of research. It is widely recognized that the HCV particle undergoes a series of intimate and well-orchestrated interactions with various receptors/coreceptors on the hepatocyte host cell surface as well as in the tight junctions, which ultimately lead to the attachment, internalization, and

http://dx.doi.org/10.5772/65470

fusion of the virion with the cellular membrane. A number of these receptor interactions are thought to be attributed to the highly lipidated nature of the HCV virion. Specifically, HCV exists as a lipo-viro particle (LVP) with a lipid composition that includes the apolipoproteins and resembles that of very low-density lipoproteins (VLDLs) and low-density lipoproteins (LDLs) [10–15]. The association with lipids on the viral particle is thought to contribute to the shielding of HCV glycoproteins from neutralization by the host antibody-mediated response. In addition, the presence of the apolipoproteins on the virion has a large influence on the production of infectious HCV and also its tissue tropism [13, 16–22].

Following circulation in the blood, the HCV viral particles reach the liver and begin the interactions with molecules at the surface of the hepatocytes (**Figure 1**). The initial contacts are with nonspecific receptor(s) including the glycosaminoglycan (GAG) heparan sulfate moieties [23–25] that can be found on the transmembrane core proteins syndecans [26, 27]. These early interactions facilitate the attachment of the HCV virion and its accumulation on the hepatocytes for subsequent binding to more specific receptors. Although the LDL receptor (LDLR) has also been suggested as a potential initial attachment factor [28–30], recent evidence suggests that it may play a more essential role in viral replication [31, 32].

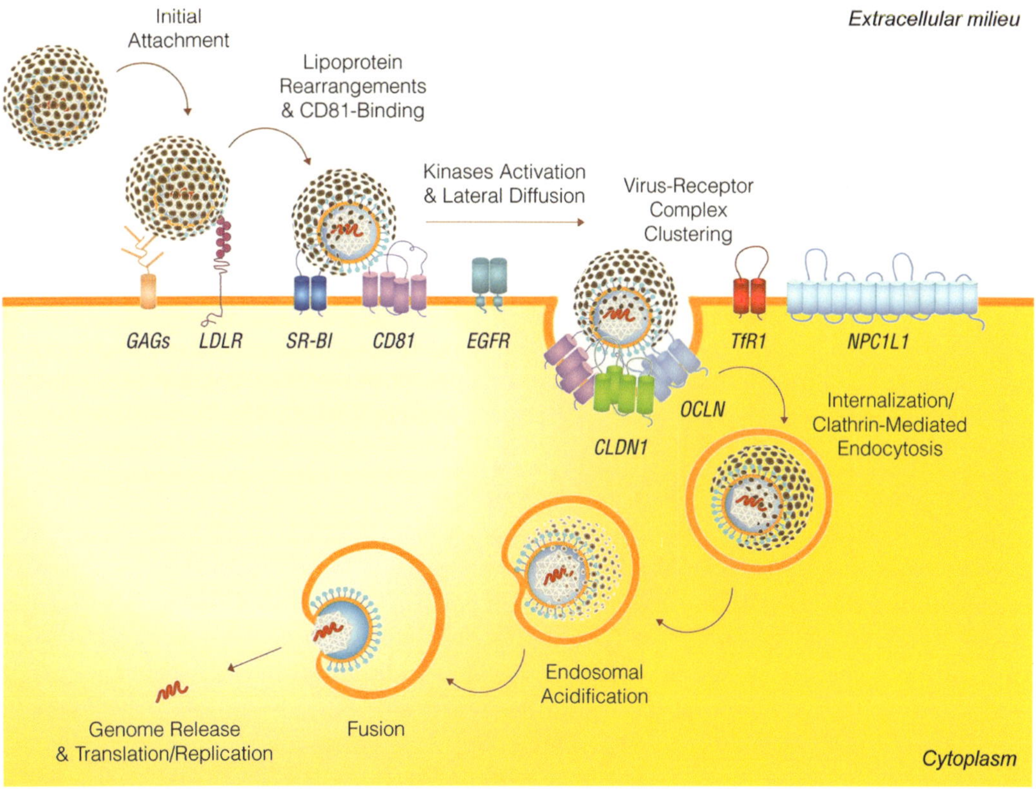

Figure 1. Overview of HCV entry.

Nevertheless, these initial interactions have been shown to be mediated via apolipoprotein E (apoE) on the virion [29, 33–36]. The capturing process of the HCV particle is finalized by its interaction with the scavenger receptor class B type I (SR-BI) [37, 38], which is able to associate with the virion's lipoproteins [37, 39] as well as the HCV E2 glycoprotein [40, 41]. Binding of HCV with SR-BI induces lipoprotein rearrangements that help prime the virion for subsequent binding to other host cell factors and promote entry. This process is proposed to occur via SR-BI's lipid transfer activity between the viral particle and the plasma membrane [37, 42] and/or by direct interaction with the hypervariable region 1 (HVR1) domain on E2 [37, 43], which ultimately leads to conformational change and the exposure of functional glycoprotein epitopes for additional receptor binding. Closely following this event is the engagement of the HCV particle with the tetraspanin receptor CD81 [44, 45], which is an important entry factor for the virus [41, 46, 47]. HCV binding to CD81 is proposed to induce a dynamic lateral diffusion of virus-receptor complexes toward the tight junction area for further interactions with additional entry factors and viral internalization [22, 48]. Specifically, CD81 forms a coreceptor complex with the tight junction protein claudin-1 (CLDN1) [49, 50] and is engaged in late events of HCV entry [51]. This re-localization and virus-receptor complex association with CLDN1 involves multiple signaling pathways (e.g., Rho GTPases, PI3K/AKT, and ERK/MAPK) [52, 53], includes the activation of host cell kinases such as the epidermal growth factor receptor (EGFR) and ephrin receptor A2 (EphA2) [54, 55], and is influenced by the absence of the CD81-associated partner EWI-2wint on the hepatocytes [56, 57]. The EWI-2wint molecule is normally bound to CD81 on most cell type surfaces and inhibits its diffusion which is required to promote HCV entry; however, it is not expressed in the hepatocytes, and hence its absence has been suggested to contribute to the restricted tropism of the virus [56]. Following interaction with the CD81/CLDN1 complex, the HCV particle is presumed to then interact with the tight junction protein occludin (OCLN) prior to viral internalization [58]. Additional proteins that take part in influencing virion entry into the hepatocyte include the transferrin receptor 1 (TfR1) [59] and the cholesterol transporter Niemann-Pick C1-like 1 (NPC1L1) [60], although their specific role and interplay with other entry factors in the HCV entry process remain to be defined. The HCV particle finally enters the cell via clathrin-mediated endocytosis [61]. The HCV-receptor complexes then migrate to endosomal compartments [62, 63] where acidification occurs to induce membrane fusion, which allows the release of viral RNA into the host cytosol.

The above sequential and multistep entry process consequently yields the successful release of the HCV genome into the host cytoplasm for direct translation and the ensuing launch of viral replication. The roles played by several of these entry factors including SR-BI, CD81, CLDN1, and OCLN not only mediate HCV entry but also presumably help to define tissue and species tropism of the virus [64–67]. The understanding of how HCV achieves viral entry has led to the possibility of antiviral targeting. From docking to virus internalization, essentially all steps are targetable to prevent HCV infection of the host cell. In addition, given the association of HCV with lipoproteins and the viral particle's interaction with lipoprotein and lipid receptors (LDLR, SR-BI, and NPC1L1), the lipidic nature of HCV virion also offers various methods of pharmacological intervention. Finally, many of the entry factors including CD81, SR-BI, CLDN1, OCLN, and NPC1L1 also play a role in mediating HCV cell-to-cell transmission between intercellular junctions [68–71], and therefore targeting these molecules could help restrict both cell-free entry and cell-to-cell spread of HCV.

3. Current development in inhibition of HCV entry

3.1. Use of monoclonal antibodies to target host cell receptors or viral antigens

Recent insight into the molecular interactions of HCV at the cellular membrane has significantly enhanced the understanding of the HCV entry paradigm and revealed potential targets for drug intervention, including the use of monoclonal antibodies (mAbs) to mask HCV entry receptors/coreceptors or viral antigens. As described below and summarized in **Table 1**, the use of mAbs targeting CD81, SR-BI, CLDN1, or the HCV E2 has been shown to have prophylactic/therapeutic effects against HCV infection in both cell culture and animal models.

3.1.1. Anti-CD81 monoclonal antibodies

CD81 is the first putative receptor identified for HCV entry [72, 73] and plays an important role in the virus infection. The molecule is a member of the tetraspanin superfamily with four transmembrane domains and two extracellular loops and is expressed in most human tissues [74]. Commercial CD81 mAb JS-81 has been applied in human liver-chimeric mouse model and shown prophylactic protection but no postexposure effect inhibiting HCV infection [75]; nonetheless, this experimental test inspired subsequent studies of anti-CD81 mAbs as antiviral agents. Of the newly generated antibodies, mAb QV-6A8-F2-C4 produced by genetic immunization could efficiently inhibit HCVcc infection and pan-genotypic HCVpp entry in a similar range as mAb JS-81 [76]. The antibody also appeared to block neutralizing antibody-resistant HCV cell-to-cell transmission and viral dissemination in a dose-dependent manner, with a less cytotoxic or antiproliferative property than JS-81 in vitro. In a recent study, another mAb K04 generated with hybridoma technique not only showed inhibitory effect against HCVpp and HCVcc infection in hepatoma cells and primary human hepatocytes (PHH), but also surprisingly blocked HCV infections in both prophylactic setting and postinfection stage in human liver-chimeric mice [77]. This is probably due to the improved intrinsic binding affinity of mAb K04 to CD81 large extracellular loop (LEL) and a different binding epitope as compared to mAb JS81. However, treatment-associated reductions in body weight and human serum albumin levels were observed in this study. Further research will be needed to determine the minimal dose of antibodies needed to provide protection and to evaluate the toxicology of anti-CD81 mAbs for long-term development.

3.1.2. Anti-SR-BI monoclonal antibodies

SR-BI is a member of the CD36 family primarily expressed in liver and non-placental steroidogenic tissues which facilitates selective cholesterol uptake [78]. The molecule has been proposed to be a horseshoe-like glycoprotein with a large extracellular loop anchored to the plasma membrane at both N- and C-termini with short extensions into the cytoplasm [79]. It was first identified as the alternative E2 receptor on HepG2 cells which efficiently recognize

Candidates	Effect(s)	Stage of Development	Reference
mAbs Against Host Entry Factors			
Anti-CD81 mAbs	Inhibit CD81-E2 interaction	Mouse model	[75–77]
Anti-SR-BI mAbs	Inhibit SR-BI-E2 interaction	Mouse model	[80–82]
Anti-CLDN1 mAbs	Inhibit E2-CD81-CLDN1 association	Mouse model	[84–87]
Passive Immunotherapy Against HCV			
Anti-E2 mAbs	Neutralize circulating virion	Phase II	[89–96]
Polyclonal IgG	Neutralize circulating virion	Phase III	[190, 192, 193]
Small Molecule Inhibitors			
Heparin, heparin-derived compounds	Heparan sulfate competitors	Cell culture	[24, 25]
Heparinases	Heparan sulfate enzyme	Cell culture	[25]
EGCG	Compete with heparan sulfate; alter viral shape; inhibit cell-to-cell spread	Cell culture	[99–101]
Delphinidin	Alter viral shape	Cell culture	[101]
SSb2	Inhibit attachment & viral fusion	Cell culture	[102]
GA	Inactivate virion	Cell culture	[103]
Hydrolysable tannins CHLA & PUG	Inactivate virion; inhibit attachment & cell-to-cell spread	Cell culture	[104]
LOD	Inactivate virion; inhibit attachment	Cell culture	[105]
DHMD	Inactivate virion; inhibit attachment	Cell culture	[106]
Curcumin	Decrease viral envelope fluidity; inhibit cell-to-cell spread	Cell culture	[107]
CV-N	E1/E2 glycan-binding protein	Cell culture	[109]
Griffithsin	E1/E2 glycan-binding protein	Mouse model	[110]
MBL	E1/E2 glycan-binding protein	Cell culture	[111]
Recombinant L-ficolin	E1/E2 glycan-binding protein	Cell culture	[112]
BA-LNCs	E2 glycan-binding protein	Cell culture	[114]
Oleanolic acid	E2 glycan-binding protein	Cell culture	[115]
CD81-derived peptides	Interact with E2	Cell culture	[116, 117]
CLDN1-derived peptide (CL58)	Interact with E1 & E2	Cell culture	[81]
E2-derived peptide	Interfere with E1/E2 hetero-dimerization	Cell culture	[119]
Terfenadine	CD81 competitor	Cell culture	[120]
ITX 5061	SR-BI inhibitor	Phase Ib	[121–124]
Aspirin	Down regulates CLDN1	Cell culture	[125]
Erlotinib	EGFR inhibitor; inhibit cell-to-cell spread	Mouse model	[54]
Dasatinib	EphA2 inhibitor; inhibit cell-to-cell spread	Cell culture	[54]

Candidates	Effect(s)	Stage of Development	Reference
Tipifarnib, sorafenib	Ras, Raf inhibitor	Cell culture	[126]
Ferristatin	TfR1 inhibitor	Cell culture	[59]
Ezetimibe	NPC1L1 inhibitor	Mouse model	[60]
PF-429242	Down regulate NPC1L1 & LDLR	Cell culture	[127]
Phenothiazines	Modulate host cell membrane	Cell culture	[128]
Chlorpromazine	Clathrin-coated pit formation inhibitor	Cell culture	[61]
Arbidol	Trap virion in clathrin-coated vesicles	Cell culture	[129]
Bafilomycin A1, concanamycin A	Disturb acidic endosomal compartments	Cell culture	[130]
Chloroquine, ammonium chloride	Disturb acidic endosomal compartments	Cell culture	[131]
RAFI dUY11	Inhibit viral fusion	Cell culture	[132]
Ferroquine	Inhibit cell-to-cell spread	Cell culture	[133]
Triazine-based compounds	Inhibit post- binding step & cell-to-cell spread	Cell culture	[134, 135]
Silibinin	Inhibit viral fusion & cell-to-cell spread	Clinical Legalon® SIL	[136–140]
Tamoxifen	Inhibit attachment & post-binding step	Cell culture	[142]
HCV II-1 (GS-563253)	Inhibit attachment & post-binding step	Cell culture	[143]
EI-1 (BJ486K)	Inhibit post-binding step	Cell culture	[144]

Table 1. Antiviral strategies to preclude HCV entry.

soluble E2 proteins but do not express CD81 on their surface [40]. As described above, both CD81 and SR-BI are considered necessary for HCV entry, since the overexpression of CD81 on HepG2 cells restores HCVpp entry in these originally poorly permissive cells [41]. Monoclonal antibodies targeting SR-BI that inhibited HCV infections include mAb C167, mAb16-71, mAb8, and mAb151. For HCV inhibitory activities in vitro, mAb C167 effectively prevented infection in hepatoma cells with HCVcc and ex vivo virus recovered from HCVcc-infected chimpanzees [80]; mAb16-71 exhibited preventive effect against HCVcc infection in both hepatoma cells and PHH [81]; mAb8 and mAb151 also prevented HCVcc infection in reporter Huh-7 cells [82]. Additionally, mAb16-71, mAb8, and mAb151 all showed their ability in blocking HCV cell-to-cell spread in vitro and in vivo. Human liver-chimeric mouse models challenged with serum-derived HCV isolates of different genotypes revealed the anti-HCV property in vivo of the three antibodies in both prophylactic and postexposure settings. Specifically, mAb16-71 showed complete blockage of infection and intrahepatic spread of HCV isolates with a prophylactic treatment, but had no effect on chronically infected chimeric mice; mAb151, on the other hand, appeared to be effective against an HCV variant escaped from adaptive immune response in a liver transplant patient and displayed better antiviral activity in inhibiting viral spread and amplification in the postexposure setup.

3.1.3. Anti-CLDN1 monoclonal antibodies

The CLDN1 tight junction protein has four transmembrane domains and is highly expressed in the liver [83]. Its role in HCV entry is proposed to occur in the post-binding steps [64]. Anti-CLDN1 antibodies directed against the CLDN1 extracellular loops were found effective in neutralizing HCV infection in hepatoma cells through disrupting CD81-CLDN1 association and therefore inhibiting E2 binding to the cell surface [84]. A CLDN1 mAb OM-7D3-B3 targeting CLDN1 extracellular loop was found to be effective in inhibiting HCV isolates in vitro [85]. Further experiments in human liver-chimeric mouse models confirmed its potency in preventing HCV infection and eliminating persistent infection in vivo [86]. Pretreatment of another anti-CLDN1 mAb 3A2 targeting CLDN1 extracellular loop also showed protective effect in a chimeric mouse model [87]. Safety profiles of these antibodies were also assessed regarding the levels of human albumin, aspartate transaminase, alanine transaminase and total bilirubin, and potential side effects on the other organs and tight junction integrity. Further studies were suggested to assess potential immune-mediated adverse effects to ensure its relevance for clinical use [86, 87].

3.1.4. Anti-HCV E2 monoclonal antibodies

Another approach to developing entry-inhibiting mAbs is to target the glycoproteins on the HCV virion surface. Albeit HCV glycoproteins exhibit high variability and are protected by glycosylation and lipids on the viral particle, neutralizing mAbs have been designed to target more conserved and accessible regions, specifically on the E2 glycoprotein [88]. Effects of E2 mAbs have been shown in vitro and in vivo [89–94]. Clinical trials have been carried out to assess the protective function of human anti-E2 mAbs HCV-Ab^{XTL}68 and MBL-HCV1 in liver transplant settings of HCV-positive patients. With a higher dose and daily infusion of HCV-Ab^{XTL}68, HCV RNA in patient serum showed transient reduction in the first week post-transplantation but not yet below the detectable limits [95]. MBL-HCV1, on the other hand, successfully suppressed the viral load from 7 to 28 days after transplantation in genotype 1a-infected patients with multiple infusions. Although the primary endpoint at day 42 was not met, the viral rebound was significantly delayed, and the magnitude of the viral load reduction was greater than the previous HCV-Ab^{XTL}68 therapy [96]. The result indicates that mAbs may be a promising class of entry inhibitors that adsorbs circulating virions to protect the new liver from reinfection after transplantation. A study of combination therapy with DAAs to prevent allograft HCV infection is currently underway [96].

Current obstacles to the development of mAbs as therapeutic antiviral agents include the high cost of production, storage, and administration, which can only be done by injection so far [88]. Nevertheless, the associated immune responses such as antibody-dependent cell-mediated cytotoxicity (ADCC) and complement-dependent cytotoxicity (CDC) may help to clear the viruses and infected cells [88, 97]. Antibodies that directly block host cell entry factors are more likely to be effective for the diverse circulating viral strains; however, due to the distribution and multiple functions of such molecules, the blockage may cause potential adverse side effects [97]. As for antibodies targeting viral antigens, designing suitable candidates may be a challenging issue due to the heterogeneity of the HCV glycoproteins [98], but such antibodies may provide a safer option for the synergistic therapy with other antivirals of different modes of action to suppress the development of resistance, particularly at the early post-transplantation stage [96]. Additional neutralizing antibodies against other entry factors have also been reported to antagonize HCV infection in vitro, such as anti-TfR1 [59] and anti-NPC1L1 [60] antibodies, suggesting they could also be potentially developed for treatments against hepatitis C.

3.2. Small-molecule inhibitors of HCV entry

In addition to the mAbs, great efforts have been put into identifying small molecules with potent antiviral effects against HCV entry. The source of such entry inhibitors includes clinically approved medications, synthetic molecules, and natural product-based compounds. These small molecules could be further evaluated for development as drug candidates or drug leads. Below is a panel of small molecules that have been investigated with their activities inhibiting HCV entry (**Table 1**).

3.2.1. Small molecules inhibiting viral attachment

The attachment step represents the primary interaction of an HCV virion with its host cell surface. Since the GAG heparan sulfate moieties dominate the capturing of HCV virions, the heparan sulfate homologue heparin and its derivatives as well as the enzyme heparinases which degrade the molecule were all shown to inhibit the viral binding to hepatoma cells [24, 25]. (-)-Epigallocatechin-3-gallate (EGCG), a green tea catechin, was speculated to exert its inhibitory effect on viral attachment [99] by competing with heparan sulfate for HCV binding [100] or altering the viral shape [101]. Delphinidin, an anthocyanidin extracted from plant pigment, was also demonstrated to inactivate HCVpp by altering its shape and was particularly potent when added concurrently with the viral inoculation [101]. The natural terpenoid saikosaponin b2 (SSb2), isolated from the root of *Bupleurum kaoi,* was observed to specifically block HCV particle binding and early viral entry without affecting other stages of the viral life cycle [102]. SSb2 could inactivate cell-free HCV particles and was suggested to target the glycoprotein E2 in mediating its antiviral effect against HCV infection. Several other natural compounds including the gallic acid (GA) extracted from *Limonium sinense* [103], the hydrolyzable tannins chebulagic acid (CHLA) and punicalagin (PUG) [104], and the hepatoprotective plant *Phyllanthus urinaria*-derived monolactone loliolide (LOD) [105] and butenolide (4R,6S)-2-dihydromenisdaurilide (DHMD) [106] were also found to efficiently inactivate cell-free HCV viral particles and impede viral attachment. Another natural compound curcumin extracted from turmeric was shown to decrease the fluidity of viral envelope and therefore prevent the binding and fusion [107], possibly by inserting into the membrane in a manner similar to cholesterol [108].

3.2.2. Small molecules blocking viral glycoproteins

A variety of broad-spectrum antiviral agents have exhibited their ability to interact with the glycans on viral glycoproteins. In the case of HCV, glycan-binding proteins interfere with the association between the E1/E2 heterodimer and the host cell receptor CD81. Lectins such as cyanovirin-N (CV-N) and griffithsin, isolated from cyanobacterium *Nostoc ellipsosporum* and the red alga *Griffithsia* sp., respectively, were reported to have such effect. CV-N was shown to interact with N-linked glycans of HCV glycoproteins and disrupt E1/E2 binding to CD81 [109]. The inhibitory effect of griffithsin on HCV entry was also quenched when N-linked high-mannose oligosaccharides were present, indicating a pattern similar to CV-N of affecting the glycoproteins-CD81 interaction [110]; pretreatment of griffithsin was shown to delay the viral infection in chimeric mouse model. Humoral lectins of the innate immune systems including the mannan-binding lectin (MBL) and L-ficolin were also considered to have analogous effect neutralizing HCV particles. MBL [111] and recombinant oligomeric L-ficolin [112] were found to interact with the glycans on the E1/E2 heterodimer in a calcium-dependent manner, thereby inhibiting the viral entry. Notably, the MBL-associated complement system was activated upon its binding to HCV E1/E2, suggesting the use of humoral lectins as viral entry inhibitors may also help facilitate viral clearance. However, the detailed mechanism and specific target of the humoral lectins remain to be defined. The boronic acid (BA)-modified nanoparticles were also found to suppress HCV entry in a way that acted similar to lectins [113], with the incorporation of lipid nanocapsule (BA-LNC) techniques enhancing their stability and solubility [114]. Chemically modified oleanolic acid, a triterpene compound originally extracted from *Dipsacus asperoides,* was found able to interrupt the E2-CD81 interaction by binding to E2 [115].

Besides the glycan-binding proteins, molecules imitating HCV host entry factors or viral glycoproteins were also developed in the attempt to block the viral entry. An imidazole-based scaffold presenting CD81 helix D amino acid side chains [116] and stapled peptides based on CD81 LEL [117] were designed to antagonize the E2-CD81 interaction by mimicking the putative E2-binding region of CD81. A CLDN1-derived peptide, CL58, was also found to inhibit HCV entry in the post-attachment stage by interacting with HCV E1 and E2 [118]. As for viral glycoprotein-based molecules, an E2-derived peptide was found able to block E1/E2-mediated fusion by targeting E1 and therefore interfere with the hetero-dimerization of the glycoproteins [119].

3.2.3. Small molecules targeting host entry factors and CD81-triggered signaling pathway

In addition to the therapeutic antibodies mentioned in the previous section, several small molecules have been suggested to exert their inhibitory activity of HCV entry by targeting cellular receptors/coreceptors. Terfenadine, an antihistamine, was found able to prevent HCV infection by competing with the CD81 antibody JS81 binding to the LEL of CD81 protein on the hepatoma cell surface [120]. ITX 5061, a clinical stage compound originally characterized as a p38 MAPK inhibitor, was identified with its capability of antagonizing SR-BI [121] and further validated for its potency of inhibiting HCV entry at post-binding step [122]. The anti-HCV effect of ITX 5061 was found additive to synergistic in combination with several standard-of-care therapeutics, and the resistant mutant was defined on the viral glycoprotein E2 [123]. A latest phase 1b clinical trial [124] revealed that the ITX 5061-treated patients, especially the genotype 1-infected patients, had a significant reduction in HCV RNA through the first week after liver transplantation and viral evolution were restricted; however, the viral RNA levels became comparable in both ITX 5061-treated and untreated patients, suggesting the need to incorporate other antiviral agents using different modes of actions to eliminate HCV infection. Aspirin, alternatively, inhibited HCV entry by downregulating CLDN1 [125].

Since the receptor tyrosine kinases are also involved in the HCV entry process, two clinically approved protein kinase inhibitors were evaluated for their ability to abrogate the viral entry. Both erlotinib, an EGFR inhibitor, and dasatinib, an EphA2 inhibitor, could successfully block HCV entry in a dose-dependent manner as well as the cell-to-cell transmission. Specifically, erlotinib was shown to inhibit the membrane fusion of hepatoma cells overexpressing HCV glycoproteins. In vivo treatment of erlotinib resulted in a significant suppression of the viral load in PHH-chimeric mouse model with HCV infection [54]. Furthermore, inhibitors of EGFR downstream kinases Ras (tipifarnib) and Raf (sorafenib) were also assessed and found effective in blocking HCV entry [126].

Inhibitors of other entry factors were also shown to be effective in hampering the viral entry. Pretreatment of ferristatin, a TfR1 inhibitor that binds to the molecule and causes its internalization and degradation, was shown to decrease HCVcc infection in vitro [59]. The NPC1L1 internalization inhibitor ezetimibe, which is also an FDA-approved cholesterol-lowering medication, diminished HCVcc foci formation before and during the viral challenge. Daily oral administration of ezetimibe starting two weeks before infection also delayed the viral growth of a genotype 1 clinical isolate in PHH-chimeric mouse model [60]. PF-429242, an SKI-1/S1P inhibitor, potentially impeded HCV entry by downregulating NPC1L1 and LDLR expression [127]. On the other hand, phenothiazines, a group of synthesized nitrogen- and sulfur-containing tricyclic compounds, inhibited HCV fusion into the cell by modulating the host cell membrane. Insertion of phenothiazines into the cholesterol-rich membrane increased its fluidity, thus possibly decreasing the local inhomogeneity of the cell required for the viral fusion [128].

3.2.4. Inhibition of clathrin-mediated endocytosis and viral fusion

Since HCV fusion has been discovered to be facilitated by clathrin-mediated endocytosis and requires an acidic environment, several reagents were assessed for their effectiveness in preventing HCV entry through blocking such pathways. Chlorpromazine, an inhibitor of clathrin-coated pit formation, was shown to inhibit both HCVpp and HCVcc infection in vitro in the validation of clathrin-mediated endocytosis pathway of HCV fusion to the host cell membrane [61]. Arbidol, a broad-spectrum antiviral agent that blocks viral entry and has been licensed in some regions for influenza, was described to trap the HCV virion in clathrin-coated vesicles, thereby hindering the release of viral genome and the following infection [129]. It was also suggested that arbidol could generally cause the intracellular accumulation of clathrin-coated structures and restrain the formation of clathrin-coated pits on the cell surface [129], possibly due to its tropism for lipid bilayers.

Small molecules disturbing the acidic endosomal compartments were also identified as HCV entry inhibitors in the discovery of the low pH-triggered entry. These include bafilomycin A1 and concanamycin A, which are inhibitors of vacuolar H+-ATPases [130]. Weak bases such as chloroquine and ammonium chloride were also found to inhibit the low pH-dependent conformational change required for the viral fusion, based on their ability to penetrate lysosomes and increase the pH [131]. Finally, dUY11, one of the rigid amphipathic fusion inhibitors (RAFIs), was suggested to inhibit HCV entry by interacting with the hydrophobic structures in virions and preventing the formation of negative curvature required for viral fusion [132]. Curcumin [107] is also able to affect the fusion step as previously mentioned.

3.2.5. *Small molecules inhibiting cell-to-cell transmission*

Besides inhibiting the HCV entry in de novo infection, blocking cell-to-cell spread of the viral particles is also important as this mode of transmission facilitates efficient spread of the virus in the liver escaping from neutralizing antibodies [68, 69]. Ferroquine was speculated to interact with HCV glycoprotein E1 and abrogate cell-to-cell spread of the virus [133]. Triazine-based compounds indicated to be closely related to the amino acids on the glycoprotein could also selectively inhibit genotype 1 HCV entry at the post-attachment step along with cell-to-cell transmission [134, 135]. Several molecules also block cell-to-cell spread in addition to their activities in hindering HCV viral entry. For instance, besides impeding viral attachment, CHLA and PUG exhibit pronounced antiviral effects at the postinfection stage, especially in restricting HCV foci expansion [104]. Others include EGCG [99], curcumin [107], erlotinib, and dasatinib [54]. Silibinin, the major component of *Silybum marianum* that has been designated as an orphan drug for the prevention of recurrent hepatitis C in liver transplant patients [136], was also suggested to possess a prominent effect blocking transmission of the viral particles between intercellular junctions [137, 138], although other studies have proposed that it may slow down clathrin-mediated endocytosis [139] as well as inhibit viral membrane fusion [140]. This could be useful since DAA-resistant HCV variants have been suggested to escape via cell-to-cell transmission route [141]. Therefore, the choice of inhibitors exhibiting mechanistic effect against both HCV cell-to-cell spread and cell-free entry, or a combination of such two types of inhibitors, should facilitate viral clearance.

3.2.6. *Additional candidate entry inhibitors*

Some other molecules were found able to prevent the infection at different steps of HCV entry. The estrogen receptor modulator tamoxifen [142] and HCV infectivity inhibitor 1 (HCV II-1 or GS-563253) [143] were shown to inhibit the HCV infection at both attachment and post-binding steps. HCV II-1 was also found capable of impeding infectious virion propagation [143]. HCV entry inhibitor 1 (EI-1 or BJ486K), a flavonoid ladanein, was shown to interrupt the viral entry at post-attachment stage [144]. The exact mechanisms of these molecules require further investigations. Other compounds such as serum amyloid A [145, 146], p7 ion channel-derived peptide H2-3 [147], amphipathic DNA polymers [148], lactoferrins [149], tellimagrandin I and its derivatives [150], indole derivatives [151], and imidazo[1,2α][1,8]naphthyridine derivatives [152] were found able to inhibit HCV entry with mechanisms that remain to be clarified.

3.3. Control of HCV infection risks in human blood-derived therapeutic products

Many viruses can contaminate human blood. HCV, along with HIV and HBV are a major cause of infectious complications of blood product transfusion therapy. HCV contamination in patients by transfusion of blood components such as red blood cells, platelets or clinical plasma, as well as industrial fractionated plasma products, has been well documented. At the time of the "tainted blood scandal," numerous recipients of blood components and hemophiliacs receiving plasma-derived factor VIII concentrates were contaminated through transfusion of nonvirally inactivated products prepared from blood products that were not HCV-tested.

HCV transmission through blood transfusion is a major medical issue, as infection can lead to high risk of liver cirrhosis and eventually cancer complications.

3.3.1. *HCV safety nets for blood components*

There are now over 100 million whole blood donations collected each year in the world. Collected blood is most often separated by "blood establishments" into red blood cell concentrates, platelet concentrates, and plasma that are transfused at nearby hospitals. Plasma, which can be obtained from whole blood collection or drawn by specialized apheresis procedures, can also be used as raw material for the production of "industrial" plasma protein products. These protein drugs include immunoglobulins G (IgGs), various coagulation factors, albumin, and many others. Industrial plasma products are manufactured from pools of plasma of several thousand liters, making them statistically more susceptible to contamination by HCV and other viruses as one highly infectious donation would contaminate the whole plasma pool and potentially the derived products.

Today in developed economies benefiting from strict regulatory oversight, several measures are in place to decrease the possibility for patients to acquire HCV by transfusion. Blood transfusion HCV safety nets for blood components rely on complementary measures encompassing (a) epidemiological control of the population, (b) individual screening of candidate blood donors to defer those identified as presenting potential risk factors, and (c) individual blood donation testing to identify and eliminate donations reactive to anti-HCV antibodies and/or HCV RNA nucleic acid test (NAT) [153]. In technology-advanced countries applying such procedures, this has allowed to decrease the risk of acquiring HCV by transfusion of single blood components down to approximately 1 per 1.8 million. The remaining risk reflects the inevitable presence of "window-phase" donations for which all markers to detect donor infection by HCV, either indirect or direct, are found nonreactive [154, 155]. Understandably, HCV transmission risks are substantially higher in less developed economies (a) lacking a safe blood donor base, (b) relying on paid or "replacement" donors to increase the blood supply, (c) with a deficient blood collection system, and (d) with a lack of reliable viral testing procedures [6]. The ultimate barrier to avoiding HCV transmission risks from blood products collected during the window-phase period relies on the implementation of dedicated viral reduction treatments. Those have been developed for industrial plasma protein products, plasma for transfusion, and platelet concentrates. Until now, however, no treatment is available commercially for whole blood and red blood cell concentrates.

3.3.2. *HCV reduction treatment of industrial plasma protein products*

Development and implementation of dedicated viral/HCV reduction treatments of industrial plasma protein products took place in the 1980s and early 1990s [156]. In the early 1980s, albumin, a relatively heat-stable protein, was the only plasma product subjected to specific HCV inactivation by heat treatment at 60 °C for 10 h in the liquid state (a process called pasteurization), in the presence of fatty acid stabilizers. From the mid-1980s to the early 1990s, heat treatment of freeze-dried coagulation factors at 60–68 °C for 24–96 h or 80 °C for 72 h were developed to inactivate HIV and HCV concomitantly [156]. Although pasteurization has successfully been adapted to several plasma products (such as antithrombin and alpha 1-antitrypsin), a milestone in the safety of industrial plasma products was the development of the solvent/detergent (S/D) incubation procedure at 20–37 °C [157] designed to dissolve the lipid envelope of viruses, including HCV, without affecting plasma protein functions. This technique is still largely used for a wide range of industrial plasma products owing to well-proven efficacy and a safety profile established by years of industrial and clinical practices [158]. Other HCV viral inactivation treatments include low pH incubation and caprylic acid precipitation/incubation of immunoglobulin products [159]. An additional milestone to enhance plasma protein product safety is nanofiltration, a procedure of filtration of protein solutions on 15–35 nm nanopore membrane devices designed to entrap and remove viruses [160]. This dedicated virus removal methodology is well established, including for HCV, and is currently applied to most plasma products [156]. Thanks to the implementation of such reduction treatments, most often combined in a complementary manner at different stages of the manufacturing process, no case of HCV transmission by industrial plasma products has been reported since 1993 [154].

3.3.3. *HCV reduction treatment applied to plasma and platelet concentrates for transfusion*

3.3.3.1. *Plasma*

Several viral inactivation treatments of clinical plasma are licensed in various countries [161]. The S/D technology was adapted to 100–500 l of pooled industrial plasma in the early 1990s [162] and demonstrated, prior to HCV identification, to efficiently inactivate non-A-non-B hepatitis virus [163]. The removal of the S/D agents is typically achieved by oil extraction and column hydrophobic interaction chromatography [162]. A miniaturized version of the S/D process using a different detergent (Triton X-45 instead of Triton X-100) has been developed allowing its implementation in single-use equipment, thereby facilitating its application in developing countries, such as Egypt, currently lacking industrial capacity [164]. The efficacy of such method to inactivate HCV has been specifically demonstrated using an in vitro culture assay [165].

A procedure consisting in adding methylene blue and illuminating acellular plasma was made available in the early 1990s [166]. The method leads to inactivation of free HCV particles through photochemical alteration of nucleic acids and incapacity of replication [154, 167].

Two other photoinactivation procedures of plasma have been licensed more recently. One combines the addition of psoralen S-59 (amotosalen) with ultraviolet light A illumination [168]. The other is based on the addition of riboflavin followed by UV irradiation [169]. These small molecules can penetrate membranes and intercalate with helical regions of HCV nucleic acids. Subsequent UV illumination irreversibly alters nucleic acids, making HCV particles unable to replicate [154, 170].

3.3.3.2. *Platelets*

Development of HCV inactivation methods in cellular blood products in general, and platelet concentrates in particular, has been more challenging due to the difficulty to inactivate intracellular viruses without affecting cell function for transfusion. The two photoinactivation methods applied to plasma could nevertheless be adapted to the inactivation of HCV and other viruses in platelet concentrates [170–172].

3.3.3.3. Cryoprecipitate

Cryoprecipitate, obtained by a freeze-thaw process of plasma, is rich in factor VIII, von Willebrand factor, and fibrinogen. This plasma fraction is still largely used in many developing countries for substitution therapy in hemophilia A, von Willebrand factor disease, or fibrinogen deficiency, respectively. The frequency of treatment of patients with congenital deficiency exposes them to a high risk of infection in countries such as Egypt with a close to 10% HCV incidence [173, 174]. Similar mini-pool methods of HCV inactivation used for clinical plasma are applied to cryoprecipitates [164].

3.3.3.4. Red blood cell concentrates and whole blood

No methodology is licensed yet for HCV inactivation in red blood cell concentrates or whole blood. However, the riboflavin/UV pathogen reduction technology is being adapted to the treatment of whole blood [175] and has been shown recently to contribute to lower the risk of malaria transmission in a clinical study in Ghana [176]. It is still uncertain whether a pathogen reduction technology can be developed to substantially inactivate HCV in whole blood or red blood cell concentrates without detrimentally affecting their transfusion quality and functionality or immunogenic potential.

3.4. Therapeutic apheresis and passive immunotherapy

Additional methods of precluding HCV infection are to remove circulating virus through therapeutic apheresis or attempting to neutralize HCV infectivity by administering plasma-derived anti-HCV immunoglobulins. These strategies are aimed at reducing the infectious viral load and have been explored in clinical trials.

3.4.1. Therapeutic apheresis for the removal of HCV virions

Therapeutic apheresis is the process of transiently circulating the blood outside the body and removing the components causing particular diseases by membrane separation and adsorption separation technologies. In the case of HCV, immunoadsorption apheresis was first applied to treat the chronic hepatitis C-related cryoglobulinemia that causes autoimmune symptoms [177]. The technique of heparin-induced extracorporeal LDL precipitation (HELP) apheresis, which could eliminate apolipoprotein B-containing lipoproteins, was then discovered to reduce HCV viral load [178]; however, the decline was found not correlated with LDL reduction in plasma and appeared to be transient due to the high turnover rate of HCV [179]. Studies using combination therapy of antiviral agents and double-filtration plasmapheresis (DFPP) that selectively removes substances with high molecular weight including HCV particles and therefore, happened to display better effects of suppressing the viral kinetics and therefore have been substantially explored during the past decade. Patients who underwent the prophylactic combination treatment of low-dose IFN, ribavirin, and

DFPP had no evidence of HCV recurrence or fibrosing cholestatic hepatitis exacerbation for more than 1 year after liver transplantation [180]. Combination of DFPP and IFN also achieved impressive SVR in difficult-to-treat patients (i.e., relapsed, nonresponder, or HIV-coinfected patients) [181–184] and may also be safe for the elderly population [185]. However, the approach of apheresis for decreasing HCV viral load requires specialty equipment and possesses potential risk of adverse events (e.g., blood pressure lowering, puncture site hematoma, or infection) [181, 185].

3.4.2. Passive immunotherapy using plasma-derived polyclonal HCV immunoglobulins

Passive immunotherapy, also known as antibody therapy, is a very well-established treatment based on the administration of polyclonal hyperimmune immunoglobulins extracted from plasma or mAbs prepared by genetic engineering technologies. One application of passive immunity is to prevent or treat infections due to viruses or to reduce the pathologies associated with bacterial or venom toxins. Human immunoglobulins for passive immunotherapy are fractionated from the plasma of immunized donors having high-titer antibodies against a particular organism or antigen. For the fractionation process, plasma donations from hundreds or thousands of donors are pooled and subjected to various purification and viral inactivation steps, as described in this chapter, to isolate an essentially pure Ig preparation [159, 186]. Current human plasma-derived hyperimmune globulin products are used for the prophylaxis and treatment of viral diseases due to hepatitis B virus (HBV), rabies virus, cytomegalovirus, hepatitis A virus, or respiratory syncytial virus [187]. Human plasma-derived polyclonal hepatitis B immunoglobulin for intravenous use has been made available commercially for over 20 years in some countries. These licensed preparations are efficacious to predictably prevent HBV recurrence after liver transplantation and vertical HBV transmission from mother to child and are used as prophylactic treatment to prevent infection following contact with HBV-contaminated body fluids [188].

The possibility to use polyclonal HCV immunoglobulin to treat or prevent HCV infection has been proposed for many years [189], but no commercial preparation is available yet as it is not proven whether such immunoglobulin can prevent HCV infection or control viremia in infected patients. The rationale in polyclonal HCV immunoglobulins made from large pool of plasma units is to have a preparation that contains neutralizing antibodies to various strains of HCV [189]. However, the presence of neutralizing antibodies has been unclear initially as their presence in plasma was just considered to reflect the occurrence of an infection. Data have suggested that HCV-neutralizing antibodies exist in anti-HCV-positive plasma, but the anti-HCV antibody titer does not correlate with neutralizing capacity [190]. In vitro and animal experiments in a mice model have nevertheless suggested the presence of neutralizing antibodies in polyclonal IgG from a patient with a long-standing HCV infection [191]. A clinical study was initiated in the USA to evaluate the capacity of polyclonal plasma-derived HCV immunoglobulins to "prevent post-transplantation HCV infection of the liver graft and related progression of HCV-related liver disease." This clinical trial was "designed to evaluate a polyclonal human hepatitis C immune globulin given during and post liver transplantation for preventing or reducing the impact of recurrent HCV infection" [192]. However the trial was terminated in 2012 after treatment of seven patients (five receiving the immunoglobulins and two standard-of-care treatment alone) and no data reported. A new trial has begun in 2013 and was recently completed [193]. It is unclear whether plasma-derived polyclonal HCV immunoglobulin will be developed. If this occurs, clear donor screening and donation testing criteria should be defined to determine the specifications of the plasma donations suitable for fractionation, as well as the fractionation methodology itself to exclude any infectious risks from the fractionation of plasma donations. It should be noted that several mAbs for clinical use in HCV-infected patients have been proposed and one has undergone a clinical trial [190]. The future will indicate whether any HCV immunoglobulin, either polyclonal or monoclonal, has a role to play in the control of HCV infection.

4. Prospects of targeting HCV entry in clinical setting

Treatment options against hepatitis C have significantly improved owing to recent advances in the development of anti-HCV therapeutics. Nevertheless, there is still much room for improvement due to potential drug resistance and possibility of viral rebound, which usually require long periods of monitoring and analysis to uncover. More importantly, there is currently no immunization or prophylactic treatment against hepatitis C. Introducing novel antivirals with a different mode of action, such as targeting viral entry using mAbs or small molecules, not only helps expand the spectrum of anti-HCV drugs but also in developing novel treatment modalities. Many of the mAbs targeting HCV receptors/coreceptors as well as small-molecule inhibitors of HCV entry impede both viral attachment and cell-to-cell transmission; this is useful in providing protection against de novo infection and at the same time in helping restrict viral spread. The inclusion of viral entry inhibitors to current DAAs has already been shown to produce synergistic treatment effect [9]. Furthermore, taking a multistep targeting approach would help elevate the genetic barrier against selection of resistant variants, thus facilitating viral clearance. Finally, the advantage of developing entry inhibitors is its potential prophylactic application against hepatitis C, which is particularly useful in protecting liver allografts from recurrent HCV infection. Other protective measures of hepatitis C transmission in clinical scenarios include implementation of viral inactivation methods for the removal of HCV infectivity in therapeutic plasma products [165]. In addition, therapeutic apheresis [180] and protective anti-HCV immunoglobulins [192, 193] have also been suggested for prevention of HCV reinfection in liver transplant patients. In the absence of an approved hepatitis C vaccine, these approaches could be explored as preventive and prophylactic measures against HCV infection. With the above-described strategies to preclude HCV entry, it is foreseeable, in a not-too-distant future, that these tactics under development will help provide a better management of chronic and recurrent hepatitis C, particularly in liver transplant setting.

Acknowledgements

CHL is a recipient of the 2016 CanHepC (Canadian Network on Hepatitis C) Summer Research Scholarship and the MOST 105 College Research Scholarship (105-2815-C-038-018-B). TB (NSC 102-2320-B-038-041-MY3) and LTL (NSC101-2320-B-038-038-MY2; MOST103-2320-B-038-031-MY3) are supported by funding from the Ministry of Science and Technology of Taiwan.

Author details

Thierry Burnouf[1], Ching-Hsuan Liu[2] and Liang-Tzung Lin[2,3]*

*Address all correspondence to: ltlin@tmu.edu.tw

1 Graduate Institute of Biomedical Materials and Tissue Engineering, College of Biomedical Engineering, Taipei Medical University, Taipei, Taiwan

2 Department of Microbiology and Immunology, School of Medicine, College of Medicine, Taipei Medical University, Taipei, Taiwan

3 Graduate Institute of Medical Sciences, College of Medicine, Taipei Medical University, Taipei, Taiwan

References

[1] U.S. Health Resources & Services Administration. Organ Procurement and Transplantation Network [Internet]. 2016. Available from: https://optn.transplant.hrsa.gov/data/view-data-reports/ [Accessed: 2016-08-15]

[2] Feeney ER, Chung RT. Antiviral treatment of hepatitis C. BMJ. 2014;**348**:g3308. DOI: 10.1136/bmj.g3308

[3] Zoulim F, Liang TJ, Gerbes AL, Aghemo A, Deuffic-Burban S, Dusheiko G, et al. Hepatitis C virus treatment in the real world: optimising treatment and access to therapies. Gut. 2015;**64**(11):1824-33. DOI: 10.1136/gutjnl-2015-310421

[4] Hoofnagle JH, Sherker AH. Therapy for hepatitis C—the costs of success. N Engl J Med. 2014;**370**(16):1552-3. DOI: 10.1056/NEJMe1401508

[5] Liang TJ, Ghany MG. Current and future therapies for hepatitis C virus infection. N Engl J Med. 2013;**368**(20):1907-17. DOI: 10.1056/NEJMra1213651

[6] Thursz M, Fontanet A. HCV transmission in industrialized countries and resource-constrained areas. Nat Rev Gastroenterol Hepatol. 2014;**11**(1):28-35. DOI: 10.1038/nrgastro.2013.179

[7] Verna EC, Brown RS, Jr. Hepatitis C and liver transplantation: enhancing outcomes and should patients be retransplanted. Clin Liver Dis. 2008;**12**(3):637-59, ix-x. DOI: 10.1016/j.cld.2008.03.010

[8] Firpi RJ, Clark V, Soldevila-Pico C, Morelli G, Cabrera R, Levy C, et al. The natural history of hepatitis C cirrhosis after liver transplantation. Liver Transpl. 2009;**15**(9):1063-71. DOI: 10.1002/lt.21784

[9] Xiao F, Fofana I, Thumann C, Mailly L, Alles R, Robinet E, et al. Synergy of entry inhibitors with direct-acting antivirals uncovers novel combinations for prevention and treatment of hepatitis C. Gut. 2015;**64**(3):483-94. DOI: 10.1136/gutjnl-2013-306155

[10] Merz A, Long G, Hiet MS, Brugger B, Chlanda P, Andre P, et al. Biochemical and morphological properties of hepatitis C virus particles and determination of their lipidome. J Biol Chem. 2011;**286**(4):3018-32. DOI: 10.1074/jbc.M110.175018

[11] Catanese MT, Uryu K, Kopp M, Edwards TJ, Andrus L, Rice WJ, et al. Ultrastructural analysis of hepatitis C virus particles. Proc Natl Acad Sci U S A. 2013;**110**(23):9505-10. DOI: 10.1073/pnas.1307527110

[12] Andre P, Komurian-Pradel F, Deforges S, Perret M, Berland JL, Sodoyer M, et al. Characterization of low- and very-low-density hepatitis C virus RNA-containing particles. J Virol. 2002;**76**(14):6919-28. DOI: 10.1128/JVI.76.14.6919-6928.2002

[13] Chang KS, Jiang J, Cai Z, Luo G. Human apolipoprotein e is required for infectivity and production of hepatitis C virus in cell culture. J Virol. 2007;**81**(24):13783-93. DOI: 10.1128/JVI.01091-07

[14] Meunier JC, Russell RS, Engle RE, Faulk KN, Purcell RH, Emerson SU. Apolipoprotein c1 association with hepatitis C virus. J Virol. 2008;**82**(19):9647-56. DOI: 10.1128/JVI.00914-08

[15] Nielsen SU, Bassendine MF, Burt AD, Martin C, Pumeechockchai W, Toms GL. Association between hepatitis C virus and very-low-density lipoprotein (VLDL)/LDL analyzed in iodixanol density gradients. J Virol. 2006;**80**(5):2418-28. DOI: 10.1128/JVI.80.5.2418-2428.2006

[16] Jiang J, Luo G. Apolipoprotein E but not B is required for the formation of infectious hepatitis C virus particles. J Virol. 2009;**83**(24):12680-91. DOI: 10.1128/JVI.01476-09

[17] Benga WJ, Krieger SE, Dimitrova M, Zeisel MB, Parnot M, Lupberger J, et al. Apolipoprotein E interacts with hepatitis C virus nonstructural protein 5A and determines assembly of infectious particles. Hepatology. 2010;**51**(1):43-53. DOI: 10.1002/hep.23278

[18] Huang H, Sun F, Owen DM, Li W, Chen Y, Gale M, Jr., et al. Hepatitis C virus production by human hepatocytes dependent on assembly and secretion of very low-density lipoproteins. Proc Natl Acad Sci U S A. 2007;**104**(14):5848-53. DOI: 10.1073/pnas.0700760104

[19] Gastaminza P, Cheng G, Wieland S, Zhong J, Liao W, Chisari FV. Cellular determinants of hepatitis C virus assembly, maturation, degradation, and secretion. J Virol. 2008;**82**(5):2120-9. DOI: 10.1128/JVI.02053-07

[20] Icard V, Diaz O, Scholtes C, Perrin-Cocon L, Ramiere C, Bartenschlager R, et al. Secretion of hepatitis C virus envelope glycoproteins depends on assembly of apolipoprotein B positive lipoproteins. PLoS One. 2009;**4**(1):e4233. DOI: 10.1371/journal.pone.0004233

[21] Hueging K, Doepke M, Vieyres G, Bankwitz D, Frentzen A, Doerrbecker J, et al. Apolipoprotein E codetermines tissue tropism of hepatitis C virus and is crucial for viral cell-

to-cell transmission by contributing to a postenvelopment step of assembly. J Virol. 2014;**88**(3):1433-46. DOI: 10.1128/JVI.01815-13

[22] Douam F, Lavillette D, Cosset FL. The mechanism of HCV entry into host cells. Prog Mol Biol Transl Sci. 2015;**129**:63-107. DOI: 10.1016/bs.pmbts.2014.10.003

[23] Barth H, Schafer C, Adah MI, Zhang F, Linhardt RJ, Toyoda H, et al. Cellular binding of hepatitis C virus envelope glycoprotein E2 requires cell surface heparan sulfate. J Biol Chem. 2003;**278**(42):41003-12. DOI: 10.1074/jbc.M302267200

[24] Barth H, Schnober EK, Zhang F, Linhardt RJ, Depla E, Boson B, et al. Viral and cellular determinants of the hepatitis C virus envelope-heparan sulfate interaction. J Virol. 2006;**80**(21):10579-90. DOI: 10.1128/JVI.00941-06

[25] Koutsoudakis G, Kaul A, Steinmann E, Kallis S, Lohmann V, Pietschmann T, et al. Characterization of the early steps of hepatitis C virus infection by using luciferase reporter viruses. J Virol. 2006;**80**(11):5308-20. DOI: 10.1128/JVI.02460-05

[26] Shi Q, Jiang J, Luo G. Syndecan-1 serves as the major receptor for attachment of hepatitis C virus to the surfaces of hepatocytes. J Virol. 2013;**87**(12):6866-75. DOI: 10.1128/JVI.03475-12

[27] Lefevre M, Felmlee DJ, Parnot M, Baumert TF, Schuster C. Syndecan 4 is involved in mediating HCV entry through interaction with lipoviral particle-associated apolipoprotein E. PLoS One. 2014;**9**(4):e95550. DOI: 10.1371/journal.pone.0095550

[28] Agnello V, Abel G, Elfahal M, Knight GB, Zhang QX. Hepatitis C virus and other flaviviridae viruses enter cells via low density lipoprotein receptor. Proc Natl Acad Sci U S A. 1999;**96**(22):12766-71. DOI: 10.1073/pnas.96.22.12766

[29] Owen DM, Huang H, Ye J, Gale M, Jr. Apolipoprotein E on hepatitis C virion facilitates infection through interaction with low-density lipoprotein receptor. Virology. 2009;**394**(1):99-108. DOI: 10.1016/j.virol.2009.08.037

[30] Molina S, Castet V, Fournier-Wirth C, Pichard-Garcia L, Avner R, Harats D, et al. The low-density lipoprotein receptor plays a role in the infection of primary human hepatocytes by hepatitis C virus. J Hepatol. 2007;**46**(3):411-9. DOI: 10.1016/j.jhep.2006.09.024

[31] Albecka A, Belouzard S, Op de Beeck A, Descamps V, Goueslain L, Bertrand-Michel J, et al. Role of low-density lipoprotein receptor in the hepatitis C virus life cycle. Hepatology. 2012;**55**(4):998-1007. DOI: 10.1002/hep.25501

[32] Syed GH, Tang H, Khan M, Hassanein T, Liu J, Siddiqui A. Hepatitis C virus stimulates low-density lipoprotein receptor expression to facilitate viral propagation. J Virol. 2014;**88**(5):2519-29. DOI: 10.1128/JVI.02727-13

[33] Jiang J, Cun W, Wu X, Shi Q, Tang H, Luo G. Hepatitis C virus attachment mediated by apolipoprotein E binding to cell surface heparan sulfate. J Virol. 2012;**86**(13):7256-67. DOI: 10.1128/JVI.07222-11

[34] Jiang J, Wu X, Tang H, Luo G. Apolipoprotein E mediates attachment of clinical hepatitis C virus to hepatocytes by binding to cell surface heparan sulfate proteoglycan receptors. PLoS One. 2013;**8**(7):e67982. DOI: 10.1371/journal.pone.0067982

[35] Xu Y, Martinez P, Seron K, Luo G, Allain F, Dubuisson J, et al. Characterization of hepatitis C virus interaction with heparan sulfate proteoglycans. J Virol. 2015;**89**(7):3846-58. DOI: 10.1128/JVI.03647-14

[36] Hishiki T, Shimizu Y, Tobita R, Sugiyama K, Ogawa K, Funami K, et al. Infectivity of hepatitis C virus is influenced by association with apolipoprotein E isoforms. J Virol. 2010;**84**(22):12048-57. DOI: 10.1128/JVI.01063-10

[37] Dao Thi VL, Granier C, Zeisel MB, Guerin M, Mancip J, Granio O, et al. Characterization of hepatitis C virus particle subpopulations reveals multiple usage of the scavenger receptor BI for entry steps. J Biol Chem. 2012;**287**(37):31242-57. DOI: 10.1074/jbc.M112.365924

[38] Catanese MT, Ansuini H, Graziani R, Huby T, Moreau M, Ball JK, et al. Role of scavenger receptor class B type I in hepatitis C virus entry: kinetics and molecular determinants. J Virol. 2010;**84**(1):34-43. DOI: 10.1128/JVI.02199-08

[39] Maillard P, Huby T, Andreo U, Moreau M, Chapman J, Budkowska A. The interaction of natural hepatitis C virus with human scavenger receptor SR-BI/Cla1 is mediated by ApoB-containing lipoproteins. FASEB J. 2006;**20**(6):735-7. DOI: 10.1096/fj.05-4728fje

[40] Scarselli E, Ansuini H, Cerino R, Roccasecca RM, Acali S, Filocamo G, et al. The human scavenger receptor class B type I is a novel candidate receptor for the hepatitis C virus. EMBO J. 2002;**21**(19):5017-25. DOI: 10.1093/emboj/cdf529

[41] Bartosch B, Vitelli A, Granier C, Goujon C, Dubuisson J, Pascale S, et al. Cell entry of hepatitis C virus requires a set of co-receptors that include the CD81 tetraspanin and the SR-B1 scavenger receptor. J Biol Chem. 2003;**278**(43):41624-30. DOI: 10.1074/jbc.M305289200

[42] Zahid MN, Turek M, Xiao F, Thi VL, Guerin M, Fofana I, et al. The postbinding activity of scavenger receptor class B type I mediates initiation of hepatitis C virus infection and viral dissemination. Hepatology. 2013;**57**(2):492-504. DOI: 10.1002/hep.26097

[43] Bankwitz D, Vieyres G, Hueging K, Bitzegeio J, Doepke M, Chhatwal P, et al. Role of hypervariable region 1 for the interplay of hepatitis C virus with entry factors and lipoproteins. J Virol. 2014;**88**(21):12644-55. DOI: 10.1128/JVI.01145-14

[44] Zeisel MB, Koutsoudakis G, Schnober EK, Haberstroh A, Blum HE, Cosset FL, et al. Scavenger receptor class B type I is a key host factor for hepatitis C virus infection required for an entry step closely linked to CD81. Hepatology. 2007;**46**(6):1722-31. DOI: 10.1002/hep.21994

[45] Kapadia SB, Barth H, Baumert T, McKeating JA, Chisari FV. Initiation of hepatitis C virus infection is dependent on cholesterol and cooperativity between CD81 and scavenger receptor B type I. J Virol. 2007;**81**(1):374-83. DOI: 10.1128/JVI.01134-06

[46] Koutsoudakis G, Herrmann E, Kallis S, Bartenschlager R, Pietschmann T. The level of CD81 cell surface expression is a key determinant for productive entry of hepatitis C virus into host cells. J Virol. 2007;**81**(2):588-98. DOI: 10.1128/JVI.01534-06

[47] Molina S, Castet V, Pichard-Garcia L, Wychowski C, Meurs E, Pascussi JM, et al. Serum-derived hepatitis C virus infection of primary human hepatocytes is tetraspanin CD81 dependent. J Virol. 2008;**82**(1):569-74. DOI: 10.1128/JVI.01443-07

[48] Feneant L, Levy S, Cocquerel L. CD81 and hepatitis C virus (HCV) infection. Viruses. 2014;**6**(2):535-72. DOI: 10.3390/v6020535

[49] Harris HJ, Davis C, Mullins JG, Hu K, Goodall M, Farquhar MJ, et al. Claudin association with CD81 defines hepatitis C virus entry. J Biol Chem. 2010;**285**(27):21092-102. DOI: 10.1074/jbc.M110.104836

[50] Harris HJ, Farquhar MJ, Mee CJ, Davis C, Reynolds GM, Jennings A, et al. CD81 and claudin 1 coreceptor association: role in hepatitis C virus entry. J Virol. 2008;**82**(10):5007-20. DOI: 10.1128/JVI.02286-07

[51] Farquhar MJ, Hu K, Harris HJ, Davis C, Brimacombe CL, Fletcher SJ, et al. Hepatitis C virus induces CD81 and claudin-1 endocytosis. J Virol. 2012;**86**(8):4305-16. DOI: 10.1128/JVI.06996-11

[52] Brazzoli M, Bianchi A, Filippini S, Weiner A, Zhu Q, Pizza M, et al. CD81 is a central regulator of cellular events required for hepatitis C virus infection of human hepatocytes. J Virol. 2008;**82**(17):8316-29. DOI: 10.1128/JVI.00665-08

[53] Liu Z, Tian Y, Machida K, Lai MM, Luo G, Foung SK, et al. Transient activation of the PI3K-AKT pathway by hepatitis C virus to enhance viral entry. J Biol Chem. 2012;**287**(50):41922-30. DOI: 10.1074/jbc.M112.414789

[54] Lupberger J, Zeisel MB, Xiao F, Thumann C, Fofana I, Zona L, et al. EGFR and EphA2 are host factors for hepatitis C virus entry and possible targets for antiviral therapy. Nat Med. 2011;**17**(5):589-95. DOI: 10.1038/nm.2341

[55] Diao J, Pantua H, Ngu H, Komuves L, Diehl L, Schaefer G, et al. Hepatitis C virus induces epidermal growth factor receptor activation via CD81 binding for viral internalization and entry. J Virol. 2012;**86**(20):10935-49. DOI: 10.1128/JVI.00750-12

[56] Rocha-Perugini V, Montpellier C, Delgrange D, Wychowski C, Helle F, Pillez A, et al. The CD81 partner EWI-2wint inhibits hepatitis C virus entry. PLoS One. 2008;**3**(4):e1866. DOI: 10.1371/journal.pone.0001866

[57] Potel J, Rassam P, Montpellier C, Kaestner L, Werkmeister E, Tews BA, et al. EWI-2wint promotes CD81 clustering that abrogates Hepatitis C Virus entry. Cell Microbiol. 2013;**15**(7):1234-52. DOI: 10.1111/cmi.12112

[58] Sourisseau M, Michta ML, Zony C, Israelow B, Hopcraft SE, Narbus CM, et al. Temporal analysis of hepatitis C virus cell entry with occludin directed blocking antibodies. PLoS Pathog. 2013;**9**(3):e1003244. DOI: 10.1371/journal.ppat.1003244

[59] Martin DN, Uprichard SL. Identification of transferrin receptor 1 as a hepatitis C virus entry factor. Proc Natl Acad Sci U S A. 2013;**110**(26):10777-82. DOI: 10.1073/pnas.1301764110

[60] Sainz B, Jr., Barretto N, Martin DN, Hiraga N, Imamura M, Hussain S, et al. Identification of the Niemann-Pick C1-like 1 cholesterol absorption receptor as a new hepatitis C virus entry factor. Nat Med. 2012;**18**(2):281-5. DOI: 10.1038/nm.2581

[61] Blanchard E, Belouzard S, Goueslain L, Wakita T, Dubuisson J, Wychowski C, et al. Hepatitis C virus entry depends on clathrin-mediated endocytosis. J Virol. 2006;**80**(14):6964-72. DOI: 10.1128/JVI.00024-06

[62] Meertens L, Bertaux C, Dragic T. Hepatitis C virus entry requires a critical postinternalization step and delivery to early endosomes via clathrin-coated vesicles. J Virol. 2006;**80**(23):11571-8. DOI: 10.1128/JVI.01717-06

[63] Coller KE, Berger KL, Heaton NS, Cooper JD, Yoon R, Randall G. RNA interference and single particle tracking analysis of hepatitis C virus endocytosis. PLoS Pathog. 2009;**5**(12): e1000702. DOI: 10.1371/journal.ppat.1000702

[64] Evans MJ, von Hahn T, Tscherne DM, Syder AJ, Panis M, Wolk B, et al. Claudin-1 is a hepatitis C virus co-receptor required for a late step in entry. Nature. 2007;**446**(7137):801-5. DOI: 10.1038/nature05654

[65] Ploss A, Evans MJ, Gaysinskaya VA, Panis M, You H, de Jong YP, et al. Human occludin is a hepatitis C virus entry factor required for infection of mouse cells. Nature. 2009;**457**(7231):882-6. DOI: 10.1038/nature07684

[66] Dorner M, Horwitz JA, Robbins JB, Barry WT, Feng Q, Mu K, et al. A genetically humanized mouse model for hepatitis C virus infection. Nature. 2011;**474**(7350):208-11. DOI: 10.1038/nature10168

[67] Da Costa D, Turek M, Felmlee DJ, Girardi E, Pfeffer S, Long G, et al. Reconstitution of the entire hepatitis C virus life cycle in nonhepatic cells. J Virol. 2012;**86**(21):11919-25. DOI: 10.1128/JVI.01066-12

[68] Timpe JM, Stamataki Z, Jennings A, Hu K, Farquhar MJ, Harris HJ, et al. Hepatitis C virus cell-cell transmission in hepatoma cells in the presence of neutralizing antibodies. Hepatology. 2008;**47**(1):17-24. DOI: 10.1002/hep.21959

[69] Brimacombe CL, Grove J, Meredith LW, Hu K, Syder AJ, Flores MV, et al. Neutralizing antibody-resistant hepatitis C virus cell-to-cell transmission. J Virol. 2011;**85**(1):596-605. DOI: 10.1128/JVI.01592-10

[70] Catanese MT, Loureiro J, Jones CT, Dorner M, von Hahn T, Rice CM. Different requirements for scavenger receptor class B type I in hepatitis C virus cell-free versus cell-to-cell transmission. J Virol. 2013;**87**(15):8282-93. DOI: 10.1128/JVI.01102-13

[71] Barretto N, Sainz B, Jr., Hussain S, Uprichard SL. Determining the involvement and therapeutic implications of host cellular factors in hepatitis C virus cell-to-cell spread. J Virol. 2014;**88**(9):5050-61. DOI: 10.1128/JVI.03241-13

[72] Pileri P, Uematsu Y, Campagnoli S, Galli G, Falugi F, Petracca R, et al. Binding of hepatitis C virus to CD81. Science. 1998;**282**(5390):938-41. DOI: 10.1126/science.282.5390.938

[73] Flint M, Maidens C, Loomis-Price LD, Shotton C, Dubuisson J, Monk P, et al. Characterization of hepatitis C virus E2 glycoprotein interaction with a putative cellular receptor, CD81. J Virol. 1999;**73**(8):6235-44.

[74] Levy S, Todd SC, Maecker HT. CD81 (TAPA-1): a molecule involved in signal transduction and cell adhesion in the immune system. Annu Rev Immunol. 1998;**16**:89-109. DOI: 10.1146/annurev.immunol.16.1.89

[75] Meuleman P, Hesselgesser J, Paulson M, Vanwolleghem T, Desombere I, Reiser H, et al. Anti-CD81 antibodies can prevent a hepatitis C virus infection in vivo. Hepatology. 2008;**48**(6):1761-8. DOI: 10.1002/hep.22547

[76] Fofana I, Xiao F, Thumann C, Turek M, Zona L, Tawar RG, et al. A novel monoclonal anti-CD81 antibody produced by genetic immunization efficiently inhibits Hepatitis C virus cell-cell transmission. PLoS One. 2013;**8**(5):e64221. DOI: 10.1371/journal.pone.0064221

[77] Ji C, Liu Y, Pamulapati C, Bohini S, Fertig G, Schraeml M, et al. Prevention of hepatitis C virus infection and spread in human liver chimeric mice by an anti-CD81 monoclonal antibody. Hepatology. 2015;**61**(4):1136-44. DOI: 10.1002/hep.27603

[78] Acton S, Rigotti A, Landschulz KT, Xu S, Hobbs HH, Krieger M. Identification of scavenger receptor SR-BI as a high density lipoprotein receptor. Science. 1996;**271**(5248):518-20. DOI: 10.1126/science.271.5248.518

[79] Krieger M. Scavenger receptor class B type I is a multiligand HDL receptor that influences diverse physiologic systems. J Clin Invest. 2001;**108**(6):793-7. DOI: 10.1172/JCI14011

[80] Catanese MT, Graziani R, von Hahn T, Moreau M, Huby T, Paonessa G, et al. High-avidity monoclonal antibodies against the human scavenger class B type I receptor efficiently block hepatitis C virus infection in the presence of high-density lipoprotein. J Virol. 2007;**81**(15):8063-71. DOI: 10.1128/JVI.00193-07

[81] Meuleman P, Catanese MT, Verhoye L, Desombere I, Farhoudi A, Jones CT, et al. A human monoclonal antibody targeting scavenger receptor class B type I precludes hepatitis C virus infection and viral spread in vitro and in vivo. Hepatology. 2012;**55**(2):364-72. DOI: 10.1002/hep.24692

[82] Lacek K, Vercauteren K, Grzyb K, Naddeo M, Verhoye L, Slowikowski MP, et al. Novel human SR-BI antibodies prevent infection and dissemination of HCV in vitro and in humanized mice. J Hepatol. 2012;**57**(1):17-23. DOI: 10.1016/j.jhep.2012.02.018

[83] Furuse M, Fujita K, Hiiragi T, Fujimoto K, Tsukita S. Claudin-1 and -2: novel integral membrane proteins localizing at tight junctions with no sequence similarity to occludin. J Cell Biol. 1998;**141**(7):1539-50. DOI: 10.1083/jcb.141.7.1539

[84] Krieger SE, Zeisel MB, Davis C, Thumann C, Harris HJ, Schnober EK, et al. Inhibition of hepatitis C virus infection by anti-claudin-1 antibodies is mediated by neutralization of E2-CD81-claudin-1 associations. Hepatology. 2010;**51**(4):1144-57. DOI: 10.1002/hep.23445

[85] Fofana I, Krieger SE, Grunert F, Glauben S, Xiao F, Fafi-Kremer S, et al. Monoclonal anti-claudin 1 antibodies prevent hepatitis C virus infection of primary human hepatocytes. Gastroenterology. 2010;**139**(3):953-64, 64 e1-4. DOI: 10.1053/j.gastro.2010.05.073

[86] Mailly L, Xiao F, Lupberger J, Wilson GK, Aubert P, Duong FH, et al. Clearance of persistent hepatitis C virus infection in humanized mice using a claudin-1-targeting monoclonal antibody. Nat Biotechnol. 2015;**33**(5):549-54. DOI: 10.1038/nbt.3179

[87] Fukasawa M, Nagase S, Shirasago Y, Iida M, Yamashita M, Endo K, et al. Monoclonal antibodies against extracellular domains of claudin-1 block hepatitis C virus infection in a mouse model. J Virol. 2015;**89**(9):4866-79. DOI: 10.1128/JVI.03676-14

[88] Flego M, Ascione A, Cianfriglia M, Vella S. Clinical development of monoclonal antibody-based drugs in HIV and HCV diseases. BMC Med. 2013;**11**:4. DOI: 10.1186/1741-7015-11-4

[89] Broering TJ, Garrity KA, Boatright NK, Sloan SE, Sandor F, Thomas WD, Jr., et al. Identification and characterization of broadly neutralizing human monoclonal antibodies directed against the E2 envelope glycoprotein of hepatitis C virus. J Virol. 2009;**83**(23):12473-82. DOI: 10.1128/JVI.01138-09

[90] Eren R, Landstein D, Terkieltaub D, Nussbaum O, Zauberman A, Ben-Porath J, et al. Preclinical evaluation of two neutralizing human monoclonal antibodies against hepatitis C virus (HCV): a potential treatment to prevent HCV reinfection in liver transplant patients. J Virol. 2006;**80**(6):2654-64. DOI: 10.1128/JVI.80.6.2654-2664.2006

[91] Ilan E, Arazi J, Nussbaum O, Zauberman A, Eren R, Lubin I, et al. The hepatitis C virus (HCV)-Trimera mouse: a model for evaluation of agents against HCV. J Infect Dis. 2002;**185**(2):153-61. DOI: 10.1086/338266

[92] Morin TJ, Broering TJ, Leav BA, Blair BM, Rowley KJ, Boucher EN, et al. Human monoclonal antibody HCV1 effectively prevents and treats HCV infection in chimpanzees. PLoS Pathog. 2012;**8**(8):e1002895. DOI: 10.1371/journal.ppat.1002895

[93] Owsianka A, Tarr AW, Juttla VS, Lavillette D, Bartosch B, Cosset FL, et al. Monoclonal antibody AP33 defines a broadly neutralizing epitope on the hepatitis C virus E2 envelope glycoprotein. J Virol. 2005;**79**(17):11095-104. DOI: 10.1128/JVI.79.17.11095-11104.2005

[94] Sabo MC, Luca VC, Prentoe J, Hopcraft SE, Blight KJ, Yi M, et al. Neutralizing monoclonal antibodies against hepatitis C virus E2 protein bind discontinuous epitopes and inhibit infection at a postattachment step. J Virol. 2011;**85**(14):7005-19. DOI: 10.1128/JVI.00586-11

[95] Schiano TD, Charlton M, Younossi Z, Galun E, Pruett T, Tur-Kaspa R, et al. Monoclonal antibody HCV-AbXTL68 in patients undergoing liver transplantation for HCV: results of a phase 2 randomized study. Liver Transpl. 2006;**12**(9):1381-9. DOI: 10.1002/lt.20876

[96] Chung RT, Gordon FD, Curry MP, Schiano TD, Emre S, Corey K, et al. Human monoclonal antibody MBL-HCV1 delays HCV viral rebound following liver transplantation: a

randomized controlled study. Am J Transplant. 2013;**13**(4):1047-54. DOI: 10.1111/ajt.12083

[97] Marasco WA, Sui J. The growth and potential of human antiviral monoclonal antibody therapeutics. Nat Biotechnol. 2007;**25**(12):1421-34. DOI: 10.1038/nbt1363

[98] Ball JK, Tarr AW, McKeating JA. The past, present and future of neutralizing antibodies for hepatitis C virus. Antiviral Res. 2014;**105**:100-11. DOI: 10.1016/j.antiviral.2014.02.013

[99] Ciesek S, von Hahn T, Colpitts CC, Schang LM, Friesland M, Steinmann J, et al. The green tea polyphenol, epigallocatechin-3-gallate, inhibits hepatitis C virus entry. Hepatology. 2011;**54**(6):1947-55. DOI: 10.1002/hep.24610

[100] Colpitts CC, Schang LM. A small molecule inhibits virion attachment to heparan sulfate- or sialic acid-containing glycans. J Virol. 2014;**88**(14):7806-17. DOI: 10.1128/JVI.00896-14

[101] Calland N, Sahuc ME, Belouzard S, Pene V, Bonnafous P, Mesalam AA, et al. Polyphenols inhibit Hepatitis C virus entry by a new mechanism of action. J Virol. 2015;**89**(19):10053-63. DOI: 10.1128/JVI.01473-15

[102] Lin LT, Chung CY, Hsu WC, Chang SP, Hung TC, Shields J, et al. Saikosaponin b2 is a naturally occurring terpenoid that efficiently inhibits hepatitis C virus entry. J Hepatol. 2015;**62**(3):541-8. DOI: 10.1016/j.jhep.2014.10.040

[103] Hsu WC, Chang SP, Lin LC, Li CL, Richardson CD, Lin CC, et al. Limonium sinense and gallic acid suppress hepatitis C virus infection by blocking early viral entry. Antiviral Res. 2015;**118**:139-47. DOI: 10.1016/j.antiviral.2015.04.003

[104] Lin LT, Chen TY, Lin SC, Chung CY, Lin TC, Wang GH, et al. Broad-spectrum antiviral activity of chebulagic acid and punicalagin against viruses that use glycosaminoglycans for entry. BMC Microbiol. 2013;**13**:187. DOI: 10.1186/1471-2180-13-187

[105] Chung CY, Liu CH, Burnouf T, Wang GH, Chang SP, Jassey A, et al. Activity-based and fraction-guided analysis of Phyllanthus urinaria identifies loliolide as a potent inhibitor of hepatitis C virus entry. Antiviral Res. 2016;**130**:58-68. DOI: 10.1016/j.antiviral.2016.03.012

[106] Chung CY, Liu CH, Wang GH, Jassey A, Li CL, Chen L, et al. (4R,6S)-2-Dihydromenisdaurilide is a Butenolide that Efficiently Inhibits Hepatitis C Virus Entry. Sci Rep. 2016;**6**:29969. DOI: 10.1038/srep29969

[107] Anggakusuma, Colpitts CC, Schang LM, Rachmawati H, Frentzen A, Pfaender S, et al. Turmeric curcumin inhibits entry of all hepatitis C virus genotypes into human liver cells. Gut. 2014;**63**(7):1137-49. DOI: 10.1136/gutjnl-2012-304299

[108] Barry J, Fritz M, Brender JR, Smith PE, Lee DK, Ramamoorthy A. Determining the effects of lipophilic drugs on membrane structure by solid-state NMR spectroscopy: the case of the antioxidant curcumin. J Am Chem Soc. 2009;**131**(12):4490-8. DOI: 10.1021/ja809217u

[109] Helle F, Wychowski C, Vu-Dac N, Gustafson KR, Voisset C, Dubuisson J. Cyanovirin-N inhibits hepatitis C virus entry by binding to envelope protein glycans. J Biol Chem. 2006;**281**(35):25177-83. DOI: 10.1074/jbc.M602431200

[110] Meuleman P, Albecka A, Belouzard S, Vercauteren K, Verhoye L, Wychowski C, et al. Griffithsin has antiviral activity against hepatitis C virus. Antimicrob Agents Chemother. 2011;**55**(11):5159-67. DOI: 10.1128/AAC.00633-11

[111] Brown KS, Keogh MJ, Owsianka AM, Adair R, Patel AH, Arnold JN, et al. Specific interaction of hepatitis C virus glycoproteins with mannan binding lectin inhibits virus entry. Protein Cell. 2010;**1**(7):664-74. DOI: 10.1007/s13238-010-0088-9

[112] Hamed MR, Brown RJ, Zothner C, Urbanowicz RA, Mason CP, Krarup A, et al. Recombinant human L-ficolin directly neutralizes hepatitis C virus entry. J Innate Immun. 2014;**6**(5):676-84. DOI: 10.1159/000362209

[113] Khanal M, Vausselin T, Barras A, Bande O, Turcheniuk K, Benazza M, et al. Phenylboronic-acid-modified nanoparticles: potential antiviral therapeutics. ACS Appl Mater Interfaces. 2013;**5**(23):12488-98. DOI: 10.1021/am403770q

[114] Khanal M, Barras A, Vausselin T, Feneant L, Boukherroub R, Siriwardena A, et al. Boronic acid-modified lipid nanocapsules: a novel platform for the highly efficient inhibition of hepatitis C viral entry. Nanoscale. 2015;**7**(4):1392-402. DOI: 10.1039/c4nr03875d

[115] Yu F, Wang Q, Zhang Z, Peng Y, Qiu Y, Shi Y, et al. Development of oleanane-type triterpenes as a new class of HCV entry inhibitors. J Med Chem. 2013;**56**(11):4300-19. DOI: 10.1021/jm301910a

[116] VanCompernolle SE, Wiznycia AV, Rush JR, Dhanasekaran M, Baures PW, Todd SC. Small molecule inhibition of hepatitis C virus E2 binding to CD81. Virology. 2003;**314**(1):371-80. DOI: 10.1016/S0042-6822(03)00406-9

[117] Cui HK, Qing J, Guo Y, Wang YJ, Cui LJ, He TH, et al. Stapled peptide-based membrane fusion inhibitors of hepatitis C virus. Bioorg Med Chem. 2013;**21**(12):3547-54. DOI: 10. 1016/j.bmc.2013.02.011

[118] Si Y, Liu S, Liu X, Jacobs JL, Cheng M, Niu Y, et al. A human claudin-1-derived peptide inhibits hepatitis C virus entry. Hepatology. 2012;**56**(2):507-15. DOI: 10.1002/hep.25685

[119] Chi X, Niu Y, Cheng M, Liu X, Feng Y, Zheng F, et al. Identification of a potent and broad-spectrum hepatitis C virus fusion inhibitory peptide from the E2 stem domain. Sci Rep. 2016;**6**:25224. DOI: 10.1038/srep25224

[120] Holzer M, Ziegler S, Albrecht B, Kronenberger B, Kaul A, Bartenschlager R, et al. Identification of terfenadine as an inhibitor of human CD81-receptor HCV-E2 interaction: synthesis and structure optimization. Molecules. 2008;**13**(5):1081-110. DOI: 10. 3390/molecules13051081

[121] Masson D, Koseki M, Ishibashi M, Larson CJ, Miller SG, King BD, et al. Increased HDL cholesterol and apoA-I in humans and mice treated with a novel SR-BI inhibitor.

Arterioscler Thromb Vasc Biol. 2009;**29**(12):2054-60. DOI: 10.1161/ATVBAHA.109.191 320

[122] Syder AJ, Lee H, Zeisel MB, Grove J, Soulier E, Macdonald J, et al. Small molecule scavenger receptor BI antagonists are potent HCV entry inhibitors. J Hepatol. 2011;**54** (1):48-55. DOI: 10.1016/j.jhep.2010.06.024

[123] Zhu H, Wong-Staal F, Lee H, Syder A, McKelvy J, Schooley RT, et al. Evaluation of ITX 5061, a scavenger receptor B1 antagonist: resistance selection and activity in combination with other hepatitis C virus antivirals. J Infect Dis. 2012;**205**(4):656-62. DOI: 10.1093/infdis/jir802

[124] Rowe IA, Tully DC, Armstrong MJ, Parker R, Guo K, Barton D, et al. Effect of scavenger receptor class B type I antagonist ITX5061 in patients with hepatitis C virus infection undergoing liver transplantation. Liver Transpl. 2016;**22**(3):287-97. DOI: 10.1002/lt.24349

[125] Yin P, Zhang L. Aspirin inhibits hepatitis C virus entry by downregulating claudin-1. J Viral Hepat. 2016;**23**(1):62-4. DOI: 10.1111/jvh.12446

[126] Zona L, Lupberger J, Sidahmed-Adrar N, Thumann C, Harris HJ, Barnes A, et al. HRas signal transduction promotes hepatitis C virus cell entry by triggering assembly of the host tetraspanin receptor complex. Cell Host Microbe. 2013;**13**(3):302-13. DOI: 10.1016/j.chom.2013.02.006

[127] Blanchet M, Sureau C, Guevin C, Seidah NG, Labonte P. SKI-1/S1P inhibitor PF-429242 impairs the onset of HCV infection. Antiviral Res. 2015;**115**:94-104. DOI: 10.1016/j.antiviral.2014.12.017

[128] Chamoun-Emanuelli AM, Pecheur EI, Simeon RL, Huang D, Cremer PS, Chen Z. Phenothiazines inhibit hepatitis C virus entry, likely by increasing the fluidity of cholesterol-rich membranes. Antimicrob Agents Chemother. 2013;**57**(6):2571-81. DOI: 10.1128/AAC.02593-12

[129] Blaising J, Levy PL, Polyak SJ, Stanifer M, Boulant S, Pecheur EI. Arbidol inhibits viral entry by interfering with clathrin-dependent trafficking. Antiviral Res. 2013;**100**(1):215-9. DOI: 10.1016/j.antiviral.2013.08.008

[130] Tscherne DM, Jones CT, Evans MJ, Lindenbach BD, McKeating JA, Rice CM. Time- and temperature-dependent activation of hepatitis C virus for low-pH-triggered entry. J Virol. 2006;**80**(4):1734-41. DOI: 10.1128/JVI.80.4.1734-1741.2006

[131] Ashfaq UA, Javed T, Rehman S, Nawaz Z, Riazuddin S. Lysosomotropic agents as HCV entry inhibitors. Virol J. 2011;**8**:163. DOI: 10.1186/1743-422X-8-163

[132] St Vincent MR, Colpitts CC, Ustinov AV, Muqadas M, Joyce MA, Barsby NL, et al. Rigid amphipathic fusion inhibitors, small molecule antiviral compounds against enveloped viruses. Proc Natl Acad Sci U S A. 2010;**107**(40):17339-44. DOI: 10.1073/pnas.1010026107

[133] Vausselin T, Calland N, Belouzard S, Descamps V, Douam F, Helle F, et al. The antimalarial ferroquine is an inhibitor of hepatitis C virus. Hepatology. 2013;**58**(1):86-97. DOI: 10.1002/hep.26273

[134] Baldick CJ, Wichroski MJ, Pendri A, Walsh AW, Fang J, Mazzucco CE, et al. A novel small molecule inhibitor of hepatitis C virus entry. PLoS Pathog. 2010;**6**(9):e1001086. DOI: 10.1371/journal.ppat.1001086

[135] Coburn GA, Fisch DN, Moorji SM, de Muys JM, Murga JD, Paul D, et al. Novel small-molecule inhibitors of hepatitis C virus entry block viral spread and promote viral clearance in cell culture. PLoS One. 2012;**7**(4):e35351. DOI: 10.1371/journal.pone.0035351

[136] European Medicines Agency. Silibinin-C-2',3-dihydrogensuccinate, disodium salt for the prevention of recurrent hepatitis C in liver transplant recipients [Internet]. 2010. Available from: http://www.ema.europa.eu/docs/en_GB/document_library/Orphan_designation/2011/01/WC500101019.pdf [Accessed: 2016-08-15]

[137] Liu CH, Lin CC, Hsu WC, Chung CY, Lin CC, Jassey A, et al. Highly bioavailable silibinin nanoparticles inhibit HCV infection. Gut. 2016. DOI: 10.1136/gutjnl-2016-312019

[138] Wagoner J, Negash A, Kane OJ, Martinez LE, Nahmias Y, Bourne N, et al. Multiple effects of silymarin on the hepatitis C virus lifecycle. Hepatology. 2010;**51**(6):1912-21. DOI: 10.1002/hep.23587

[139] Blaising J, Levy PL, Gondeau C, Phelip C, Varbanov M, Teissier E, et al. Silibinin inhibits hepatitis C virus entry into hepatocytes by hindering clathrin-dependent trafficking. Cell Microbiol. 2013;**15**(11):1866-82. DOI: 10.1111/cmi.12155

[140] Wagoner J, Morishima C, Graf TN, Oberlies NH, Teissier E, Pecheur EI, et al. Differential in vitro effects of intravenous versus oral formulations of silibinin on the HCV life cycle and inflammation. PLoS One. 2011;**6**(1):e16464. DOI: 10.1371/journal.pone.0016464

[141] Xiao F, Fofana I, Heydmann L, Barth H, Soulier E, Habersetzer F, et al. Hepatitis C virus cell-cell transmission and resistance to direct-acting antiviral agents. PLoS Pathog. 2014;**10**(5):e1004128. DOI: 10.1371/journal.ppat.1004128

[142] Murakami Y, Fukasawa M, Kaneko Y, Suzuki T, Wakita T, Fukazawa H. Selective estrogen receptor modulators inhibit hepatitis C virus infection at multiple steps of the virus life cycle. Microbes Infect. 2013;**15**(1):45-55. DOI: 10.1016/j.micinf.2012.10.003

[143] Bush CO, Pokrovskii MV, Saito R, Morganelli P, Canales E, Clarke MO, et al. A small-molecule inhibitor of hepatitis C virus infectivity. Antimicrob Agents Chemother. 2014;**58**(1):386-96. DOI: 10.1128/AAC.02083-13

[144] Haid S, Novodomska A, Gentzsch J, Grethe C, Geuenich S, Bankwitz D, et al. A plant-derived flavonoid inhibits entry of all HCV genotypes into human hepatocytes. Gastroenterology. 2012;**143**(1):213-22 e5. DOI: 10.1053/j.gastro.2012.03.036

[145] Lavie M, Voisset C, Vu-Dac N, Zurawski V, Duverlie G, Wychowski C, et al. Serum amyloid A has antiviral activity against hepatitis C virus by inhibiting virus entry in a cell culture system. Hepatology. 2006;**44**(6):1626-34. DOI: 10.1002/hep.21406

[146] Cai Z, Cai L, Jiang J, Chang KS, van der Westhuyzen DR, Luo G. Human serum amyloid A protein inhibits hepatitis C virus entry into cells. J Virol. 2007;**81**(11):6128-33. DOI: 10.1128/JVI.02627-06

[147] Hong W, Lang Y, Li T, Zeng Z, Song Y, Wu Y, et al. A p7 ion channel-derived peptide inhibits hepatitis C virus infection in vitro. J Biol Chem. 2015;**290**(38):23254-63. DOI: 10.1074/jbc.M115.662452

[148] Matsumura T, Hu Z, Kato T, Dreux M, Zhang YY, Imamura M, et al. Amphipathic DNA polymers inhibit hepatitis C virus infection by blocking viral entry. Gastroenterology. 2009;**137**(2):673-81. DOI: 10.1053/j.gastro.2009.04.048

[149] El-Fakharany EM, Sanchez L, Al-Mehdar HA, Redwan EM. Effectiveness of human, camel, bovine and sheep lactoferrin on the hepatitis C virus cellular infectivity: comparison study. Virol J. 2013;**10**:199. DOI: 10.1186/1743-422X-10-199

[150] Tamura S, Yang GM, Yasueda N, Matsuura Y, Komoda Y, Murakami N. Tellimagrandin I, HCV invasion inhibitor from Rosae Rugosae Flos. Bioorg Med Chem Lett. 2010;**20**(5):1598-600. DOI: 10.1016/j.bmcl.2010.01.084

[151] Han Z, Liang X, Wang Y, Qing J, Cao L, Shang L, et al. The discovery of indole derivatives as novel hepatitis C virus inhibitors. Eur J Med Chem. 2016;**116**:147-55. DOI: 10.1016/j.ejmech.2016.03.062

[152] Wang H, Wang S, Cheng L, Chen L, Wang Y, Qing J, et al. Discovery of imidazo[1,2-alpha][1,8]naphthyridine derivatives as potential HCV entry inhibitor. ACS Med Chem Lett. 2015;**6**(9):977-81. DOI: 10.1021/acsmedchemlett.5b00159

[153] WHO. Guidelines on good manufacturing practices for blood establishments. Annex 4. WHO Technical Report Series. 2011;**961**:148-214.

[154] Busch MP, Glynn SA, Stramer SL, Strong DM, Caglioti S, Wright DJ, et al. A new strategy for estimating risks of transfusion-transmitted viral infections based on rates of detection of recently infected donors. Transfusion. 2005;**45**(2):254-64. DOI: 10.1111/j.1537-2995.2004.04215.x

[155] Dodd RY. Current risk for transfusion transmitted infections. Curr Opin Hematol. 2007;**14**(6):671-6. DOI: 10.1097/MOH.0b013e3282e38e8a

[156] Burnouf T, Radosevich M. Reducing the risk of infection from plasma products: specific preventative strategies. Blood Rev. 2000;**14**(2):94-110. DOI: 10.1054/blre.2000.0129

[157] Horowitz B, Wiebe ME, Lippin A, Stryker MH. Inactivation of viruses in labile blood derivatives. I. Disruption of lipid-enveloped viruses by tri(n-butyl)phosphate detergent combinations. Transfusion. 1985;**25**(6):516-22. DOI: 10.1046/j.1537-2995.1985.25686071422.x

[158] Dichtelmuller HO, Biesert L, Fabbrizzi F, Gajardo R, Groner A, von Hoegen I, et al. Robustness of solvent/detergent treatment of plasma derivatives: a data collection from Plasma Protein Therapeutics Association member companies. Transfusion. 2009;**49** (9):1931-43. DOI: TRF02222 [pii]10.1111/j.1537-2995.2009.02222.x

[159] Burnouf T. Modern plasma fractionation. Transfus Med Rev. 2007;**21**(2):101-17. DOI: 10.1016/j.tmrv.2006.11.001

[160] Burnouf T, Radosevich M. Nanofiltration of plasma-derived biopharmaceutical products. Haemophilia. 2003;**9**(1):24-37. DOI: 10.1046/j.1365-2516.2003.00701.x

[161] Reesink HW, Panzer S, McQuilten ZK, Wood EM, Marks C, Wendel S, et al. Pathogen inactivation of platelet concentrates. Vox Sanguinis. 2010;**99**(1):85-95. DOI: 10.1111/j.1423-0410.2010.01319.x

[162] Horowitz B, Bonomo R, Prince AM, Chin SN, Brotman B, Shulman RW. Solvent/detergent-treated plasma: a virus-inactivated substitute for fresh frozen plasma. Blood. 1992;**79**(3):826-31.

[163] Piet MP, Chin S, Prince AM, Brotman B, Cundell AM, Horowitz B. The use of tri(n-butyl) phosphate detergent mixtures to inactivate hepatitis viruses and human immunodeficiency virus in plasma and plasma's subsequent fractionation. Transfusion. 1990;**30** (7):591-8. DOI: 10.1046/j.1537-2995.1990.30790385516.x

[164] El-Ekiaby M, Sayed MA, Caron C, Burnouf S, El-Sharkawy N, Goubran H, et al. Solvent-detergent filtered (S/D-F) fresh frozen plasma and cryoprecipitate minipools prepared in a newly designed integral disposable processing bag system. Transfus Med. 2010;**20** (1):48-61. DOI: 10.1111/j.1365-3148.2009.00963.x

[165] Chou ML, Burnouf T, Chang SP, Hung TC, Lin CC, Richardson CD, et al. TnBPTriton X-45 treatment of plasma for transfusion efficiently inactivates hepatitis C virus. PLoS One. 2015;**10**(2):e0117800. DOI: 10.1371/journal.pone.0117800

[166] Mohr H, Pohl U, Lambrecht B, Wieding JU, Schmitt H. [Methylene blue/light treatment of virus inactivated human plasma: production and clinical experience]. Infusionsther Transfusionsmed. 1993;**20 Suppl 2**:19-24.

[167] Steinmann E, Gravemann U, Friesland M, Doerrbecker J, Muller TH, Pietschmann T, et al. Two pathogen reduction technologies–methylene blue plus light and shortwave ultraviolet light–effectively inactivate hepatitis C virus in blood products. Transfusion. 2013;**53**(5):1010-8. DOI: 10.1111/j.1537-2995.2012.03858.x

[168] de Alarcon P, Benjamin R, Dugdale M, Kessler C, Shopnick R, Smith P, et al. Fresh frozen plasma prepared with amotosalen HCl (S-59) photochemical pathogen inactivation: transfusion of patients with congenital coagulation factor deficiencies. Transfusion. 2005;**45**(8):1362-72. DOI: 10.1111/j.1537-2995.2005.00216.x

[169] Hornsey VS, Drummond O, Morrison A, McMillan L, MacGregor IR, Prowse CV. Pathogen reduction of fresh plasma using riboflavin and ultraviolet light: effects on plasma

coagulation proteins. Transfusion. 2009;**49**(10):2167-72. DOI: 10.1111/j.1537-2995.2009.02272.x

[170] Ruane PH, Edrich R, Gampp D, Keil SD, Leonard RL, Goodrich RP. Photochemical inactivation of selected viruses and bacteria in platelet concentrates using riboflavin and light. Transfusion. 2004;**44**(6):877-85. DOI: 10.1111/j.1537-2995.2004.03355.x

[171] Dodd RY, Moroff G, Wagner S, Dabay MH, Dorfman E, George V, et al. Inactivation of viruses in platelet suspensions that retain their in vitro characteristics: comparison of psoralen-ultraviolet A and merocyanine 540-visible light methods. Transfusion. 1991;**31**(6):483-90. DOI: 10.1046/j.1537-2995.1991.31691306242.x

[172] Lin L, Cook DN, Wiesehahn GP, Alfonso R, Behrman B, Cimino GD, et al. Photochemical inactivation of viruses and bacteria in platelet concentrates by use of a novel psoralen and long-wavelength ultraviolet light. Transfusion. 1997;**37**(4):423-35. DOI: 10.1046/j.1537-2995.1997.37497265344.x

[173] Attia MA. Prevalence of hepatitis B and C in Egypt and Africa. Antivir Ther. 1998;**3**(Suppl 3):1-9.

[174] Reker C, Islam KM. Risk factors associated with high prevalence rates of hepatitis C infection in Egypt. Int J Infect Dis. 2014. DOI: 10.1016/j.ijid.2014.02.003

[175] Marschner S, Goodrich R. Pathogen reduction technology treatment of platelets, plasma and whole blood using riboflavin and UV light. Transfus Med Hemother. 2011;**38**(1):8-18. DOI: 10.1159/000324160

[176] Allain JP, Owusu-Ofori AK, Assennato SM, Marschner S, Goodrich RP, Owusu-Ofori S. Effect of Plasmodium inactivation in whole blood on the incidence of blood transfusion-transmitted malaria in endemic regions: the African Investigation of the Mirasol System (AIMS) randomised controlled trial. Lancet. 2016;**387**(10029):1753-61. DOI: 10.1016/S0140-6736(16)00581-X

[177] Stefanutti C, Di Giacomo S, Mareri M, De Lorenzo F, D'Alessandri G, Angelico F, et al. Immunoadsorption apheresis (Selesorb) in the treatment of chronic hepatitis C virus-related type 2 mixed cryoglobulinemia. Transfus Apher Sci. 2003;**28**(3):207-14. DOI: 10.1016/S1473-0502(03)00055-7

[178] Schettler V, Monazahian M, Wieland E, Ramadori G, Grunewald RW, Thomssen R, et al. Reduction of hepatitis C virus load by H.E.L.P.-LDL apheresis. Eur J Clin Invest. 2001;**31**(2):154-5. DOI: 10.1046/j.1365-2362.2001.00758.x

[179] Schettler V, Monazahian M, Wieland E, Thomssen R, Muller GA. Effect of heparin-induced extracorporeal low-density lipoprotein precipitation (HELP) apheresis on hepatitis C plasma virus load. Ther Apher. 2001;**5**(5):384-6. DOI: 10.1046/j.1526-0968.2001.00374.x

[180] Taniguchi M, Furukawa H, Shimamura T, Suzuki T, Yamashita K, Ota M, et al. Impact of double-filtration plasmapheresis in combination with interferon and ribavirin in living

donor liver transplant recipients with hepatitis C. Transplantation. 2006;**81**(12):1747-9. DOI: 10.1097/01.tp.0000226075.04938.43

[181] Fujiwara K, Kaneko S, Kakumu S, Sata M, Hige S, Tomita E, et al. Double filtration plasmapheresis and interferon combination therapy for chronic hepatitis C patients with genotype 1 and high viral load. Hepatol Res. 2007;**37**(9):701-10. DOI: 10.1111/j.1872-034X.2007.00117.x

[182] Ishikawa T, Higuchi K, Kubota T, Seki K, Honma T, Yoshida T, et al. Complete early virological response was highly achieved by double filtration plasmapheresis plus IFN-beta induction therapy for HCV-1b patients with relapse or no response after previous IFN therapy. Ther Apher Dial. 2011;**15**(4):400-5. DOI: 10.1111/j.1744-9987.2011.00965.x

[183] Mednikov RV, Rabinovich VI, Kizlo SN, Belyakov NA, Sokolov AA. Double Filtration Plasmapheresis in Treatment of Patients With Co-Infection of Hepatitis C and Human Immunodeficiency Virus. Ther Apher Dial. 2016. DOI: 10.1111/1744-9987.12396

[184] Sugimoto K, Kim SR, El-Shamy A, Imoto S, Fujioka H, Kim KI, et al. Outcome of double-filtration plasmapheresis plus interferon treatment in nonresponders to pegylated interferon plus ribavirin combination therapy. Dig Dis. 2013;**31**(5-6):434-9. DOI: 10.1159/000355241

[185] Kaneko S, Sata M, Ide T, Yamashita T, Hige S, Tomita E, et al. Efficacy and safety of double filtration plasmapheresis in combination with interferon therapy for chronic hepatitis C. Hepatol Res. 2010;**40**(11):1072-81. DOI: 10.1111/j.1872-034X.2010.00708.x

[186] Radosevich M, Burnouf T. Intravenous immunoglobulin G: trends in production methods, quality control and quality assurance. Vox Sang. 2010;**98**(1):12-28. DOI: 10.1111/j.1423-0410.2009.01226.x

[187] Sawyer LA. Antibodies for the prevention and treatment of viral diseases. Antiviral Res. 2000;**47**(2):57-77. DOI: 10.1016/S0166-3542(00)00111-X

[188] Congly SE, Burak KW, Coffin CS. Hepatitis B immunoglobulin for prevention of hepatitis B virus infection and recurrence after liver transplantation. Expert Rev Clin Immunol. 2011;**7**(4):429-36. DOI: 10.1586/eci.11.30

[189] Piazza M, Sagliocca L, Tosone G, Guadagnino V, Stazi MA, Orlando R, et al. Prophylaxis of hepatitis C with intramuscular immunoglobulin: clinical and economic appraisal. BioDrugs. 1999;**12**(4):291-300. DOI: 10.2165/00063030-199912040-00006

[190] Borgia G. Specific immunoglobulin against HCV: new perspectives. IDrugs. 2004;**7**(6):570-4.

[191] Vanwolleghem T, Bukh J, Meuleman P, Desombere I, Meunier JC, Alter H, et al. Polyclonal immunoglobulins from a chronic hepatitis C virus patient protect human liver-chimeric mice from infection with a homologous hepatitis C virus strain. Hepatology. 2008;**47**(6):1846-55. DOI: 10.1002/hep.22244

[192] ClinicalTrials.gov: A service of the U.S. National Institutes of Health. Randomized Phase II Study of Hepatitis C Immune Globulin Intravenous (Human), Civacir(TM), in Liver Transplantation [Internet]. 2007. updated May 7 2012. Available from: https://clinicaltrials.gov/ct2/show/study/NCT00473824 [Accessed: 2016-08-15]

[193] ClinicalTrials.gov: A service of the U.S. National Institutes of Health. Civacir® Polyclonal Immune Globulin (IgG) to Prevent Hepatitis C Virus (HCV) Recurrence in Liver Transplant Patients [Internet]. 2013. updated April 20 2016. Available from: https://www.clinicaltrials.gov/ct2/show/NCT01804829 [Accessed: 2016-08-15]

Chapter 14

Hepatitis C Virus Infection Treatment: Recent Advances and New Paradigms in the Treatment Strategies

Imran Shahid, Waleed H. AlMalki,

Mohammed W. AlRabia, Muhammad H. Hafeez and

Muhammad Ahmed

Additional information is available at the end of the chapter

http://dx.doi.org/10.5772/65873

Abstract

The advancement in hepatitis C virus (HCV) therapeutics has been profoundly enhanced by an improved understanding of viral life cycle in host cells, development of novel direct-acting antivirals (DAAs), and exploring other emerging treatment paradigms on the horizon. The approvals of first-, second-, and next-wave direct-acting antivirals highlight the swift pace of progress in the successful development of an expanding variety of therapeutic regimens for use in patients with chronic hepatitis C virus infection. Triple or quadruple therapies based on a combination of different direct-acting antivirals with or without pegylated interferon (IFN) and ribavirin (RBV) have raised the hopes to improve the current treatment strategies for other difficult-to-treat individuals. The development of more efficacious, well-tolerated, and cost-effective interferons with a low frequency of adverse events and short treatment durations is also in the pipeline. An experimental protective vaccine against hepatitis C virus demonstrated promise in preliminary human safety trials, and a larger phase II clinical trials are under consideration to further determine the efficacy of the vaccine. This pragmatic book chapter discusses the current state of knowledge in hepatitis C virus therapeutics and provides a conceptual framework of emerging and investigational treatment strategies directed against this silent epidemic.

Keywords: HCV medications, direct-acting antivirals, NS3/4A serine protease inhibitors, NS5A inhibitors, polymerase inhibitors, antiviral resistance, all oral interferon-free antivirals, triple or quadruple therapies, interferon lambda, anti-HCV vaccine model

1. Introduction

Afflicting around 170 million people worldwide, hepatitis C virus (HCV) infection represents a disease of significant global impact. The regional prevalence for HCV varies substantially around the world, where the infection presents the state of universal coverage in East and South Asia (e.g., in Egypt, the prevalence is as high as 22 %) to no access at all to others (i.e., some North American and European countries) [1, 2]. The new incidents of chronic HCV infection are increasing 3–4 million every year without previous ascertainment of HCV risk, and it seems tough to determine because many acute HCV cases are not noticed clinically [2, 3]. Analogously, acute HCV infection, a multifaceted disease is often asymptomatic or sometimes linked with nonspecific symptoms that lead to chronic hepatitis C in 80 % of infected individuals [4]. Chronic HCV-infected patients may at high risk of developing HCV-associated liver diseases (fibrosis, cirrhosis, and hepatocellular carcinoma) if not treated timely, and infection persists for an extended time [5]. The morbidity and the mortality rate is rising unexpectedly in developing world and even in resource-replete countries (e.g., the United States and the United Kingdom), where more patients are now dying from HCV and associated hepatic diseases (e.g., hepatocellular carcinoma) than HIV [6].

Pegylated interferon alpha (PEG-IFNα) and weight-based nucleoside analog ribavirin (RBV) were recommended as "gold standard of care" more than a decade and still considered an integral part of some newly developed anti-HCV direct-acting antiviral therapeutic regimens [2]. The therapy is used in combination to attain a sustained virologic response rate (SVR; HCV RNA undetectable after 6-month treatment completion) in acute and chronic HCV-infected individuals [2, 7]. The SVR rates achieve up to 80 % in HCV genotype 3-infected patients and not more than 50–60 % of genotype 1- and 4-infected patients [2, 7]. At present, less than 10 % of patients with chronic HCV have been treated successfully because of the failure of risk-based screening to identify all infected patients and the low efficacy and high rate of side effects from regimens based on IFN and RBV [2, 8]. By this token then, PEG-IFN/RBV has proven an ineffective means of managing the HCV infection burden. It is highly significant then that we stand today, at the cusp of a pharmacological revolution.

The current therapeutic approaches in the pipeline to coup HCV infection are the development of novel direct-acting antivirals (DAAs), which directly target viral genome via covalent or non-covalent interactions and disrupt HCV replication and translation [9]. The most widely studied direct-acting antivirals are protease inhibitors (PIs), NS5A inhibitors, and polymerase inhibitors which inhibit HCV translation and replication, respectively, by achieving higher sustained virologic response rates (SVR) with or without PEG-IFNα/RBV in treated patients (**Table 1**) [10]. Two first-generation protease inhibitors (i.e., telaprevir (TLV) and boceprevir (BOC)) were approved by the United States (US) Food and Drug Administration (FDA) in 2011 to treat chronic HCV genotype 1 infection [11]. Simeprevir classified as second-generation protease inhibitor got approval in 2013 to treat chronic HCV genotype 1 populations, and sofosbuvir (SOF) (a viral RNA-dependent RNA polymerase inhibitor) was also recommended in the same year to treat chronic HCV genotype 1-, 2-, 3 and 4-infected patients [11]. These innovative treatment regimens have revolutionized the field of HCV medicine and

http://dx.doi.org/10.5772/65873

Drug name	Drug efficacy[a]	Drug-resistance barrier[b]	Pan-genotype coverage[c]	Adverse effects[d]	Drug-drug interactions[e]	Development phase	Target site
(1) Protease inhibitors							
Telaprevir	++	+	+	+++	+++	Discontinued	NS3/4A Serine protease
Boceprevir	++	+	+	++	++	Discontinued	NS3/4A Serine protease
Simeprevir	+++	++	++	+	++	Approved	NS3/4A Serine protease
Simeprevir plus sofosbuvir	+++	++	++	+	++	Approved	NS3/4A Serine protease/NS5B Inhibitor
Faldaprevir	++	+++	++	+ +	+	Withdraw	NS3/4A Serine protease
Asunaprevir	++	+++	+	++	+	Phase III clinical trials	NS3/4A Serine protease
Danoprevir	++	++	+	++	+	Phase III clinical trials	NS3/4A Serine protease
Vaniprevir	++	+	+	++	+	Phase III clinical trials	NS3/4A Serine protease
(2) NS5A inhibitors							
Daclatasvir	+++	++	++	+	+	Approved	NS5A inhibitors
Daclatasvir plus sofosbuvir	+++	++	++	+	+	Approved	NS5A inhibitors/ NS5B inhibitors
(3) RNA-dependent RNA polymerase inhibitors (NS5B inhibitors)							
(3.1) Nucleoside analog inhibitors (NIs)							
Sofosbuvir	+++	+++	+++	+	+	Approved	NS5B inhibitors
Sofosbuvir plus ledipasvir	+++	+++	+++	+	+	Approved	NS5B inhibitors/ NS5A inhibitors
Sofosbuvir plus velpatasvir	+++	+++	+++	+	+	Approved	NS5B inhibitors/ NS5A inhibitors
Elbasvir plus grazoprevir	+++	++	+++	++	++	Approved	NS3-4A Serine protease/NS5A Inhibitor
Mericitabine	+++	+++	++	+	+	Phase III clinical trials	NS5B inhibitors
Paritaprevir ombitasvir-ritonavir and dasabuvir combination	+++	+++	++	+	+	Approved	NS3-4A Serine protease/NS5A Inhibitor/NNIs

Drug name	Drug efficacy[a]	Drug-resistance barrier[b]	Pan-genotype coverage[c]	Adverse effects[d]	Drug-drug interactions[e]	Development phase	Target site
(3.2) Non-nucleoside analog inhibitors (NNIs)							
Tegobuvir	++	+	++	++	+	Phase II clinical trials	NS5B/NNI site 1/ thumb 1
Setrobuvir	++	+++	+	+	+	Phase II clinical trials	NS5B/NNI site 1/ thumb 1
Filibuvir	++	++	+	+	+	Phase II clinical trials	NS5B/NNI site 2/ thumb 2
BMS-791325	++	++	+	+	+	Phase II clinical trials	NS5B/NNI site 4/ palm 1
(4) Interferon derivatives							
Consensus interferon	+	-	++	+++	–	Approved	Type 1 interferon
Interferon lambda	+++	–	–	+	+	Phase II clinical trials	Type 1 interferon receptors
(5) HCV vaccines							
ChronVac-C	–	–	–	–	–	Phase I/II clinical trials	–
GI-5005	–	–	–	–	–	Phase II clinical trials	–
TG4040	–	–	–	–	–	Phase I clinical trials	–
ChAd3/MVA	–	–	–	–	–	Phase I/II clinical trials	–

[a] Drug efficacy profile was based on the overall SVR rates achieved in phase II/III clinical trials where SVRs > 95 % = high profile, SVRs > 90 % = average profile, and SVRs > 85–90 % = low profile.

[b] Drug-resistance barrier profile is based upon the clinical data registered to clinicaltrials.gov.

[c] Pan-genotypic coverage was based on the fact that the DAA combination was therapeutically effective against 1–6 genotypes = high profile, two/three genotypes = average profile, and one genotype > = low profile.

[d] Adverse event (AE) profile was accomplished on the basis of percentage occurrence of adverse effects in phase II/III clinical trials which caused treatment discontinuation in treated individuals, where 10 % AEs > high profile, 10→5 % AEs > average profile, and 5→0 % AEs > low profile.

[e] Drug-drug interaction profile was established on the basis of the DAA ability to induce/inhibit hepatic cytochrome P450 system, P-glycoprotein (P-gp), and organic anion-transporting polypeptide (OATP) induction/inhibition. CYP 450, P-gp, and OATP induction/inhibition = high profile, P-gp and OATP induction/inhibition = average profile, and one or none of these CYP 450 or P-gp or OATP inductions/inhibitions = low profile.

High profile = +++, average profile = ++, and low profile = +

Table 1. The most promising direct-acting antivirals against HCV with their therapeutic activity profile, current stage of development, and targeted active sites.

provided optimism that cure rates in chronically infected HCV patients have much improved with these new drugs.

From 2015, HCV therapy has achieved higher response rates, fewer contraindications, shorter durations, and greater tolerability after the approval of interferon-free antiviral therapies. All oral interferon-free therapeutic regimens directed against hepatitis C virus are shown to be highly effective in the entire spectrum of patient populations, including the previously difficult-to-treat "special" situations (e.g., HCV subtype 1a patients with resistance-associated amino acid variants (RAVs), partial or null responders to first-generation protease and PEG-IFN/RBV-based triple therapies, decompensated cirrhosis, IL28 polymorphism, chronic kidney diseases, and HCV/HIV-coinfected patients). These revolutionary drug strategies now incorporate a cocktail of agents blended to take advantage of the synergistic mechanism of action. With these patient-friendlier attributes, the demand for treatment will conceivably reach unprecedented heights, but will health services be able to match this demand with supply? HCV antiviral therapy is not cheap; the current going rate, which new therapies are likely to exceed, stands at approximately US $ 80,000–100,000 per treatment course. So with more than 170 million people living with chronic infection around the world, clearly we cannot afford at least immediately to treat everyone.

On the other hand, treatment-emergent adverse events (e.g., risk of developing hepatocellular carcinoma and adverse cardiovascular effects) in treated individuals are also posing some serious challenges to the newly developed DAAs. The developers of prophylactic or protective vaccines have faced the most difficult challenges of rapid mutation rate (10^{-5} to 10^{-4} nucleotides per HCV replication cycle) and remarkable genetic heterogeneity of the virus in experimental trials [12,13]. It is beyond the scope of this article to cover every anti-HCV drug studies in details, so we primarily focus on FDA-approved direct-acting antivirals whose clinical efficacies have proven against chronic HCV both in vitro and in vivo (**Table 1**). We also highlight some interferon derivatives and investigational HCV vaccine models which mark the recent trends and new paradigms in the treatment strategies against HCV (**Table 1**).

2. Potential active sites for anti-HCV agents

HCV replication and translation into the cytoplasm of host cells facilitate the direct exposure of direct-acting antivirals to their targeted active sites [14]. Moreover, the direct-acting antivirals are structure specific to their targeted active sites (**Figure 1**) [15]. Viral-encoded proteases (e.g., NS3/4A serine protease), HCV replication complex (NS5A), and viral RNA-dependent RNA polymerase (RdRp; NS5B) enzyme are the core targeted sites for the first-, second-, and next-wave direct-acting antivirals (**Figure 1**) [16]. Viral attachment and entry into the host cell, viral assembly, packaging, and virion release are the less specific anti-HCV drug targets but still important to develop novel anti-HCV compounds with promising therapeutic activity (**Figure 1**) [17]. NS3/4A inhibitors inhibit viral translation by disrupting the downstream polyprotein processing of HCV genome. NS5B inhibitors obstruct HCV replication by blocking the addition of further nucleotide in growing mRNA chain (**Figure 1**) [15]. NS5A inhibitors prevent the formation of a membranous web structure which is crucial for HCV replication [16]. Viral assembly and packaging are disturbed by host-targeting agents which target a host-encoded enzyme responsible for viral assembly [18]. Cyclophilin (nonimmune suppressive cyclosporins) inhibitors block the interaction of cyclophilin (a family of a highly conserved cellular peptidylprolyl isomerase involved in protein folding and trafficking) with other HCV proteins to prevent the formation of a functional replication complex (**Figure 1**) [17]. α-Glucosidase inhibitors interrupt the release of newly formed viral particles from the host cells [17]. Some immunoglobulins (i.e., monoclonal and polyclonal antibodies) prevent the viral attachment and entry into host cells, but their therapeutic benefits are not highly significant [11].

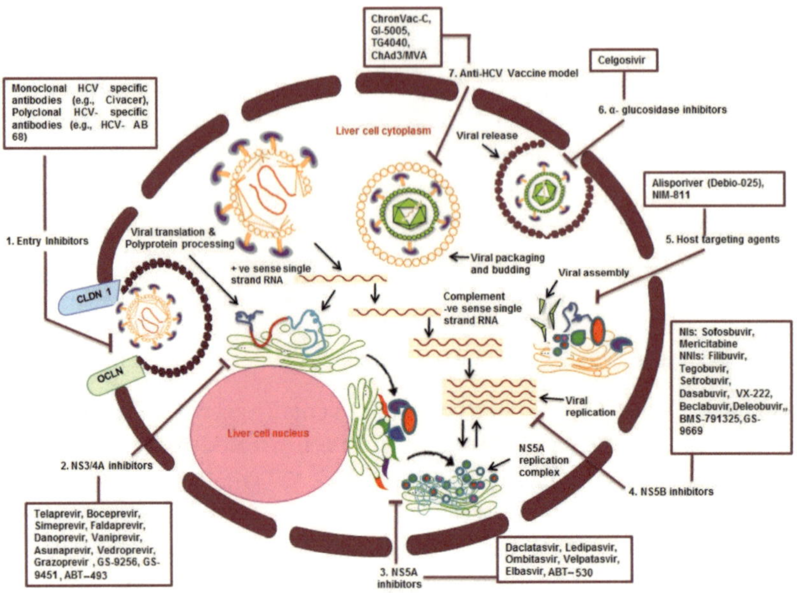

Figure 1. Potential active sites for direct-acting antivirals against hepatitis C virus. NS3/4A serine protease, NS5A replication complex, and RNA-dependent RNA polymerase are the key targeted sites for anti-HCV drug development. Some other anti-HCV drug targets have also been demonstrated by the investigators including viral attachment and entry into host cells, host-targeting agents, and α-glucosidase. However, these drug targets are less specific but still significant to develop novel anti-HCV agents. Direct-acting antivirals according to their target specificity are also enlisted in and rectangular square boxes in the figure. NIs, nucleoside analog inhibitors; NNIs, non-nucleoside analog inhibitors; CLDN1, claudin 1; OCLN, occludin.

3. NS3-4A serine protease inhibitors

3.1. First-generation protease inhibitors

Telaprevir and boceprevir represent the first in class of direct-acting antivirals or more correctly the first-generation protease inhibitors which were approved by the US FDA in 2011 for the treatment of genotype 1 hepatitis C infection. Telaprevir (TLV, Incivek®) is an orally bioavailable, a peptidomimetic NS3-4A protease inhibitor, which forms a reversible covalent bond with NS3/4A serine protease and impedes downstream HCV polyprotein processing [19]. The therapy was recommended along with PEG-IFN α and RBV for treatment-naïve genotype 1 adult patients with associated liver diseases, in null responders (i.e., HCV RNA decline <2 $\log_{10}$ at week 12 during PEG-IFN α plus RBV therapy), in poor or partial responders (HCV RNA decline ≥2 log10 at week 12 but positive at week 24 during PEG-IFN α plus RBV therapy), and in the relapsers (HCV RNA negative at the end of treatment but recurrence of HCV RNA during the follow-up of 6 months) of PEG-IFN α plus RBV dual therapy [20]. The therapeutic efficacy was evaluated in a series of multicenter phase II and III clinical trials named as PROVE 1, PROVE 2, PROVE 3, ADVANCE, ILLUMINATE, and REALIZE (**Table 2**) [20]. The overall SVR rates were achieved from 60 to 90 % in treated patients. However, TLV monotherapy and suboptimal doses resulted in

http://dx.doi.org/10.5772/65873

Referenced clinical studies	Trials name/phase	±PEG-IFN/RBV	Treatment-naïve patient	Treatment-experienced	Genotype coverage	NCT#	Overall SVR
(1) NS3-4A serine protease inhibitors							
(1.1) Ketoamide derivative inhibitors							
Telaprevir							
McHutchison *et al.*, [116]	PROVE-1	+	+	–	1	NCT00336479	PROVE-1 = 61 %
Hezode *et al.*, [115]	PROVE-2	+	+	–	1	NCT00372385	PROVE-2 = 69 %
McHutchison *et al.*, [117]	PROVE-3	+	–	+	1	NCT00420784	PROVE-3 = 53 %
Jacobson *et al.*, [118]	ADVANCE	+	+	–	1	NCT00627926	ADVANCE = 69 %
Sherman *et al.*, [119]	ILLUMINATE	+	+	–	1	NCT00758043	ILLUMINATE = 92 %
Zeuzem *et al.*, [120]	REALIZE	+	–	+	1	NCT00703118	REALIZE = 66 %
Boceprevir							
Kwo *et al.*, [121]	SPRINT-1	+	–	+	1	NCT00423670	SPRINT-1 = 75 %
Poordad *et al.*, [122]	SPRINT-2	+	+	–	1	NCT00705432	SPRINT-2 = 68 %
Bacon *et al.*, [123]	RESPOND-2	+	–	+	1	NCT00708500	RESPOND-2 = 65 %
(1.2) Tripeptide or macrocyclic inhibitors							
Simeprevir							
Jacobson *et al.* [21]	QUEST-1	+	+	–	1	NCT01289782	QUEST-1 = 80–90 %
Manns *et al.*, [124]	QUEST-2	+	+	–	1	NCT01290679	QUEST-2 = 67–80 %
Forns *et al.*, [125]	PROMISE	+	–	+	1	NCT01281839	PROMISE = 79 %
Moreno *et al.*, [126]	RESTORE	+	+	+	4	NCT01567735	RESTORE = 66 %
Simeprevir and sofosbuvir combination							
Lawitz *et al.*, [109]	COSMOS	±RBV	+	+	1	NCT01466790	Overall SVR = 90–94 %
Kwo *et al.* [22]	OPTIMIST-1	-	+	+	1	NCT02114177	Overall SVR = 97 %
Lawitz *et al.* [23]	OPTIMIST-2	–	+	+	1	NCT02114151	Overall SVR = 83 %

Referenced clinical studies	Trials name/phase	±PEG-IFN/RBV	Treatment-naïve patient	Treatment-experienced	Genotype coverage	NCT#	Overall SVR
(2) NS5A inhibitors							
Daclatasvir							
	Phase III	+	+	+	1-6	–	Overall SVRs = 59–100 %
Hezode *et al.* [24]	COMMAND-1	+	+	–	1/4	NCT01125189	GT1 (20 mg) = 65 %
							GT1 (60 mg) = 90 %
							GT4 (20 mg) = 75 %
							GT4 (60 mg) = 100 %
Hezode *et al.* [24]	COMMAND-4	+	+	–	4	NCT01448044	COMMAND-4 = 82–86 %
Daclatasvir and sofosbuvir combination							
Poordad *et al.* [25]	ALLY-1	±RBV	+	+	1/3	NCT02032875	GT1 (cirrhotics) = 83 %
							GT1(posttransplant) = 95 %
							GT3 = 88%
Sulkowski *et al.*, [110]	A1444040	±RBV	+	+	1/3	NCT01359644	GT3 T.N = 89 %
							GT2 T.N = 92 %
							GT1 T. N = 98 %
							GT1T. E = 98 %
Wyles *et al.* [26]	ALLY-2	–	+	+	1/4	NCT02032888	GT1/4 T.N (12 weeks) = 97 %
							GT1/4 T.N (8 weeks) = 76 %
							GT1/4 T.E (12 weeks) = 98 %
Nelson *et al.* [27]	ALLY-3	–	+	+	3	NCT02032901	GT3 T. N = 90 %
							GT3 T. E = 86 %
Leroy *et al.* [28]	ALLY-3+	±RBV	+	+	3	–	GT3 T. N (12 weeks) = 88 %
							GT3 T. E (16 weeks) = 92 %
Daclatasvir asunaprevir and beclabuvir combination							
Poordad *et al.* [29]	UNITY-1	–	+	+	1	NCT01979939	GT1 T.N = 92 %

Referenced clinical studies	Trials name/phase	±PEG-IFN/RBV	Treatment-naïve patient	Treatment-experienced	Genotype coverage	NCT#	Overall SVR
							GT1 T.E = 89 %
Muir *et al.* [30]	UNITY-2	±RBV	+	+	1	NCT01973049	GT1 T.N = 93–98 %
							GT1 T.E = 87–93 %
Ledipasvir and sofosbuvir combination							
Afdhal *et al.* [31]	ION-1	±RBV	+	–	1	NCT01701401	ION-1 = 97–99 %
Afdhal *et al.* [31]	ION-2	±RBV	–	+	1	NCT01768286	ION-2 = 94–96 %
Kowdely *et al.*, [111]	ION-3	±RBV	+	–	1	NCT01851330	ION-3 = 93–95 %
Naggie *et al.*, [112]	ION-4	–	+	+	1/4	NCT02073656	ION-4 = 96 %
(3) RNA-dependent RNA polymerase inhibitors (NS5B inhibitors)							
(3.1) Nucleoside analog inhibitors (NIs)							
Sofosbuvir							
Lawitz *et al.* [32]	NEUTRINO	+	+	–	1/4/5/6	NCT01641640	NEUTRINO = 90 %
Lawitz *et al.* [33]	FISSION	+RBV	+	–	2/3	NCT01497366	FISSION = 67 %
Jacobson *et al.* [34]	POSITRON	+RBV	–	+	2/3	NCT01542788	POSITRON = 78 %
Jacobson *et al.* [35]	FUSION	+RBV	–	+	2/3	NCT01604850	FUSION = 50–73 %
Sofosbuvir and velpatasvir combination							
Feld *et al.* [36]	ASTRAL-1	–	+	+	1/2/4/5/6	NCT02201940	ASTRAL-1 = 99 %
Foster *et al.*, [113]	ASTRAL-3	–	+	+	3	NCT02201953	ASTRAL-3 = 95 %
Foster *et al.*, [113]	ASTRAL-2	–	+	+	2	NCT02220998	ASTRAL-2 = 99 %
Curry *et al.*, [114]	ASTRAL-4	–	+	+	1-6	NCT02201901	ASTRAL-4 = 83 %
Wyles *et al.*, [127]	ASTRAL-5	–	+	+	1-6	NCT02480712	ASTRAL-5 = 95 %
Elbasvir and grazoprevir combination							
Dore *et al.* [37]	C-EDGE CO-STAR	–	+	–	1/4/6	NCT02105688	Overall SVR = 95 %

Referenced clinical studies	Trials name/phase	±PEG-IFN/RBV	Treatment-naïve patient	Treatment-experienced	Genotype coverage	NCT#	Overall SVR
Rockstroh *et al.* [38]	C-EDGE coinfection	–	+	–	1/4/6	NCT02105662	Overall SVR = 96 %
Kwo *et al.* [39]	C-EDGE T. E	±RBV	–	+	1/4/6	NCT02105701	C-EDGE + RBV(12) = 94 % C-EDGE-RBV(12) = 92 % C-EDGE + RBV(16) = 97 % C-EDGE-RBV(16) = 92 %
Zeuzem *et al.* [40]	C-EDGE T. N	–	+	–	1/4/6	NCT02105467	C-EDGE T. N = 95 %
Roth *et al.* [41]	C-SURFER	–	+	–	1	NCT02092350	C-SURFER = 99 %
Paritaprevir-ombitasvir-ritonavir and dasabuvir combination							
Feld *et al.* [42]	SAPPHIRE I	+RBV	+	–	1	NCT01716585	Overall SVR = 96 %
Zeuzem *et al.* [43]	SAPPHIRE II	+RBV	–	+	1	NCT01715415	Overall SVR = 96 %
Sulkowski *et al.* [44]	TURQUOISE I	+RBV	+	+	1/HIV	NCT01704755	Overall SVR = 91–94 %
Poordad *et al.* [45]	TURQUOISE II	+RBV	+	+	1	NCT01939197	Overall SVR = 92–96 %
Andreone *et al.* [46]	PEARL II	±RBV	–	+	1b	NCT01674725	Overall SVR = 96–100 %
Ferenci *et al.* [47]	PEARL III	±RBV	+	–	1b	NCT01767116	Overall SVR = 99–99.5 %
Ferenci *et al.* [47]	PEARL IV	±RBV	+	–	1a	NCT01833533	Overall SVR = 90–97 %
Paritaprevir-ombitasvir-and ritonavir combination							
Hezode *et al.* [24]	PEARL-I	±RBV	+	+	4	NCT01685203	Overall SVR = 91–100 %
Asselah *et al.*, [129]	AGATE-I	+RBV	+	+	4	NCT02265237	Overall SVR = 97–98 %
Waked *et al.*, [128]	AGATE-II	+RBV	+	+	4	NCT02247401	Overall SVR = 93–97 %

[a] Only those clinical studies/trials were referenced which were considered by the US FDA for the approval of anti-HCV compounds and which were registered to clinicaltrials.gov. Similarly, the clinical trial data regarding the inclusion of patients, genotype coverage, and SVR rates were extracted only from FDA, NCBI, and clinicaltrials.gov websites. + = included, - = not included, ± = with or without, T.N = treatment-naïve, T.E = treatment-experienced, RBV = ribavirin, GT = genotype, SVR = sustained virologic response

Table 2. The most promising phase II and III clinical trials for novel direct-acting antivirals with overall SVRs in HCV-infected patients[a].

the rapid emergence of viral escape mutants followed by viral breakthrough (HCV RNA remains lower limit of quantification but increased to ≥100 IU/ml or ≥1 $\log_{10}$ during telaprevir therapy) in some patients during therapy and significantly in all the patients after treatment completion [48]. The addition of PEG-IFN α plus RBV reduced the frequency of viral escape mutants and achieved higher SVR rates in both treatment-naive and treatment-experienced patients in phase II and III clinical trials than PEG-IFN α plus RBV therapy alone [49]. Similarly, some studies also describe that telaprevir is not equally useful for difficult-to-treat populations (i.e., patients with decompensated liver diseases, IL28B polymorphism, HCV genotype 3, 4, 5, and 6 infections) as compared with HCV genotype 1 infection [48]. For such HCV-infected patients, interferon-free antiviral combination therapies are the best treatment options. Boceprevir (BOC; Victrelis®) another first-generation protease inhibitor shares the similar pharmacokinetics and pharmacodynamics like telaprevir to confer anti-HCV activity. The clinical efficacy of boceprevir-based triple therapy (along with PEG-IFN α plus RBV) was evaluated in phase III clinical trials both in treatment-naïve (SPRINT-2 clinical trial) and poor responders to PEG-IFN α and RBV therapy (RESPOND-2 clinical trial) patients (**Table 2**) [50–52]. The overall cure rates were almost equivalent to telaprevir-based triple therapy. However, the treatment-naïve patients achieved higher SVR rates than treatment-experienced patients (**Table 2**). Telaprevir or boceprevir monotherapy seems effective in treatment-naïve HCV genotype 1-infected patients. However, administration of telaprevir or boceprevir as monotherapy in infected individuals is not a suitable option because of the early emergence of viral escape mutants during therapy and followed by viral breakthrough after treatment completion [53]. The minor resistant populations exist at baseline in all HCV-infected individuals and are selected rapidly with telaprevir or boceprevir monotherapy (**Table 3**) [51]. Consequently, the first-generation DAAs/PIs still require a platform of PEG-IFN α and RBV to prevent the emergence of viral escape mutants and also to achieve significantly higher SVR rates [54]. Similarly, notable drug-drug interactions with many HIV antiretrovirals and calcineurin inhibitors also decrease the therapeutic activity of telaprevir and boceprevir monotherapy [54]. Drug toxicities and unusual adverse event profile (anemia, rashes, dysgeusia, and depression) of first-generation protease inhibitors also limit their clinical efficacy in treated patients [54]. These adverse effects result in treatment withdrawal in the majority of treated individuals, and this ratio is 10 % much higher in telaprevir- or boceprevir-based triple therapy vs. PEG-IFNα and RBV therapy alone [50, 52]. The physicians and hepatologists do not recommend telaprevir or boceprevir monotherapy or even in combination with PEG-IFN/RBV due to the harsh adverse event profile and the emergence of viral escape mutants. Similarly, premature treatment discontinuation and mandatory intake of food have heightened the adherence concern related to first-generation protease inhibitors. The treatment has already discontinued in the United States and expected to be stopped from other parts of the world after the approval of interferon-free therapeutic regimens.

3.2. Second-generation protease inhibitors

Telaprevir and boceprevir were found more effective in treatment-naive HCV genotype 1 patients and had to be administered three times daily [54]. The situation demanded to

Drug name	Resistance amino acid variants
Telaprevir	V36A/M; T54S/A; R155K/T/Q; A156S; B156T/V
Boceprevir	V36A/M; T54S/A; V55A; R155K/T/Q; A156S; B156T/V; V170A/T
Simeprevir	Q80R/K; R155K/T/Q; B156T/V; D168A/V/T/H
Faldaprevir	R155K/T/Q; D168A/V/T/H
Danoprevir	R155K/T/Q; D168A/V/T/H
Asunaprevir	Q80R/K; R155K/T/Q; D168A/V/T/H
ABT-450	R155K/T/Q; D168A/V/T/H
Daclatasvir	M28; Q30; L31; Y93Y/H
Sofosbuvir	282 T
Ledipasvir	K24R, M28T/V, Q30R/H/K/L, L31M, Y93H/N
Velpatasvir	Q30R, Y93H/N, L31M
Elbasvir	A156T, D168A/Y, R155K
Grazoprevir	M28, Q30, L31, Y93
Paritaprevir	V36A/M/T, F43L, V55I, Y56H, Q80L, I132V, R155K, A156G
Ombitasvir	K24R, M28A/T/V, Q30E/K/R, H/Q54Y, H58D/P/R, Y93C/H/N
Dasabuvir	G307R, C316Y, M414I/T, E446K/Q, A450V, Y561H

Table 3. Resistance amino acid variants (RAVs) associated with antiviral drug resistance to direct-acting antivirals.

develop the regimens, which must be effective against other difficult-to-treat HCV populations with an improved dosing schedule. Simeprevir (Olysio®) was approved by the US FDA to treat chronic HCV genotype 1 infection in 2013 (www.hcvonline.org/page/treatment/drugs/simeprevir-drug) [55, 56]. The drug was approved along with PEG-IFN α-2a or 2b and RBV for treatment-naive HCV genotype 1-infected patients [35], for patients with compensated liver diseases (fibrosis and cirrhosis), and for those who are relapsers and nonresponders to interferon-based therapy [32,57]. Simeprevir 150 mg once daily along with PEG-IFN/RBV achieved overall SVR rates approximately 80–90 % in treatment-naïve and relapsers [56] and 67–80 % of previously treated and null responders to interferon-based therapy (**Table 2**) (QUEST-1 and QUEST-2 clinical trials). The therapy seems to be more efficient than telaprevir/boceprevir-based triple therapies; however, there are certain disadvantages. For example, SVR rates were lower at the start of antiviral therapy in patients with advanced hepatic fibrosis as well as in patients with Q80R/K polymorphism of NS3 protein [58]. It is a naturally occurring amino acid substitution at NS3 codon 80, where glutamine is replaced to lysine. The Q80K polymorphism exists naturally in HCV genotype 1a (30–50 %)- and 1b (0.5 %)-infected patients [56]. It substantially reduces the efficacy of simeprevir-based triple therapy in HCV genotype 1a-infected patients. In QUEST-1 clinical studies, SVR rates were demonstrated 20 % lower in HCV genotype 1a-infected individuals than 1b [21, 56]. Furthermore, approximately one-third HCV genotype 1a patients were found with Q80K NS3 protein mutation at baseline [21]. Interestingly, the mutation was infrequent, was nonexistent, and did not impact the SVR rates significantly in HCV genotype 1b patients [56, 59]. HCV genotype 1a-infected patients are strongly recommended for Q80K polymorphism screening and NS3 genotype test before the start of treatment and to avoid any complications during therapy. The mutations associated with NS3 protease inhibitors may detect by reverse transcribing HCV RNA, followed by PCR amplification and then DNA sequencing of NS3 gene [21, 60]. Some institute/laboratories in the United States have launched the tests for Q80K polymorphism (Quest Diagnostics®) and HCV drug-resistance test for NS3/4A protease inhibitors (LabCorp®). Treatment withdrawal and alternative treatment strategies may adopt for the patients found with a Q80K polymorphism in NS3 genotype analysis. Skin rashes, itching, nausea, and photosensitivity reactions are the most commonly observed adverse events with simeprevir-based triple therapies [56]. Sunscreen creams and lotions are highly recommended to use while taking the drug [61].

In 2014, simeprevir was approved in combination with sofosbuvir to treat chronic HCV genotype 1 patients with or without cirrhosis. The combination regimen (150/400 mg q.d.) without PEG-IFN/RBV was found almost equally effective in both patient arms; however, relatively better in treatment-naïve than treatment-experienced patients (OPTIMIST-1 and OPTIMIST-2 clinical trials) (**Table 2**) [22, 23]. Similarly, the therapeutic outcome was much significant in subtype 1a patients without Q80K polymorphism and in noncirrhotics as compared to those with cirrhosis and Q80K polymorphism (**Table 2**). The frequency of treatment-emergent adverse events was similar in both clinical trials, and the drug combination was well tolerated and safe even in patients with Q80K polymorphism as compared to simeprevir and PEG-IFN/RBV-based triple therapies.

4. NS5A inhibitor-based direct-acting antivirals

Daclatasvir (Daklinza®) is the first in a new class of direct-acting antivirals, which inhibit the action of NS5A, a protein essential to play a diverse role in HCV replication, assembly, and release [62]. The US FDA approved initially daclatasvir and sofosbuvir combination to treat chronic HCV genotype 3-infected patients in July 2015. However, the indications were modified and expanded to treat HCV genotype 1- and 3-infected patients, patients with decompensated cirrhosis, patients with post-liver transplantation, and HCV/HIV-coinfected patients in February 2016 [63]. Daclatasvir monotherapy along with PEG-IFN/RBV leads initially to higher SVR rates in treated patients, but viral escape mutants occur rapidly indicating its relatively lower genetic barrier to resistance (COMMAND-1 and COMMAND-4 clinical trials) (**Table 2**) [64]. To overcome the emergence of viral escape mutants and to achieve high SVR rates, the treatment is recommended along with sofosbuvir and with or without ribavirin. Higher SVR rates were documented in HCV genotype

1 and 3 treatment-naive patients when administered to daclatasvir and sofosbuvir combination [24]. Other multi-series clinical trials also demonstrate high clinical efficacy and well tolerability of daclatasvir-sofosbuvir with or without RBV against HCV genotype 1–6 infected patients (ALLY 1–3 clinical trial) (**Table 2**) [25–28]. Similarly, higher SVR rates (87–98 %) were achieved in HCV genotype 1-infected patients treated with a combination of daclatasvir, asunaprevir, and beclabuvir for 12 weeks (UNITY 1–2 clinical trial) (**Table 2**) [29, 30]. Headache, nausea, and vomiting were the most commonly noticed adverse effects, and the adverse event profile was almost similar in all genotype-treated patients and managed during or after the treatment completion [62]. The viral-resistant mutants were found commonly at residue M28, Q30, L31, and Y93 of NS5A region in HCV genotype 1a patients (**Table 3**) [25, 28]. However, viral-resistant mutants were reported less frequently at position L31 and Y93 in HCV genotype 1b patients [64]. Some experimental studies demonstrate that these mutations are responsible for increasing the EC_{50} (i.e., the concentration of a drug which produces therapeutic response halfway between the baseline and maximum after a certain period of time) of daclatasvir in treated patients [64]. In contrast to NS3 protease, viral-resistant mutants against NS5A inhibitors do not impair replication fitness and do not disappear during follow-up examinations at the end of treatment. One-year follow-up studies predict the persistence of NS5A-resistance mutants, but no cross-resistance has reported between daclatasvir and other direct-acting antivirals as yet [65]. The approval of daclatasvir monotherapy and daclatasvir with other different regimens is expected soon.

5. HCV polymerase inhibitor-based therapeutic regimens

Sofosbuvir (Sovaldi®; SOF) was approved by the US FDA in 2013 to treat treatment-naïve and treatment-experienced HCV genotype 1–6-infected patients [66]. SOF is a uridine nucleotide analog inhibitor, which exerts its antiviral activity by competing with endogenous uridine triphosphate of the growing HCV mRNA chain incorporated by HCV polymerase enzyme [66,67]. After incorporation into growing mRNA chain, no further nucleotides can be added, and mRNA chain is terminated [67]. The drug is active against all HCV genotypes (1–6) as well as difficult-to-treat HCV populations [68]. The approval was momentous and based on the results of four registration studies in phase III clinical trials (FISSION, POSITRON, FUSION, and NEUTRINO clinical trials) where the therapy endpoint was to achieve a sustained virologic response rate at week 12 after stopping the active treatment (i.e., SVR12) (**Table 2**) [69]. Sofosbuvir in combination with ribavirin presented very promising clinical efficacy data against HCV genotype 1–4-treated patients (**Table 2**) [33, 34]. The relapse rate was only 9 % among all the four phase III drug registration studies [34]. No major side effects or severe cardiac adverse events were reported during SOF plus RBV dual therapy. However, the adverse event profiles of sofosbuvir monotherapy and even in combination with RBV are not sufficiently addressed because of the lack of controlled trials [66]. Meaningful historical controls, as well as ribavirin monotherapy arm as a comparator, are not available due to which we may not draw conclusions about the eventual adverse effects of sofosbuvir [33, 34]. However, adverse events associated with sofosbuvir-related therapies are not frequent and severe in nature. Antiviral resistance was only observed in a single patient after sofosbuvir monotherapy, which was successfully re-treated with SOF plus RBV dual therapy [69].

Sofosbuvir in combination with ledipasvir (Harvoni®; the first fixed-dose drug combination claims to "two firsts") with or without RBV was approved in 2014 for HCV genotype 1 infection treatment. Later on, the approval was expanded to treat HCV genotype 4-, 5-, 6-, and HCV/HIV-coinfected patients in 2015. Recently, the US FDA has extended the treatment recommendation to liver transplant genotype 1 and 4 patients with compensated cirrhosis and in genotype 1 patients with decompensated cirrhosis (http://www.hepatitisc.uw.edu/page/treatment/drugs/ledipasvir-sofosbuvir#drug-summary) [31, 70]. Ledipasvir (90 mg) and sofosbuvir (400 mg) have formulated as a single coformulated pill [31]. However, ledipasvir (an NS5A inhibitor) monotherapy is not approved by the US FDA to treat the infection as yet. This combo drug seems very efficient to achieve SVR rates more than 90 % of HCV genotype 1- and 4-treated patients without cirrhosis when administered to 8, 12, or 24 weeks (**Table 2**) [31, 71]. Cirrhotic patients may also achieve higher SVR rates with 12- or 24-week treatment schedule [72]. Severe adverse events are rare and manageable during or after the therapy. The inclusion of ribavirin does not affect the therapeutic efficacy and achievement of higher SVR rates. Consequently, the addition of RBV does not seem prerequisite in every all-oral DAA combinations against HCV. RBV results in hemolytic anemia and is highly teratogenic [11], and for this reason, RBV-sparing regimens are considerably advantageous and eagerly awaited in the future.

6. Treatment paradigms for difficult-to-treat populations

As the treatment success in HCV-infected patients mainly depends on HCV genotype, previous treatment history, cirrhosis or fibrosis score, and the high barrier to antiviral drug resistance, the combination of experimental drug velpatasvir and sofosbuvir might simplify the treatment strategies in "difficult-to-treat subgroups" in the future. Velpatasvir (An NS5A inhibitor) and sofosbuvir in a fixed-dose combination (100 mg/400 mg) exhibit the pan-genotypic coverage with a simple 12-week regimen in treatment-naïve, treatment-experienced, as well as in cirrhotic patients as determined in multicentered clinical trials (i.e., ASTRAL 1–5) conducted at 81 sites including the United States, Canada, and Europe in 2014 (**Table 2**) [36]. The adverse event profile was almost similar to each clinical trials, and headache, nausea, and vomiting were the most common ones. However, overall the drug combination was well tolerated and safe in treated patients. The US FDA has approved the fixed-dose combination of velpatasvir and sofosbuvir (Epclusa®) in June 2016 to treat chronic HCV genotype 1–6-infected adult patients.

The discovery and development of elbasvir/grazoprevir fixed-dose combination have shifted the treatment paradigm for genotype 1 and 4 patients with stage 4–5 chronic kidney disease (CKD) and HCV/HIV coinfection [40, 41]. The US FDA has approved elbasvir/grazoprevir (50/100 mg q.d.) (Zepatier®) combination for HCV genotype 1 and 4 infection with chronic kidney diseases and HCV/HIV coinfection with some specific clinical requirements (i.e., viral genotype, prior treatment experience, NS5A-associated RAVs at position M28, Q30,

L31, or Y93) (http://www.hepatitisc.uw.edu/page/treatment/dugs/elbasvir-grazoprevir#drug-summary) [73, 74]. Similarly, the treatment regimen is prescribed with many precautions in subtype 1a patient with prior testing of NS5A-associated RAVs, because it determines the overall treatment duration and the inclusion of ribavirin to therapy (**Table 3**) [38, 40, 41]. The FDA approval was granted on the findings of a series of multicenter phase III clinical trials (C-EDGE and C-SURFER) in treatment-naïve, treatment-experienced, and other difficult-to-cure populations (i.e., HCV/HIV coinfection, stage 4/5 CKD including hemodialysis patients) where overall SVR rates were highly promising (i.e., 92–99 %) (**Table 2**) [37–41]. The adverse event profile was not serious in the treatment groups, and the renal system adverse effects were comparable without significant changes in estimated glomerular filtration rate (eGFR) value and creatinine levels [38, 40, 41]. Headache, nausea, and fatigue were the most commonly observed adverse events with an elevation in alanine aminotransferase (ALT) levels five times more than the normal one [38, 40, 41]. However, most of the adverse effects resolved at or after the treatment completion.

The first 3D regimen, "Viekira Pak®" (i.e., a combination of three direct-acting antivirals: ombitasvir, paritaprevir, and dasabuvir) along with ritonavir, to treat chronic HCV genotype 1 infection was approved by the US FDA in 2014 (http://www.hepatitisc.uw.edu/page/treatment/drugs/3d#drug-summary) [75]. The drug combination is prescribed to genotype 1-compensated cirrhotic patients, however, still contraindicated to decompensated cirrhotics [42]. The approval was based on phase II/III multicenter clinical trials (**Table 2**) involving more than 2300 patients with chronic HCV 1 infection, some of whom had cirrhosis [43–47, 76]. Cure rates across the various groups were ranged from 91 % to 100 % (**Table 2**). The therapeutic outcomes demonstrated that the drug combination was safe with no significant adverse effects in a population with compensated cirrhosis [47]; however, the drug combination is forbidden in decompensated cirrhotic patients.

A recent ongoing clinical trial conducted in HCV genotype 4 noncirrhotic patients showed the promising therapeutic activity of ombitasvir, paritaprevir, and ritonavir with or without RBV for a 12-week course (PEARL-I clinical studies) [24]. Similarly, the therapeutic regimen along with RBV was also found highly effective to treat genotype 4, cirrhotic patients, as shown by the results of AGATE-I and AGATE-II ongoing clinical studies. PEARL-I, phase 2 open-label, randomized, and multicentre clinical trials were conducted in Europe, Turkey, and the United States [24]. The treatment-naïve patients included in the study received the ombitasvir, paritaprevir, and ritonavir combination with or without RBV; however, all treatment-experienced patients (i.e., previously treated with PEG-IFN/RBV) received the active treatment with RBV. Interestingly, dasabuvir was not included in the treatment regimen as it does not show therapeutic activity against HCV genotype 4. The overall SVR rates were achieved 91 % (40/44) in treatment-naïve patients who received active treatment without RBV and 100 % (42/42) in those who took RBV along with the regimen. All treatment-experienced patients achieved SVR12 at the treatment completion (49/49, 100 %) (**Table 2**). Viral relapse occurred in two patients, and the virologic breakthrough was experienced in one patient. The adverse event profile was almost negligible including headache and decreased hemoglobin level (i.e., 100 g/L, anemic state), but no treatment discontinuation was attributed to active regimen except the dose modification of RBV to nullify anemic state [24].

The AGATE-I open-label phase 3 multicenter and randomized clinical trial revealed the therapeutic outcome of ombitasvir, paritaprevir, and ritonavir plus RBV in HCV genotype 4 patients with compensated cirrhosis [77]. The study was conducted in both treatment-naïve and treatment-experienced patients (PEG-IFN/RBV treated) at different locations in Europe and the United States. Overall, 120 adult patients were enrolled in the study of which 59 patients received 12-week treatment (i.e., ombitasvir, paritaprevir, and ritonavir plus RBV) and 61 patients were assigned to take 16 weeks of the same treatment regimen. The overall SVR rates were achieved 97 % (57/59) in the 12-week group and 98 % (60/61) in the 16-week group. The adverse event frequency was significantly higher, mixed in both patient arms, and noticed in more than 10 % of all patients including asthenia, fatigue, headache, anemia, pruritus, nausea, and dizziness more common ones. However, virologic breakthrough was reported in one patient, and one patient discontinued the treatment at day 1 in the 12-week treatment group, and one missed the posttreatment week 12 visit in the 16-week group [77].

The AGATE-II open label and partly randomized clinical studies were conducted in native Egyptian population infected with HCV genotype 4 [77]. Overall 182 patients both treatment-naïve and treatment-experienced (previously treated to PEG-IFN/RBV-based dual therapies) anticipated in the clinical trial of whom 160 were eligible for inclusion criteria. 100 patients had no cirrhosis and received active regimen and RBV for 12 weeks. The remaining 60 having cirrhosis were randomly assigned to 12-week active treatment (n = 31) or 24-week treatment group (n = 29). The SVR rates were achieved 94 % in the noncirrhotic 12-week patient arm (94/100), 97 % in cirrhotic patients (30/31) enrolled in the 12-week treatment group, and 93 % (27/29) in cirrhotic patients administered for 24-week active treatment (**Table 2**). The adverse event profile was significantly higher particularly in noncirrhotic patients including headache and fatigue the most common (i.e., 41 % and 35 %, respectively) ones than the cirrhotic ones (29–38 %, respectively). However, no treatment discontinuation was related to drug side effects or active treatment itself [77].

The findings of the ongoing PEARL-I, AGATE-I, and AGATE-II clinical trials are promising while treating HCV genotype 4 cirrhotic and noncirrhotic patients; however, no additional benefits were reported in terms of higher SVR, when treatment duration was extended for cirrhotic patients from 12 weeks to 16 weeks or even 24 weeks in native Egyptian population. Similarly, a small number of patients enrolled in the clinical trials limit the comprehensive determination of the drug side effects. Further studies are eagerly awaited in this prospect, and as a precaution, any HCV cirrhotic patients using such combination therapeutic regimens should be hepatically intact for any hepatic complications/comorbidities because the patients in clinical trials are often very carefully monitored than patients in real-world clinical practice [40].

7. Interferon derivatives

Over the years, the principal objectives to develop novel interferon formulations include the replacement of conventional interferon with the new ones, to reduce the adverse effects of current interferon and ease of administration with an improved dosing schedule [78].

The treatment success for HCV is primarily dependent on the patient adherence to therapy so that the development of unique IFN formulations with improved pharmacokinetics is a prime objective of HCV therapeutics nowadays. The main advantage of this approach may seem to maintain viral suppression across the longer dose interval, avoid of inter-dose trough, and reduce dosage frequencies (twice or even once per month as compared to once per week for the current PEG-IFN and consensus interferons). Although the development of new interferon formulations primarily focuses on HCV genotype 1 patients, their administration can also be prized for HCV genotype 2- and 3-infected individuals [79]. Similarly, the duration of treatment can also be reduced in easy-to-treat populations (HCV genotype 2- and 3-infected patients) up to 12 weeks if a rapid virologic response achieves earlier [79]. This approach may suggest a very convenient therapeutic regimen of only three injections if long-acting IFNs are used in treated patients.

7.1. Interferon lambda

Interferon lambda (IFN-λ) is still promising and may be beneficial as an adjuvant therapy to treat HCV infection in combination with other DAAs in the near future. It has also raised the hopes to replace the conventional interferons (IFN-α 2a, IFN-α 2b, PEG-IFN α) to reduce the frequency of side effects and treatment discomfort during and after the treatment completion in infected individuals. The discovery of three interferon-λ cytokines (i.e., interferons $\lambda 1$, $\lambda 2$, and $\lambda 3$ encoded by IL29, IL28A, and IL28B, respectively) in 2003 has suggested their plausible role in suppression of HCV replication [80]. This fact was supported by the identification of common genetic variants in IL28B genome, which are highly associated with responses to PEG-IFN α/RBV treatment for chronic HCV infection [81]. Similarly, genome-wide association studies and in vitro studies also demonstrate an interactive and complementary relationship between IFN-α and IFN-λ for suppressing HCV replication [82]. IFN-λ like another type 3 interferons binds to different host cell receptors than type 1 interferons (e.g., IFN-α 2a, 2b) to trigger the JAK-STAT antiviral pathways (**Figure 2**). However, the downstream cell signaling pathways are largely comparable to interferon-α which upregulate several hundreds of interferon-stimulated genes to initiate antiviral activity [80]. IFN-λ binds mainly to IL28 receptors, which are positioned only to hepatocytes, plasmacytoid dendritic cells, peripheral B cells, and epithelial cells [83]. This restricted distribution of IL28 receptors for interferon-λ facilitates its targeted hepatic delivery, better tolerability, and increase safety profile than the conventional interferons [83]. IFN-λ may also escalate the subsaturating levels of IFN-α and increase its antiviral efficacy. In vitro studies reveal that IFN-α induces the expression of IFN-λ genes that upregulate a distinct pattern of signal transduction and interferon-stimulated genes than IFN-α to abort HCV replication [84]. Consequently, the combination of IFN-λ and IFN-α may provide additive therapeutic effects due to the complementary roles of two types of cytokines. Interferon-λ has been pegylated and phase I clinical trials with or without ribavirin have been completed [85]. Subsequent phase II clinical trials demonstrated that the administration of PEG-IFN λ (240 μg, 180 μg, or 120 μg once weekly) showed 10 % higher rapid virologic response (RVR; HCV RNA negative after 4 weeks of therapy) rates and 20 % higher extended rapid virologic response (eRVR; HCV RNA negative at the lower limit of detection but not the lower limit of quantification between week 4 and week 12 during PEG-IFN therapy) rates

http://dx.doi.org/10.5772/65873

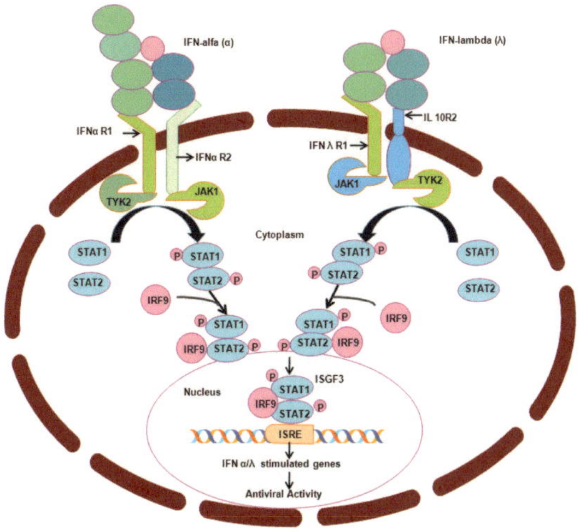

Figure 2. Interferon-lambda (λ) cell signaling pathways to induce anti-HCV activity. Interferon lambda binds to different cell receptors than IFN alpha to activate JAK-STAT pathways and initiate the antiviral activity by upregulating a distinct pattern of signal transduction. IFN, interferon; IL, interleukin; R, receptor; JAK, Janus kinase; TYK, tyrosine kinase; STAT, signal transducer and activator of transcription; IRF, interferon regulatory factor; P, phosphate; ISRE, interferon-stimulated response element.

than PEG-IFN α-2a in treatment-naïve patients [86]. IFN-λ is associated with less adverse event profile, including less hematologic toxicity, flu-like symptoms, and muscular pain, but increased aminotransferase and bilirubin levels in treated patients [86]. Now, full phase III clinical trials of interferon-λ with other DAAs (i.e., in combination with daclatasvir and asunaprevir plus RBV) are under consideration [87].

8. HCV vaccine technology

8.1. Barriers to developing prophylactic and protective HCV vaccines

The tendency of acute HCV infection to develop into chronic infection and optimal outcomes of the current therapies in the majority of treated patients underscores an urgent need to search and develop potential anti-HCV vaccine molecules. Interestingly, the efforts to develop HCV vaccines are facing real challenges due to some reasons. First, despite the consistent efforts by the researchers, still now there is no permissive cell culture system available where HCV can replicate persistently at high enough levels to evaluate antibodies which may neutralize [88]. Second, there is no authenticated and handy animal model available which is susceptible to HCV and can tackle the candidate vaccine challenge studies [88]. Although the chimpanzee model is the first choice for the investigators in HCV replication and candidate vaccine studies, it is expensive, endangered, and difficult to handle [89]. Third, genome variations in HCV genotypes, subtypes, and quasispecies nature of HCV may require the construction of polyvalent vaccines, which protect against a significant number of closely related epitopes [90]. In fact, the genetic heterogeneity of HCV in an infected individual and immune responses selected for neutralization of escape mutants within the hypervariable regions (HVR1) of E1 envelope glycoprotein as well as cytotoxic T lymphocytes (CTL) escape mutants may limit the effectiveness and utility of any HCV vaccine model [91]. Fourth, it is unclear that either HCV envelope glycoproteins contain all the antigenic determinants require for effective neutralization or not [92]. Fifth, acute HCV infection persists in the majority of infected individuals, even though innate and acquired immune responses accelerate against nearly all of the HCV-encoded polyproteins [93]. T-cell responses immediately accelerate to clear HCV in acutely infected individuals; therefore, a successful anti-HCV vaccine has to elicit both CD^{4+} and CD^{8+} T-cell responses in infected individuals [94]. Sixth, HCV may associate with immunoglobulin or β-lipoprotein in the blood, which may "mask" the virus and reduce the efficiency of neutralization [95].

8.2. Current anti-HCV vaccine models

Due to the above-mentioned qualms, the development of prophylactic or protective HCV vaccine is a highly challenging task and fraught with barriers. Anyhow, the advancement in vaccinology has inspired the researchers to work out different models of protective HCV candidate vaccines (**Table 1**). In this vein, the principle goal of an anti-HCV vaccine design should be to wipe out the chronic infection in exposed individuals or remove the virus from already infected individuals by boosting the innate and acquired host immune responses, which also seems an uphill task [94]. In this context, the strategy paradigms have been shifted from the production of traditional recombinant envelope proteins to the engineering of complex viral vectors directing the expression of multiple hepatitis C viral antigens (i.e., Core, NS3, NS4, and NS5B) [94]. We briefly describe here the recent advancement in HCV vaccine technology, which may consider as the role models for the successful development of an effective preventive/protective vaccine in the future.

An HCV immunoglobulin (Civacir) has studied for its therapeutic effects on recurrent hepatitis C following liver transplantation in phase II clinical trials, but the SVR data from these trials are not yet available [96]. Similarly, the high-dose monoclonal antibodies were evaluated against HCV glycoprotein E2 in genotype 1a patients undergoing liver transplantation in phase II clinical trials [97]. Although the strategy was not effective to prevent the recurrence of HCV infection, the reappearance of viremia in liver transplant patients significantly delayed as compared to the placebo control population [97]. Now, this regimen along with a direct-acting antiviral is under consideration for further clinical trials.

Currently, a DNA vector-based vaccine (ChronVac-C) is in clinical development against chronic HCV genotype 1 infection [98]. By using DNA electroporation, the gene-encoding HCV NS3/4A protein was introduced into the patient skeletal muscle. The skeletal muscle expressed NS3/4A protein, which in turn stimulated the particular host innate and acquired immune responses against HCV. The clinical efficacy of ChronVac-C was evaluated in 12 treatment-naïve HCV genotype 1-infected patients with four different doses given monthly for four months in phase I/II clinical trials [98]. T-cell responses were detected in one patient, and viral load reduction up to 1.2 log10–2.4 log10 was reported in two out of three patients with the highest dose [98]. Further clinical trials of this candidate vaccine are under consideration.

8.3. T-cell-based vaccines

Vaccines based on robust T-cell responses are vital and crucial because such vaccine triggers both antibodies and cytotoxic T-cell responses against an insidious virus [11]. The HCV-infected cells display the viral surface and internal particles/molecules (i.e., HCV genome) to the immune system of the body, especially to CD^{4+} and CD^{8+} killer cells, which induce the host innate and acquired immune responses against the virus surface particles as well as the HCV genome [11]. CD^{8+} T-cell immunity induced by CD^{4+} T cells is mainly responsible for HCV viral infection control in human as well as in chimpanzee challenge studies [11]. Recently researchers have evaluated heterologous T-cell vaccine (ChAd3/MVA) targeting HCV non-structural proteins in HCV genotype 1b-infected individuals [13]. The vaccine is a combination of replication-defective chimpanzee adenovirus (ChAd3) and modified vaccinia Ankara (MVA) vectors so named as ChAd3/MVA [13]. The vaccine induced higher magnitude of T-cell responses in most infected individuals against all six nonstructural (from NS2 to NS5B) antigenic pools in phase I clinical studies [13]. CD^{8+} memory T cells were also generated, and CD^{8+} T-cell polyfunctionality was also increased in vaccinated individuals [13]. There were no signs of regulatory T-cell induction which might suppress an anti-HCV immune response [13]. The viral heterogeneity and high mutation rate of HCV are always potential biological barriers to developing protective HCV vaccine. ChAd3/MVA vaccine generates cross-reactive T-cell responses between heterologous viral genotypes so may be tested in diverse HCV populations [13]. Now, this vaccine is under consideration for a larger phase II clinical trials to further determine the efficacy of the vaccine.

Another therapeutic T-cell-based vaccine (GI-5005) is in clinical development which contains a fusion of HCV structural "core" and nonstructural "NS3" protein in yeast vector. The therapeutic efficacy of the vaccine was tested in both treatment-naïve and prior null responders to PEG-IFNα/RBV treatment in phase IIb clinical trials [99, 100]. Overall, 133 HCV genotype 1-infected patients (96 treatment-naïve patients) were administered to once monthly dose of vaccine along with PEG-IFNα plus RBV vs. placebo (PEG-IFNα/RBV) for 48 weeks [100]. SVR rates were reported slightly higher in vaccinated patient's arm than the patients in placebo (47 % vs. 35 %, respectively) [100]. However, the achieved SVR rates were not statistically significant. The same trends in SVR rates were reported for the patients who were stratified by their prior treatment status. In that case, the previous null responders of PEG-IFNα plus RBV therapy achieved SVR rates only 17 % upon vaccination as compared to control studies who received PEG-IFN/RBV (SVR 5 % only) [101]. At subtype levels, treatment-naïve patients with unfavorable IL28B TT polymorphism met SVR24 in vaccinated patient's arm as compared to those who treated with PEG- IFNα plus RBV alone [100]. The study was further expanded to 17 additional treatment-naïve patients with IL28B TT polymorphism, and the results were compared to the original 10 IL28B TT patients from the first cohort [100]. An undetectable HCV RNA level at the end of treatment was reported in 10 out of 16 patients (63 %) who received GI-5005 as compared to 3 out of 11 patients (27 %) who were treated with PEG-IFNα plus RBV alone [100].

Another recombinant poxvirus vaccine (TG-4040) expressing HCV nonstructural proteins (NS3, NS4, and NS5B) is in phase I clinical trials and demonstrated significantly higher SVR rates in treated patients [102]. Some other potential anti-HCV vaccine models are also in the pipeline, including T-cell-based peptide vaccines, recombinant HCV subunit vaccines, and pseudo-viral particles expressing HCV glycoproteins (E1 and E2) [103, 104]. Preclinical studies of some of these vaccine models have shown spectacular results, but a lot of further clinical studies are required to evaluate their therapeutic outcomes.

8.4. Clinical issues regarding HCV vaccine trials

No doubt, much work is being done on the development of an effective anti-HCV vaccine model, but all the efforts revolve around HCV genotype 1 infection. We know very well that more than 100 million people worldwide are infected with HCV genotype 3, 4, 5, and 6 infections, and in some countries like Egypt, the infection is almost an endemic [11]. It may indicate that the cross-reactive protective immunity induced by a proposed HCV vaccine model against one genotype would not be sufficient for selecting the best candidate HCV vaccine for the whole world. The other potential challenge is the lack of vaccine clinical trials in a high-risk population where some other factors are responsible for HCV transmission. In the United States and the Western world, where only 1–2 % general population are infected with HCV, more than 100,000 infected individuals have to be enrolled in clinical trials to determine vaccine efficacy[94]. The situation is different in developing world where HCV prevalence depends on various predisposing factors including injection drug users (IDUs), blood transfusion without screening anti-HCV antibodies, unsterilized medical instruments use, piercing of ears and nose, unprotected sexual act, and healthcare workers. Such regions represent an alternative place to conduct HCV vaccine clinical trials. Similarly, in a highly endemic area (e.g., Egypt, where almost 22 % of the country's population have afflicted with HCV), preventive or protective vaccine trials may initiate. Unfortunately, the test results would be genotype specific in that area (i.e., HCV genotype 4 is the most prevalent genotype in Egypt and the Middle East) and may not apply to the other parts of the world. The lack of basic health infrastructure and intrinsic ethical and drug regulatory issues are also potential challenges in developing countries to initiate vaccine clinical trials.

Designing of vaccine clinical trials in some concrete and high-risk populations also depends on certain crucial factors including HCV prevalence, exposure frequency of the infection, viral infectivity, and infection chronicity. The infection rate should be reduced up to 50 % in the appropriate population size for the acceptable vaccine efficacy. By assigning a certain value to the above mentioned parameters in a high-risk population, at least, 500–10,000 individuals are required in vaccine clinical trials [105]. Although this number can be managed easily with the high-risk population and in HCV endemic area, but the testing and handling of large candidate vaccines pose particular challenges in this context. The ultimate success and realistic goal of HCV vaccines must be to prevent the chronic infection in infected individuals. To achieve this objective, the term "chronic HCV infection" must be clearly defined and should not rely on the classical definition based on chronic HBV infection (i.e., the persistence of HCV viral replication more than 6 months detected quantitatively by polymerase chain reaction). Some studies have demonstrated that during acute HCV infection, viral RNA fluctuates markedly from undetectable limit to a higher level of quantification (10^6 IU/ml) [106]. In such acutely infected individuals, the viral clearance may not occur until 1 year later. Consequently, the clinical trials for HCV vaccines need longer test duration (approximately 2 years). Withholding therapy is another ethical issue while treating acutely infected patients with PEG-IFNα and RBV after a close follow-up of 6–9 months [107]. Development of surrogate biomarkers and their validation to evaluate vaccine efficacy is also challenging. In all clinical trials, a standard methodology should be applied to compare the vaccine efficacy results with each other especially in high-risk populations.

One of the big concerns which is always debatable among doctors, researchers, public healthcare workers, policy makers, and patient groups is how to implement a successful vaccine program when once effective vaccines would be available in the future. In this scenario, cost-effective analysis, careful monitoring of the adverse effects, and compliance with futility rules must be extensively scrutinized before issuing public health policies regarding mass vaccination program [108]. Implementation of a universal HCV vaccination program instead of targeting high-risk populations would be more appropriate and have a profound impact in some developing countries where HCV is highly prevalent.

9. Conclusions

The development of novel direct-acting antivirals has simplified the treatment paradigm for chronically infected and difficult-to-treat HCV genotype populations around the globe. These game changer regimens have revolutionized the HCV therapeutics regarding pan-genotypic coverage, low pill burden, fewer drug-drug interactions, improved adverse event profile, and high barrier to drug resistance. However, the treatment cost and accessibility of the drugs to infected patients are major issues which must be resolved to get full therapeutic benefits of such therapeutic regimens. Interferon lambda is promising as more efficacious, well tolerated, and short treatment of duration and has been entered into phase III clinical trials with several direct-acting antivirals. It may be beneficial as an adjuvant therapy in IFN-α-intolerant patients as well as in individuals where IL28B genetic polymorphism is highly associated to lower SVR rates. The steadily improved DAAs are playing a frontline role to surmount the burden of HCV around the globe, but the development and implementation of a successful HCV vaccine program would be mandatory to win an uphill battle against this silent epidemic. In this context, the core knowledge of intricate interplays between molecular and cellular immune responses toward HCV, viral clearance and persistence, and long-lasting immune responses would play a significant role to develop an effective protective HCV vaccine model. Adenovirus-based vector vaccines have shown promising results while generating durable, broad, sustained, and balanced innate and acquired immune response in chimpanzees and humans. A heterologous T-cell vaccine (ChAd3/MVA) has also shown very high levels of T-cell responses against multiple HCV antigens in HCV genotype 1b patients. If HCV vaccines are available in the near future, then mass vaccination program in high-risk populations would probably have a profound impact on eradicating HCV infection. The technology and scientific innovation definitely play its part, but the role of scientific community, implementation of controlled HCV healthcare policies, applications of risk prediction tools, collective will, and public health notes will galvanize the efforts to a proper ending of this silent epidemic from the world. Thus, this two-pronged attack on HCV—a variety of novel direct-acting antivirals and the possibility of a vaccine—suggests the global eradication of HCV. Overall, the achievements and improvements in the field of HCV medicine predict that the future of HCV therapeutics is bright and becoming brighter every day.

Author details

Imran Shahid[1,2]*, Waleed H. AlMalki[1], Mohammed W. AlRabia[3], Muhammad H. Hafeez[4] and Muhammad Ahmed[1]

*Address all correspondence to: iyshahid@uqu.edu.sa

[1] Department of Pharmacology and Toxicology, College of Pharmacy, Umm Al-Qura University, Makkah, Saudi Arabia

[2] Applied and Functional Genomics Laboratory, Center of Excellence in Molecular Biology (CEMB), University of the Punjab, Lahore, Pakistan

[3] Department of Medical Microbiology, College of Medicine, King Abdul Aziz University, Jeddah, Saudi Arabia

[4] Department of Gastroenterology and Hepatology, Fatima Memorial College of Medicine and Dentistry, Shadman, Lahore, Pakistan

References

[1] Davis GL, Alter MJ, El-Serag H, Poynard T, Jennings LW: Aging of hepatitis C virus (HCV)-infected persons in the United States: a multiple cohort model of HCV prevalence and disease progression. *Gastroenterology* 2010, **138**(2):513-521, 521 e511-516.

[2] Innes H, Goldberg D, Dillon J, Hutchinson SJ: Strategies for the treatment of Hepatitis C in an era of interferon-free therapies: what public health outcomes do we value most? *Gut* 2015, **64**(11):1800-1809.

[3] Shahid I, Gull S, Ijaz B, Ahmad W, Ansar M, Asad S, Kausar H, Sarwar MT, Khan MK, Hassan S: Stable Huh-7 cell lines expressing non-structural proteins of genotype 1a of hepatitis C virus. *J Virol Methods* 2013, **189**(1):65-69.

[4] Attaullah S, Khan S, Ali I: Hepatitis C virus genotypes in Pakistan: a systemic review. *Virol J* 2011, **8**:433.

[5] Ahmad W, Ijaz B, Gull S, Asad S, Khaliq S, Jahan S, Sarwar MT, Kausar H, Sumrin A, Shahid I *et al*: A brief review on molecular, genetic and imaging techniques for HCV fibrosis evaluation. *Virol J* 2011, **8**:53.

[6] Kabiri M, Jazwinski AB, Roberts MS, Schaefer AJ, Chhatwal J: The changing burden of hepatitis C virus infection in the United States: model-based predictions. *Ann Intern Med* 2014, **161**(3):170-180.

[7] Ascione A, De Luca M, Tartaglione MT, Lampasi F, Di Costanzo GG, Lanza AG, Picciotto FP, Marino-Marsilia G, Fontanella L, Leandro G: Peginterferon alfa-2a plus ribavirin is more effective than peginterferon alfa-2b plus ribavirin for treating chronic hepatitis C virus infection. *Gastroenterology* 2010, **138**(1):116-122.

[8] Manns M, Zeuzem S, Sood A, Lurie Y, Cornberg M, Klinker H, Buggisch P, Rossle M, Hinrichsen H, Merican I *et al*: Reduced dose and duration of peginterferon alfa-2b and weight-based ribavirin in patients with genotype 2 and 3 chronic hepatitis C. *J Hepatol* 2011, **55**(3):554-563.

[9] Yuan XL, Li MY, Zhang DZ: Efficacy and safety of a protease inhibitor with pegylated interferon and ribavirin in patients with untreated chronic hepatitis C: a meta analysis. *Zhonghua Gan Zang Bing Za Zhi* 2012, **20**(5):357-362.

[10] Summa V, Ludmerer SW, McCauley JA, Fandozzi C, Burlein C, Claudio G, Coleman PJ, Dimuzio JM, Ferrara M, Di Filippo M *et al*: MK-5172, a selective inhibitor of hepatitis C virus NS3/4a protease with broad activity across genotypes and resistant variants. *Antimicrob Agents Chemother* 2012, **56**(8):4161-4167.

[11] Shahid I, ALMaki WH, Hafeez MH, Hassan S: Hepatitis C virus infection treatment: An era of game changer direct acting antivirals and novel treatment strategies. *Crit Rev Microbiol* 2014, 42 (4):1-13.

[12] Schaefer M, Capuron L, Friebe A, Diez-Quevedo C, Robaeys G, Neri S, Foster GR, Kautz A, Forton D, Pariante CM: Hepatitis C infection, antiviral treatment and mental health: a European expert consensus statement. *J Hepatol* 2012, **57**(6):1379-1390.

[13] Swadling L, Capone S, Antrobus RD, Brown A, Richardson R, Newell EW, Halliday J, Kelly C, Bowen D, Fergusson J *et al*: A human vaccine strategy based on chimpanzee adenoviral and MVA vectors that primes, boosts, and sustains functional HCV-specific T cell memory. *Sci Transl Med* 2014, **6**(261):261ra153.

[14] Tran TT: A review of standard and newer treatment strategies in hepatitis C. *Am J Manag Care* 2012, **18**(14 Suppl):S340-349.

[15] Wahid A, Dubuisson J: Virus-neutralizing antibodies to hepatitis C virus. *J Viral Hepat* 2013, **20**(6):369-376.

[16] Gutierrez JA, Lawitz EJ, Poordad F: Interferon-free, direct-acting antiviral therapy for chronic hepatitis C. *J Viral Hepat* 2015, **22**(11):861-870.

[17] Ascher DB, Wielens J, Nero TL, Doughty L, Morton CJ, Parker MW: Potent hepatitis C inhibitors bind directly to NS5A and reduce its affinity for RNA. *Sci Rep* 2014, **4**:4765.

[18] Gaudieri S, Rauch A, Pfafferott K, Barnes E, Cheng W, McCaughan G, Shackel N, Jeffrey GP, Mollison L, Baker R *et al*: Hepatitis C virus drug resistance and immune-driven adaptations: relevance to new antiviral therapy. *Hepatology* 2009, **49**(4):1069-1082.

[19] Perry CM: Telaprevir: a review of its use in the management of genotype 1 chronic hepatitis C. *Drugs* 2012, **72**(5):619-641.

[20] Kong Y, Wang X, Shang Y, Schroder PM, Liang W, Ling X, Guo Z, He X: Efficacy and tolerability of telaprevir for chronic hepatitis virus C genotype 1 infection: a meta-analysis. *PLoS One* 2012, **7**(12):e52158.

[21] Jacobson IM, Dore GJ, Foster GR, Fried MW, Radu M, Rafalsky VV, Moroz L, Craxi A, Peeters M, Lenz O *et al*: Simeprevir with pegylated interferon alfa 2a plus ribavirin in treatment-naive patients with chronic hepatitis C virus genotype 1 infection (QUEST-1): a phase 3, randomised, double-blind, placebo-controlled trial. *Lancet* 2014, **384**(9941):403-413.

[22] Kwo P, Gitlin N, Nahass R, Bernstein D, Etzkorn K, Rojter S, Schiff E, Davis M, Ruane P, Younes Z *et al*: Simeprevir Plus Sofosbuvir (12 and 8 Weeks) in HCV genotype 1-infected patients without cirrhosis: OPTIMIST-1, a phase 3, randomized study. *Hepatology* 2016.

[23] Lawitz E, Matusow G, DeJesus E, Yoshida EM, Felizarta F, Ghalib R, Godofsky E, Herring RW, Poleynard G, Sheikh A *et al*: Simeprevir plus sofosbuvir in patients with chronic hepatitis C virus genotype 1 infection and cirrhosis: A Phase 3 study (OPTIMIST-2). *Hepatology* 2015.

[24] Hezode C, Asselah T, Reddy KR, Hassanein T, Berenguer M, Fleischer-Stepniewska K, Marcellin P, Hall C, Schnell G, Pilot-Matias T *et al*: Ombitasvir plus paritaprevir plus ritonavir with or without ribavirin in treatment-naive and treatment-experienced patients with genotype 4 chronic hepatitis C virus infection (PEARL-I): a randomised, open-label trial. *Lancet* 2015, **385**(9986):2502-2509.

[25] Poordad F, Schiff ER, Vierling JM, Landis C, Fontana RJ, Yang R, McPhee F, Hughes EA, Noviello S, Swenson ES. Daclatasvir with sofosbuvir and ribavirin for HCV infection with advanced cirrhosis or post-liver transplant recurrence. Hepatology. 2016, doi:10.1002/hep.28446.

[26] Wyles DL, Ruane PJ, Sulkowski MS, Dieterich D, Luetkemeyer A, Morgan TR, Sherman KE, Dretler R, Fishbein D, Gathe JC, Jr., Henn S, Hinestrosa F, Huynh C, McDonald C, Mills A, Overton ET, Ramgopal M, Rashbaum B, Ray G, Scarsella A, Yozviak J, McPhee F, Liu Z, Hughes E, Yin PD, Noviello S, Ackerman P, Investigators A. Daclatasvir plus sofosbuvir for HCV in patients coinfected with HIV-1. N Engl J Med 2015, **373**:714-725.

[27] Nelson DR, Cooper JN, Lalezari JP, Lawitz E, Pockros PJ, Gitlin N, Freilich BF, Younes ZH, Harlan W, Ghalib R, Oguchi G, Thuluvath PJ, Ortiz-Lasanta G, Rabinovitz M, Bernstein D, Bennett M, Hawkins T, Ravendhran N, Sheikh AM, Varunok P, Kowdley KV, Hennicken D, McPhee F, Rana K, Hughes EA, Team A-S. All-oral 12-week treatment with daclatasvir plus sofosbuvir in patients with hepatitis C virus genotype 3 infection: ALLY-3 phase III study. Hepatology. 2015, 61:1127-1135.

[28] Leroy V, Angus P, Bronowicki JP, Dore GJ, Hezode C, Pianko S, Pol S, Stuart K, Tse E, McPhee F, Bhore R, Jesus Jimenez-Exposito M, Thompson AJ. Daclatasvir, sofosbuvir, and ribavirin for hepatitis C virus genotype 3 and Advanced liver disease: a randomized phase III study (ALLY-3+). Hepatology. 2016, doi:10.1002/hep.28473.

[29] Poordad F, Sievert W, Mollison L, Bennett M, Tse E, Brau N, Levin J, Sepe T, Lee SS, Angus P, Conway B, Pol S, Boyer N, Bronowicki JP, Jacobson I, Muir AJ, Reddy KR, Tam E, Ortiz-Lasanta G, de Ledinghen V, Sulkowski M, Boparai N, McPhee F, Hughes E, Swenson ES, Yin PD, Group U-S. Fixed-dose combination therapy with daclatasvir, asunaprevir, and beclabuvir for noncirrhotic patients with HCV genotype 1 infection. JAMA. 2015, 313:1728-1735.

[30] Muir AJ, Poordad F, Lalezari J, Everson G, Dore GJ, Herring R, Sheikh A, Kwo P, Hezode C, Pockros PJ, Tran A, Yozviak J, Reau N, Ramji A, Stuart K, Thompson AJ, Vierling J, Freilich B, Cooper J, Ghesquiere W, Yang R, McPhee F, Hughes EA, Swenson ES, Yin PD. Daclatasvir in combination with asunaprevir and beclabuvir for hepatitis C virus genotype 1 infection with compensated cirrhosis. JAMA. 2015, **313**:1736-1744.

[31] Afdhal N, Zeuzem S, Kwo P, Chojkier M, Gitlin N, Puoti M, Romero-Gomez M, Zarski JP, Agarwal K, Buggisch P *et al*: Ledipasvir and sofosbuvir for untreated HCV genotype 1 infection. *N Engl J Med* 2014, **370**(20):1889-1898.

[32] Lawitz E FX, Zeuzem S, et al.: Simeprevir (TMC435) with Peginterferon/Ribavirin for Treatment of Chronic HCV Genotype 1 Infection in Patients who Relapsed After Previous Interferon-Based Therapy: Results from PROMISE, a Phase III trial. In. Edited by Week PaDD. 18–21 May; 2013.

[33] Lawitz E, Mangia A, Wyles D, Rodriguez-Torres M, Hassanein T, Gordon SC, Schultz M, Davis MN, Kayali Z, Reddy KR *et al*: Sofosbuvir for previously untreated chronic hepatitis C infection. *N Engl J Med* 2013, **368**(20):1878-1887.

[34] Jacobson IM, Gordon SC, Kowdley KV, Yoshida EM, Rodriguez-Torres M, Sulkowski MS, Shiffman ML, Lawitz E, Everson G, Bennett M *et al*: Sofosbuvir for hepatitis C genotype 2 or 3 in patients without treatment options. *N Engl J Med* 2013, **368**(20):1867-1877.

[35] Jacobson I DG, Foster GR, et al.: Simeprevir (TMC435) with peginterferon/ribavirin for chronic HCV genotype 1 infection in treatment-nave patients: results from QUEST-1, a phase III trial. In. Edited by International Liver Congress. Amsterdam; 2013.

[36] Feld JJ, Jacobson IM, Hezode C, Asselah T, Ruane PJ, Gruener N, Abergel A, Mangia A, Lai CL, Chan HL *et al*: Sofosbuvir and Velpatasvir for HCV Genotype 1, 2, 4, 5, and 6 Infection. *N Engl J Med* 2015, **373**(27):2599-2607.

[37] Dore G, Altice F, Litwin AH, et al. C-EDGE CO-STAR: efficacy of grazoprevir and elbasvir in persons who inject drugs (PWID) receiving opioid agonist therapy. Presented at the 2015 Annual Meeting of the American Association for the Study of Liver Diseases, San Francisco; Abstract 40. **2015**.

[38] Rockstroh JK, Nelson M, Katlama C, Lalezari J, Mallolas J, Bloch M, Matthews GV, Saag MS, Zamor PJ, Orkin C et al.: Efficacy and safety of grazoprevir (MK-5172) and elbasvir (MK-8742) in patients with hepatitis C virus and HIV co-infection (C-EDGE CO-INFECTION): a non-randomised, open-label trial. Lancet HIV 2015, 2(8):319-327.

[39] Kwo P, Gane E, Peng CY, et al. Efficacy and safety of grazoprevir/elbasvir+/– RBV for 12 or 16 weeks in patients with HCV G1, G4, or G6 infection who previously failed peginterferon/RBV: C-EDGE treatment experienced. Presented at the 50th Annual meeting of the European Association for the Study of the Liver, Vienna; Abstract P0886. 2015

[40] Zeuzem S, Ghalib R, Reddy KR, Pockros PJ, Ben Ari Z, Zhao Y, Brown DD, Wan S, DiNubile MJ, Nguyen BY *et al*: Grazoprevir-elbasvir combination therapy for treatment-naive cirrhotic and noncirrhotic patients with chronic hepatitis C virus genotype 1, 4, or 6 infection: a randomized trial. *Ann Intern Med* 2015, **163**(1):1-13.

[41] Roth D, Nelson DR, Bruchfeld A, Liapakis A, Silva M, Monsour H, Jr., Martin P, Pol S, Londono MC, Hassanein T *et al*: Grazoprevir plus elbasvir in treatment-naive and treatment-experienced patients with hepatitis C virus genotype 1 infection and stage 4-5 chronic kidney disease (the C-SURFER study): a combination phase 3 study. *Lancet* 2015, **386**(10003):1537-1545.

[42] Feld JJ, Jacobson IM, Jensen DM, Foster GR, Pol S, Tam E, Jablkowski M, Berak H, Vierling JM, Yoshida EM et al.: Randomized study of danoprevir/ritonavir-based therapy for HCV genotype 1 patients with prior partial or null responses to peginterferon/ribavirin. J Hepatol 2014, 62(2):294-302.

[43] Zeuzem S, Jacobson IM, Baykal T, Marinho RT, Poordad F, Bourliere M, Sulkowski MS, Wedemeyer H, Tam E, Desmond P *et al*: Retreatment of HCV with ABT-450/r-ombitasvir and dasabuvir with ribavirin. *N Engl J Med* 2014, **370**(17):1604-1614.

[44] Sulkowski MS, Eron JJ, Wyles D, Trinh R, Lalezari J, Wang C, Slim J, Bhatti L, Gathe J, Ruane PJ *et al*: Ombitasvir, paritaprevir co-dosed with ritonavir, dasabuvir, and ribavirin for hepatitis C in patients co-infected with HIV-1: a randomized trial. *JAMA* 2015, **313**(12):1223-1231.

[45] Poordad F, Hezode C, Trinh R, Kowdley KV, Zeuzem S, Agarwal K, Shiffman ML, Wedemeyer H, Berg T, Yoshida EM et al.: ABT-450/r-ombitasvir and dasabuvir with ribavirin for hepatitis C with cirrhosis. N Engl J Med 2014, 370(21):1973-1982.

[46] Andreone P, Colombo MG, Enejosa JV, Koksal I, Ferenci P, Maieron A, Mullhaupt B, Horsmans Y, Weiland O, Reesink HW *et al*: ABT-450, ritonavir, ombitasvir, and dasabuvir achieves 97% and 100% sustained virologic response with or without ribavirin in treatment-experienced patients with HCV genotype 1b infection. *Gastroenterology* 2014, **147**(2):359-365 e351.

[47] Ferenci P, Bernstein D, Lalezari J, Cohen D, Luo Y, Cooper C, Tam E, Marinho RT, Tsai N, Nyberg A *et al*: ABT-450/r-ombitasvir and dasabuvir with or without ribavirin for HCV. *N Engl J Med* 2014, **370**(21):1983-1992.

[48] Hayashi N, Okanoue T, Tsubouchi H, Toyota J, Chayama K, Kumada H: Efficacy and safety of telaprevir, a new protease inhibitor, for difficult-to-treat patients with genotype 1 chronic hepatitis C. *J Viral Hepat* 2012, **19**(2):e134-142.

[49] Foster GR, Hezode C, Bronowicki JP, Carosi G, Weiland O, Verlinden L, van Heeswijk R, van Baelen B, Picchio G, Beumont M: Telaprevir alone or with peginterferon and ribavirin reduces HCV RNA in patients with chronic genotype 2 but not genotype 3 infections. *Gastroenterology* 2011, **141**(3):881-889 e881.

[50] Manns MP, Markova AA, Calle Serrano B, Cornberg M: Phase III results of Boceprevir in treatment naive patients with chronic hepatitis C genotype 1. *Liver Int* 2012, **32** Suppl 1:27-31.

[51] Camma C, Petta S, Cabibbo G, Ruggeri M, Enea M, Bruno R, Capursi V, Gasbarrini A, Alberti A, Craxi A *et al*: Cost-effectiveness of boceprevir or telaprevir for previously treated patients with genotype 1 chronic hepatitis C. *J Hepatol* 2013, **59**(4):658-666.

[52] Flamm SL, Lawitz E, Jacobson I, Bourliere M, Hezode C, Vierling JM, Bacon BR, Niederau C, Sherman M, Goteti V *et al*: Boceprevir with peginterferon alfa-2a-ribavirin is effective for previously treated chronic hepatitis C genotype 1 infection. *Clin Gastroenterol Hepatol* 2013, **11**(1):81-87 e84; quiz e85.

[53] Sarrazin C, Kieffer TL, Bartels D, Hanzelka B, Muh U, Welker M, Wincheringer D, Zhou Y, Chu HM, Lin C *et al*: Dynamic hepatitis C virus genotypic and phenotypic changes in patients treated with the protease inhibitor telaprevir. *Gastroenterology* 2007, **132**(5):1767-1777.

[54] Jacobson IM, Pawlotsky JM, Afdhal NH, Dusheiko GM, Forns X, Jensen DM, Poordad F, Schulz J: A practical guide for the use of boceprevir and telaprevir for the treatment of hepatitis C. *J Viral Hepat* 2012, **19** Suppl 2:1-26.

[55] http://www.hcvonline.org/page/treatment/drugs/simeprevir-drug.Pdf [Accessed: 2016-06-08].

[56] Jacobson IM DG, Foster GR, et al.: Simeprevir (TMC435) with peginterferon/ribavirin for treatment of chronic HCV genotype 1 infection in treatment-naïve patients: efficacy in difficult-to-treat patient sub-populations in the QUEST 1 and 2 phase III trials. In. Edited by AASLD; 2013.

[57] You DM, Pockros PJ: Simeprevir for the treatment of chronic hepatitis C. *Expert Opin Pharmacother* 2013, **14**(18):2581-2589.

[58] Lenz O, de Bruijne J, Vijgen L, Verbinnen T, Weegink C, Van Marck H, Vandenbroucke I, Peeters M, Simmen K, Fanning G *et al*: Efficacy of re-treatment with TMC435 as combination therapy in hepatitis C virus-infected patients following TMC435 monotherapy. *Gastroenterology* 2012, **143**(5):1176-1178 e1171-1176.

[59] Manns M MP, Poordad FP, et al.: Simeprevir (TMC435) with peginterferon/ribavirin for treatment of chronic HCV genotype -1 infection in treatment-naïve patients: results from QUEST-2, a phase III trial. In. Edited by International Liver Congress Amsterdam; 2013.

[60] Pawlotsky JM: Treatment of chronic hepatitis C: current and future. *Curr Top Microbiol Immunol* 2013, **369**:321-342.

[61] Vermehren J, Sarrazin C: The role of resistance in HCV treatment. *Best Pract Res Clin Gastroenterol* 2012, **26**(4):487-503.

[62] Hezode C, Hirschfield GM, Ghesquiere W, Sievert W, Rodriguez-Torres M, Shafran SD, Thuluvath PJ, Tatum HA, Waked I, Esmat G *et al*: Daclatasvir plus peginterferon alfa and ribavirin for treatment-naive chronic hepatitis C genotype 1 or 4 infection: a randomised study. *Gut* 2014.

[63] Gao M, Nettles RE, Belema M, Snyder LB, Nguyen VN, Fridell RA, Serrano-Wu MH, Langley DR, Sun JH, O'Boyle DR, 2nd *et al*: Chemical genetics strategy identifies an HCV NS5A inhibitor with a potent clinical effect. *Nature* 2010, **465**(7294):96-100.

[64] FFridell RA, Wang C, Sun JH, O'Boyle DR, 2nd, Nower P, Valera L, Qiu D, Roberts S, Huang X, Kienzle B *et al*: Genotypic and phenotypic analysis of variants resistant to hepatitis C virus nonstructural protein 5A replication complex inhibitor BMS-790052 in humans: in vitro and in vivo correlations. *Hepatology* 2011, **54**(6):1924-1935.

[65] Lok AS, Gardiner DF, Lawitz E, Martorell C, Everson GT, Ghalib R, Reindollar R, Rustgi V, McPhee F, Wind-Rotolo M *et al*: Preliminary study of two antiviral agents for hepatitis C genotype 1. *N Engl J Med* 2012, **366**(3):216-224.

[66] Gane EJ, Stedman CA, Hyland RH, Ding X, Svarovskaia E, Symonds WT, Hindes RG, Berrey MM: Nucleotide polymerase inhibitor sofosbuvir plus ribavirin for hepatitis C. *N Engl J Med* 2013, **368**(1):34-44.

[67] Sofia MJ, Bao D, Chang W, Du J, Nagarathnam D, Rachakonda S, Reddy PG, Ross BS, Wang P, Zhang HR *et al*: Discovery of a beta-d-2'-deoxy-2'-alpha-fluoro-2'-beta-C-methyluridine nucleotide prodrug (PSI-7977) for the treatment of hepatitis C virus. *J Med Chem* 2010, **53**(19):7202-7218.

[68] Lam AM, Espiritu C, Bansal S, Micolochick Steuer HM, Niu C, Zennou V, Keilman M, Zhu Y, Lan S, Otto MJ *et al*: Genotype and subtype profiling of PSI-7977 as a nucleotide inhibitor of hepatitis C virus. *Antimicrob Agents Chemother* 2012, **56**(6):3359-3368.

[69] Osinusi A, Meissner EG, Lee YJ, Bon D, Heytens L, Nelson A, Sneller M, Kohli A, Barrett L, Proschan M *et al*: Sofosbuvir and ribavirin for hepatitis C genotype 1 in patients with unfavorable treatment characteristics: a randomized clinical trial. *JAMA* 2013, **310**(8):804-811.

[70] http://www.hepatitisc.uw.edu/page/treatment/drugs/ledipasvir-sofosbuvir#drug-summary.Pdf [Accessed: 2016-06-10].

[71] Afdhal N, Reddy KR, Nelson DR, Lawitz E, Gordon SC, Schiff E, Nahass R, Ghalib R, Gitlin N, Herring R *et al*: Ledipasvir and sofosbuvir for previously treated HCV genotype 1 infection. *N Engl J Med* 2014, **370**(16):1483-1493.

[72] Gane EJ, Stedman CA, Hyland RH, Ding X, Svarovskaia E, Subramanian GM, Symonds WT, McHutchison JG, Pang PS: Efficacy of nucleotide polymerase inhibitor sofosbuvir plus the NS5A inhibitor ledipasvir or the NS5B non-nucleoside inhibitor GS-9669 against HCV genotype 1 infection. *Gastroenterology* 2014, **146**(3):736-743 e731.

[73] http://www.hepatitisc.uw.edu/page/treatment/dugs/elbasvir-grazoprevir#drug-summary.Pdf [Accessed: 2016-06-12].

[74] http://www.hepatitisc.uw.edu/page/treatment/dugs/elbasvir-grazoprevir#drug-summary.Pdf [Accessed: 2016-06-14].

[75] http://www.hepatitisc.uw.edu/page/treatment/drugs/3d#drug-summary.Pdf [Accessed: 2016-06-16].

[76] Feld JJ, Kowdley KV, Coakley E, Sigal S, Nelson DR, Crawford D, Weiland O, Aguilar H, Xiong J, Pilot-Matias T *et al*: Treatment of HCV with ABT-450/r-ombitasvir and dasabuvir with ribavirin. *N Engl J Med* 2014, **370**(17):1594-1603.

[77] Keating GM: Ombitasvir/paritaprevir/ritonavir: a review in chronic HCV genotype 4 infection. *Drugs* 2016, **76**(12):1203-1211.

[78] Clark V, Nelson DR: Novel interferons for treatment of hepatitis C virus. *Clin Liver Dis* 2009, **13**(3):351-363.

[79] Ramos EL: Preclinical and clinical development of pegylated interferon-lambda 1 in chronic hepatitis C. *J Interferon Cytokine Res* 2010, **30**(8):591-595.

[80] Kotenko SV, Gallagher G, Baurin VV, Lewis-Antes A, Shen M, Shah NK, Langer JA, Sheikh F, Dickensheets H, Donnelly RP: IFN-lambdas mediate antiviral protection through a distinct class II cytokine receptor complex. *Nat Immunol* 2003, **4**(1):69-77.

[81] Grebely J, Petoumenos K, Hellard M, Matthews GV, Suppiah V, Applegate T, Yeung B, Marks P, Rawlinson W, Lloyd AR *et al*: Potential role for interleukin-28B genotype in treatment decision-making in recent hepatitis C virus infection. *Hepatology* 2010, **52**(4):1216-1224.

[82] Marcello T, Grakoui A, Barba-Spaeth G, Machlin ES, Kotenko SV, MacDonald MR, Rice CM: Interferons alpha and lambda inhibit hepatitis C virus replication with distinct signal transduction and gene regulation kinetics. *Gastroenterology* 2006, **131**(6):1887-1898.

[83] Dickensheets H, Sheikh F, Park O, Gao B, Donnelly RP: Interferon-lambda (IFN-lambda) induces signal transduction and gene expression in human hepatocytes, but not in lymphocytes or monocytes. *J Leukoc Biol* 2013, **93**(3):377-385.

[84] Freeman J, Baglino S, Friborg J, Kraft Z, Gray T, Hill M, McPhee F, Hillson J, Lopez-Talavera JC, Wind-Rotolo M: Pegylated interferons Lambda-1a and alfa-2a display different gene induction and cytokine and chemokine release profiles in whole blood, human hepatocytes and peripheral blood mononuclear cells. *J Viral Hepat* 2014, **21**(6):e1-9.

[85] Muir AJ, Shiffman ML, Zaman A, Yoffe B, de la Torre A, Flamm S, Gordon SC, Marotta P, Vierling JM, Lopez-Talavera JC *et al*: Phase 1b study of pegylated interferon lambda 1 with or without ribavirin in patients with chronic genotype 1 hepatitis C virus infection. *Hepatology* 2010, **52**(3):822-832.

[86] Muir AJ, Arora S, Everson G, Flisiak R, George J, Ghalib R, Gordon SC, Gray T, Greenbloom S, Hassanein T *et al*: A randomized phase 2b study of peginterferon lambda-1a for the treatment of chronic HCV infection. *J Hepatol* 2014, **61**(6):1238-1246.

[87] Friborg J, Levine S, Chen C, Sheaffer AK, Chaniewski S, Voss S, Lemm JA, McPhee F: Combinations of lambda interferon with direct-acting antiviral agents are highly efficient in suppressing hepatitis C virus replication. *Antimicrob Agents Chemother* 2013, **57**(3):1312-1322.

[88] Asad S, Ijaz B, Ahmad W, Kausar H, Sarwar MT, Gull S, Shahid I, Khan MK, Hassan S: Development of persistent HCV genotype 3a infection cell culture model in huh-7 cell. *Virol J* 2012, **9**:11.

[89] Choo QL, Kuo G, Ralston R, Weiner A, Chien D, Van Nest G, Han J, Berger K, Thudium K, Kuo C *et al*: Vaccination of chimpanzees against infection by the hepatitis C virus. *Proc Natl Acad Sci U S A* 1994, **91**(4):1294-1298.

[90] Weiner AJ, Brauer MJ, Rosenblatt J, Richman KH, Tung J, Crawford K, Bonino F, Saracco G, Choo QL, Houghton M *et al*: Variable and hypervariable domains are found in the regions of HCV corresponding to the flavivirus envelope and NS1 proteins and the pestivirus envelope glycoproteins. *Virology* 1991, **180**(2):842-848.

[91] Weiner AJ, Geysen HM, Christopherson C, Hall JE, Mason TJ, Saracco G, Bonino F, Crawford K, Marion CD, Crawford KA *et al*: Evidence for immune selection of hepatitis C virus (HCV) putative envelope glycoprotein variants: potential role in chronic HCV infections. *Proc Natl Acad Sci U S A* 1992, **89**(8):3468-3472.

[92] Chien DY, Choo QL, Ralston R, Spaete R, Tong M, Houghton M, Kuo G: Persistence of HCV despite antibodies to both putative envelope glycoproteins. *Lancet* 1993, **342**(8876):933.

[93] Walker CM: Adaptive immunity to the hepatitis C virus. *Adv Virus Res* 2010, **78**:43-86.

[94] Liang TJ: Current progress in development of hepatitis C virus vaccines. *Nat Med* 2013, **19**(7):869-878.

[95] Thomssen R, Bonk S, Thiele A: Density heterogeneities of hepatitis C virus in human sera due to the binding of beta-lipoproteins and immunoglobulins. *Med Microbiol Immunol* 1993, **182**(6):329-334.

[96] Davis GL, Nelson DR, Terrault N, Pruett TL, Schiano TD, Fletcher CV, Sapan CV, Riser LN, Li Y, Whitley RJ *et al*: A randomized, open-label study to evaluate the safety and pharmacokinetics of human hepatitis C immune globulin (Civacir) in liver transplant recipients. *Liver Transpl* 2005, **11**(8):941-949.

[97] Chung RT, Gordon FD, Curry MP, Schiano TD, Emre S, Corey K, Markmann JF, Hertl M, Pomposelli JJ, Pomfret EA *et al*: Human monoclonal antibody MBL-HCV1 delays HCV viral rebound following liver transplantation: a randomized controlled study. *Am J Transplant* 2013, **13**(4):1047-1054.

[98] Sallberg M, Frelin L, Diepolder H, et al. A first clinical trial of therapeutic vaccination using naked DNA delivered by in vivo electroporation shows antiviral effects in patients with chronic hepatitis C. Presented at the 44th Annual Meeting of the European Association for the Study of the Liver. Copenhagen, Denmark; abstract #43. 2009.

[99] Pockros P, Jacobson I, Boyer TD, et al.: GI-5005 therapeutic vaccine plus PEG-IFN/ribavirin improves sustained virologic response versus PEG-IFN/ribavirin in piror non-responders with genotype 1 chronic HCV infection. Hepatology; 2010, 52:404A.

[100] Shiffman ML MA, Vierling JM, et al.: GI-5005 therapeutic vaccine enhances virologic clearance by Peg-IFN/ribavirin in naïve HCV genotype 1 patients with IL28B genotype T/T. Presented at the 63rd Annual Meeting of the American Association for the Study of Liver Diseases. In. Boston, MA; 2012.

[101] Shiffman ML: Treatment of hepatitis C in 2011: what can we expect? *Curr Gastroenterol Rep* 2010, **12**(1):70-75.

[102] Habersetzer F, Honnet G, Bain C, Maynard-Muet M, Leroy V, Zarski JP, Feray C, Baumert TF, Bronowicki JP, Doffoel M *et al*: A poxvirus vaccine is safe, induces T-cell responses, and decreases viral load in patients with chronic hepatitis C. *Gastroenterology* 2011, **141**(3):890-899 e891-894.

[103] Folgori A, Capone S, Ruggeri L, Meola A, Sporeno E, Ercole BB, Pezzanera M, Tafi R, Arcuri M, Fattori E *et al*: A T-cell HCV vaccine eliciting effective immunity against heterologous virus challenge in chimpanzees. *Nat Med* 2006, **12**(2):190-197.

[104] Elmowalid GA, Qiao M, Jeong SH, Borg BB, Baumert TF, Sapp RK, Hu Z, Murthy K, Liang TJ: Immunization with hepatitis C virus-like particles results in control of hepatitis C virus infection in chimpanzees. *Proc Natl Acad Sci U S A* 2007, **104**(20):8427-8432.

[105] Strickland GT, El-Kamary SS, Klenerman P, Nicosia A: Hepatitis C vaccine: supply and demand. *Lancet Infect Dis* 2008, **8**(6):379-386.

[106] Heller T, Rehermann B: Acute hepatitis C: a multifaceted disease. *Semin Liver Dis* 2005, **25**(1):7-17.

[107] Ghany MG, Strader DB, Thomas DL, Seeff LB, American Association for the Study of Liver D: Diagnosis, management, and treatment of hepatitis C: an update. *Hepatology* 2009, **49**(4):1335-1374.

[108] Krahn MD, John-Baptiste A, Yi Q, Doria A, Remis RS, Ritvo P, Friedman S: Potential cost-effectiveness of a preventive hepatitis C vaccine in high risk and average risk populations in Canada. *Vaccine* 2005, **23**(13):1549-1558.

[109] Lawitz E, Sulkowski MS, Ghalib R, Rodriguez-Torres M, Younossi ZM, Corregidor A, DeJesus E, Pearlman B, Rabinovitz M, Gitlin N *et al*: Simeprevir plus sofosbuvir, with or without ribavirin, to treat chronic infection with hepatitis C virus genotype 1 in non-responders to pegylated interferon and ribavirin and treatment-naive patients: the COSMOS randomised study. *Lancet* 2014, **384**(9956):1756-1765.

[110] Sulkowski MS, Gardiner DF, Rodriguez-Torres M, Reddy KR, Hassanein T, Jacobson I, Lawitz E, Lok AS, Hinestrosa F, Thuluvath PJ *et al*: Daclatasvir plus sofosbuvir for previously treated or untreated chronic HCV infection. *N Engl J Med* 2014, **370**(3):211-221.

[111] Kowdley KV, Gordon SC, Reddy KR, Rossaro L, Bernstein DE, Lawitz E, Shiffman ML, Schiff E, Ghalib R, Ryan M *et al*: Ledipasvir and sofosbuvir for 8 or 12 weeks for chronic HCV without cirrhosis. *N Engl J Med* 2014, **370**(20):1879-1888.

[112] Naggie S, Cooper C, Saag M, Workowski K, Ruane P, Towner WJ, Marks K, Luetkemeyer A, Baden RP, Sax PE *et al*: Ledipasvir and Sofosbuvir for HCV in Patients Coinfected with HIV-1. *N Engl J Med* 2015, **373**(8):705-713.

[113] Foster GR, Afdhal N, Roberts SK, Brau N, Gane EJ, Pianko S, Lawitz E, Thompson A, Shiffman ML, Cooper C *et al*: Sofosbuvir and Velpatasvir for HCV Genotype 2 and 3 Infection. *N Engl J Med* 2015, **373**(27):2608-2617.

[114] Curry MP, O'Leary JG, Bzowej N, Muir AJ, Korenblat KM, Fenkel JM, Reddy KR, Lawitz E, Flamm SL, Schiano T *et al*: Sofosbuvir and Velpatasvir for HCV in Patients with Decompensated Cirrhosis. *N Engl J Med* 2015, **373**(27):2618-2628.

[115] Hezode C, Forestier N, Dusheiko G, Ferenci P, Pol S, Goeser T, Bronowicki JP, Bourliere M, Gharakhanian S, Bengtsson L *et al*: Telaprevir and peginterferon with or without ribavirin for chronic HCV infection. *N Engl J Med* 2009, **360**(18):1839-1850.

[116] McHutchison JG, Everson GT, Gordon SC, Jacobson IM, Sulkowski M, Kauffman R, McNair L, Alam J, Muir AJ, Team PS: Telaprevir with peginterferon and ribavirin for chronic HCV genotype 1 infection. *N Engl J Med* 2009, **360**(18):1827-1838.

[117] McHutchison JG, Manns MP, Muir AJ, Terrault NA, Jacobson IM, Afdhal NH, Heathcote EJ, Zeuzem S, Reesink HW, Garg J *et al*: Telaprevir for previously treated chronic HCV infection. *N Engl J Med* 2010, **362**(14):1292-1303.

[118] Jacobson IM, McHutchison JG, Dusheiko G, Di Bisceglie AM, Reddy KR, Bzowej NH, Marcellin P, Muir AJ, Ferenci P, Flisiak R *et al*: Telaprevir for previously untreated chronic hepatitis C virus infection. *N Engl J Med* 2011, **364**(25):2405-2416.

[119] Sherman KE, Flamm SL, Afdhal NH, Nelson DR, Sulkowski MS, Everson GT, Fried MW, Adler M, Reesink HW, Martin M *et al*: Response-guided telaprevir combination treatment for hepatitis C virus infection. *N Engl J Med* 2011, **365**(11):1014-1024.

[120] Zeuzem S, Andreone P, Pol S, Lawitz E, Diago M, Roberts S, Focaccia R, Younossi Z, Foster GR, Horban A *et al*: Telaprevir for retreatment of HCV infection. *N Engl J Med* 2011, **364**(25):2417-2428.

[121] Kwo PY, Lawitz EJ, McCone J, Schiff ER, Vierling JM, Pound D, Davis MN, Galati JS, Gordon SC, Ravendhran N *et al*: Efficacy of boceprevir, an NS3 protease inhibitor, in combination with peginterferon alfa-2b and ribavirin in treatment-naive patients with genotype 1 hepatitis C infection (SPRINT-1): an open-label, randomised, multicentre phase 2 trial. *Lancet* 2010, **376**(9742):705-716.

[122] Poordad F, McCone J, Jr., Bacon BR, Bruno S, Manns MP, Sulkowski MS, Jacobson IM, Reddy KR, Goodman ZD, Boparai N *et al*: Boceprevir for untreated chronic HCV genotype 1 infection. *N Engl J Med* 2011, **364**(13):1195-1206.

[123] Bacon BR, Gordon SC, Lawitz E, Marcellin P, Vierling JM, Zeuzem S, Poordad F, Goodman ZD, Sings HL, Boparai N *et al*: Boceprevir for previously treated chronic HCV genotype 1 infection. *N Engl J Med* 2011, **364**(13):1207-1217.

[124] Manns M, Marcellin P, Poordad F, de Araujo ES, Buti M, Horsmans Y, Janczewska E, Villamil F, Scott J, Peeters M *et al*: Simeprevir with pegylated interferon alfa 2a or 2b plus ribavirin in treatment-naive patients with chronic hepatitis C virus genotype 1 infection (QUEST-2): a randomised, double-blind, placebo-controlled phase 3 trial. *Lancet* 2014, **384**(9941):414-426.

[125] Forns X, Lawitz E, Zeuzem S, Gane E, Bronowicki JP, Andreone P, Horban A, Brown A, Peeters M, Lenz O *et al*: Simeprevir with peginterferon and ribavirin leads to high rates of SVR in patients with HCV genotype 1 who relapsed after previous therapy: a phase 3 trial. *Gastroenterology* 2014, **146**(7):1669-1679 e1663.

[126] Moreno C, Hezode C, Marcellin P, Bourgeois S, Francque S, Samuel D, Zoulim F, Grange JD, Shukla U, Lenz O *et al*: Efficacy and safety of simeprevir with PegIFN/ribavirin in naive or experienced patients infected with chronic HCV genotype 4. *J Hepatol* 2015, **62**(5):1047-1055.

[127] Wyles D, Brau N, Kottilil S, et al. Sofosbuvir/velpatasvir fixed dose combination for 12 weeks in patients co-infected with HCV and HIV-1: the phase 3 ASTRAL-5 study. Presented at the 51st Annual Meeting of the European Association for the Study of the Liver, Barcelona, April 13-17, 2016. Abstract PS104.

[128] Waked I, Shiha G, Qaqish BR, Esmat G, Yosry A, Hassany M, Soliman R, Mohey AM, Allam N, Zayed N et al: Ombitasvir, paritaprevir, and ritonavir plus ribavirin for chronic hepatitis C virus genotype 4 infection in Egyptian patients with or without compensated cirrhosis (AGATE-II): a multicentre, phase 3, partly randomised open-label trial. *Lancet* 2016, S2468-1253(16)30002-4.

[129] Asselah T, Hézode C, Qaqish BR, ElKhashab M, Hassanein T, Papatheodoridis G, Feld JJ, Moreno C, Zeuzem S, Ferenci P et al: Ombitasvir, paritaprevir, and ritonavir plus ribavirin in adults with hepatitis C virus genotype 4 infection and cirrhosis (AGATE-I): a multicentre, phase 3, randomised open-label trial. Lancet 2016, S2468-1253(16)30001-2.

Chapter 15

Importance of MicroRNAs in Hepatitis B and C Diagnostics and Treatment

Mateja M. Jelen and Damjan Glavač

Additional information is available at the end of the chapter

http://dx.doi.org/10.5772/66498

Abstract

MicroRNAs (miRNAs) are small-sized RNAs with ability to regulate gene expression and have been recently discovered as promising diagnostic and therapeutic biomarkers in the field of clinical medicine and microbiology, specifically in viral diseases. Infections with hepatitis B virus (HBV) or hepatitis C virus (HCV) often lead to chronic infections and development of liver hepatocellular carcinoma (HCC). Challenges in early diagnosis of HCC and rapid development of novel HCV antivirals call for identification of novel miRNA biomarkers. An extensive selection of single miRNAs and miRNA panels has been provided by accumulating studies, discovering miRNA potentials in HBV and HCV diagnostics and treatment. Currently, the diagnostic potential of miRNAs in HBV and HCV has not been established yet. However, a promising HCV treatment drug Miravirsen, a locked nucleic acid, complementary to miRNA-122, has entered a human clinical trial recently. In this review, we outline the role of miRNAs in HBV and HCV pathogenesis and differences in up- and downregulation of miRNAs upon HBV and HCV infection and HCC development.

Keywords: microRNA, hepatitis B virus, hepatitis C virus, diagnosis, treatment

1. Introduction

Hepatitis B and C viruses (HBV and HCV) are globally spread hepatotropic pathogens and major etiological factors of liver cirrhosis and hepatocellular carcinoma (HCC), infecting millions of people worldwide. HBV and HCV significantly differ in structure, genomic characteristics, and pathogenesis [1, 2].

MicroRNAs (miRNAs) are small noncoding RNAs that control gene expression and participate in complex cellular pathways and pathogenesis of various viral infections and cancers [3–5].

Despite the availability of prophylactic HBV vaccine and recently improved HCV therapy strategies, early diagnosis of HBV/HCV-related HCC, viral reactivation, resistance, drug interactions, and viral interferences in HBV/HCV co-infected patients remain major obstacles in currently available HBV and HCV diagnostics and treatments [6, 7].

Multiple studies have proposed specific miRNA or miRNA panels to be used as biomarkers for HBV/HCV-related liver disease, staging of liver disease progression, and anti-HBV/HCV therapeutic options.

In this chapter, we briefly outline the HBV and HCV biology and basis of miRNA expression in liver and HCC. Subsequently, we summarize recently described and proposed miRNAs for HBV- and HCV-associated diagnostics, particularly HBV/HCV-related HCC.

2. Hepatitis B virus

Hepatitis B virus is an enveloped, partially double-stranded DNA virus, classified in the *Hepadnaviridae* family. HBV genome is approximately 3.2 kb long and contains four RNA transcripts (P, S, C, and X), of which the S transcript encodes the surface antigen HBsAg, the main indicator of HBV infection [1]. Upon infection, cellular polymerase converts HBV DNA into covalently closed circular DNA (cccDNA), which represents a constant template for pregenomic RNA and mRNA transcription. Due to the stable state of HBV cccDNA in hepatocytes, HBV can reactivate after immunosuppression [1, 8].

HBV is classified into eight genotypes (designated A through H). Most chronic infections are related to infection with HBV genotypes B and C; however, in Europe, genotype D has been shown to be more often associated with active liver disease [1].

Globally, two billion people are infected with HBV, with majority of HBV infections occurring in South-Eastern Asia and sub-Saharan Africa [9, 10]. Approximately, one-fourth of HBV-infected individuals suffer from liver cirrhosis and 70–90% of HCC develop from cirrhotic liver [1, 10]. In developing countries, HBV infection accounts for about 60% of the total liver cancer and in developed countries for about 23% [11]. In endemic areas, HBV infections occur mostly by vertical and perinatal transmission and in more than 90% lead to chronic HBV infections. In low prevalence countries, HBV infections occur mostly through a horizontal transfer (sexual transmission), which in more than 90% lead to acute HBV infections with spontaneous viral clearance [10]. Despite improved HBV antiviral therapy over the past two decades, and the prophylactic anti-HBV vaccine, available since 1981, prenatal maternal HBeAg seropositivity in endemic countries remains significantly connected to HCC and elimination of cccDNA remains the major challenge in HBV-related treatment strategies [1, 12, 13].

http://dx.doi.org/10.5772/66498

3. Hepatitis C virus

Hepatitis C virus has a positive-sense single-stranded RNA genome of approximate length of 9.6 kb and is classified in the family *Flaviviridae*. The HCV genome encodes a polyprotein that is cleaved into three structural and seven nonstructural proteins. Based on HCV genomic sequence diversity, HCV is classified into seven genotypes and more than 60 subtypes are identified [2, 14]. Genotypes 1, 2, and 3 are globally distributed and cause most of HCV infections in North America and Europe. In Middle East and North and Central Africa, genotype 4 prevails generally, in South Africa genotype 5, in Asia genotype 6, while a recently discovered genotype 7 originates from Central Africa [2, 15].

Currently, no vaccine is available for the prevention of HCV infection. Most HCV transmissions occur by intravenous drug abuse, sexual transmission, and occupational exposure to HCV-infected blood [2]. Potential long-term outcomes in chronically HCV-infected people are liver cirrhosis and HCC, which remain the leading cause for liver transplantation. HCV is globally infecting over 150 million individuals [16–18]. Recent estimate on global anti-HCV prevalence is 115 million-infected individuals, of whom 80 million are actively viremic [19].

A recent study by Sibley et al. [20] forecasted changes in HCV-related disease up to 2030 and concluded that HCV-related morbidity and mortality are estimated to increase due to an aging of the HCV-infected population and currently available treatment will be inadequate if reductions in HCV-related disease of this magnitude are to be achieved [20].

4. MicroRNAs

Micro-ribonucleic acids (microRNAs/miRNAs) are noncoding RNAs of 18–25 nucleotides in length that complementarily target the 3′-untranslated regions (3′ UTRs), or less commonly 5′-untranslated regions (5′ UTRs) of messenger RNAs (mRNAs) [3]. Genes encoding miRNAs are located in intragenic regions or introns of mRNAs or noncoding RNAs [21]. MiRNAs are transcribed from the genome by the RNA polymerase II into primary-miRNA (pri-miRNA) hairpins, which are processed by Drosha (class III RNase) into pre-miRNAs. Pre-miRNAs are exported from the nucleus to the cytoplasm, where they are processed by a second RNaseIII Dicer into short double-stranded mature miRNAs, consisting of 5′ and 3′ arms. Finally, single-stranded miRNAs are assembled with specific proteins and form a RNA-induced-silencing complex (RISC). At least two to seven nucleotide complementarities with the target sequence are required for RISC-mediated target silencing [22–24].

The binding of miRNAs in posttranscriptional or translational level provides a rapid and sensitive mechanism of gene expression regulation, either by suppressing the translation of mRNA or by promoting mRNA degradation [25]. Gene silencing by a full complementary miRNA sequence directs cleavage of the target mRNA, while partial complementary miRNA sequence suppresses mRNA translation [26, 27]. Currently, more than 2,588 mature miRNAs are reported in a human genome [28, 29] and due to sufficient partial complementarity to the target sequence it has been shown that one type of miRNA could affect up to 200 genes, and over a 100 different targets can be involved in approximately 100 different biochemical pathways [30, 31].

4.1. MiRNAs mechanism

MiRNAs are participating in various cellular processes such as cell development, differentiation, proliferation, metabolism, immune responses, apoptosis, and oncogenesis [32, 33]. Estimates in humans suggest that 60–70% of all genes are regulated by miRNAs [4]. Being involved in numerous biological pathways, their expression and regulation reflect in various diseases, stages of the particular disease, especially in cancer development [34, 35].

MiRNAs are cell-free-circulating molecules that can be detected in almost every body fluid. Their high stability and accessibility make them ideal noninvasive markers for the early diagnosis of different pathophysiological processes. Indeed, a large amount of evidence suggests that miRNA profiles could provide a classification system for various tumors, as well as an important tool for the diagnosis and treatment of cancer and viral diseases [36–41]. Accordingly, cellular miRNAs have an ability to regulate pathogenesis of viral infections, and at the same time viruses manipulate with host cellular machinery, including miRNAs [42, 43].

Increased interest in hepatitis B and hepatitis C disease pathogenesis and diagnostics has lead to the emergence of various studies over the last 15 years that have tried to evaluate plasma and tissue levels of miRNAs in order to provide or improve the diagnosis of HBV and HCV infections as well as HBV- and HCV-related HCC [5].

5. MiRNAs in normal liver

Liver consists of various cell types, mainly divided in the parenchymal cells (hepatocytes) and non-parenchymal cells (biliary epithelial cells and lymphoid cells, etc.). Each cell type expresses its unique miRNA profile. While miRNAs are up- or downregulated in almost every stage of hepatic development, they accelerate or inhibit liver proliferation and play the major role in regulation of diverse liver functions [44]. It has been shown that a total of 277 miRNAs are expressed in the liver, with miR-122 being one of the most abundant and liver-specific miRNAs [45, 46]. Besides miR-192, miR-199a/b-3p, miR-101, miR-99a, and let-7a/b/c/f (let-7 family), which account for 80% of the total miRNA in liver, miR-122 accounts for 70% of the total liver miRNAs [45, 47]. Expression of miRNAs in the normal liver has been established by microarray systems and library sequencing [47–49].

5.1. Function of miRNAs in normal liver

The function of miR-122 has been explored in a variety of *in vivo* studies, including the miR-122 gene knockdown or silencing of miR-122 with antagomirs [50–52]. In the miR-122 gene knockdown mice, it has been shown that the deletion of the miR-122 gene resulted in hepatosteatosis, hepatitis, and the development of liver tumors [52]. Beyond that, studies implicate miR-122 as a key regulator of cholesterol and fatty-acid metabolism [50]. However, results of studies evaluating up- and downregulated miRNA profiles in differentiating liver cells are not consistent. Besides various technical issues, including differences in clinical samples and different miRNA matrices in miRNA assays, different degrees of miRNA expression among studies suggest that the miRNA profile is also influenced by the origin of the progenitor cell and that it is difficult to compare miRNA profiles in different cellular developmental stages [53].

However, it has been shown in two studies by Liu et al. [54] and Tzur et al. [55] that embryonic liver mainly contains miRNAs-122, -192, -194, -451, and -483-3p, whereas miR-122 can be detected in embryonic stem cells as well as in hepatocytes and continues to be expressed in the adulthood. Studies of hepatic malignancy pathologies have shown that miRNAs have specific targets in specific disease states [44, 53, 56]. Interestingly, a biphasic pattern of miRNA expression was observed in rats after liver surgical resection [57]. In the first 18 h after hepatectomy, about 40% of miRNAs were upregulated, whereas by 24 h there was a negative feedback mechanism which downregulated about 70% of all miRNAs [57]. These negative feedback loops are postulated to play an important role in liver regeneration processes, required for recovery of liver cells after injury; however, the abundance of miRNAs does not directly correlate with the predictable role of specific cells.

Since essential knowledge on liver regeneration processes has been delivered from rodent model studies, further studies are warranted to confirm post-hepatectomy miRNA level changes in humans [4, 57]. Investigation of miRNA levels in specific stages of liver organogenesis may reveal potential biomarkers for liver disease states.

6. miRNA and HBV- and HCV-related liver disease

HCC is the fifth most common cancer worldwide. Deregulation of miRNA expression could be one of the key factors in the development of liver pathology, including viral hepatitis and HCC [11]. Evidence is rapidly growing that specific miRNAs could be used as potential biomarkers for HCC, tumor progression, and response to therapeutic targets [4].

Infection with HBV and HCV can lead to chronic hepatitis, liver cirrhosis, or even HCC. Approximately 50–80% of HCC cases are associated with chronic HBV or HCV infection [10]. In the past several years, the involvement of miRNA in the pathogenesis of HBV-/HCV-related liver diseases has been well documented [53]. Since miRNAs can be directly involved in antiviral immune-pathological events, it is inevitable that miRNA target sequences in viral populations remained conserved, providing relevant evidence of the biological significance of potential miRNA-based antiviral interventions [58]. For the time being, no HBV- or HCV-encoded miRNAs have been reported. Using computational approaches, one candidate HBV miRNA has been found but its function remains undetermined [59].

It should be noted that miRNA dysregulation has been studied in various experimental settings, mainly involving *in vitro* systems, HBV-/HCV-replication-supporting cell lines, transgenic mice, cultured hepatocytes (mouse/rat/human), circulating blood cells or serum of HBV-/HCV-infected individuals, and liver tissue samples. MiRNA expression in model systems has been measured mainly with qualitative real time-polymerase chain reactions (RT-PCRs) and/or miRNA microarrays and less frequently with next-generation sequencing (NGS) (for review, see [23, 60]).

6.1. MiRNAs and HBV infection

It is well known that numerous cellular miRNAs are able to promote or repress the HBV lifecycle, either by directly targeting HBV transcripts or by indirectly targeting cellular mediators, involved in the HBV pathogenesis. Alternatively, HBV infection dysregulates cellular miRNAs and in this manner controls the host gene expression to promote its replication [60].

A variety of miRNAs have been reported in regulation of HBV replication namely miR-122, let-7 family, miR-199 family, miR-15 family, miR-125 family, and miR-17-92 cluster (extensively reviewed in [60]). Reported effects of the most abundant liver miRNA, miR-122, on HBV lifecycle remain mixed. Whereas some studies reported miRNAs as inhibitors of HBV replication [61–64], others have failed to even identify miR-122 as a regulator of the HBV lifecycle [65]. For example, in a study by Qiu et al. [63], in comparison to the control system, co-transfection of Huh7 cells with miR-122 inhibitor, and a plasmid encoding the HBV genome, the production of HBsAg and HBeAg increased, suggesting a negative regulatory effect of miR-122 on HBV lifecycle.

The study of Wang et al. [64] reported downregulation of miR-122 expression in liver of patients with HBV infection, in comparison to healthy controls, and showed that the miR-122 levels were negatively correlated with intrahepatic viral load and hepatic inflammation. Researchers concluded that HBV-induced miR-122 downregulation enhances HBV replication through cyclin G1-modulated P53 activity and that HBV mRNAs harboring complementary sites to miR-122 sequester miR-122 and contribute to viral persistence and carcinogenesis [61, 64].

Guo et al. [66] showed that members of the miRs-371-372-373 (miRs-371-3) gene cluster were co-upregulated in HBV-producing HepG2.2.15 cells and revealed that miRs-372/373 promotes HBV expression by targeting the transcription factor NFIB. Furthermore, Zhang et al. [65] reported that miR-1 promotes HBV replication, transcription, and antigen expression by indirect modulation of host genes expression in HCC cell line. In addition, they have shown that miR-1 arrested cell cycle, inhibited proliferation, and therefore reversed the cancer cell phenotype, which is in contradiction with HBV-induced carcinogenesis, since HBV infection promotes hepatocellular proliferation [65].

Jin et al. [67] have shown that downregulation of miR-501 in HepG2.2.15 cells could significantly inhibit HBV replication, thus representing a potential therapeutic target. They suggested that miR-501 promotes HBV replication through inhibition of the HBXIP, which interacts with HBx protein and normally represses HBV replication [67]. In a mouse model, Dai et al. [68] reported that miR-15b promoted HBV replication by direct inhibition of hepatocyte nuclear factor HNF1α.

On the other hand, miR-125 family members, miR-125a and miR-125b, have been reported to suppress the HBV lifecycle. In the PLC/PRF/5 cell line, miR-125a-5p was identified as a down-regulator of HBsAg expression by directly targeting HBV RNAs [69], while miR-125b inhibited HBV in HepG2.2.15 cells [70]. The miR-22 has been reported as a regulatory molecule which inhibits HBV infection [71]. Furthermore, miR-199a-3p and miR-210 were shown to repress the HBV replication in HepG2.2.15 cells by directly targeting the HBV S protein-coding region [72], while inhibition of miR-20 and miR-92a-1 increased levels of HBV RNAs in HepAD38 hepatoma cells [73]. Hu et al. [74] demonstrated that miR-141 suppresses HBV replication by reducing HBV promoter activities and two separate studies suggested upregulation of miR-181a in HBV-infected hepatoma cells, implying an important role in the development of HCC [75, 76].

6.2. MiRNAs and HCV infection

HCV lifecycle is influenced by host miRNAs in all stages: entry, translation, replication, and assembly [43]. As the HCV genome is single-stranded RNA, it serves as a template for its replication and direct binding site for host miRNAs. Among high number of miRNAs reported to be involved in the regulation of HCV infection and replication, most miRNAs have been documented to directly target the HCV genome: miR-1, miR-30, miR-122, miR-128, miR-196, miR-296, miR-351, miR-431, and miR-448 [77, 78].

Microarray analysis on human hepatoma cells has revealed changed expression profiles of 108 human miRNAs after HCV infection [79]. Furthermore, Liu et al. [79] showed that after acute HCV infection, miR-122 was downregulated, whereas miR-296 and miR-351 were significantly upregulated. In addition, it has been shown that HCV infection upregulated the expression of miR-192, miR-194, and miR-215, whereas the expression of miR-320 and miR-491 was downregulated [80]. It was reported that miR-192/miR-215 and miR-491 could enhance HCV replication [80].

For the most abundant miRNA in the liver, miR-122, it has been demonstrated that it promotes HCV replication by direct binding to the less commonly used UTR-binding site, the 5′ UTR site of the HCV RNA, which leads to Argonaute (Ago) protein complex recruitment, stabilization of the viral RNA, and activation of the RNA translation [77, 81, 82]. *In vitro* studies have shown that miR-122 is essential for HCV replication [81].

On the other hand, it has been shown that miR-122 exhibits anti-inflammatory and anti-tumorigenic properties in mice knockdown studies [52]. Mixed results exist on expression levels of miR-122 and development of HCC- or HCV-induced HCC. Coulouarn et al. [83] have shown that the loss of miR-122 expression in liver cancer correlated with HCC progression, whereas in another study, the upregulation of miR-122 promoted the HCV-related HCC [84].

The increased expression of miR-155 in HCV-infected patients promotes hepatocarcinogenesis and inhibits apoptosis of hepatocytes [85]. Furthermore, the direct effect on HCV replication cycle has been determined in the cell culture system for the miR-196b, which is complementary to the NS5A region of the HCV genome and is downregulated in HCV-infected patients. MiR-196b inhibits HCV replication directly by targeting HCV RNA or indirectly by increasing the expression of HMOX1. It has anti-inflammatory, antioxygenic, and hepatoprotective properties [86].

Some miRNAs can facilitate HCV lifecycle by targeting host proteins involved in innate immunity-signaling pathways. For example, HCV induced upregulation of miR-130 blocks expression of interferon stimulatory gene IFITM1, which promotes HCV entry into host cells [87]. Furthermore, miR-491 promotes HCV replication through inhibition of the PI3 kinase/ Akt pathway, one of the pathways leading to cancerous properties [80]. Studies analyzing circulating miRNA profiles in serum provide novel insights on miRNA expression in HCV pathogenesis [88, 89]. In a study by Shwetha et al. [89], it has been shown that the expression of miR-134, miR-198, miR-320c, and miR-483-5p was upregulated in patients infected with HCV 1 and HCV 3 genotypes.

Complex correlation between hepatic expression of abundant liver miRNAs, miR-122, miR-126, miR-136, and miR-181a, and histopathological and clinical characteristic of HCV-infected patients has been reported by Boštjančič et al. [31]. The study included liver biopsies of patients infected with different genotypes (1, 1a, 1b, 3, and 4) and provided an important insight into miRNA expression patterns in different stages and grades of liver disease and revealed association among specific miRNA deregulation and patient gender, serum HCV viral load, presence of steatosis, and mode of HCV transmission [31].

By contrast, another study by Elhelw et al. [90] has demonstrated upregulation of miR-181a in serum samples of HCV genotype 4-infected individuals and downregulation in HCV-infected Huh7 cells. In addition, the inverse correlation between miR-181a serum levels, viral load, and liver enzymes was observed. Due to complexity of viral and host factors involved in HCV infection and progression to HCV-induced HCC, multiple clinical parameters should be considered and controlled for in the future studies. A systematic approach was recently reported by Oliveira et al. [91]. The study evaluated liver and serum expression of miR-122 in patients infected with HCV genotypes 1 and 3 to identify possible associations between miR-122 expression and lipid profiles, HCV viral load, apolipoproteins, and liver enzymes [91].

7. MiRNAs as biomarkers in diagnostics and treatment of HBV and HCV

Early diagnosis and treatment of HCC remain challenging due to the lack of early detection methods, limited access to diagnosis, expensive medications and the presence of comorbidities, coinfections, and contraindications due to different host and viral factors. Most of HBV-/HCV-infected individuals remain undiagnosed before they seek medical help due to advanced HCC [10, 92].

The gold standard for the etiology of liver diseases is liver biopsy, an invasive method being replaced recently by serological methods and imaging technologies. Current diagnostic techniques for HCC, which are generally divided into radiological (first-line diagnostic method is ultrasound) and serological methods (serological marker alpha-fetoprotein, AFP, and des-gamma-carboxy prothrombin), provide limited reliability [93, 94].

7.1. MiRNAs as biomarkers in body fluids

MiRNAs can be detected in various body fluids, such as plasma, serum, urine, and infected or diseased tissue and may exhibit host responses to the pathogen or other inflammatory processes; however, miRNA levels in body fluids may not necessarily reflect the miRNA level in the infected/diseased tissue, and second, the same miRNA may be upregulated in one state of disease and downregulated in another. To provide optimal management of HBV- and HCV-related diseases, novel surrogate miRNA biomarkers should be considered [41]. A great amount of studies provide promising information on miRNAs as potential diagnostic biomarkers of HBV or HCV infection as well as potential diagnostic and treatment tool in HBV-/HCV-related HCC. According to specific miRNA targets and up- or downregulation of miRNA expression, potential imitating or antagonistic characteristics of miRNAs could be used in HBV-/HCV-related therapy.

7.2. HBV miRNA biomarkers

Currently used markers in the diagnostics of HBV can serve as indicators of specific HBV infection phases; however, none of them can be used to predict the HBV infection outcome [41].

Several studies suggest that the use of miRNA panels in serum or liver tissue could improve the specificity of HBV diagnostics. For example, Li et al. [41] have reported that their 13-miRNA-based biomarker panel could accurately discriminate between HBV cases from healthy controls and HCV cases, as well as HBV-positive HCC cases from healthy controls and HBV-infected patients. The panel of 13 miRNA consisted of the following miRNAs: miR-375, miR-92a, miR-10a, miR-223, miR-423, miR-23b/a, miR-342-3p, miR-99a, miR-122a, miR-125b, miR-150, and let-7c [41] (**Table 1**).

In order to reliably differentiate HCC from chronic HBV infection, cirrhosis, and healthy subjects, plasma panel of seven miRNAs (miR-122, miR-192, miR-21, miR-223, miR-26a, miR-27a, and miR-801) has been investigated by Zhou et al. [104]. Mizuguchi et al. [107] employed sequencing-based miRNA clustering and showed that the panel of miRNAs was more effective for the detection of high-risk patients for HBV-related HCC recurrence after liver surgery, in comparison to investigation of a single miRNA. MiR-122, miR-21, and miR-34a were identified as potential biomarkers for the prediction of HBV-related HCC.

The miR-34a is a direct target of the P53 and it has been shown that the expression of miR-34a is downregulated in several human cancers, and when overexpressed, miR-34a can repress several oncogenes and induces apoptosis and arrest of the cell cycle. Deletion of gene region encoding miR-34a has been well detected in breast, lung, cervical, and prostate cancers (reviewed by Agostini and Knight [111]). A mimic miR-34a (MRX34) became a promising therapeutic tool for HCC and has reached a clinical trial, phase 1 in 2013 [111].

Individual miRNAs or combination of miRNA and serological markers for HCC have been examined and proposed. While an upregulated oncogenic miRNA-27a has been suggested as a therapeutic target in HBV-related HCC patients [108] and miR-101 as a potential noninvasive biomarker to differentiate HBV-related HCC from HBV liver cirrhosis [97, 112], a combination of circulating miR-126 and AFP has been proposed as a promising noninvasive-specific diagnostic biomarker for HBV-related HCC. Furthermore, combinations of miR-126/AFP AFP and miR-142-3p/AFP showed higher efficiency rather than AFP alone in discriminating HCC from non-HCC patients [99].

miRNA	Deregulation	Type of sample	Type of method	Clinical relevance	Reference
miR-101	Up/down	HepG2 and HepG2.2.15, HBV-HCC tissue, Hep3B, and L02, HBVHCC-related serum	Microarray, qRT-PCR	Biomarker for monitoring the progression of tumor development in HBV-related HCC	Zhang et al. [95], Wei et al. [96], Fu et al. [97]
miR-106b-25 cluster (miR-106b, miR-93, miR-25)	Up	HBV-infected HCC patients	Microarray, qRT-PCR,	Decrease in survival time, increase in the recurrence rate and HCC differentiation in HBV-related HCC	Yen et al. [98]
miR-122a	Up	HBV-infected serum, liver tissue of HBV-related HCC	qRT-PCR, NGS	HCC differentiation from healthy, chronic hepatitis and cirrhosis	Li et al. [41]
miR-126	Up	Plasma of HBV HCC, liver tissue of HCC	Microarray	Potential biomarker for HBV-related HCC	Ghosh et al. [99]
miR-132-3p	Up	Plasma of HBV-related HCC patients	qRT-PCR	Potential biomarker for HBV-related HCC	Wen et al. [100]
miR-141-3p	Up	Serum of HBV-related HCC patients	NGS, qRT-PCR	Clinical value in HBV-related HCC diagnostics	Tan et al. [101]
miR-142-3p	Up	Plasma and liver tissue of HBV-related HCC	Microarray	Potential biomarker for HBV-related HCC	Ghosh et al. [99]
miR-146a	Up/down	HepG2 and HepG2.2.15, HBV-related HCC and serum	Microarray and Northern blotting	Involved in chronicity of HBV infection	Liu et al. [75], Gui et al. [102], Zhang et al. [95]
miR-146b-5p	Up/down	HepG2 and HepG2.2.15, HBV-related HCC, HBV-infected serum	Microarray, qRT-PCR, NGS	Potential research interest in chronic HBV infections and HBV-induced HCC	Hou et al. [47], Zhang et al. [95]
miR-155	Up	HepG2, H7402	qRT-PCR	Inhibits HBV infection in human hepatoma cells	Su et al. [103]
miR-181a/b	Up	HepG2 and HepG2.2.15	Microarray, Northern blotting, qRT-PCR	Important role in HBV-induced HCC development	Liu et al. [75], Zou et al. [76]
miR-185-5p	Up	Plasma of HBV-related HCC patients	qRT-PCR	Potential biomarker for HBV-related HCC	Wen et al. [100]
miR-192	Up	HBV-related HCC plasma	qRT-PCR, microarray	HCC differentiation from healthy, chronic hepatitis and cirrhosis	Zhou et al. [104]

miRNA	Deregulation	Type of sample	Type of method	Clinical relevance	Reference
miR-1228-5p	Up	Serum of HBV-related HCC patients	NGS, qRT-PCR	Clinical value in HBV-related HCC diagnostics	Tan et al. [101]
miR-20a/20a-5p	Up/down	HepG2 and HepG2.2.15, plasma of HBV-related HCC	Microarray, qRT-PCR	Potential research interest in chronic HBV infections and HBV-induced HCC	Wen et al. [100], Zhang et al. [95]
miR-21	Up/down	HepG2, HepG2.2.15, Hep3B, HBV-related HCC, plasma of HBV HCC, liver tissue of HCC	qRT-PCR, stem-loop RT-qPCR, microarray, NGS, clone count	HCC differentiation from healthy, chronic hepatitis and cirrhosis	Hou et al. [47], Zhou et al. [104], Gao et al. [105], Bandopadhyay et al. [106], Ghosh et al. [99], Mizuguchi et al. [107]
miR-23a/b	Up	HBV-infected serum	qRT-PCR, NGS	Biomarker to differentiate HBV-related HCC from controls	Li et al. [41]
miR-25/25-3p	Up	HBV-infected serum, HepG2 and HepG2.2.15, plasma of HBV-related HCC	qRT-PCR, microarray, NGS	Biomarker to differentiate HBV-related HCC from controls	Li et al. [41], Zhang et al. [95], Wen et al. [100]
miR-27a	Up/down	HBV-related HCC, HepG2 and Huh7, HBV-related HCC plasma	qRT-PCR, microarray	HCC differentiation from healthy, chronic hepatitis and cirrhosis	Zhou et al. [104], Wu et al. [108]
miR-200b	Up	HepG2, HepG2.2.15	microarray, Northern blotting	involved in chronicity of HBV infection	Liu et al. [75]
miR-206	Up	Serum of HBV-related HCC patients	NGS, qRT-PCR	Clinical value in HBV-related HCC diagnostics	Tan et al. [101]
miR-221	Up/down	HepG2, HepG2.2.15, Hep3B, HBV-related HCC	Microarray, Stem-loop RT-qPCR	Potential research interest in chronic HBV infections and HBV-induced HCC	Gao et al. [105], Zhang et al. [95]
miR-222	Up/down	HepG2 and HepG2.2.15	Microarray, qRT-PCR	Promotes cell growth and migration	Bandopadhyay et al. [106], Zhang et al., 2011 [95]
miR-223	Up/down	HBV-infected serum, plasma	qRT-PCR, microarray, NGS	HCC differentiation from healthy, chronic hepatitis and cirrhosis	Zhou et al. [104], Li et al. [41]
miR-224	Up/down	Hep3B and HepG2	Stem-loop RT-qPCR	Significantly upregulated in HCC	Gao et al. [105], Zhang 2011 [95]

miRNA	Deregulation	Type of sample	Type of method	Clinical relevance	Reference
miR-30a-5p	Up	Plasma of HBV-related HCC	qRT-PCR	Potential biomarker for HBV-related HCC	Wen et al. [100]
miR-34a	Up	HBV-related liver samples	NGS, clone count	Expressed aberrantly in liver cancer	Mizuguchi et al. [107]
miR-320a	Up	Plasma of HBV HCC	qRT-PCR	Potential biomarker for HBV-related HCC	Wen et al. [100]
miR-324-3p	Up	Plasma of HBV HCC	qRT-PCR	Potential biomarker for HBV-related HCC	Wen et al. [100]
miR-342-3p	Up	HBV-infected serum	qRT-PCR, NGS	Biomarker for differentiation of HBV-positive HCC from controls	Li et al. [41]
miR-375	Up	HBV-infected serum	qRT-PCR, NGS	Biomarker for differentiation of HBV-positive HCC from controls	Li et al. [41]
miR-423	Up	HBV-infected serum	qRT-PCR, NGS	Biomarker for differentiation of HBV-positive HCC from controls	Li et al. [41]
miR-433-3p	Up	Serum of HBV-related HCC patients	NGS, qRT-PCR	Clinical value in HBV-related HCC diagnostics	Tan et al. [101]
miR-801	Up	HBV-related HCC plasma	qRT-PCR, microarray	HCC differentiation from healthy, chronic hepatitis and cirrhosis	Zhou et al. [104]
miR-92a/92a-3p	Up	HBV-infected serum, plasma of HBV HCC	qRT-PCR, microarray, NGS	Potential biomarker for HBV-related HCC	Wen et al. [100], Hou et al. [47], Li et al. [41]
let-7f	Up	HBV-infected serum	qRT-PCR, NGS	Biomarker for differentiation of HBV-positive HCC from controls	Li et al. [41]
miR-15a	Up/down	HepG2 and HepG2.2.15, plasma of HBV-related HCC, liver tissue of HCC	Microarray and Northern blotting	Involved in chronicity of HBV infection	Liu et al. [75], Ghosh et al. [99]
miR-18a/b	Up/down	HepG2 and HepG2.2.15, HBV-related HCC serum	Microarray, NGS, Northern blotting, qRT-PCR	Potential research interest in chronic HBV infections and HBV-induced HCC	Zhang et al. [95], Li et al. [109]
miR-100	Down	HBV-related HCC	qRT-PCR	Important deregulated miRNA in HCC	Hou et al. [47]
miR-106a	Down	HepG2 and HepG2.2.15	Microarray	Potential research interest in chronic HBV infections and HBV-induced HCC	Zhang et al. [95]

miRNA	Deregulation	Type of sample	Type of method	Clinical relevance	Reference
miR-122	Down	HepG2.2.15, HBV infected HCC tissue, HBV-related HCC plasma	Microarray, qRT-PCR, NGS, clone count	Potential biomarker for HCC detection	Zhou et al. [104], Li et al. [61], Fan et al. [62], Mizuguchi et al. [107]
miR-122-5p	Down	Serum of HBV-related HCC patients	NGS, qRT-PCR	Clinical value in HBV-related HCC diagnostics	Tan et al. [101]
miR-125b-5p	Up/down	HBV-related HCC, HBV positive plasma	qRT-PCR, microarray, NGS	Potential biomarker for HBV-related HCC	Hou et al. [47], Giray et al. [110]
miR-143	Down	HepG2 and HepG2.2.15	qRT-PCR, microarray, NGS	Potential research interest in chronic HBV infections and HBV-induced HCC	Hou et al. [47], Zhang et al. [95]
miR-145	Down	HepG2, Hep3B. HBV-related HCC, HBV-infected serum	Stem-loop RT-qPCR	Candidate tumor-suppressor miRNA	Gao et al. [105], Bandopadhyay et al. [106]
miR-192-5p	Down	Serum of HBV-related HCC patients	NGS, qRT-PCR	Clinical value in HBV-related HCC diagnostics	Tan et al. [101]
miR-199a-5p	Down	Serum of HBV-related HCC patients	NGS, qRT-PCR	Clinical value in HBV-related HCC diagnostics	Tan et al. [101], Zhang et al. [95]
miR-199a/b-3p	Down	HBV-related HCC	qRT-PCR, microarray, NGS	Important deregulated miRNA in HCC	Hou et al. [47]
miR-199b-5p	Down	HepG2, HepG2.2.15, Hep3B. HBV-related HCC	miRNA microarray, Stem-loop RT-qPCR	Potential research interest in chronic HBV infections and HBV-induced HCC	Gao et al. [105], Zhang et al. [95]
miR-22	Down	HepG2 and HBV-related HCC	qRT-PCR	Inhibits viral gene expression	Shi et al. [71]
miR-26a	Down	HBV-related HCC plasma	qRT-PCR, microarray	HCC differentiation from healthy, chronic hepatitis and cirrhosis	Zhou et al. [104]
miR-26a-5p	Down	Serum of HBV-related HCC patients	NGS, qRT-PCR	Clinical value in HBV-related HCC diagnostics	Tan et al. [101]
miR-29c	Down	HBV-related HCC	qRT-PCR, microarray, NGS	Tumor- suppressive miRNA	Hou et al. [47]
let-7a/b/c/d	Down	HBV-related HCC	qRT-PCR, microarray, NGS	Important deregulated miRNA in HCC	Hou et al. [47]

Abbreviations: HCC, hepatocellular carcinoma; NGS, next-generation sequencing; ND, no data available; qRT-PCR, quantitative real-time polymerase chain reaction.

Table 1. Studies reporting on miRNA deregulation in HBV-infected patients with HCC or in HBV-expressing cell lines.

Serum miRNAs could serve as biomarkers for the detection of liver pathologies [102]. Serum HBV-related miRNAs for HBV-related HCC diagnosis have been investigated by Tan et al. [101]. The study identified eight miRNAs (miR-206, miR-141-3p, miR-433-3p, miR-1228-5p, miR-199a-5p, miR-122-5p, miR-192-5p, and miR-26a-5p) and constructed a miRNA set that provided high diagnostic accuracy for HBV-related HCC [101]. The study published by Winther et al. [113] presented a panel of circulating plasma miRNAs that are differentially expressed in immunological phases of chronically HBV-infected children and positively correlated with the quantity of HBsAg.

A multicenter study was conducted by Wen et al. [100] to discover a panel of plasma miRNAs to discriminate HBV-related HCC patients from healthy controls. The study revealed that four miRNAs (miR-20a-5p, miR-320a, miR-324-3p, and miR-375) (alone or combined with AFP) could be used as preclinical biomarkers in HCC screening, while the expression profile of eight miRNAs (miR-20a-5p, miR-25-3p, miR-30a-5p, miR-92a-3p, miR-132-3p, miR-185-5p, miR-320a, and miR-324-3p) can discriminate HCC patients from noncancerous controls [100]. Some of the described miRNAs were studied as well by Zhang et al. [95]. MiR-18a, miR-125b-5p, and miR-223-3p were well described as potential biomarkers for HBV-related HCC [109, 110].

Hou et al. [47] performed an extensive study of miRNomes in human normal liver, hepatitis liver, and HCC. Researchers presented 15 deregulated miRNAs in 40 HBV-related HCC samples in comparison to healthy controls. Additionally, the consistent decline of miR-199a/b-3p in HCC and its significant correlation with poor prognosis of HCC patients has been elucidated, suggesting miR-199a/b-3p as a potential HBV therapeutic target. Gao et al. [105] investigated the expression of cancer-related miRNA profiles in early stages of HBV-related HCC development and observed altered miRNA expression at various pre-malignant stages of HCC and persistent downregulation of miR-145 and miR-199b and upregulation of miR-244 throughout the HCC development. The miR-145 has been suggested as a candidate tumor-suppressive miRNA due to suppression of cell proliferation caused by overexpression of miR-145 precursor in HepG2 cell lines and abundant expression of miR-145 in non-tumorous livers as well as pre-malignant low-grade dysplastic nodules.

Several studies have suggested the role of HBx protein in miRNA expression during HBV infection [67, 96, 98, 106]. For example, the recent study, conducted on 120 patients with HBV-related HCC, has shown that the expression of miR-106b was significantly higher in HBV-related HCC patients in comparison to non-HBV/non-HCV-related HCC patients and suggested that HBx enhances miR-106b transcription and therefore promotes tumor progression in HBV-related HCC [98]. Transfection with the HBx expression plasmid has been recently used in an additional study by Yu et al. [114] to investigate HBx-related regulation of miR-19a, miR-122, and miR-223 in malignant hepatocytes. The study has shown that the expression of miRNAs was regulated by HBx protein, which enhanced the proliferation of HBx-transfected HepG2 cells.

7.3. HCV miRNA biomarkers

Apart from a variety of published studies focusing on the identification of HCV infection miRNA biomarkers [88], our review focused more on difference in miRNAs profiles between HCV-infected cancerous liver cells and HCV-infected cells without progression to HCC. Despite the fact that treatment for most common HCV genotype 1 has been evolving rapidly in the past 10 years, no effective and safe anti-HCV vaccine is available and only approximately 50% of patients, infected with HCV genotype 1 (the more common genotype in USA and Western Europe), reach sustained viral response (SVR) while treated with most accessible treatment, the interferon. Therefore, the management of HCV-induced liver disease remains problematic [115].

Antagonism of miR-122 by locked nucleic acid is a promising tool for the treatment of HCV. The current most advanced research on miR-122 antagonist Miravirsen is discussed in the following section. Likewise, the therapeutic potential of mimic miR-196b is presented by Kaluzna [30], reviewing studies which confirmed the ability of miR-196b to inhibit HCV replication and revealed that interferon-induced overexpression of miR-196b decreases inflammation and leads to a better response in interferon-based HCV therapy.

Circulating serum levels of miR-122 and miR-222 have been shown to be useful potential diagnostic biomarkers for chronic HCV infection in Egyptian patients [116–118], whereas in another study miR-122, miR-199a, and miR-16 have been implicated as potential early diagnostic biomarkers for HCC in Egyptian patients, chronically infected with HCV [118] (**Table 2**).

Of note, miR-222 and miR-224 have been reported to be upregulated in both, HBV and HCV infections [95, 105, 116, 121]. However, Bandopadhyay et al. [106] and Zhang et al. [95] reported downregulation of miR-222 and miR-224 in HBV-infected patients, respectively. As expression profiles of circulating serum biomarkers became a subject of interest in different disease studies, serum miRNAs possibly involved in HCV-related HCC have been investigated in several studies. Oksuz et al. [119] examined HCV-infected patients with chronic infection, cirrhosis, and HCC and compared them with control group samples. When all groups of samples were compared, the study revealed deregulation of miR-30c-5p, miR-223-3p, miR-302c-3p, and miR-17-5p in cirrhosis and HCC, suggesting possible novel noninvasive biomarkers for HCC.

Using whole-genome expression profiling, Abdalla and Haj-Ahmad [120] identified 10 potential HCV-induced HCC biomarker candidates in urine; five of which were upregulated in HCC: miR-335, miR-618, miR-625, miR-532, and miR-7, and five downregulated: miR-323, miR-449, miR-520d, miR-516-5p, and miR-650. The proposed tandem signature of downregulated miR-650 and upregulated miR-618 showed improved sensitivity and specificity for HCC detection, in comparison to the traditional AFP-level-based detection method.

Increased expression of miR-155 in hepatocytes of patients infected with HCV has been confirmed *in vitro* and *in vivo* by Zhang et al. [85]. In addition, the study revealed that overexpression of miR-155 inhibits apoptosis, and promotes hepatocyte proliferation and tumorigenesis, which suggested miR-155 could be a negative prognostic biomarker for HCC (reviewed by Kaluzna [30]). In addition, miR-155 has been shown to be upregulated in HBV-infected human hepatoma cells, where it inhibits HBV infection [103] (**Figure 1**).

MiRNA	Deregulation	HCV genotype	Type of sample	Method	Clinical relevance	Reference
miR-10a	Up	ND	HCV-related HCC	qRT-PCR	Increased expression in HCV-related HCC	Varnholt et al. [84]
miR-15a	Up	ND	HCV-related HCC	qRT-PCR	Increased expression in HCV-related HCC	Varnholt et al. [84]
miR-16	Up/down	ND	HCV-related HCC, serum of HCV chronic infections	qRT-PCR, stem loop qRT-PCR	Associated with progression of HCC	Varnholt et al. [84], El-Abd et al. [118]
miR-17-5p	Up	ND	Plasma of HCV-related HCC	qRT-PCR	Noninvasive biomarker of HCV-positive HCC	Oksuz et al. [119]
miR-100	Up	ND	HCV-related HCC	qRT-PCR	Increased expression in HCV-related HCC	Varnholt et al. [84]
miR-122	Up/down	ND	Serum of HCV patients serum of patients with chronic HCV infection, HCV-related HCC	RT-PCR, qRT-PCR, stem loop qRT-PCR, microarray	Detection of HCC in HCV-chronic patients	El-Garem et al. [117], Motawi et al. [116], El-Abd et al. [118], Varnholt et al. [84]
miR-125b	Up	ND	HCV-related HCC	qRT-PCR	Increased expression in HCV-related HCC	Varnholt et al. [84]
miR-155	Up	ND	HCV-infected patients	Stem loop qRT-PCR	Promotes hepatocarcinogenesis	Zhang et al. [85]
miR-192	Up	Chimera of 1a/2	Huh7, Huh-RepSI	Microarray	Relevant to carcinogenesis	Ishida et al. [80]
miR-194	Up	Chimera of 1a/2	Huh7, Huh-RepSI	Microarray	Relevant to carcinogenesis	Ishida et al. [80]
miR-200a	Up	4	Urine of HCV-related HCC	Microarray, qRT-PCR	Potential HCC biomarker	Abdalla et al. [120]
miR-215	Up	Chimera of 1a/2	Huh7, Huh-RepSI	Microarray	Relevant to carcinogenesis	Ishida et al. [80]
miR-221	Up	ND	HCV-related HCC	Microarray	Exclusively expressed in HCV-associated HCC	Diaz et al. [121]
miR-222-3p	Up	ND	HCV-related HCC	Microarray	Exclusively expressed in HCV-associated HCC	Diaz et al. [121]
miR-224-3p	Up	ND	HCV-related HCC	Microarray	Exclusively expressed in HCV-associated HCC	Diaz et al. [121]

http://dx.doi.org/10.5772/66498

MiRNA	Deregulation	HCV genotype	Type of sample	Method	Clinical relevance	Reference
miR-224-5p	Up	ND	HCV-related HCC	Microarray	Exclusively expressed in HCV-associated HCC	Diaz et al. [121]
miR-299	Up	ND	HCV-related HCC	qRT-PCR	Increased expression in HCV-related HCC	Varnholt et al. [84]
miR-30c-5p	Up	ND	Plasma of HCV-related HCC patients	qRT-PCR	Noninvasive biomarker of HCV-positive HCC	Oksuz et al. [119]
miR-302c-3p	Up	ND	Plasma of HCV-related HCC patients	qRT-PCR	Noninvasive biomarker of HCV-positive HCC	Oksuz et al. [119]
miR-326	Up	ND	HCV-related HCC tumors	qRT-PCR	Increased expression in HCV-related HCC	Varnholt et al. [84]
miR-335	Up	4	Urine of HCV-related HCC patients	Microarray, qRT-PCR	Potential HCC biomarker	Abdalla et al. [120]
miR-370	Up	ND	HCV-related HCC	qRT-PCR	Increased expression in HCV-related HCC	Varnholt et al. [84]
miR-452	Up	ND	HCV-related HCC	Microarray	Exclusively expressed in HCV-associated HCC	Diaz et al. [121]
miR-520a*	Up	4	Urine of HCV-related HCC patients	Microarray, qRT-PCR	Potential HCC biomarker	Abdalla et al. [120]
miR-521	Up	4	Urine of HCV-related HCC patients	Microarray, qRT-PCR	Potential HCC biomarker	Abdalla et al. [120]
miR-522-3p	Up	ND	HCV-related HCC	Microarray	Exclusively expressed in HCV-associated HCC	Diaz et al. [121]
miR-532	Up	4	Urine of HCV-related HCC patients	Microarray, qRT-PCR	Potential HCC biomarker	Abdalla et al. [120]
miR-618	Up	4	Urine of HCV-related HCC patients	Microarray, qRT-PCR	miR-618/650 in tandem to detect HCC among HCV-positive patients	Abdalla et al. [120]
miR-625	Up	4	Urine of HCV-related HCC patients	Microarray, qRT-PCR	Potential HCC biomarker	Abdalla et al. [120]

MiRNA	Deregulation	HCV genotype	Type of sample	Method	Clinical relevance	Reference
miR-640	Up	4	Urine of HCV-related HCC patients	Microarray, qRT-PCR	Potential HCC biomarker	Abdalla et al. [120]
miR-7	Up	4	Urine of HCV-related HCC patients	Microarray, qRT-PCR	Potential HCC biomarker	Abdalla et al. [120]
miR-765	Up	4	Urine of HCV-related HCC patients	Microarray, qRT-PCR	Potential HCC biomarker	Abdalla et al. [120]
miR-9	Up	ND	HCV-related HCC	qRT-PCR	Increased expression in HCV-related HCC	Varnholt et al. [84]
miR-1269	Up	ND	HCV-related HCC	Microarray	Exclusively expressed in HCV-associated HCC	Diaz et al. [121]
let-7g	Up	ND	HCV-related HCC	qRT-PCR	Increased expression in HCV-related HCC	Varnholt et al. [84]
miR-16-5p	Down	ND	HCV-related HCC	Microarray	Exclusively expressed in HCV-associated HCC	Diaz et al. [121]
miR-104	Down	ND	HCV-related HCC tumors	qRT-PCR	Decreased expression in HCV-related HCC	Varnholt et al. [84]
miR-106a	Down	ND	HCV-related HCC tumors	qRT-PCR	Decreased expression in HCV-related HCC	Varnholt et al. [84]
miR-122a	Down	ND	Mainly HCV-related HCC	Microarray	Deregulated in HCV-related HCC	Gramantieri et al. [122]
miR-125a-5p	Down	ND	HCV-related HCC	Microarray	Exclusively expressed in HCV-associated HCC	Diaz et al. [121]
miR-125b-5p	Down	ND	HCV-related HCC	Microarray	Exclusively expressed in HCV-associated HCC	Diaz et al. [121]
miR-130a	Down	ND	HCV-related HCC	Microarray	Exclusively expressed in HCV-associated HCC	Diaz et al. [121]
miR-134	Down	ND	HCV-related HCC tumors	qRT-PCR	Decreased expression in HCV-related HCC	Varnholt et al. [84]
miR-137	Down	ND	HCV-related HCC tumors	qRT-PCR	Decreased expression in HCV-related HCC	Varnholt et al. [84]

http://dx.doi.org/10.5772/66498

MiRNA	Deregulation	HCV genotype	Type of sample	Method	Clinical relevance	Reference
miR-139-3p	Down	ND	HCV-related HCC	Microarray	Exclusively expressed in HCV-associated HCC	Diaz et al. [121]
miR-139-5p	Down	ND	HCV-related HCC	Microarray	Exclusively expressed in HCV-associated HCC	Diaz et al. [121]
miR-145	Down	ND	HCV-related HCC tumors	qRT-PCR	Decreased expression in HCV-related HCC	Varnholt et al. [84]
miR-147	Down	ND	HCV-related HCC tumors	qRT-PCR	Decreased expression in HCV-related HCC	Varnholt et al. [84]
miR-159a	Down	ND	HCV-related HCC tumors	qRT-PCR	Decreased expression in HCV-related HCC	Varnholt et al. [84]
miR-181a	Up/down	4	Huh7, blood, serum liver biopsies from chronically infected HCV patients	RT-PCR	Disparity in expression between serum and liver tissue. Upregulation in serum-good prognosis, downregulation-progression to HCC	Elhelw et al. [90]
miR-185	Down	ND	HCV-related HCC	qRT-PCR	Decreased expression in HCV-related HCC	Varnholt et al. [84]
miR-195	Down	ND	HCV-related HCC	Microarray	Exclusively expressed in HCV-associated HCC	Diaz et al. [121]
miR-198	Down	ND	HCV-related HCC	qRT-PCR	Decreased expression in HCV-related HCC	Varnholt et al. [84]
miR-199a/-3p	Down	ND	HCV-related HCC, serum of chronically HCV infected	Microarray, qRT-PCR, stem loop qRT-PCR	Exclusively expressed in HCV-associated HCC	Diaz et al. [121], El-Abd et al. [118]
miR-199a-5p	Down	ND	HCV-related HCC	Microarray	Exclusively expressed in HCV-associated HCC	Diaz et al. [121]
miR-199b	Down	ND	HCV-related HCC	qRT-PCR	Decreased expression in HCV-related HCC	Varnholt et al. [84]
miR-199b-3p	Down	ND	HCV-related HCC	Microarray	Exclusively expressed in HCV-associated HCC	Diaz et al. [121]

MiRNA	Deregulation	HCV genotype	Type of sample	Method	Clinical relevance	Reference
miR-29c	Down	ND	HCV-related HCC	qRT-PCR	Decreased expression in HCV-related HCC	Varnholt et al. [84]
miR-204	Down	ND	HCV-related HCC	qRT-PCR	Decreased expression in HCV-related HCC	Varnholt et al. [84]
miR-214	Down	ND	HCV-related HCC	Microarray	Exclusively expressed in HCV-associated HCC	Diaz et al. [121]
miR-218	Down	ND	HCV-related HCC	qRT-PCR	Decreased expression in HCV-related HCC	Varnholt et al. [84])
miR-221	Down	ND	Serum chronic HCV patients	RT-PCR, qRT-PCR	Potential noninvasive biomarker for HCV-related HCC	El-Garem et al. [117]
miR-223-3p	Down	ND	Plasma of HCV-related HCC	qRT-PCR	Noninvasive biomarker of HCV-positive HCC	Oksuz et al. [119]
miR-301a-3p	Down	ND	HCV-related HCC	Microarray	Exclusively expressed in HCV-associated HCC	Diaz et al. [121]
miR-302b	Down	ND	HCV-related HCC	qRT-PCR	Decreased expression in HCV-related HCC	Varnholt et al. [84]
miR-320	Down	Chimera of 1a/2	Huh7, Huh-RepSI	Microarray	Relevant to carcinogenesis	Ishida et al. [80]
miR-323	Down	4	Urine of HCV-related HCC patients	Microarray, qRT-PCR	Potential HCC biomarker	Abdalla et al. [120]
miR-330	Down	ND	HCV-related HCC	qRT-PCR	Decreased expression in HCV-related HCC	Varnholt et al. [84]
miR-368	Down	ND	HCV-related HCC	qRT-PCR	Decreased expression in HCV-related HCC	Varnholt et al. [84]
miR-424-3p	Down	ND	HCV-related HCC	Microarray	Exclusively expressed in HCV-associated HCC	Diaz et al. [121]
miR-449	Down	4	Urine of HCV-related HCC patients	Microarray, qRT-PCR	Potential HCC biomarker	Abdalla et al. [120]
miR-491	Down	chimera of 1a/2	Huh7, Huh-RepSI	Microarray	Relevant to carcinogenesis	Ishida et al. [80]

MiRNA	Deregulation	HCV genotype	Type of sample	Method	Clinical relevance	Reference
miR-497	Down	ND	HCV-related HCC	Microarray	Exclusively expressed in HCV-associated HCC	Diaz et al. [121]
miR-516-5p	Down	4	Urine of HCV-related HCC patients	Microarray, qRT-PCR	Potential HCC biomarker	Abdalla et al. [120]
miR-520d	Down	4	Urine of HCV-related HCC patients	Microarray, qRT-PCR	Potential HCC biomarker	Abdalla et al. [120]
miR-650	Down	4	Urine of HCV-related HCC patients	Microarray, qRT-PCR	miR-618/650 in tandem to detect HCC among HCV-positive patients	Abdalla et al. [120]
miR-761	Down	ND	HCV-related HCC	Microarray	Exclusively expressed in HCV-associated HCC	Diaz et al. [121]
miR-9*	Down	ND	HCV-related HCC	qRT-PCR	Decreased expression in HCV-related HCC	Varnholt et al. [84]
miR-95	Down	ND	HCV-related HCC	qRT-PCR	Decreased expression in HCV-related HCC	Varnholt et al. [84]
let-7 family	Down	ND	Mainly HCV-related HCC	Microarray	Deregulated in HCV-related HCC	Gramantieri et al. [122]

Abbreviations: HCC, hepatocellular carcinoma; NGS, next-generation sequencing; ND, no data available; qRT-PCR, quantitative real-time polymerase chain reaction.

* Different mature miRNA from the same stem loop.

Table 2. Studies reporting on miRNA deregulation in HCV-infected patients with HCC- or in HCV-expressing cell lines.

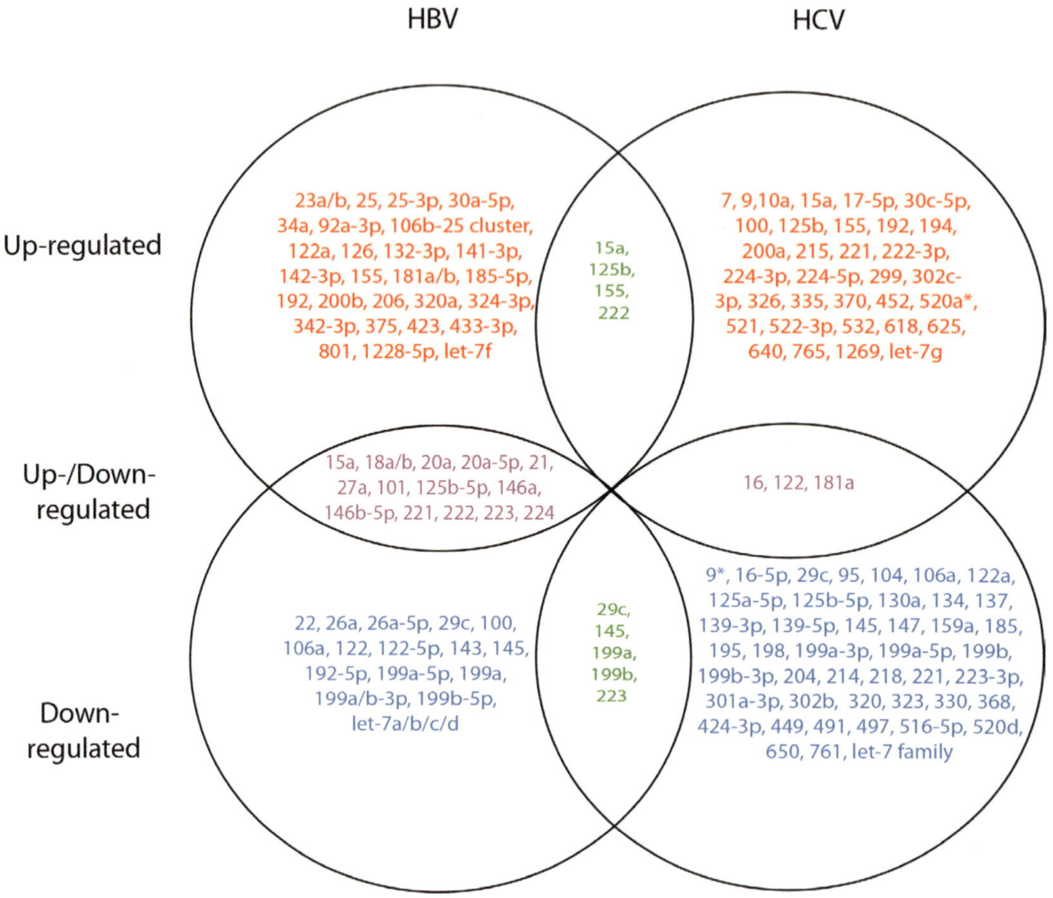

Figure 1. miRNAs deregulated in HBV- and HCV-related HCC or HBV/HCV-expression cell lines. miRNAs upregulated in HBV and HCV infections are presented in red color, miRNAs downregulated in HBV and HCV infections are presented in blue color, while miRNAs that were shown to be up- and downregulated in different studies are presented in violet color. MiRNAs reported to be up- or downregulated in HBV and HCV infections are presented in green color.

Despite the fact that several studies examined the expression of miRNAs in HCC, discrepancies exist among published data. Diaz et al. [121] assumed that non-concordance may be the result of differences in selection of noncancerous control samples or commonly included HCC samples without prior confirmation of possible HBV or HCV infection. In some previous studies, Diaz et al. [121] investigated the expression of miRNAs in HCV-induced HCC, in comparison to a wide range of liver samples and identified 18 miRNAs exclusively expressed in HCV-induced HCC. Several other studies have as well examined subsets of miRNAs potentially involved in hepatocellular changes, advancing to HCC [80, 84, 122].

According to an increasing amount of miRNAs identified and examined throughout various stages Of HBV/HCV infection and HCC development (**Tables 1** and **2**), miRNAs not specifically presented in this review should be as well included as a subject of interest in future studies.

http://dx.doi.org/10.5772/66498

7.4. MiRNA-122 in HBV and HCV

The levels of liver-specific miRNA-122 (miR-122) are down- and upregulated in HBV and HCV, respectively. The miR-122 promotes the replication of HCV and blocks the replication of HBV. It has been shown recently that HBV inhibits the miR-122 expression, suggesting a possibility of miR-122 replacement therapy in HBV-infected individuals [61, 64]. The study by Fan et al. [62] showed that miR-122 inhibited the expression of the NDRG3 protein, which subsequently inhibited malignant cell transformation and presented the miR-122 and its target NDRG3 as key diagnostic markers and potential therapeutic targets in HBV-related HCC. On the other hand, in HCV infections, it has been shown *in vitro* and *in vivo* that antagonistic utility of miR-122 inhibits HCV replication cycle and reduces viral load, and thus represents an effective treatment of HCV infection. A model of Miravirsen interaction with miR-122 is shown in **Figure 2** [77, 123].

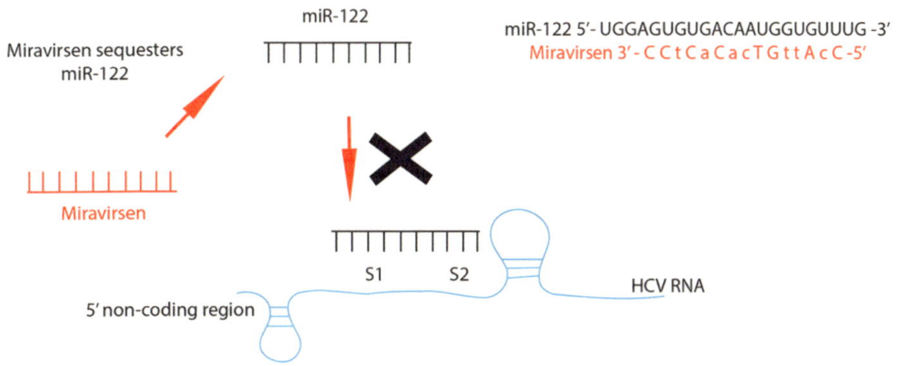

Figure 2. Miravirsen interaction with miR-122 inhibits binding between miR-122 and the 5′ UTR of the HCV RNA. The most abundant liver miRNA-miRNA-122 binds with two seed sites in the 5′ UTR of the HCV genome. Miravirsen sequesters mature miR-122 and suppresses HCV.

Recently, the safety and efficacy of the Miravirsen, a locked nucleic acid form of antisense-miR-122 that sequesters miR-122, has been evaluated in a phase 2a clinical study, which included 36 patients with chronic HCV genotype 1 infection from seven international sites [40]. The study observed that treatment with Miravirsen prolonged dose-dependent reductions in HCV RNA, without evidence of viral resistance [40]. Moreover, a recent study, conducted on 51 HCV-infected Japanese patients, treated with interferon, presented miR-122 as an independent predictor of SVR [124]. Unfortunately, no single miRNA representing a promising treatment option in HBV infections has been pointed out as yet.

Nevertheless, therapies that silence HBV RNAs are emerging. Multiple cell-line-based studies and *in vivo* studies on mouse models have evaluated synthetically engineered or chemically modified small RNAs that complementarily target HBV transcripts and lead to RNA degradation and thus to the inhibition of HBV replication. However, due to short duration of their activity, the lack of applicable animal model for testing in clinical trials, and subsequent pharmacokinetic difficulties, further investigations are warranted to evaluate RNA-interference-based approaches to clinical practice (reviewed by Ivacik et al. [125]).

HBV/HCV dual infection is not an uncommon event, occurring in approximately 2–10% of chronically infected HCV patients and in 5–20% of chronically infected HBV patients [126]. Dual HBV/HCV infection has prognosis of a more aggressive clinical course of liver disease than either mono-infection. Despite the fact that compiling evidence exists on reciprocal inhibition between HBV and HCV and that miR-122 represents a crucial host gene involved in pathogenesis of both viruses, the role of miR-122 in HBV/HCV dual infection has not been defined so far [127].

8. Conclusion

Cellular miRNAs contribute to HBV and HCV pathogenesis by direct or indirect interactions with viral genome or proteins and molecules critical for regulation of the cell cycle. Regulation of miRNAs expression upon HBV and HCV infection significantly differs between both viruses. Reports summarized in this chapter indicate that miRNAs represent an effective, noninvasive biomarker tools for early diagnosis of HBV and HCV infection, early diagnosis of liver disease and its progressive stages, particularly HCC. Mimic and antagonistic effects of cellular miRNAs have been considered in diagnostic and treatment of HBV/HCV-related liver disease, with miR-122 representing a promising treatment option for chronic infection with HCV genotype 1. Because most studies identified and validated miRNAs in heterogenic tumors and because miRNA targets were validated mostly in the already-transformed cell culture systems, transfected with plasmids encoding HBV or HCV genome or parts of their genome, discrepancies exist in candidate biomarker miRNAs across published studies. Due to an extensive number of miRNA targets and other clinical factors considered in significant number of studies published in the last 10 years, efforts should be made to establish a specific, repetitive, and easy-to-operate method to identify reliable panels of miRNA biomarkers for early diagnosis and treatment of HBV-HCV-related diseases. Suitable reference miRNA targets and positive and negative controls should be included in such profiling applications. The application of novel techniques such as next-generation sequencing, development of synthetic small RNAs, and hepatoma cell lines will impact the subsequent advances in miRNA studies related to HBV and HCV pathogenesis as well as miRNA deregulation in other pathological conditions.

Author details

Mateja M. Jelen and Damjan Glavač*

*Address all correspondence to: damjan.glavac@mf.uni-lj.si

Department of Molecular Genetics, Institute of Pathology, Faculty of Medicine, University of Ljubljana, Ljubljana, Slovenia

References

[1] Horvat RT TR. Hepatitis B and D viruses. 2015. In: Manual of Clinical Microbiology (eds. Jorgensen JH, Pfaller MA, Carroll KC, Funke G, Landry5 ML, Richter SS, Warnock DW). Washington DC: ASM Press. 11st. [1841–58].

[2] Forman MS VA. Hepatitis C virus. 2015. In: Manual of Clinical Microbiology (eds. Jorgensen JH, Pfaller MA, Carroll KC, Funke G, Landry5 ML, Richter SS, Warnock DW). Washington DC: ASM Press. 11st. [1599–840].

[3] Lytle JR, Yario TA, Steitz JA. Target mRNAs are repressed as efficiently by microRNA-binding sites in the 5′ UTR as in the 3′ UTR. Proceedings of the National Academy of Sciences of the United States of America. 2007;104(23):9667–72.

[4] Mahgoub A, Steer CJ. MicroRNAs in the evaluation and potential treatment of liver diseases. Journal of Clinical Medicine. 2016;5(5) (doi: 10.3390/jcm5050052).

[5] Fiorino S, Bacchi-Reggiani ML, Visani M, Acquaviva G, Fornelli A, Masetti M, et al. MicroRNAs as possible biomarkers for diagnosis and prognosis of hepatitis B- and C-related-hepatocellular-carcinoma. World Journal of Gastroenterology. 2016;22(15): 3907–36.

[6] Majumdar A, Kitson MT, Roberts SK. Systematic review: current concepts and challenges for the direct-acting antiviral era in hepatitis C cirrhosis. Alimentary Pharmacology & Therapeutics. 2016;43(12):1276–92.

[7] EASL clinical practice guidelines: Management of chronic hepatitis B virus infection. Journal of Hepatology. 2012;57(1):167–85.

[8] Sundaram V, Kowdley K. Management of chronic hepatitis B infection. BMJ. 2015;351:h4263 (doi: 10.1136/bmj.h4263).

[9] Te HS, Jensen DM. Epidemiology of hepatitis B and C viruses: a global overview. Clinics in Liver Disease. 2010;14(1):1–21.

[10] Mittal S, El-Serag HB. Epidemiology of hepatocellular carcinoma: consider the population. Journal of Clinical Gastroenterology. 2013;47 Suppl:S2–6 (doi: 10.1097/MCG.0b013e3182872f29).

[11] Jemal A, Bray F, Center MM, Ferlay J, Ward E, Forman D. Global cancer statistics. CA: A Cancer Journal for Clinicians. 2011;61(2):69–90.

[12] Chang MH, You SL, Chen CJ, Liu CJ, Lee CM, Lin SM, et al. Decreased incidence of hepatocellular carcinoma in hepatitis B vaccines: a 20-year follow-up study. Journal of the National Cancer Institute. 2009;101(19):1348–55.

[13] McMahon BJ, Dentinger CM, Bruden D, Zanis C, Peters H, Hurlburt D, et al. Antibody levels and protection after hepatitis B vaccine: results of a 22-year follow-up study and response to a booster dose. The Journal of Infectious Diseases. 2009;200(9):1390–6.

[14] Smith DB, Bukh J, Kuiken C, Muerhoff AS, Rice CM, Stapleton JT, et al. Expanded classification of hepatitis C virus into 7 genotypes and 67 subtypes: updated criteria and genotype assignment web resource. Hepatology. 2014;59(1):318–27.

[15] Murphy DG, Sablon E, Chamberland J, Fournier E, Dandavino R, Tremblay CL. Hepatitis C virus genotype 7, a new genotype originating from central Africa. Journal of Clinical Microbiology. 2015;53(3):967–72.

[16] Mohd Hanafiah K, Groeger J, Flaxman AD, Wiersma ST. Global epidemiology of hepatitis C virus infection: new estimates of age-specific antibody to HCV seroprevalence. Hepatology. 2013;57(4):1333–42.

[17] Kim WR, Stock PG, Smith JM, Heimbach JK, Skeans MA, Edwards EB, et al. OPTN/SRTR 2011 Annual Data Report: liver. American Journal of Transplantation: Official Journal of the American Society of Transplantation and the American Society of Transplant Surgeons. 2013;13 Suppl 1:73–102.

[18] WHO. Guidelines for the screening, care and treatment of persons with hepatitis C infection. Switzerland: WHO Press; 2014. ISBN 978 92 4 154875 5. Available at: http://apps.who.int/iris/bitstream/10665/111747/1/9789241548755_eng.pdf?ua

[19] Gower E, Estes C, Blach S, Razavi-Shearer K, Razavi H. Global epidemiology and genotype distribution of the hepatitis C virus infection. Journal of Hepatology. 2014;61(Suppl 1):S45-57.

[20] Sibley A, Han KH, Abourached A, Lesmana LA, Makara M, Jafri W, et al. The present and future disease burden of hepatitis C virus infections with today's treatment paradigm—volume 3. Journal of Viral Hepatitis. 2015;22(Suppl 4):21–41.

[21] Rodriguez A, Griffiths-Jones S, Ashurst JL, Bradley A. Identification of mammalian microRNA host genes and transcription units. Genome Research. 2004;14(10a):1902–10.

[22] Cai X, Hagedorn CH, Cullen BR. Human microRNAs are processed from capped, polyadenylated transcripts that can also function as mRNAs. RNA 2004;10(12):1957–66.

[23] Borel F, Konstantinova P, Jansen PL. Diagnostic and therapeutic potential of miRNA signatures in patients with hepatocellular carcinoma. Journal of Hepatology. 2012;56(6):1371–83.

[24] Starega-Roslan J, Koscianska E, Kozlowski P, Krzyzosiak WJ. The role of the precursor structure in the biogenesis of microRNA. Cellular and Molecular Life Sciences: CMLS. 2011;68(17):2859–71.

[25] Rajewsky N. microRNA target predictions in animals. Nature Genetics. 2006;38 Suppl:S8–13.

[26] Yekta S, Shih IH, Bartel DP. MicroRNA-directed cleavage of HOXB8 mRNA. Science. 2004;304(5670):594–6.

[27] Zeng Y, Wagner EJ, Cullen BR. Both natural and designed micro RNAs can inhibit the expression of cognate mRNAs when expressed in human cells. Molecular Cell. 2002;9(6):1327–33.

[28] miRBase. miRBase 2014 [updated 22.07.2016]. 2004. Available from: http://www.mirbase.org.

[29] Kozomara A, Griffiths-Jones S. miRBase: annotating high confidence microRNAs using deep sequencing data. Nucleic Acids Research. 2014;42(Database issue):D68–73.

[30] Kaluzna EM. MicroRNA-155 and microRNA-196b: promising biomarkers in hepatitis C virus infection? Reviews in Medical Virology. 2014;24(3):169–85.

[31] Bostjancic E, Bandelj E, Luzar B, Poljak M, Glavac D. Hepatic expression of miR-122, miR-126, miR-136 and miR-181a and their correlation to histopathological and clinical characteristics of patients with hepatitis C. Journal of Viral Hepatitis. 2015;22(2):146–57.

[32] Lewis BP, Burge CB, Bartel DP. Conserved seed pairing, often flanked by adenosines, indicates that thousands of human genes are microRNA targets. Cell. 2005;120:15–20.

[33] Ebert MS, Sharp PA. Roles for microRNAs in conferring robustness to biological processes. Cell. 2012;149(3):515–24.

[34] Croce CM. Causes and consequences of microRNA dysregulation in cancer. Nature Reviews Genetics. 2009;10(10):704–14.

[35] Volinia S, Calin GA, Liu CG, Ambs S, Cimmino A, Petrocca F, et al. A microRNA expression signature of human solid tumors defines cancer gene targets. Proceedings of the National Academy of Sciences of the United States of America. 2006;103(7):2257–61.

[36] Gasparini P, Cascione L, Landi L, Carasi S, Lovat F, Tibaldi C, et al. microRNA classifiers are powerful diagnostic/prognostic tools in ALK-, EGFR-, and KRAS-driven lung cancers. Proceedings of the National Academy of Sciences of the United States of America. 2015;112(48):14924–9.

[37] Lu J, Getz G, Miska EA, Alvarez-Saavedra E, Lamb J, Peck D, et al. MicroRNA expression profiles classify human cancers. Nature. 2005;435(7043):834–8.

[38] Geisler A, Fechner H. MicroRNA-regulated viral vectors for gene therapy. World Journal of Experimental Medicine. 2016;6(2):37–54.

[39] Kaboli PJ, Rahmat A, Ismail P, Ling KH. MicroRNA-based therapy and breast cancer: A comprehensive review of novel therapeutic strategies from diagnosis to treatment. Pharmacological Research. 2015;97:104–21.

[40] Janssen HL, Reesink HW, Lawitz EJ, Zeuzem S, Rodriguez-Torres M, Patel K, et al. Treatment of HCV infection by targeting microRNA. The New England Journal of Medicine. 2013;368(18):1685–94.

[41] Li LM, Hu ZB, Zhou ZX, Chen X, Liu FY, Zhang JF, et al. Serum microRNA profiles serve as novel biomarkers for HBV infection and diagnosis of HBV-positive hepatocarcinoma. Cancer Research. 2010;70(23):9798–807.

[42] Skalsky RL, Cullen BR. Viruses, microRNAs, and host interactions. Annual Review of Microbiology. 2010;64:123–41.

[43] Li H, Jiang JD, Peng ZG. MicroRNA-mediated interactions between host and hepatitis C virus. World Journal of Gastroenterology. 2016;22(4):1487–96.

[44] Kim N, Kim H, Jung I, Kim Y, Kim D, Han YM. Expression profiles of miRNAs in human embryonic stem cells during hepatocyte differentiation. Hepatology Research. 2011;41(2):170–83.

[45] Xu H, He JH, Xiao ZD, Zhang QQ, Chen YQ, Zhou H, et al. Liver-enriched transcription factors regulate microRNA-122 that targets CUTL1 during liver development. Hepatology. 2010;52(4):1431–42.

[46] Gamazon ER, Innocenti F, Wei R, Wang L, Zhang M, Mirkov S, et al. A genome-wide integrative study of microRNAs in human liver. BMC Genomics. 2013;14:395 (doi: 10.1186/1471-2164-14-395).

[47] Hou J, Lin L, Zhou W, Wang Z, Ding G, Dong Q, et al. Identification of miRNomes in human liver and hepatocellular carcinoma reveals miR-199a/b-3p as therapeutic target for hepatocellular carcinoma. Cancer Cell. 2011;19(2):232–43.

[48] Landgraf P, Rusu M, Sheridan R, Sewer A, Iovino N, Aravin A, et al. A mammalian microRNA expression atlas based on small RNA library sequencing. Cell. 2007;129(7):1401–14.

[49] Barad O, Meiri E, Avniel A, Aharonov R, Barzilai A, Bentwich I, et al. MicroRNA expression detected by oligonucleotide microarrays: system establishment and expression profiling in human tissues. Genome Research. 2004;14(12):2486–94.

[50] Esau C, Davis S, Murray SF, Yu XX, Pandey SK, Pear M, et al. miR-122 regulation of lipid metabolism revealed by in vivo antisense targeting. Cell Metabolism. 2006;3(2): 87–98.

[51] Krutzfeldt J, Rajewsky N, Braich R, Rajeev KG, Tuschl T, Manoharan M, et al. Silencing of microRNAs in vivo with 'antagomirs'. Nature. 2005;438(7068):685–9.

[52] Hsu SH, Wang B, Kota J, Yu J, Costinean S, Kutay H, et al. Essential metabolic, anti-inflammatory, and anti-tumorigenic functions of miR-122 in liver. The Journal of Clinical Investigation. 2012;122(8):2871–83.

[53] Finch ML, Marquardt JU, Yeoh GC, Callus BA. Regulation of microRNAs and their role in liver development, regeneration and disease. The International Journal of Biochemistry & Cell Biology. 2014;54:288–303.

[54] Liu D, Fan J, Zeng W, Zhou Y, Ingvarsson S, Chen H. Quantitative analysis of miRNA expression in several developmental stages of human livers. Hepatology Research. 2010;40(8):813–22.

[55] Tzur G, Israel A, Levy A, Benjamin H, Meiri E, Shufaro Y, et al. Comprehensive gene and microRNA expression profiling reveals a role for microRNAs in human liver development. PloS One. 2009;4(10):e7511 (doi: 10.1371/journal.pone.0007511).

[56] Cui L, Zhou X, Li J, Wang L, Wang J, Li Q, et al. Dynamic microRNA profiles of hepatic differentiated human umbilical cord lining-derived mesenchymal stem cells. PloS One. 2012;7(9):e44737 (doi: 10.1371/journal.pone.0044737).

[57] Shu J, Kren BT, Xia Z, Wong PY, Li L, Hanse EA, et al. Genome wide microRNA down-regulation as a negative feedback mechanism in the early phases of liver regeneration. Hepatology. 2011;54(2):609–19.

[58] Russo A, Potenza N. Antiviral effects of human microRNAs and conservation of their target sites. FEBS Letters. 2011;585(16):2551–5.

[59] Jin WB, Wu FL, Kong D, Guo AG. HBV-encoded microRNA candidate and its target. Computational Biology and Chemistry. 2007;31(2):124–6.

[60] Lamontagne J, Steel LF, Bouchard MJ. Hepatitis B virus and microRNAs: Complex interactions affecting hepatitis B virus replication and hepatitis B virus-associated diseases. World Journal of Gastroenterology. 2015;21(24):7375–99.

[61] Li C, Wang Y, Wang S, Wu B, Hao J, Fan H, et al. Hepatitis B virus mRNA-mediated miR-122 inhibition upregulates PTTG1-binding protein, which promotes hepatocellular carcinoma tumor growth and cell invasion. Journal of Virology. 2013;87(4):2193–205.

[62] Fan CG, Wang CM, Tian C, Wang Y, Li L, Sun WS, et al. miR-122 inhibits viral replication and cell proliferation in hepatitis B virus-related hepatocellular carcinoma and targets NDRG3. Oncology Reports. 2011;26(5):1281–6.

[63] Qiu L, Fan H, Jin W, Zhao B, Wang Y, Ju Y, et al. miR-122-induced down-regulation of HO-1 negatively affects miR-122-mediated suppression of HBV. Biochemical and Biophysical Research Communications. 2010;398(4):771–7.

[64] Wang S, Qiu L, Yan X, Jin W, Wang Y, Chen L, et al. Loss of microRNA 122 expression in patients with hepatitis B enhances hepatitis B virus replication through cyclin G(1) -modulated P53 activity. Hepatology. 2012;55(3):730–41.

[65] Zhang X, Zhang E, Ma Z, Pei R, Jiang M, Schlaak JF, et al. Modulation of hepatitis B virus replication and hepatocyte differentiation by MicroRNA-1. Hepatology. 2011;53(5):1476–85.

[66] Guo H, Liu H, Mitchelson K, Rao H, Luo M, Xie L, et al. MicroRNAs-372/373 promote the expression of hepatitis B virus through the targeting of nuclear factor I/B. Hepatology. 2011;54(3):808–19.

[67] Jin J, Tang S, Xia L, Du R, Xie H, Song J, et al. MicroRNA-501 promotes HBV replication by targeting HBXIP. Biochemical and Biophysical Research Communications. 2013;430(4):1228–33.

[68] Dai X, Zhang W, Zhang H, Sun S, Yu H, Guo Y, et al. Modulation of HBV replication by microRNA-15b through targeting hepatocyte nuclear factor 1alpha. Nucleic Acids Research. 2014;42(10):6578–90.

[69] Potenza N, Papa U, Mosca N, Zerbini F, Nobile V, Russo A. Human microRNA hsa-miR-125a-5p interferes with expression of hepatitis B virus surface antigen. Nucleic Acids Research. 2011;39(12):5157–63.

[70] Zhang Z, Chen J, He Y, Zhan X, Zhao R, Huang Y, et al. miR-125b inhibits hepatitis B virus expression in vitro through targeting of the SCNN1A gene. Archives of Virology. 2014;159(12):3335–43.

[71] Shi C, Xu X. MicroRNA-22 is down-regulated in hepatitis B virus-related hepatocellular carcinoma. Biomedicine & Pharmacotherapy = Biomedicine & Pharmacotherapy. 2013;67(5):375–80.

[72] Zhang GL, Li YX, Zheng SQ, Liu M, Li X, Tang H. Suppression of hepatitis B virus replication by microRNA-199a-3p and microRNA-210. Antiviral Research. 2010;88(2):169–75.

[73] Jung YJ, Kim JW, Park SJ, Min BY, Jang ES, Kim NY, et al. c-Myc-mediated overexpression of miR-17-92 suppresses replication of hepatitis B virus in human hepatoma cells. Journal of Medical Virology. 2013;85(6):969–78.

[74] Hu W, Wang X, Ding X, Li Y, Zhang X, Xie P, et al. MicroRNA-141 represses HBV replication by targeting PPARA. PLoS One. 2012;7(3):e34165 (doi: 10.1371/journal.pone.0034165).

[75] Liu Y, Zhao JJ, Wang CM, Li MY, Han P, Wang L, et al. Altered expression profiles of microRNAs in a stable hepatitis B virus-expressing cell line. Chinese Medical Journal. 2009;122(1):10–4.

[76] Zou C, Li Y, Cao Y, Zhang J, Jiang J, Sheng Y, et al. Up-regulated MicroRNA-181a induces carcinogenesis in hepatitis B virus-related hepatocellular carcinoma by targeting E2F5. BMC Cancer. 2014;14:97 (doi: 10.1186/1471-2407-14-97).

[77] Jopling CL, Yi M, Lancaster AM, Lemon SM, Sarnow P. Modulation of hepatitis C virus RNA abundance by a liver-specific MicroRNA. Science. 2005;309(5740):1577–81.

[78] Pedersen IM, Cheng G, Wieland S, Volinia S, Croce CM, Chisari FV, et al. Interferon modulation of cellular microRNAs as an antiviral mechanism. Nature. 2007;449(7164):919–22.

[79] Liu X, Wang T, Wakita T, Yang W. Systematic identification of microRNA and messenger RNA profiles in hepatitis C virus-infected human hepatoma cells. Virology. 2010;398(1):57–67.

[80] Ishida H, Tatsumi T, Hosui A, Nawa T, Kodama T, Shimizu S, et al. Alterations in microRNA expression profile in HCV-infected hepatoma cells: involvement of miR-491 in regulation of HCV replication via the PI3 kinase/Akt pathway. Biochemical and Biophysical Research Communications. 2011;412(1):92–7.

[81] Jopling CL. Regulation of hepatitis C virus by microRNA-122. Biochemical Society Transactions. 2008;36(Pt 6):1220–3.

[82] Shimakami T, Yamane D, Jangra RK, Kempf BJ, Spaniel C, Barton DJ, et al. Stabilization of hepatitis C virus RNA by an Ago2-miR-122 complex. Proceedings of the National Academy of Sciences of the United States of America. 2012;109(3):941–6.

[83] Coulouarn C, Factor VM, Andersen JB, Durkin ME, Thorgeirsson SS. Loss of miR-122 expression in liver cancer correlates with suppression of the hepatic phenotype and gain of metastatic properties. Oncogene. 2009;28(40):3526–36.

[84] Varnholt H, Drebber U, Schulze F, Wedemeyer I, Schirmacher P, Dienes HP, et al. MicroRNA gene expression profile of hepatitis C virus-associated hepatocellular carcinoma. Hepatology. 2008;47(4):1223–32.

[85] Zhang Y, Wei W, Cheng N, Wang K, Li B, Jiang X, et al. Hepatitis C virus-induced up-regulation of microRNA-155 promotes hepatocarcinogenesis by activating Wnt signaling. Hepatology. 2012;56(5):1631–40.

[86] Hou W, Tian Q, Zheng J, Bonkovsky HL. MicroRNA-196 represses Bach1 protein and hepatitis C virus gene expression in human hepatoma cells expressing hepatitis C viral proteins. Hepatology. 2010;51(5):1494–504.

[87] Bhanja Chowdhury J, Shrivastava S, Steele R, Di Bisceglie AM, Ray R, Ray RB. Hepatitis C virus infection modulates expression of interferon stimulatory gene IFITM1 by upregulating miR-130A. Journal of Virology. 2012;86(18):10221–5.

[88] Zhang S, Ouyang X, Jiang X, Gu D, Lin Y, Kong SK, et al. Dysregulated Serum MicroRNA Expression Profile and Potential Biomarkers in Hepatitis C Virus-infected Patients. International Journal of Medical Sciences. 2015;12(7):590–8.

[89] Shwetha S, Gouthamchandra K, Chandra M, Ravishankar B, Khaja MN, Das S. Circulating miRNA profile in HCV infected serum: novel insight into pathogenesis. Scientific Reports. 2013;3:1555.

[90] Elhelw DS, Mekky RY, El-Ekiaby N, Ahmed R, Eldin MA, El-Sayed M, et al. Predictive prognostic role of with discrepancy in the liver and serum of genotype 4 hepatitis C virus patients. Biomedical Reports. 2014;2(6):843–8.

[91] Oliveira KG, Malta FM, Nastri AC, Widman A, Faria PL, Santana RA, et al. Increased hepatic expression of miRNA-122 in patients infected with HCV genotype 3. Medical Microbiology and Immunology. 2016;205(2):111–7.

[92] Callaway E. Hepatitis C drugs not reaching poor. Nature. 2014;508:295–6.

[93] Patel M, Shariff MI, Ladep NG, Thillainayagam AV, Thomas HC, Khan SA, et al. Hepatocellular carcinoma: diagnostics and screening. Journal of Evaluation in Clinical Practice. 2012;18(2):335–42.

[94] Murakami Y, Kawada N. MicroRNAs in hepatic pathophysiology. Hepatology Research. 2017;7(1):60–9.

[95] Zhang ZZ, Liu X, Wang DQ, Teng MK, Niu LW, Huang AL, et al. Hepatitis B virus and hepatocellular carcinoma at the miRNA level. World Journal of Gastroenterology. 2011;17(28):3353–8.

[96] Wei X, Xiang T, Ren G, Tan C, Liu R, Xu X, et al. miR-101 is down-regulated by the hepatitis B virus x protein and induces aberrant DNA methylation by targeting DNA methyltransferase 3A. Cellular Signalling. 2013;25(2):439–46.

[97] Fu Y, Wei X, Tang C, Li J, Liu R, Shen A, et al. Circulating microRNA-101 as a potential biomarker for hepatitis B virus-related hepatocellular carcinoma. Oncology Letters. 2013;6(6):1811–5.

[98] Yen CS, Su ZR, Lee YP, Liu IT, Yen CJ. miR-106b promotes cancer progression in hepatitis B virus-associated hepatocellular carcinoma. World Journal of Gastroenterology. 2016;22(22):5183–92.

[99] Ghosh A, Datta S, Dasgupta D, Das S, Ray S, Gupta S, et al. Hepatic miR-126 is a potential plasma biomarker for detection of hepatitis B virus infected hepatocellular carcinoma. International Journal of Cancer. 2016;138(11):2732–44.

[100] Wen Y, Han J, Chen J, Dong J, Xia Y, Liu J, et al. Plasma miRNAs as early biomarkers for detecting hepatocellular carcinoma. International Journal of Cancer. 2015;137(7):1679–90.

[101] Tan Y, Ge G, Pan T, Wen D, Chen L, Yu X, et al. A serum microRNA panel as potential biomarkers for hepatocellular carcinoma related with hepatitis B virus. PloS One. 2014;9(9):e107986 (doi: 10.1371/journal.pone.0107986).

[102] Gui J, Tian Y, Wen X, Zhang W, Zhang P, Gao J, et al. Serum microRNA characterization identifies miR-885-5p as a potential marker for detecting liver pathologies. Clinical Science. 2011;120(5):183–93.

[103] Su C, Hou Z, Zhang C, Tian Z, Zhang J. Ectopic expression of microRNA-155 enhances innate antiviral immunity against HBV infection in human hepatoma cells. Virology Journal. 2011;8:354 (doi: 10.1186/1743-422x-8-354).

[104] Zhou J, Yu L, Gao X, Hu J, Wang J, Dai Z, et al. Plasma microRNA panel to diagnose hepatitis B virus-related hepatocellular carcinoma. Journal of Clinical Oncology: 2011;29(36):4781–8.

[105] Gao P, Wong CC, Tung EK, Lee JM, Wong CM, Ng IO. Deregulation of microRNA expression occurs early and accumulates in early stages of HBV-associated multistep hepatocarcinogenesis. Journal of Hepatology. 2011;54(6):1177–84.

[106] Bandopadhyay M, Banerjee A, Sarkar N, Panigrahi R, Datta S, Pal A, et al. Tumor suppressor micro RNA miR-145 and onco micro RNAs miR-21 and miR-222 expressions are differentially modulated by hepatitis B virus X protein in malignant hepatocytes. BMC Cancer. 2014;14:721 (doi: 10.1186/1471-2407-14-721).

[107] Mizuguchi Y, Mishima T, Yokomuro S, Arima Y, Kawahigashi Y, Shigehara K, et al. Sequencing and bioinformatics-based analyses of the microRNA transcriptome in hepatitis B-related hepatocellular carcinoma. PLoS One. 2011;6(1):e15304 (doi: 10.1371/journal.pone.0015304).

[108] Wu XJ, Li Y, Liu D, Zhao LD, Bai B, Xue MH. miR-27a as an oncogenic microRNA of hepatitis B virus-related hepatocellular carcinoma. Asian Pacific Journal of Cancer Prevention: APJCP. 2013;14(2):885–9.

[109] Li L, Guo Z, Wang J, Mao Y, Gao Q. Serum miR-18a: a potential marker for hepatitis B virus-related hepatocellular carcinoma screening. Digestive Diseases and Sciences. 2012;57(11):2910–6.

[110] Giray BG, Emekdas G, Tezcan S, Ulger M, Serin MS, Sezgin O, et al. Profiles of serum microRNAs; miR-125b-5p and miR223-3p serve as novel biomarkers for HBV-positive hepatocellular carcinoma. Molecular Biology Reports. 2014;41(7):4513–9.

[111] Agostini M, Knight RA. miR-34: from bench to bedside. Oncotarget. 2014;5(4):872–81.

[112] Xie Y, Yao Q, Butt AM, Guo J, Tian Z, Bao X, et al. Expression profiling of serum microRNA-101 in HBV-associated chronic hepatitis, liver cirrhosis, and hepatocellular carcinoma. Cancer Biology & Therapy. 2014;15(9):1248–55.

[113] Winther TN, Heiberg IL, Bang-Berthelsen CH, Pociot F, Hogh B. Hepatitis B surface antigen quantity positively correlates with plasma levels of microRNAs differentially expressed in immunological phases of chronic hepatitis B in children. PLoS One. 2013;8(11):e80384 (doi: doi: 10.1371/journal.pone.0080384).

[114] Yu G, Chen X, Chen S, Ye W, Hou K, Liang M. MiR-19a, miR-122 and miR-223 are differentially regulated by hepatitis B virus X protein and involve in cell proliferation in hepatoma cells. Journal of Translational Medicine. 2016;14(1):122 (doi: 10.1186/s12967-016-0888-7).

[115] Webster DP, Klenerman P, Dusheiko GM. Hepatitis C. Lancet. 2015;385(9973):1124–35.

[116] Motawi TM, Sadik NA, Shaker OG, Ghaleb MH. Elevated serum microRNA-122/222 levels are potential diagnostic biomarkers in Egyptian patients with chronic hepatitis C but not hepatic cancer. Tumour Biology. 2016;37(7):9865–74.

[117] El-Garem H, Ammer A, Shehab H, Shaker O, Anwer M, El-Akel W, et al. Circulating microRNA, miR-122 and miR-221 signature in Egyptian patients with chronic hepatitis C related hepatocellular carcinoma. World Journal of Hepatology. 2014;6(11):818–24.

[118] El-Abd NE, Fawzy NA, El-Sheikh SM, Soliman ME. Circulating miRNA-122, miRNA-199a, and miRNA-16 as biomarkers for early detection of hepatocellular carcinoma in egyptian patients with chronic Hepatitis C virus infection. Molecular Diagnosis & Therapy. 2015;19(4):213–20.

[119] Oksuz Z, Serin MS, Kaplan E, Dogen A, Tezcan S, Aslan G, et al. Serum microRNAs; miR-30c-5p, miR-223-3p, miR-302c-3p and miR-17-5p could be used as novel non-invasive biomarkers for HCV-positive cirrhosis and hepatocellular carcinoma. Molecular Biology Reports. 2015;42(3):713–20.

[120] Abdalla MA, Haj-Ahmad Y. Promising candidate urinary microRNA biomarkers for the early detection of hepatocellular carcinoma among high-risk hepatitis C virus Egyptian patients. Journal of Cancer. 2012;3:19–31.

[121] Diaz G, Melis M, Tice A, Kleiner DE, Mishra L, Zamboni F, et al. Identification of microRNAs specifically expressed in hepatitis C virus-associated hepatocellular carcinoma. International Journal of Cancer. 2013;133(4):816–24.

[122] Gramantieri L, Ferracin M, Fornari F, Veronese A, Sabbioni S, Liu CG, et al. Cyclin G1 is a target of miR-122a, a microRNA frequently down-regulated in human hepatocellular carcinoma. Cancer Research. 2007;67(13):6092–9.

[123] Lanford RE, Hildebrandt-Eriksen ES, Petri A, Persson R, Lindow M, Munk ME, et al. Therapeutic silencing of microRNA-122 in primates with chronic hepatitis C virus infection. Science. 2010;327(5962):198–201.

[124] Kamo Y, Ichikawa T, Miyaaki H, Uchida S, Yamaguchi T, Shibata H, et al. Significance of miRNA-122 in chronic hepatitis C patients with serotype 1 on interferon therapy. Hepatology Research: 2015;45(1):88–96.

[125] Ivacik D, Ely A, Arbuthnot P. Countering hepatitis B virus infection using RNAi: how far are we from the clinic? Reviews in Medical Virology. 2011;21(6):383–96.

[126] Chu CJ, Lee SD. Hepatitis B virus/hepatitis C virus coinfection: epidemiology, clinical features, viral interactions and treatment. Journal of Gastroenterology and Hepatology. 2008;23(4):512–20.

[127] Song K, Han C, Dash S, Balart LA, Wu T. MiR-122 in hepatitis B virus and hepatitis C virus dual infection. World Journal of Hepatology. 2015;7(3):498–506.

Chapter 16

Can Proteomic Profiling Identify Biomarkers and/or Therapeutic Targets for Liver Fibrosis?

Seyma Katrinli, H. Levent Doganay, Kamil Ozdil and
Gizem Dinler-Doganay

Additional information is available at the end of the chapter

http://dx.doi.org/10.5772/65608

Abstract

Liver fibrosis is a serious disease that affects around 350–400 million people worldwide. The main approach for fibrosis staging is liver biopsy, which is an invasive procedure that is not endured pretty well by patients. Currently, some serum-based biomarker panels are available for diagnosis and staging of liver fibrosis. Recent high-throughput proteomic studies are also very promising for identification of novel biomarkers for diagnosis and/or treatment of liver fibrosis. We hereby review the application of proteomic profiling studies for identification of fibrosis biomarkers with their advantages and drawbacks.

Keywords: proteome profiling, liver fibrosis, biomarkers, therapeutic markers

1. Liver fibrosis

Liver fibrosis results from chronic damage to the liver and causes accumulation of excessive matrix or scar. This scar tissue may inhibit blood flow due to the contraction of liver that results progressive liver damage and cirrhosis (the most advanced stage of liver fibrosis) or even hepatocellular carcinoma (HCC) [1]. Liver fibrosis is prominently observed in chronic liver diseases such as viral hepatitis, alcoholic steatohepatitis, nonalcoholic fatty liver disease (NAFLD), toxic liver injury, auto-immune diseases, and some genetic diseases [2]. From these chronic liver diseases, chronic hepatitis B (CHB) and chronic hepatitis C are major global health problems, and despite national vaccination programs, around 350–400 million people are infected with hepatitis B virus (HBV) and 130–150 million people are infected with hepatitis C virus (HCV) worldwide [3, 4]. Chronic HBV (CHB) infection results in liver fibrosis that can further develop into cirrhosis or HCC, both being the major causes of liver-related death [5]. The annual incidence of cirrhosis in patients infected with HBV has been evaluated at 1.3–2.4% [6], and although the cumulative 5-year-old survival rate for patients with compensated cirrhosis is 84% [7], in patients with decompensated cirrhosis, this survival rate decreases to 14–35% [7, 8].

Regeneration of liver is an extremely complex process, but recent studies in human and animal models have indicated that liver fibrosis could be reversible in specific cases [9, 10]. It is hoped that deeper understanding of the etiology of liver fibrosis will contribute to improved diagnostic tools and potential therapeutic approaches for liver fibrosis and cirrhosis. Even though curing the underlying disease may reverse fibrosis progression, currently, the most effective treatment that prolongs survival in advanced cirrhotic patients is liver transplantation [11]. However, this approach is limited because of the shortages of organs, the presence of concurrent disease affecting other tissues, and recurrence of the original disease in transplant patients [12]. Despite the advancement in noninvasive tests, liver biopsy still remains as the gold standard test for evaluation of liver disease severity [13–16]. However, it has several disadvantages such as invasive character, sampling errors and limitations for effective surveillance, and follow-up [17–19]. Upon antiviral treatment, HCV-infected patients may clear HCV RNA from their bloodstream [5]. For the treatment of CHB, current therapies do not accomplish complete eradication of HBV infection. HBV remains in infected hepatocytes in the form of covalently closed circular DNA (cccDNA) even if the patient clears HBsAg, and this cccDNA can possibly be reactivated with the right stimulus [20]. Hence, the therapeutic strategy for CHB is to prevent liver fibrosis and the other complications of advanced liver disease that can further develop cirrhosis and HCC. Therefore, recent studies focus on the search of biomarkers for noninvasive diagnosis and staging of liver fibrosis and for discovery of new therapeutic targets to prevent HBV-related liver fibrosis.

Proteomics, which studies the complex protein mixtures in a biological system, is a valuable tool to investigate cellular pathways, protein–protein interactions, and identify target proteins [21]. No requirement of a priori knowledge of protein identities present in a biological system makes proteomic profiling an ideal tool for screening the most discerning set of biomarkers [22].

In this review, we will focus on the advances in the proteomic research concerning liver fibrosis and evaluate whether proteomic profiling studies are applicable in the search of protein biomarkers and/or therapeutic targets for this condition with a focus on HBV and HCV infection.

2. Pathogenesis and staging of liver fibrosis

Hepatic fibrosis develops as a result of wound healing response of the liver to chronic injury in conjunction with the deposition of extracellular matrix (ECM) proteins [23]. Deposition of ECM proteins forms a fibrous scar that alters hepatic architecture, and subsequent formation of nodules of regenerating hepatocytes results in cirrhosis [24]. After an acute liver damage (e.g., HBV and HCV infection), parenchymal cells regenerate and substitute the necrotic and apoptotic cells. This process is accompanied with an inflammatory response and minor accumulation of ECM. Following persistent damage, eventually liver regeneration declines, and hepatocytes are replaced with abundant ECM, including fibrillar collagen. Origin of liver injury determines the distribution of this fibrous material. While in chronic hepatitis and chronic cholestatic disorders, the localization of fibrotic tissue is around portal tracts, in alcohol-induced liver diseases, its localization is in pericentral and perisinusoidal areas [25].

In the fibrotic liver, the main ECM-producing cells are hepatic stellate cells (HSCs) [26]. In the healthy liver, HSCs are found in the space of Disse and act as the major repository sites of vitamin A. Following sustained injury, HSCs activate or transdifferentiate into myofibroblast-like cells that have contractile, proinflammatory, and fibrogenic characteristics [27, 28]. Activated HSCs, which migrate and accumulate at the wound repair locations, secrete bulk amounts of ECM and mediate ECM degradation [29].

Some other hepatic cells, besides HSCs, may show fibrogenic properties. One of them is myofibroblasts derived from small portal vessels which reproduce around biliary tracts in cholestatis-induced liver fibrosis to induce collagen accumulation [30, 31]. The origin of the liver injury may determine the relative significance of each cell type in liver fibrogenesis. For instance, while HSCs exert the main fibrogenic activity in alcohol-induced liver fibrosis, portal myofibroblasts may be the most crucial fibrogenic cell types in viral hepatitis or chronic cholestatic disorders [1]. Thus, origin of liver injury may determine the molecular pathway differentiation in the formation of each liver disease, affecting the final proteomic outcome.

During fibrosis development, a complex interaction occurs between different hepatic cell types [32]. Most of the hepatoxic agents such as hepatitis viruses, alcohol metabolites, and bile acids target hepatocytes [33]. Injured hepatocytes secrete reactive oxygen species (ROS) and fibrogenic mediators, which triggers the activation of lymphocytes by inflammatory cells. Apoptosis of these injured hepatocytes further induces the fibrogenic actions of liver myofibroblasts [34]. Inflammatory cells such as lymphocytes and polymorphonuclear cells stimulate HSCs for collagen synthesis [35]. Activated HSCs also release inflammatory chemocines, secrete cell adhesion molecules, and mediate activation of lymphocytes [36]. Thus, a fierce cycle in which inflammatory and fibrogenic cells induce each other likely appears [37]. Kupffer cells, which are the local macrophages of liver, also greatly participate in liver inflammation by secreting ROS and cytokines [38, 39]. In conclusion, fibrogenesis is directly activated by alterations in the ECM composition and this altered ECM can serve as a repository for MMPs, growth factors, and inflammatory cytokines [1, 40].

Fibrosis progression is generally evaluated by two different accepted scoring systems: Ishak (modified Knodell score) and METAVIR scores. While in METAVIR, only interface hepatitis and lobular necrosis are used to determine the grade of activity, in Ishak, portal infiltrate and confluent necrosis are included with the two previous parameters [41]. Generally, fibrosis begins to develop as expansion of portal tracts occurring with interface hepatitis. As fibrosis advances, portal-portal linkage develops in conjunction with septa formation. At the end, fibrous tissue completely surrounds hepatocyte nodules. While complete cirrhosis develops generally in several years in some circumstances such as in the case of viral hepatitis, following liver transplantation cirrhosis may develop much more rapidly. Parenchymal fibrosis can also be observed in the presence of lobular inflammation, especially in areas of bridging necrosis [42]. This may be the cause of portal-central septa formation, which has been considered as more crucial process in the development of cirrhosis than portal-portal linkages [43]. In the terminology of liver fibrosis, septa indicate expansion of portal tract edges without formation of bridges or actual connection between portal areas or portal area and central vein. On the other hand, the term bridge is used to assess actual fibrous connection between two portal areas or portal area and central vein [44]. It is important to consider these mentioned staging systems in a descriptive sense that a patient with stage 2 fibrosis cannot be assumed to have sustained twice as much liver damage as one with stage 1 fibrosis, nor half as much as one with stage 4 fibrosis because numerical stages are not evenly distributed along the progression of fibrosis, and also transition from one stage to the next one is not linear. Nonetheless, pathologists' interobserver agreement in fibrosis staging among one stage is approximately 90% [45, 46].

3. Biomarkers of liver fibrosis

An optimal biomarker of liver fibrosis would not get affected by functional distress in liver or kidneys and only be specific to liver, also be easily observed with simple, inexpensive, and noninvasive assays [13]. Liver enzymes that are routinely measured in serum such as alanine transaminase (ALT) and aspartate transaminase (AST) are not suitable biomarkers of liver fibrosis as they have poor correlation with liver fibrosis. Studies demonstrated that 20% of the biopsy-proven cirrhotic patients' ALT levels are in normal range [47]. Unfortunately, canonical markers of liver synthetic dysfunction [e.g., albumin, platelet count (PLT), prothrombin time (PT)] are shown to be unsuccessful in the detection of early fibrotic stages [48]. Currently, novel serum proteins have been observed with altered expression in progressing liver fibrosis such as apolipoprotein A1 (ApoA1), serum transferrin, and alpha 2 macroglobulin [49–51]. Biomarker panels that incorporate combination of these individual markers are also applicable for improved accuracy of fibrotic stage assessment [46]. The most currently used biomarker panels are AST to platelet ratio index [52], FibroTest that includes apolipoprotein A1 (ApoA1), haptoglobin (HPT), gamma-glutamyl transpeptidase (γGT), γ-globin, total bilirubin, and alanine aminotransferase as biomarkers [53], and FibroIndex that combines PLT, AST, and γGT [54]. These noninvasive biomarker panels have shown to achieve good negative predictive scores in patients with low fibrosis stages and good positive predictive scores in those with advanced stages. However, intermediate fibrotic stages are not successfully interpreted by these combined biomarkers [53]. Unfortunately, this setback limits the use of current available biomarker panels for routine clinical assessments of liver fibrosis [55].

4. Current proteomic profiling methodologies

Proteomics, which is a swiftly developing area, is currently preferred in discovery of novel disease biomarkers due to its potential to surpass the drawbacks of traditional screening methods. The first step of the proteomic biomarker screening research is to separate and profile whole proteome of the biological fluid (e.g., serum, whole blood, saliva) or tissue of interest. Then, protein profile of the diseased sample is compared with a relevant control to identify the differentially expressed proteins related to that disease. Several different techniques based on in-gel separation and/or mass spectrometry are currently used for protein separation.

Mass spectrometry (MS) is the common technique in proteomic profiling methodologies. The basic concept of mass spectrometry is to evaluate the mass-to-charge (m/z) ratio for determination of the exact mass of the protein. The components of a mass spectrometry are an ion source, a mass analyzer, and a mass detector. Ionization of proteins is done either with matrix-assisted laser desorption/ionization (MALDI) or electrospray ionization (ESI). Following ionization, proteins pass through one or two mass analyzers that measure their m/z ratio (MS or versus tandem MS/MS). Time-of-flight (TOF) that measures the time spent by the protein through the vacuum tube in an electric field can be coupled with one or two quadrupoles (Q-TOF or Q-Q-TOF) with oscillating electric field that enables molecules with specific m/z ratios to travel without collision [56, 57].

4.1. Two-dimensional gel electrophoresis (2D-PAGE)

The 2D-PAGE technique separates protein according to two independent parameters, isoelectric point and molecular weight, and therefore provides the best resolution possible in protein separation currently [58, 59]. Following staining and digitalization with specific softwares, protein quantitation is performed by evaluation of spot intensities. 2D-PAGE also enables detection of posttranslational modifications, such as phosphorylation, or presence of different protein isoforms due to the emerging shifts in protein mass or isoelectric point [46]. In addition, two-dimensional difference gel electrophoresis (2D-DIGE) presents various advances including reproducibility, detection sensitivity, and credibility of analysis [60–62]. In 2D-DIGE, different samples are labeled with charge- and mass-matched fluorescent cyanine dyes, Cy3 and Cy5. The internal standard prepared by mixing equal amounts of all samples is labeled by Cy2. The Cy3 and Cy5 labeled samples and Cy2 labeled internal standard are then mixed and co-separated on the same 2-DE gel, providing accurate spot detection and intra-gel matching with reduced experimental variations. Running internal standard within all gels also improves gel-to-gel spot matching and enables for statistically strong comparisons between protein samples [63]. At the end, protein spots cut from 2D gels were identified by mass spectrometry [64].

4.2. Liquid chromatography coupled mass spectrometry (LC-MS)

Gel-based techniques such as 2D-PAGE are not very successful and reliable for profiling of small (>10 kDa) or hydrophobic proteins; besides, the evaluation of large numbers of samples is time-consuming and expensive. LC-MS, which couples a prefractionation stage with different types of mass spectrometry, is a relatively new gel-free proteomic methodology for proteomic profiling. One of the highly used MS methods is MALDI-TOF. In this technique, first, protein mixtures are fractionated by their physicochemical characteristics such as hydrophobicity or isoelectric point by liquid chromatography. Then, bound proteins are vaporized and ionized by a laser. Finally, peptide mass is computed from the time spend to reach the detector ("time-of-flight"). Another frequently applied method is LC-MS/MS which efficiently profiles large numbers of samples with the analysis of extremely small volume samples (i.e., <75 μl) by evaluating proteins with masses ranging from 2 to 200 kDa with tremendous efficiency and reasonable reproducibility [65]. In addition, SELDI-TOF MS, which couples a prefractination stage with MALDI-TOF, is currently used for proteomic profiling studies. In SELDI, protein mixtures that selectively bind to an array with a specified characteristic are analyzed. This methodology requires very low amount of crude sample, such as serum or needle biopsy samples, and it is very efficient in analysis of low molecular weight proteins. Considering the minimal labor required for SELDI application, this technique is very useful for high-throughput screening. However, higher cost of SELDI still limits its large clinical scale usage [66–68].

5. Proteomic profiling studies in search of biomarkers for liver fibrosis

Proteomic studies on liver fibrosis mainly focus on cirrhosis and HCC, which are the very end and morbid stage of liver fibrosis. One of the earlier studies has compared tumor tissue and surrounding nontumor tissue from eight HCC patients and has showed overexpression of 14-3-3γ protein in HCC [69]. Another study has investigated the proteomic differences between tumor and adjacent nontumor tissue samples of 12 HBV-associated HCC patients and has found out upregulation of members of the heat shock protein 70 and 90 families and downregulation of metabolism-associated mitochondrial and peroxisomal proteins in HCC [70]. A recent study has analyzed sera of 40 HCC patients and 47 healthy controls and has discovered leucine-rich α2-glycoprotein (LRG) and haptoglobin (HPT) between HCV- and HBV-related HCC [71]. Molleken and Sitek (72) also have analyzed cirrhotic septa and liver parenchyma of seven cirrhotic patients and discovered an increase in cell structure-associated proteins, which are actin, prolyl 4-hydroxylase, tropomyosin, calponin, transgelin, and human microfibril-associated protein 4 (MFAP-4). However, all these studies investigate the alterations occurring at the very end stage of fibrosis and did not give information about the proteomic changes during fibrosis progression.

To identify therapeutic targets and their involved pathways in fibrosis, the proteomic changes between different fibrotic stages should be investigated. There are several studies that focus on proteomic changes between different fibrotic stages. One of these studies has investigated serum protein profiles of HCV-infected patients and has showed that Mac-2-binding protein, α-2-macroglobin, and hemopexin were increased in cirrhosis, and α-1-antitrypsin, LRG, and fetuin-A (also named as alpha-2-HS-glycoprotein) were decreased in cirrhosis [73]. A recent research, which has enrolled sera of 16 healthy controls and 45 HCV patients with different fibrotic stages graded due to METAVIR, has found out that α-2-macroglobin (A2M) was increased, while vitamin D-binding protein (VDBP) and apolipoprotein A1 (ApoA1) were decreased in late fibrosis [51]. One of the studies examining serum samples of seven healthy controls and 27 HBV-infected patients with different stages of fibrosis has shown that fibrinogen, collagen, A2M, hemopexin, α-1-antitrypsin, transthyretin, and thiredoxin peroxidase were upregulated, while HPT, serotransferrin, CD5 antigen-like protein, clusterin, ApoA1, and LRG were downregulated along with fibrogenesis [74]. A recent study has analyzed sera of 19 CHB, six HBV-related cirrhotic patients, and five healthy controls and observed increased plasma myeloperoxidase levels in cirrhotic patients and decreased transthyretin, ceruloplasmin, and α-1-antitrypsin levels in both CHB- and HBV-related cirrhosis patients and downregulation of ApoA1 in HBV-related cirrhosis [75]. These studies about liver fibrosis have revealed the proteomic changes of serum samples throughout fibrogenesis. There are few studies that investigated proteomic changes in HCV-associated fibrogenesis. Diamond et al. demonstrated the effect of oxidative stress proteins to fibrosis progression in biopsy samples of HCV-infected patients [76]. The same group recently analyzed proteomic mechanisms of HCV-mediated liver fibrosis in posttransplant recipients by LC-MS (liquid chromatography coupled mass spectrometry) and demonstrated once again the important role of enhanced oxidative stress in the rapid fibrosis progression observed in HCV-infected liver transplant patients [77]. Ferrin et al. studied liver biopsies of HCV-infected alcoholic patients with cirrhosis for altered proteins in the progression of HCC and observed deregulation of ceruloplasmin (CP), paraoxanase (PON1), complement component 4a (CD4a), and fibrinogen-α (FGA) expression [78]. Another study investigated the differences in the protein profiles between liver samples from HBV-infected transgenic mouse and nontransgenic mouse and demonstrated increased aldehyde dehydrogenase 2 (ALDH2), protein disulfide isomerase precursor (PRDX1), actin, 78 kDa glucose-regulated protein (GRP78), tumor rejection antigen (GRP94), keratin 18 (KRT18), and decreased glutamate dehydrogenease 1 (GLUD1) and high mobility group 1 (HMGB1) protein levels [79]. An extensive list of potential biomarkers emerging from these studies is listed in **Table 1**.

Currently, studies also focused on understanding whether proteomic alterations may predict the treatment response in chronic hepatitis C. Hence, the effect of pegylated interferon (PegIFN) plus ribavirin (RBV) therapy, which is the common HCV treatment, may be understood better. When the serum samples from patients with chronic hepatitis C were subjected to metabolomics analysis to investigate the pretreatment and posttreatment characteristics of their metabolites by using capillary electrophoresis and liquid chromatography coupled mass spectrometry, tryptophan has been found to be associated with response to PegIFN/RBV therapy [82]. Moreover, identification of factors that predict virological response to antiviral therapy may improve treatment response through patient-specific treatment strategy. Recent studies revealed significant variances in proteome profiles throughout longitudinal serum samples in virological responders, in patients with mild fibrosis, and in those with mild necroinflammation [83]. In the current phase 2 studies (PROVE1, PROVE2, and PROVE3) of the direct-acting antiviral drug telaprevir, serum samples from responders and nonresponders to HCV treatment were analyzed by proteomic profiling and 15 differentially expressed proteins, with seven of them belonging to focal adhesion proteins or other macromolecular assemblies that constitute structural links between integrins and the actin cytoskeleton, were observed [84]. The ultimate goal of performing pretreatment serum proteome profiling prior to treatment is to predict sustained virological response (SVR) and nonresponse (NR) to antiviral drugs in chronic HCV infection and design suitable treatments for each patient.

Protein	Proteomic Analysis	Sample	Disease	Positive or Nagative Marker[a]	Reference
5′-3′ exoribonuclease 1	LC-MS	Liver biopsy	HCV	+	[77]
78 kDa glucose regulated protein, GRP78	2D-DIGE	Mouse liver tissue	HBV	+	[79]
A-1-antitrypsin	2D-PAGE	Serum	HCV	-	[73]
	2D-DIGE	Serum	HBV	+	[74]
Actin	2D-PAGE	Liver tissue	HCV	+	[72]
	2D-DIGE	Mouse liver tissue	HBV	+	[79]
Aldehyde dehydrogenase 2	2D-DIGE	Mouse liver tissue	HBV	+	[79]
Apolipoprotein A1	2D-PAGE	Serum	CHB	-	[75]
	2D-DIGE	Serum	HBV	-	[74]
	2D-DIGE	Serum	HCV	-	[51]
Aryl sulfotransferase 1A3	LC-MS	Liver biopsy	HCV	+	[77]
Bone martr stromal cell antigen 2	LC-MS	Liver biopsy	HCV	+	[77]
Calponin	LC-MS	Liver biopsy	HCV	+	[80]
	2D-PAGE	liver tissue	HCV	+	[72]
Carboxymethylenebutenolisade homologue	LC-MS	Liver biopsy	HCV	-	[77]
CD44 antigen	LC-MS	Liver biopsy	HCV	+	[77]
CD5 antigen like protein	2D-DIGE	Serum	HBV	-	[74]
Ceruloplasmin	2D-DIGE	Serum	HCV	+	[78]
Clusterin	2D-DIGE	Serum	HBV	-	[74]
Collagen	2D-DIGE	Serum	HBV	+	[74]
	LC-MS	Liver biopsy	HCV	+	[80]
Complement component 4a	2D-DIGE	Serum	HCV	+	[78]
Cystathione beta synthase	LC-MS	Liver biopsy	HCV	-	[77]
Cysteine and glycine rich protein 2	LC-MS	Liver biopsy	HCV	+	[80]
Cytochrome b-245 beta	LC-MS	Liver biopsy	HCV	+	[77]
Cytochrome c	LC-MS	Liver biopsy	HCV	+	[76]
Fetuin A	2D-PAGE	Serum	HCV	-	[73]
Fibrinogen	2D-DIGE	Serum	HCV	+	[78]
	2D-DIGE	Serum	HBV	+	[74]
Fibulin-5	LC-MS	Liver biopsy	HCV	+	[80]
FK506 binding protein 14	LC-MS	Liver biopsy	HCV	-	[77]
Gelsolin	2D-PAGE	Serum	HBV	-	[81]
Glutamate dehydrogenase 1	2D-DIGE	Mouse liver tissue	HBV	-	[79]
Gluthatione-S-transferases	LC-MS	Liver biopsy	HCV	-	[77]
Haptoglobin	2D-PAGE	Serum	HCV	-	[73]
	2D-DIGE	Serum	HBV	-	[74]
Hemopexin	2D-PAGE	Serum	HCV	+	[73]
	2D-DIGE	Serum	HBV	+	[74]
High mobility group 1	2D-DIGE	Mouse liver tissue	HBV	-	[79]

http://dx.doi.org/10.5772/65608

Protein	Proteomic Analysis	Sample	Disease	Positive or Nagative Marker[a]	Reference
Human leukocyte antigen class 2 antigen DR beta 1	LC-MS	Liver biopsy	HCV	+	[77]
Human leukocyte antigen class I antigen C	LC-MS	Liver biopsy	HCV	+	[77]
Keratin 18	2D-DIGE	Mouse liver tissue	HBV	+	[79]
Leucine-rich α-2-glycoprotein	2D-PAGE	Serum	HCV	-	[73]
	2D-DIGE	Serum	HBV	-	[74]
Leukotriene	LC-MS	Liver biopsy	HCV	+	[77]
Lumican	LC-MS	Liver biopsy	HCV	+	[80]
Mac-2-binding protein	2D-PAGE	Serum	HCV	+	[73]
Macroglobin	2D-PAGE	Serum	HCV	+	[73]
	2D-DIGE	Serum	HBV	+	[74]
	2D-DIGE	serum	HCV	+	[51]
Microfibril-associated glycoprotein 4	LC-MS	Liver biopsy	HCV	+	[80]
	2D-PAGE	liver tissue	HCV	+	[72]
Paraoxanase 1	2D-DIGE	Serum	HCV	+	[78]
Peroxiredoxin 1	2D-DIGE	Mouse liver tissue	HBV	+	[79]
Peroxiredoxin 2	2D-DIGE	Serum	HBV	-	[74]
Peroxiredoxin 5	LC-MS	Liver biopsy	HCV	+/-	[76]
Plasma myeloperoxidase	2D-PAGE	Serum	CHB	+	[75]
Prealbumin	2D-DIGE	Serum	HBV	+	[74]
Pre-angiotensionogen	LC-MS	Liver biopsy	HCV	+/-	[77]
Prolyl 4-hydroxylase	2D-PAGE	liver tissue	HCV	+	[72]
Protein disulfide isomerase precursor	2D-DIGE	Mouse liver tissue	HBV	+	[79]
Proteosome beta subunit type 4	LC-MS	Liver biopsy	HCV	+	[77]
Retinal dehydrogenase	LC-MS	Liver biopsy	HCV	+/-	[76]
Serotransferrin	2D-DIGE	Serum	HBV	-	[74]
Serum amyloid A1	LC-MS	Liver biopsy	HCV	+/-	[77]
Superoxide dismutase 1	LC-MS	Liver biopsy	HCV	-	[77]
Thioredoxin reductase 1	LC-MS	Liver biopsy	HCV	+	[77]
Transgelin	LC-MS	Liver biopsy	HCV	+	[80]
	2D-PAGE	liver tissue	HCV	+	[72]
Tropomyosin	2D-PAGE	liver tissue	HCV	+	[72]
Tumor rejection antigen, GRP94	2D-DIGE	Mouse liver tissue	HBV	+	[79]
Vitamin D binding protein	2D-DIGE	serum	HCV	-	[51]

[a] Proteins up- (+) or downregulated (S) in liver fibrosis, as detected in proteomic studies.
[b] When multiple comparisons have been performed between individual fibrosis stages certain proteins might have been reported as positive and negative markers.

Table 1. Candidate biomarkers of liver fibrosis identified from proteomic studies.

6. Limitations of proteomics

Proteomics have been shown as a promising tool in the evaluation of the molecular insights of liver fibrosis and in complementing previously known fibrosis biomarkers. Proteomic research is prone to unexpected and sometimes unpredictable biases [85]. Especially in analysis with multiple testing, extensive care should be given to assure that alterations observed are biologically significant and associated with the target disease [86]. Moreover, the unstable nature of biological samples makes them prone to degradation and alteration during sample processing [87]. Low-abundant proteins such as some stress expressed proteins and transcription factors are quite hard to be detected by proteomic screening.

Over 90% of the total serum protein concentration is constituted by some abundant proteins such as albumin and immunoglobins. Therefore, these abundant proteins may prevent detection of low-abundant proteins [88]. Depletion of serum from high-abundant proteins may increase the resolution and detection of low-abundance proteins [89]. However, while depleting serum from albumin, some potentially important proteins may bind to albumin and be lost for the upcoming analysis [90].

For the tissue samples, the diagnostic quality of biopsied tissue is limited for the evaluation of liver fibrosis. Presentation of only a very small part of the liver (approximately 1/50,000) by needle biopsy causes high sampling variability [91, 92]. Especially since fibrotic tissue is not distributed homogeneously inside the liver, sampling errors form 10% of false-negative diagnoses [91]. Moreover, interobserver agreement is not very high for particularly intermediate fibrosis stages. By considering these facts altogether, proteomic studies of liver fibrosis carry a robust characteristic.

7. Future directions and concluding remarks

Future studies in search of biomarkers for liver fibrosis should involve an adequate reference standard. Moreover, it is fairly possible that each chronic liver disease (CLD) could have its etiology-specific biomarkers, and further research should cover the identification of optimal biomarker sets for each cause of CLD (such as HBV, HCV, NASH, alcohol abuse). Serum proteomic studies might be combined with imaging techniques such as MALDI imaging to improve the performance of noninvasive techniques [93].

In summary, proteomic studies offer a great insight into differentially expressed proteins in plasma and hepatic tissue of patients with liver fibrosis. The results of this proteomic knowledge present researchers a better understanding about the pathobiology of liver fibrosis and lead to the discovery of the best set of biomarkers for the noninvasive assessment of the clinical stage of patients.

Author details

Seyma Katrinli[1], H. Levent Doganay[2], Kamil Ozdil[2] and Gizem Dinler-Doganay[1*]

*Address all correspondence to: gddoganay@itu.edu.tr

1 Molecular Biology and Genetics Department, Istanbul Technical University, Maslak, Istanbul, Turkey

2 Department of Gastroenterology, Umraniye Teaching and Research Hospital, Umraniye, Istanbul, Turkey

References

[1] Bataller R, Brenner DA. Liver fibrosis. J Clin Investig. 2005; 115(2): 209–18.

[2] Hannivoort RA, Hernandez-Gea V, Friedman SL. Genomics and proteomics in liver fibrosis and cirrhosis. Fibrogenesis Tissue Repair. 2012; 5(1): 1.

[3] Lavanchy D. Hepatitis B virus epidemiology, disease burden, treatment, and current and emerging prevention and control measures. J Viral Hepat. 2004; 11(2): 97–107.

[4] World Health Organization Fact Sheet [Internet]. 2016 [cited 2016-07-28]. Available from: http://www.who.int/mediacentre/factsheets/fs164/en/.

[5] Calvaruso V, Craxi A. Fibrosis in chronic viral hepatitis. Best Pract Res Clin Gastroenterol. 2011; 25(2): 219–30.

[6] Liaw YF, Tai DI, Chu CM, Chen TJ. The development of cirrhosis in patients with chronic type B hepatitis: a prospective study. Hepatology. 1988; 8(3): 493–6.

[7] de Jongh FE, Janssen HL, de Man RA, Hop WC, Schalm SW, van Blankenstein M. Survival and prognostic indicators in hepatitis B surface antigen-positive cirrhosis of the liver. Gastroenterology. 1992; 103(5): 1630–5.

[8] Fattovich G, Giustina G, Schalm SW, Hadziyannis S, Sanchez-Tapias J, Almasio P, Christensen E, Krogsgaard K, Degos F, Carneiro de Moura M, et al. Occurrence of hepatocellular carcinoma and decompensation in western European patients with cirrhosis type B. The EUROHEP Study Group on Hepatitis B Virus and Cirrhosis. Hepatology. 1995; 21(1): 77–82.

[9] Desmet VJ, Roskams T. Cirrhosis reversal: a duel between dogma and myth. J Hepatol. 2004; 40(5): 860–7.

[10] Iredale JP, Benyon RC, Pickering J, McCullen M, Northrop M, Pawley S, Hovell C, Arthur MJ. Mechanisms of spontaneous resolution of rat liver fibrosis. Hepatic stellate

cell apoptosis and reduced hepatic expression of metalloproteinase inhibitors. J Clin Investig. 1998; 102(3): 538–49.

[11] Fallowfield JA, Iredale JP. Targeted treatments for cirrhosis. Expert Opin Ther Targets. 2004; 8(5): 423–35.

[12] Xu R, Zhang Z, Wang FS. Liver fibrosis: mechanisms of immune-mediated liver injury. Cell Mol Immunol. 2012; 9(4): 296–301.

[13] Afdhal NH, Nunes D. Evaluation of liver fibrosis: a concise review. Am J Gastroenterol. 2004; 99(6): 1160–74.

[14] European Association for Study of Liver; Asociacion Latinoamericana para el Estudio del Higado. EASL-ALEH Clinical Practice Guidelines: non-invasive tests for evaluation of liver disease severity and prognosis. J Hepatol. 2015; 63(1): 237–64.

[15] Kaswala DH, Lai M, Afdhal NH. Fibrosis assessment in nonalcoholic fatty liver disease (NAFLD) in 2016. Dig Dis Sci. 2016; 61(5): 1356–64.

[16] Fukui H, Saito H, Ueno Y, Uto H, Obara K, Sakaida I, Shibuya A, Seike M, Nagoshi S, Segawa M, Tsubouchi H, Moriwaki H, Kato A, Hashimoto E, Michitaka K, Murawaki T, Sugano K, Watanabe M, Shimosegawa T. Evidence-based clinical practice guidelines for liver cirrhosis 2015. J Gastroenterol. 2016; 51(7): 629–50.

[17] Thampanitchawong P, Piratvisuth T. Liver biopsy:complications and risk factors. World J Gastroenterol. 1999; 5(4): 301–4.

[18] Regev A, Berho M, Jeffers LJ, Milikowski C, Molina EG, Pyrsopoulos NT, Feng ZZ, Reddy KR, Schiff ER. Sampling error and intraobserver variation in liver biopsy in patients with chronic HCV infection. Am J Gastroenterol. 2002; 97(10): 2614–8.

[19] Poynard T, Imbert-Bismut F, Munteanu M, Messous D, Myers RP, Thabut D, Ratziu V, Mercadier A, Benhamou Y, Hainque B. Overview of the diagnostic value of biochemical markers of liver fibrosis (FibroTest, HCV FibroSure) and necrosis (ActiTest) in patients with chronic hepatitis C. Comp Hepatol. 2004; 3(1): 8.

[20] Feld JJ, Wong DK, Heathcote EJ. Endpoints of therapy in chronic hepatitis B. Hepatology. 2009; 49(5 Suppl): S96–102.

[21] Cravatt BF, Simon GM, Yates JR, 3rd. The biological impact of mass-spectrometry-based proteomics. Nature. 2007; 450(7172): 991–1000.

[22] Liotta LA, Ferrari M, Petricoin E. Clinical proteomics: written in blood. Nature. 2003; 425(6961): 905.

[23] Friedman SL. Liver fibrosis—from bench to bedside. Journal of hepatology. 2003; 38 Suppl 1: S38–53.

[24] Poynard T, Ratziu V, Benhamou Y, Opolon P, Cacoub P, Bedossa P. Natural history of HCV infection. Baillieres Best Pract Res Clin Gastroenterol. 2000; 14(2): 211–28.

[25] Pinzani M. Liver fibrosis. Springer Semin Immunopathol. 1999; 21(4): 475–90.

[26] Gabele E, Brenner DA, Rippe RA. Liver fibrosis: signals leading to the amplification of the fibrogenic hepatic stellate cell. Front Biosci. 2003; 8: d69–77.

[27] Milani S, Herbst H, Schuppan D, Kim KY, Riecken EO, Stein H. Procollagen expression by nonparenchymal rat liver cells in experimental biliary fibrosis. Gastroenterology. 1990; 98(1): 175–84.

[28] Lindquist JN, Parsons CJ, Stefanovic B, Brenner DA. Regulation of alpha1(I) collagen messenger RNA decay by interactions with alphaCP at the 3'-untranslated region. J Biol Chem. 2004; 279(22): 23822–9.

[29] Lindquist JN, Marzluff WF, Stefanovic B. Fibrogenesis. III. Posttranscriptional regulation of type I collagen. Am J Physiol Gastrointest Liver Physiol. 2000; 279(3): G471–6.

[30] Kinnman N, Housset C. Peribiliary myofibroblasts in biliary type liver fibrosis. Front Biosci. 2002; 7: d496–503.

[31] Magness ST, Bataller R, Yang L, Brenner DA. A dual reporter gene transgenic mouse demonstrates heterogeneity in hepatic fibrogenic cell populations. Hepatology. 2004; 40(5): 1151–9.

[32] Kmiec Z. Cooperation of liver cells in health and disease. Adv Anat Embryol Cell Biol. 2001; 161: III–XIII, 1–151.

[33] Higuchi H, Gores GJ. Mechanisms of liver injury: an overview. Curr Mol Med. 2003; 3(6): 483–90.

[34] Canbay A, Friedman S, Gores GJ. Apoptosis: the nexus of liver injury and fibrosis. Hepatology. 2004; 39(2): 273–8.

[35] Casini A, Ceni E, Salzano R, Biondi P, Parola M, Galli A, Foschi M, Caligiuri A, Pinzani M, Surrenti C. Neutrophil-derived superoxide anion induces lipid peroxidation and stimulates collagen synthesis in human hepatic stellate cells: role of nitric oxide. Hepatology. 1997; 25(2): 361–7.

[36] Vinas O, Bataller R, Sancho-Bru P, Gines P, Berenguer C, Enrich C, Nicolas JM, Ercilla G, Gallart T, Vives J, Arroyo V, Rodes J. Human hepatic stellate cells show features of antigen-presenting cells and stimulate lymphocyte proliferation. Hepatology. 2003; 38(4): 919–29.

[37] Maher JJ. Interactions between hepatic stellate cells and the immune system. Semin Liver Dis. 2001; 21(3): 417–26.

[38] Naito M, Hasegawa G, Ebe Y, Yamamoto T. Differentiation and function of Kupffer cells. Med Electron Microsc. 2004; 37(1): 16–28.

[39] Thurman RG. II. Alcoholic liver injury involves activation of Kupffer cells by endotoxin. Am J Physiol. 1998; 275(4 Pt 1): G605–11.

[40] Olaso E, Ikeda K, Eng FJ, Xu L, Wang LH, Lin HC, Friedman SL. DDR2 receptor promotes MMP-2-mediated proliferation and invasion by hepatic stellate cells. J Clin Investig. 2001; 108(9): 1369–78.

[41] Shiha G and Zalata K (2011). Ishak versus METAVIR: Terminology, Convertibility and Correlation with Laboratory Changes in Chronic Hepatitis C. In: Takahashi H, editor. Liver Biopsy: InTech; Croatia. ISBN: 978-953-307-644-7. Available from: http://www.intechopen.com/books/howtoreference/liver-biopsy/ishak-versus-metavir-terminology-convertibility-and-correlation-with-laboratory-changes-in-chronic-h

[42] Cooksley WG, Bradbear RA, Robinson W, Harrison M, Halliday JW, Powell LW, Ng HS, Seah CS, Okuda K, Scheuer PJ, et al. The prognosis of chronic active hepatitis without cirrhosis in relation to bridging necrosis. Hepatology. 1986; 6(3): 345–8.

[43] Desmet VJ, Gerber M, Hoofnagle JH, Manns M, Scheuer PJ. Classification of chronic hepatitis: diagnosis, grading and staging. Hepatology. 1994; 19(6): 1513–20.

[44] Ishak K, Baptista A, Bianchi L, Callea F, De Groote J, Gudat F, Denk H, Desmet V, Korb G, MacSween RN, et al. Histological grading and staging of chronic hepatitis. J Hepatol. 1995; 22(6): 696–9.

[45] Westin J, Lagging LM, Wejstal R, Norkrans G, Dhillon AP. Interobserver study of liver histopathology using the Ishak score in patients with chronic hepatitis C virus infection. Liver. 1999; 19(3): 183–7.

[46] Cowan ML, Rahman TM, Krishna S. Proteomic approaches in the search for biomarkers of liver fibrosis. Trends Mol Med. 2010; 16(4): 171–83.

[47] Stanley AJ, Haydon GH, Piris J, Jarvis LM, Hayes PC. Assessment of liver histology in patients with hepatitis C and normal transaminase levels. Eur J Gastroenterol Hepatol. 1996; 8(9): 869–72.

[48] Poynard T, Bedossa P. Age and platelet count: a simple index for predicting the presence of histological lesions in patients with antibodies to hepatitis C virus. METAVIR and CLINIVIR Cooperative Study Groups. J Viral Hepat. 1997; 4(3): 199–208.

[49] Abdollahi M, Pouri A, Ghojazadeh M, Estakhri R, Somi M. Non-invasive serum fibrosis markers: a study in chronic hepatitis. Bioimpacts. 2015; 5(1): 17–23.

[50] Cho HJ, Kim SS, Ahn SJ, Park JH, Kim DJ, Kim YB, Cho SW, Cheong JY. Serum transferrin as a liver fibrosis biomarker in patients with chronic hepatitis B. Clin Mol Hepatol. 2014; 20(4): 347–54.

[51] Ho AS, Cheng CC, Lee SC, Liu ML, Lee JY, Wang WM, Wang CC. Novel biomarkers predict liver fibrosis in hepatitis C patients: alpha 2 macroglobulin, vitamin D binding protein and apolipoprotein AI. J Biomed Sci. 2010; 17: 58.

[52] Wai CT, Greenson JK, Fontana RJ, Kalbfleisch JD, Marrero JA, Conjeevaram HS, Lok AS. A simple noninvasive index can predict both significant fibrosis and cirrhosis in patients with chronic hepatitis C. Hepatology. 2003; 38(2): 518–26.

[53] Imbert-Bismut F, Ratziu V, Pieroni L, Charlotte F, Benhamou Y, Poynard T, Group M. Biochemical markers of liver fibrosis in patients with hepatitis C virus infection: a prospective study. Lancet. 2001; 357(9262): 1069–75.

[54] Koda M, Matunaga Y, Kawakami M, Kishimoto Y, Suou T, Murawaki Y. FibroIndex, a practical index for predicting significant fibrosis in patients with chronic hepatitis C. Hepatology. 2007; 45(2): 297–306.

[55] Guha IN. Back to the future with noninvasive biomarkers of liver fibrosis. Hepatology. 2009; 49(1): 9–11.

[56] Aebersold R, Mann M. Mass spectrometry-based proteomics. Nature. 2003; 422(6928): 198–207.

[57] Schwartz JC, Senko MW, Syka JE. A two-dimensional quadrupole ion trap mass spectrometer. J Am Soc Mass Spectrom. 2002; 13(6): 659–69.

[58] O'Farrell PH. High resolution two-dimensional electrophoresis of proteins. J Biol Chem. 1975; 250(10): 4007–21.

[59] Gorg A, Postel W, Gunther S. The current state of two-dimensional electrophoresis with immobilized pH gradients. Electrophoresis. 1988; 9(9): 531–46.

[60] Unlu M, Morgan ME, Minden JS. Difference gel electrophoresis: a single gel method for detecting changes in protein extracts. Electrophoresis. 1997; 18(11): 2071–7.

[61] Tonge R, Shaw J, Middleton B, Rowlinson R, Rayner S, Young J, Pognan F, Hawkins E, Currie I, Davison M. Validation and development of fluorescence two-dimensional differential gel electrophoresis proteomics technology. Proteomics. 2001; 1(3): 377–96.

[62] Zhou G, Li H, DeCamp D, Chen S, Shu H, Gong Y, Flaig M, Gillespie JW, Hu N, Taylor PR, Emmert-Buck MR, Liotta LA, Petricoin EF, 3rd, Zhao Y. 2D differential in-gel electrophoresis for the identification of esophageal scans cell cancer-specific protein markers. Mol Cell Proteom MCP. 2002; 1(2): 117–24.

[63] Alban A, David SO, Bjorkesten L, Andersson C, Sloge E, Lewis S, Currie I. A novel experimental design for comparative two-dimensional gel analysis: two-dimensional difference gel electrophoresis incorporating a pooled internal standard. Proteomics. 2003; 3(1): 36–44.

[64] Magdeldin S, Zhang Y, Xu B, Yoshida Y, Yamamoto T (2012). Two-Dimensional Polyacrylamide Gel Electrophoresis - A Practical Perspective. In: Magdeldin S, editor. Gel Electrophoresis: InTech; Croatia. ISBN: 978-953-51-0458-2. Available from: http://www.intechopen.com/books/gel-electrophoresis-principles-and-basics/two-dimensional-polyacrylamidegel-electrophoresis-a-practical-perspective

[65] Gil GC, Brennan J, Throckmorton DJ, Branda SS, Chirica GS. Automated analysis of mouse serum peptidome using restricted access media and nanoliquid chromatography-tandem mass spectrometry. J Chromatogr B Analyt Technol Biomed Life Sci. 2011; 879(15–16): 1112–20.

[66] Hutchens TA. Automaticity and reading in learning-disabled college students. Ann N Y Acad Sci. 1993; 682: 357–8.

[67] Issaq HJ, Veenstra TD, Conrads TP, Felschow D. The SELDI-TOF MS approach to proteomics: protein profiling and biomarker identification. Biochem Biophys Res Commun. 2002; 292(3): 587–92.

[68] De Bock M, de Seny D, Meuwis MA, Chapelle JP, Louis E, Malaise M, Merville MP, Fillet M. Challenges for biomarker discovery in body fluids using SELDI-TOF-MS. J Biomed Biotechnol. 2010; 2010: 906082.

[69] Lee IN, Chen CH, Sheu JC, Lee HS, Huang GT, Yu CY, Lu FJ, Chow LP. Identification of human hepatocellular carcinoma-related biomarkers by two-dimensional difference gel electrophoresis and mass spectrometry. J Proteome Res. 2005; 4(6): 2062–9.

[70] Sun W, Xing B, Sun Y, Du X, Lu M, Hao C, Lu Z, Mi W, Wu S, Wei H, Gao X, Zhu Y, Jiang Y, Qian X, He F. Proteome analysis of hepatocellular carcinoma by two-dimensional difference gel electrophoresis: novel protein markers in hepatocellular carcinoma tissues. Mol Cell Proteomics MCP. 2007; 6(10): 1798–808.

[71] Sarvari J, Mojtahedi Z, Taghavi SA, Kuramitsu Y, Shamsi Shahrabadi M, Ghaderi A, Nakamura K. Differentially expressed proteins in chronic active hepatitis, cirrhosis, and HCC related to HCV infection in comparison with HBV infection: a proteomics study. Hepatitis. 2013; 13(7): e8351.

[72] Molleken C, Sitek B, Henkel C, Poschmann G, Sipos B, Wiese S, Warscheid B, Broelsch C, Reiser M, Friedman SL, Tornoe I, Schlosser A, Kloppel G, Schmiegel W, Meyer HE, Holmskov U, Stuhler K. Detection of novel biomarkers of liver cirrhosis by proteomic analysis. Hepatology. 2009; 49(4): 1257–66.

[73] Cheung KJ, Tilleman K, Deforce D, Colle I, Van Vlierberghe H. The HCV serum proteome: a search for fibrosis protein markers. J Viral Hepat. 2009; 16(6): 418–29.

[74] Lu Y, Liu J, Lin C, Wang H, Jiang Y, Wang J, Yang P, He F. Peroxiredoxin 2: a potential biomarker for early diagnosis of hepatitis B virus related liver fibrosis identified by proteomic analysis of the plasma. BMC Gastroenterol. 2010; 10: 115.

[75] Mohamadkhani A, Jazii FR, Sayehmiri K, Jafari-Nejad S, Montaser-Kouhsari L, Poustchi H, Montazeri G. Plasma myeloperoxidase activity and apolipoprotein A-1 expression in chronic hepatitis B patients. Arch Iran Med. 2011; 14(4): 254–8.

[76] Diamond DL, Jacobs JM, Paeper B, Proll SC, Gritsenko MA, Carithers RL, Jr., Larson AM, Yeh MM, Camp DG, 2nd, Smith RD, Katze MG. Proteomic profiling

of human liver biopsies: hepatitis C virus-induced fibrosis and mitochondrial dysfunction. Hepatology. 2007; 46(3): 649–57.

[77] Diamond DL, Krasnoselsky AL, Burnum KE, Monroe ME, Webb-Robertson BJ, McDermott JE, Yeh MM, Dzib JF, Susnow N, Strom S, Proll SC, Belisle SE, Purdy DE, Rasmussen AL, Walters KA, Jacobs JM, Gritsenko MA, Camp DG, Bhattacharya R, Perkins JD, Carithers RL, Jr., Liou IW, Larson AM, Benecke A, Waters KM, Smith RD, Katze MG. Proteome and computational analyses reveal new insights into the mechanisms of hepatitis C virus-mediated liver disease posttransplantation. Hepatology. 2012; 56(1): 28–38.

[78] Ferrin G, Rodriguez-Peralvarez M, Aguilar-Melero P, Ranchal I, Llamoza C, Linares CI, Gonzalez-Rubio S, Muntane J, Briceno J, Lopez-Cillero P, Montero-Alvarez JL, de la Mata M. Plasma protein biomarkers of hepatocellular carcinoma in HCV-infected alcoholic patients with cirrhosis. PloS One. 2015; 10(3): e0118527.

[79] Spano D, Cimmino F, Capasso M, D'Angelo F, Zambrano N, Terracciano L, Iolascon A. Changes of the hepatic proteome in hepatitis B-infected mouse model at early stages of fibrosis. J Proteome Res. 2008; 7(7): 2642–53.

[80] Bracht T, Schweinsberg V, Trippler M, Kohl M, Ahrens M, Padden J, Naboulsi W, Barkovits K, Megger DA, Eisenacher M, Borchers CH, Schlaak JF, Hoffmann AC, Weber F, Baba HA, Meyer HE, Sitek B. Analysis of disease-associated protein expression using quantitative proteomics-fibulin-5 is expressed in association with hepatic fibrosis. J Proteome Res. 2015; 14(5): 2278–86.

[81] Marrocco C, Rinalducci S, Mohamadkhani A, D'Amici GM, Zolla L. Plasma gelsolin protein: a candidate biomarker for hepatitis B-associated liver cirrhosis identified by proteomic approach. Blood Transfus. 2010; 8(Suppl. 3): s105–12.

[82] Saito T, Sugimoto M, Igarashi K, Saito K, Shao L, Katsumi T, Tomita K, Sato C, Okumoto K, Nishise Y, Watanabe H, Tomita M, Ueno Y, Soga T. Dynamics of serum metabolites in patients with chronic hepatitis C receiving pegylated interferon plus ribavirin: a metabolomics analysis. Metabolism. 2013; 62(11): 1577–86.

[83] Yen YH, Wang JC, Hung CH, Lu SN, Wang JH, Hu TH, Kee KM, Hsiao CC, Lee CM. Serum proteome predicts virological response in chronic hepatitis C genotype 1b patients treated with pegylated interferon plus ribavirin. J Formos Med Assoc. 2015; 114(7): 652–8.

[84] Hare BJ, Haseltine E, Fleming M, Chelsky D, McIntosh L, Allard R, Botfield M. A signature for immune response correlates with HCV treatment outcome in Caucasian subjects. J Proteomics. 2015; 116: 59–67.

[85] Ransohoff DF. Bias as a threat to the validity of cancer molecular-marker research. Nat Rev Cancer. 2005; 5(2): 142–9.

[86] Ransohoff DF. Rules of evidence for cancer molecular-marker discovery and validation. Nat Rev Cancer. 2004; 4(4): 309–14.

[87] Banks RE, Stanley AJ, Cairns DA, Barrett JH, Clarke P, Thompson D, Selby PJ. Influences of blood sample processing on low-molecular-weight proteome identified by surface-enhanced laser desorption/ionization mass spectrometry. Clin Chem. 2005; 51(9): 1637–49.

[88] Verrills NM. Clinical proteomics: present and future prospects. Clin Biochem Rev. 2006; 27(2): 99–116.

[89] Bjorhall K, Miliotis T, Davidsson P. Comparison of different depletion strategies for improved resolution in proteomic analysis of human serum samples. Proteomics. 2005; 5(1): 307–17.

[90] Geho DH, Liotta LA, Petricoin EF, Zhao W, Araujo RP. The amplified peptidome: the new treasure chest of candidate biomarkers. Curr Opin Chem Biol. 2006; 10(1): 50–5.

[91] Bedossa P, Dargere D, Paradis V. Sampling variability of liver fibrosis in chronic hepatitis C. Hepatology. 2003; 38(6): 1449–57.

[92] Ratziu V, Charlotte F, Heurtier A, Gombert S, Giral P, Bruckert E, Grimaldi A, Capron F, Poynard T, Group LS. Sampling variability of liver biopsy in nonalcoholic fatty liver disease. Gastroenterology. 2005; 128(7): 1898–906.

[93] Castera L, Vergniol J, Foucher J, Le Bail B, Chanteloup E, Haaser M, Darriet M, Couzigou P, De Ledinghen V. Prospective comparison of transient elastography, fibrotest, APRI, and liver biopsy for the assessment of fibrosis in chronic hepatitis C. Gastroenterology. 2005; 128(2): 343–50.

Chapter 17

New Strategy Treating Hepatitis B Virus (HBV) Infection: A Review of HBV Infection Biology

Yong-Yuan Zhang

Additional information is available at the end of the chapter

http://dx.doi.org/10.5772/66083

Abstract

Chronic hepatitis B virus (HBV) infection affects 240 million people worldwide and represents a significant burden on public health. Current antiviral treatment of chronic hepatitis B mainly focuses on inhibiting viral replication. A main deficiency of the current treatment is unable to protect uninfected liver cells or hepatocytes that cleared HBV from next rounds of infection. HBV infection biology shows that natural clearance of HBV cccDNA from infected cells frequently occurs, HBV infection including chronic HBV infection is established and maintained by multiround infection, and the course of HBV infection is largely determined by the number of round of infection. Thus, an effective treatment of HBV infection must block new rounds of infection. A proposed new strategy for treating chronic HBV infection aims to immediately interrupt infection course and to achieve HbsAg seroconversion as early as possible. Under this strategy, a main target of antiviral treatment is extracellular viruses, and an effective therapeutics is specific neutralizing (anti-HBs) antibodies. A difference in tempo and efficiency of treating HBV infection between current antivirals and neutralizing antibody is that the antivirals inhibit viral infection only after cells are virus infected while the neutralizing antibody clears viruses before the infection of cells takes place.

Keywords: hepatitis B virus, acute hepatitis B, chronic HBV infection, HBV infection biology, antivirals, neutralizing antibody, anti-HBs

1. Introduction: why we need a better understanding of HBV infection biology?

Chronic hepatitis B virus (HBV) infection affects 240 million people worldwide [1]. Estimated 4.5 million of new HBV infection occurs each year [2]. A significant portion of new HBV infections occurs in infants borne to HBV-positive mothers despite a fully scheduled HBV immunization. More than 90% of HBV-infected infants will become chronic [3–5], resulting in constant expansion of chronic HBV-infected population.

Chronic HBV infection can induce severe or repeated liver injury, which can lead to advanced liver diseases including cirrhosis [6, 7] and hepatocellular carcinoma [8]. The disease burden of HBV infection is enormous, and WHO reports that 780,000 people die of HBV-related liver diseases or complications annually [9]. In addition, as many as 70% of chronic HBV-infected patients who have persistently normal ALT already experienced significant alterations in liver histology [10–13]. We need to provide more effective treatment to chronic HBV-infected patients.

Current antiviral treatment is recommended for chronic HBV-infected patients who have evidence of liver injury related to HBV infection [14, 15]. Antivirals that mainly consist of nucleos/tide analogues can potently inhibit HBV replication, mitigate liver injury and slow-down progression of necroinflammation in the liver [16, 17]. However, the current treatment rarely clears chronic HBV infection. Majority of chronic HBV-infected patients are not suitable for current antiviral treatment. Untreated patients, despite normal ALT history, can experience unpredictable flare-ups of liver injury [18, 19]. Exacerbation insults, if occurred in patients with chronic liver injury or significant alterations in liver histology despite normal ALT, can trigger acute chronic liver failure with up to 70% mortality [20, 21].

Clearly, the current antiviral treatment strategy and available antivirals do not meet clinical needs.

Here, we briefly discuss a number of limitations of current antiviral strategy and antivirals.

1.1. Current treatment strategy does not protect virus-cleared cells or uninfected cells from new rounds of infection

Current antiviral therapy is guided by belief and strategy that a viral infection can be cleared by directly inhibiting viral replication. This approach certainly mitigates viral diseases associated with viral replication, even clears viral infection under certain circumstances, for instance, a significant portion of chronic HCV infection can be cleared with a relatively short course of direct-acting antiviral agents [22, 23]. However, it does not take consideration of viral infection biology, which is featured with multiround infection (see below). This is why current antiviral strategy cannot clear chronic HBV infection. The NA-based antiviral therapy for chronic HBV infection, even with early generation of NAs like lamivudine, can clear HBV from HBV-infected cells, evidence includes wild-type (WT) virus, or early viral population was eliminated and replaced with drug-related mutant (MT) virus [24, 25]. Additional evidence consists of 5–6 logs reduction of serum HBV DNA level [26, 27–29] and 100-fold reduction of intracellular total HBV DNA and cccDNA levels in treated animals and patients [30–32]. However, during the same period, serum HBsAg level is only reduced by two- to three fold [33], suggesting HBsAg level remains constantly high. The enduring high level of HBsAg keeps depleting the limited amount of endogenous neutralizing antibodies and leaves HBV virions that are produced by infected cells in the same livers, unneutralized and infectious, which continue to cause new rounds of infection. Under the current antiviral strategy, virus-cleared cells can immediately become infected again, gains in clearing viral infection are continuously reversed, and it is extremely difficult to establish permanent and complete viral clearance under current antiviral strategy because virus-cleared cells and uninfected cells are not protected.

1.2. Antivirals target viral replication in infected cells and do not directly act against extracellular viruses

Two events occur simultaneously during antiviral therapy. One is viral replication is inhibited intracellularly, and the other is new rounds of infection continue as long as there are unneutralized extracellular viruses and susceptible cells that are not protected. Antivirals only suppress viral replication in infected cells, reducing production of new viruses that will lower level of extracellular viruses, which eventually lead to reducing new rounds of infection. Once no more viruses available for new rounds of infection, the infection course is actually interrupted, which brings the infection course to the end. Thus, the direct impact of treatment with antivirals is to reduce viral replication while an indirect impact is leading to limiting spread of infection, which really matters in containing and clearing viral infection. However, the antivirals do not directly act against extracellular viruses that may continuously cause new rounds of infection and compromise antiviral efficacy. This feature determines relatively ineffectiveness of direct antivirals in treating chronic HBV infection.

1.3. Effectiveness of antivirals depends on HBV replication efficiency

The third issue is that antivirals do not inhibit or kill viruses that were already produced. They only inhibit producing new viruses upon replication. Antivirals will not function if there was no active viral replication. Actual effectiveness of an antiviral in treating hepatitis B is largely determined by HBV replication efficiency. In clinic, a link between HBV replication level and antiviral response has been indicated. For instance, in patients with long-term entecavir therapy, a full virological response rate was 59, 84, 90, 93, and 95% after 48, 96, 144, 192, and 240 weeks of therapy, respectively [27]. Clearly, 59% of treated patients achieved the full virological response to entecavir in the first 48 weeks, but only 16, 6, 3 and 2% of net increased response were, respectively, achieved when the therapy was extended from 48 to 96, 144, 192 and 240 weeks. The net increased response rate was progressively declined along with extending therapy period since the viral replication was increasingly depressed to very low level. The replication-dependent effectiveness determines the direct antivirals are not effective against HBV infection with inactive replication, for instance in anti-HBe–positive patients with low HBV DNA level or only HBsAg positive patients.

1.4. Ineffective against severe acute HBV diseases

Direct antivirals would not be effective in treating severe acute hepatitis B since they take a few days or longer to significantly reduce viral replication or serum viral load (a log or greater) [34–37]. They would take much longer time to mitigate pathologic injury and to improve clinical manifestations [38]. Relatively slow action and no direct inhibition of extracellular viruses highlight potential ineffectiveness of antivirals in treating fulminant hepatitis B and acute severe exacerbation of chronic HBV infection-induced liver injury, both of which induce rapidly deteriorated clinic course and high mortality [39–41].

1.5. Antivirals alone cannot completely clear viral infection

Antivirals may be no longer effective once the viral replication was inhibited to low level. Residual viruses can be secreted out, or released by turnovers of infected cells, leading to clearing infection or infected cells. The released residual viruses are small in quantity and can be completely neutralized if there is relatively sufficient amount of endogenous neutralizing antibodies, which lead to stopping the course of viral infection by blocking new rounds of infection. This scenario likely happens to clearing chronic hepatitis C virus infection with direct antivirals.

The released residual viruses following potent inhibition of virus production will still be capable of causing new rounds of infection if there were no sufficient neutralizing antibodies, prolonging the course of chronic infection. This scenario likely happens to antivirals-treated HBV-infected patients.

Clearly, antivirals alone cannot complete clearing viral infection,which requires the presence of sufficient neutralizing antibodies.

What we need is new treatment strategies and new therapeutics that can improve current treatment approach and antivirals in treating chronic HBV infection.

We believe we can find effective solutions to current problems in treating chronic HBV infection through a better understanding of HBV infection biology, which will also accelerate developing new prophylactics and therapeutics.

2. Understanding HBV infection biology

2.1. Natural course of HBV infection

Infection biology is science illustrating fundamentals of infection, which is centered on understanding how a productive infection is established and maintained. Understanding of infection biology starts with understanding natural course of infection. In this review, we only focus on the natural course of HBV infection that causes hepatitis. The natural course of hepatitis B consists of initial infection, incubation period and clinical phase (**Figure 1**).

http://dx.doi.org/10.5772/66083

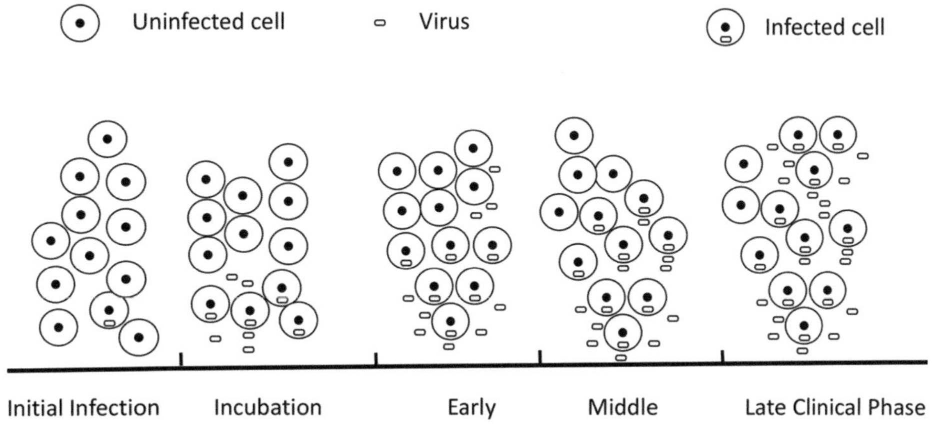

Figure 1. Schematic illustration of a typical course of infection that consists of initial infection, incubation and clinical phases. Progression of infection course is directly driven by new rounds of infections. It also suggests the infection course can be ended at any stage as long as extracellular pathogens are completely neutralized.

2.1.1. Initial HBV infection

Initial infection represents beginning of an infection and it provides seed of infection and usually consists of a few or small clusters of infected cells in the liver. The initial infection is important, but it cannot become a full-blown infection without incubation period.

2.1.2. Incubation period

The incubation refers to a period between initial infection and appearance of clinical symptoms. Length of the incubation varies considerably from individual to individual, but it is required for every HBV infection that causes hepatitis, which suggests the number of virus involved in the initial infection is so small that cannot immediately cause significant injury or clinical manifestations. Likely sequential events during the incubation include that infected HBV replicates in initial infected cells, progeny viruses are released through secretion or/and cytopathic destruction of infected cells, resulting in new rounds of infection of more cells, most likely in neighboring areas because short distances between viruses and susceptible cells favor higher efficiency of infection. Continuously released viruses keep initiating new rounds of infections, infecting more cells and extending the scope of infection. When the number of destructed cells reached an extent that causes clinical symptoms, the incubation is progressing to clinical phase.

Requirement of incubation period in full-blown HBV infection provides evidence that more than one round infection is required to establish and maintain a full-blown infection or hepatitis B (**Figure 1**). Thus, acute hepatitis B is caused by multiround of infection.

A main factor that allows multiround of infection is that there is no sufficient amount of endogenous neutralizing antibodies to neutralize the released viruses.

New rounds of infections inevitably occur during the infection course as long as there are unneutralized extracellular viruses and susceptible cells.

2.1.3. Clinical phase of acute HBV infection

Acute HBV infection in adults is a self-limiting disease, and 95% of them will be recovered without treatment [42]. A unique kinetics of serum HBV DNA level during acute HBV infection includes a rapid fall of HBV DNA level after the peak (**Figure 2**), suggesting HBV infection is being progressively cleared from the liver, as evidenced by rising ALT level (a result of destructing the infected cells) at the same time frame. Critically, it also suggests no new rounds of HBV infection, implying a block of new rounds of infection is required for clearing HBV infection. A mechanism behind these changes is called "HBsAg seroconversion," a hallmark for resolving HBV infection.

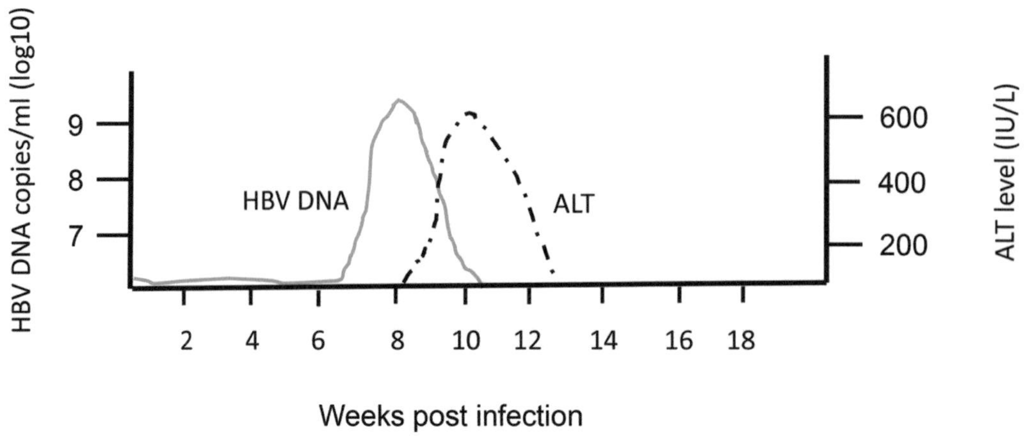

Figure 2. Kinetics of serum HBV DNA and ALT levels during acute hepatitis B. HBV DNA quickly falls after the peak, which coincides with rising ALT level. The rapid fall of HBV DNA suggests no new round infection.

When destruction of the infected cells is started during acute HBV infection, it will initially cause transit elevation of serum HBsAg and HBV DNA levels by releasing viral particles. However, the serum HBsAg and HBV DNA levels will then keep falling because the number of infected cells that supply and replenish serum HBsAg and HBV virion is progressively reduced by the liver injury (the supply reduced) while the removal or the half-life of viral particles from/in circulation should be at a constant rate, contributing to rapidly significant reduction of serum HBsAg and HBV levels. At certain point, the relative ratio between amounts of HBV particles (both viral and subviral particles) and anti-HBs antibodies will be reversed from the former greatly exceeding the latter, to the latter exceeding the former (HBsAg seroconversion). This conversion creates a sufficient anti-HBs capacity to clear serum HBsAg and to block new round infection, which allows uninfected cells and cells that cleared HBV infection permanently stay infection free. This process highlights an indispensable requirement of anti-HBs antibodies in blocking new rounds of HBV infection and resolving HBV infection.

Different impacts of liver injury on outcomes of infection are expected if occurred at different frequencies. For instance, continuous or progressive liver injury at moderate or medium scale, as is in acute hepatitis B, or at massive scale as is in fulminant hepatitis can lead to complete clearance of HBV infection because of successful reversal of the ratio of serum HBsAg and anti-HBs. On the other hand, if occurred intermittently, it unlikely leads to a complete viral clearance as is in chronic hepatitis B because of no reversal of the ratio of HBsAg and anti-HBs. The different outcomes once again emphasize that HBsAg seroconversion is critically required for completely clearing HBV infection.

A HBV infection can be ended at any stage if subsequently released viruses were completely neutralized by endogenous neutralizing antibodies. Most of HBV infections are aborted during the incubation period without developing into a full-blown infection because relative amount of infected viruses is still low. Those individuals who ended the HBV infection before clinical stage only show detectable anti-HBs and anti-HBc antibodies without clinical manifestations and noticeable HBV infection history [43, 44].

Thus, a natural strategy to clear viral infection or end infection course utilized by the host is to include producing neutralizing antibodies to block new rounds of infection with newly released viruses [45]. However, in minority cases, the infection will advance to clinical stage or viral disease will be aggravated or clinical stage will be prolonged if the amount of endogenous neutralizing antibodies produced in the host is not high enough to neutralize all specific viruses during the incubation or clinical stage of infection. This is how acute and chronic infections are established.

Cellular immunity consists of two major functional mechanisms in controlling viral infection [46–48], one is to kill infected cells by cytotoxic T cells that not only contribute to pathological changes of viral disease, but also release viruses for new rounds of infection if not neutralized. The impacts of killing infected cells by the specific immunity are similar to cytopathic effects of viruses. The other is to inhibit replication of viruses in the infected cells by cytokines, which will reduce the number of released viruses. From controlling infection point of view, the cellular immunity can be counterproductive or helpful dependent on net effect of two actions (the amount of virions released) as well as the level of specific neutralizing antibodies. A difference in tempo of clearing viral infection between cellular and humoral immunity is that the cellular immunity clears viral infection only after cells are virus infected while the neutralizing antibody clears viruses before the infection takes place, one step ahead of the cellular immunity (**Figure 3**). Humoral immunity of neutralizing antibody is direct, decisively effective and required for controlling viral infection. Once new rounds of infection were completely blocked by sufficient amount of neutralizing antibodies, the viral infection in the already infected cells will be cleared by virus secretion, cytopathic effects of viral replication, cell turnover or the cellular immunity. Alternatively, the viral infection will be restricted to those already infected cells if the infected cells were long-lived, implying that viral infection has been brought under control with the neutralizing antibody.

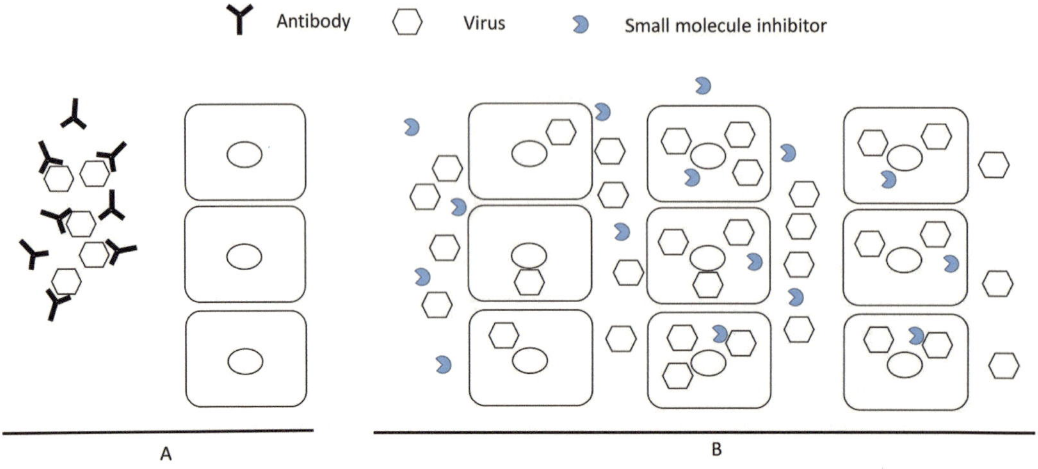

Figure 3. Differences in tempo and efficiency of clearing viral infection between neutralizing antibody and antivirals. (A) Administrated neutralizing antibody immediately neutralizes extracellular viruses and protect uninfected cells; (B) administrated small molecule inhibitor first allows virus to infect cells then starts inhibiting viral replication in infected cells. It cannot immediately and completely remove viremia.

A chronic HBV infection is usually maintained by new rounds of infection. The chronic infection can be spontaneously cleared if the level of endogenous neutralizing antibodies is high and can neutralize all released viruses to stop new rounds of infection. For instance, spontaneous clearance of chronic HBV infection occurs at annual rates of 1–2% and is featured with seroconversion of HBsAg to anti-HBs antibody [49, 50].

2.1.4. A main risk that will prolong HBV infection course is extracellular viruses, and a main target in treating viral diseases is extracellular viruses

Clearly, to cure HBV infection, it is essential and also efficient to interrupt infection course that consists of repeated rounds of infection.

There are three consequent scenarios during the course of hepatitis B: one is the infected cells become lost, resulting in releasing more virions as a consequence of cytopathic effects of infected HBV, cell turnover or destruction by cellular immunity; the second one is the infection is spontaneously cleared from infected cells by virus secretion or/and cellular immunity that reduces production and release of viruses, a same outcome as inhibiting viral replication by antivirals, and the third one is the infected cells are relatively long-lived (non-cytopathic infection) and producing and releasing low or high level of viruses. A shared main consequence produced by each scenario is releasing viruses. Thus, a main target in treating HBV infection should be the extracellular viruses, which cause new rounds of infection. Direct antivirals like NAs are not agents that can directly counter the extracellular viruses. Overall effectiveness of treating chronic HBV infection will be significantly improved if neutralizing antibodies are employed.

2.2. HBV infection course and persistence

HBV infection is known for long incubation period that may last up to 6 months (average 2–3 months) [51, 52] before occurrence of clinical symptoms of acute HBV infection. We believed that multiround infection occurs during the incubation period. Duck hepatitis B virus (DHBV) experimental infection was utilized to verify this understanding of HBV infection dynamics during the incubation period. Ducklings were inoculated with high DHBV inoculation dose, and three animals were daily sacrificed for 7 days after inoculation. Viral core protein was stained on liver sections, and DHBV DNA was detected in liver tissues [45]. As shown in **Figure 4A** and **B**, DHBV infection rapidly expanded from a few clusters of initially infected cells in the infected livers and reached a full-blown infection in 7 days, showing there were repeatedly new rounds of infection that expanded the infection scope in the livers, even under the circumstances of experimental infection that used a very large inoculum.

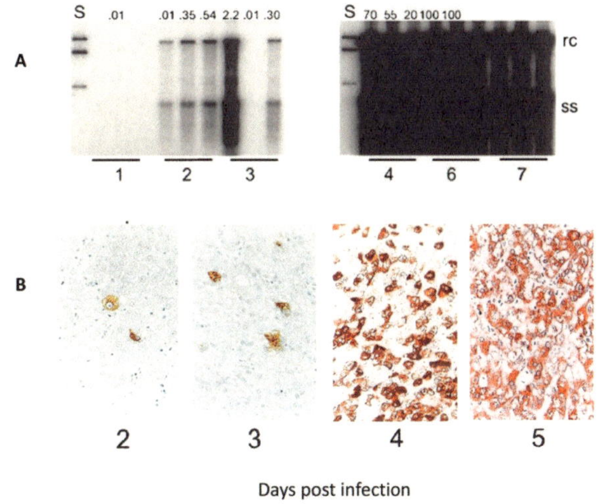

Figure 4. Multiround infection during the incubation period of DHBV infection. Viral replicative intermediates (A) and antigen-staining cells (B) were detected in livers of DHBV-infected ducks. Three ducks were sacrificed at the indicated days postinfection, and replicative intermediates were extracted from the liver. The viral DNA was detected by hybridization. The percent antigen-staining hepatocytes in some of the samples is indicated at the top of the lanes.

Are there continuously new rounds of infections after the full-blown HBV infection was established?

Current theory views that chronic HBV infection is a consequence of the host's insufficient T-cell immunity that cannot kill all HBV-infected cells or cannot clear HBV infection from infected cells [53, 54], implying chronic HBV infection is a simple extension of the initial or early HBV infection; the hepatocytes, once infected with HBV, are long-lived and constantly infected with the same initial viruses during chronic course.

However, such view is not supported by experimental and clinical evidence.

To investigate whether DHBV infection and DHBV-infected cell populations are stable after liver was fully infected, 3-day-old ducklings were inoculated with a large inoculum containing both DHBV 3 and 16 viruses at 1:1 ratio. The first biopsy was conducted at day 11 by which the liver was fully infected, and then, series of liver biopsies were performed every 3 weeks. Distinct genetic markers in two viral genomes allowed us to monitor kinetic changes in DHBV 3 and 16 singly and dually infected populations by determining cccDNA genotypes at single nucleus level. It was found that majority of hepatocytes were singly infected and nearly 20% of cells exhibited dual infection with both viruses at day 11 postinfection (p.i.) (**Figure 5**). We detected new rounds of infections at each of 5 time points after day 11 because the fraction of DHBV3-infected cells was expanding, but the expansion occurred in only singly infected fashion, suggesting that already infected cells resisted superinfection while the new rounds of infection were occurring. It also suggested occurrence of viral clearance in DHBV-infected liver, which generated uninfected cells for new rounds of infection. This viral clearance conclusion is consistent with data showing that the fraction of DHBV16-infected cells was decreased from 80% at day 32, to about 40% at day 131 p.i., and at least 40% of DHBV16-infected cells either cleared the infection or were eliminated, which triggered regeneration of hepatocytes. Either of two scenarios would produce uninfected cells targeted by new rounds of infection. The results suggest DHBV infection even after the full infection was established in the liver remains dynamic and is featured with new rounds of infections.

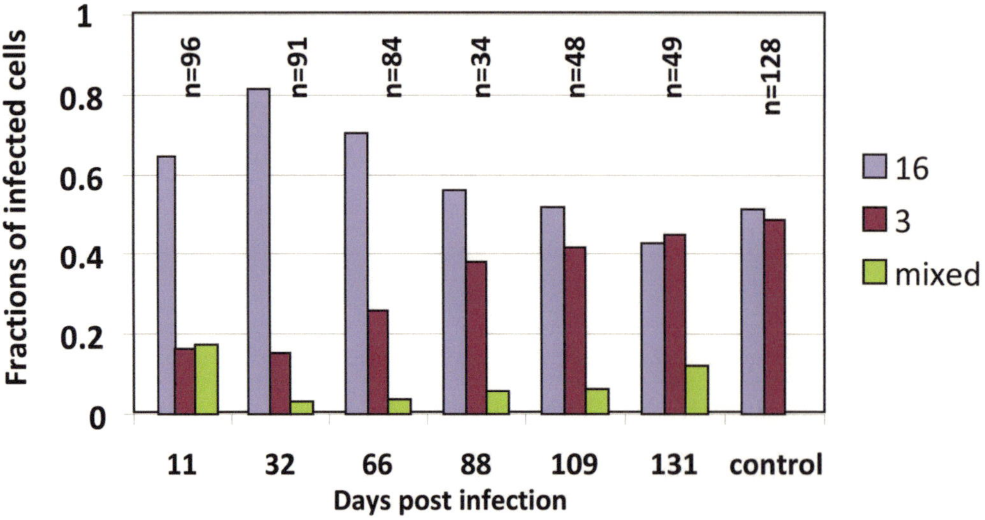

Figure 5. Repeated new rounds of infection after a liver was fully infected. Three-day-old ducklings (n = 20) were infected with an inoculum containing both DHBV3 and 16. Six biopsies were performed on one animal at day 11, 32, 66, 88, 109 and 131 days postinfection (shown in this figure). cccDNA genotypes were determined by sequencing PCR products amplified from cccDNA released from single individual nuclei. DHBV3-infected cells were expanding, while DHBV16-infected cells were decreasing during the period of six times of biopsies, suggesting ongoing viral clearance and new rounds of infection. As a quality control for our procedure, the same number of nuclei isolated from DHBV3 and DHBV16 singly infected livers was mixed and single individual nucleus was sorted into individual well of 96-well plates for PCR amplification and sequencing. No dual infections were detected in 128 mixed nuclei, suggesting that our procedure for detection is valid.

The results on clearing of DHBV16 cccDNA and new establishing of DHBV3 cccDNA pool from new rounds of infection are consistent with the early reports, in which a replication defective pre-core mutant or revertants successfully spread infection and became the predominant viral population following elimination of wild type (WT) or the initially inoculated viruses (**Figure 6**) [55, 56]. Taken together, all results suggest that a chronic DHBV infection is not a simple extension of the initial infection because the initial infection was cleared and the early cccDNA genotypes were replaced. Rather chronic DHBV infection course is dynamic and consists of viral clearance and new rounds of infection. Thus, repeatedly new rounds of infection maintain the persistence of viral cccDNA and prolong the course of chronic infection.

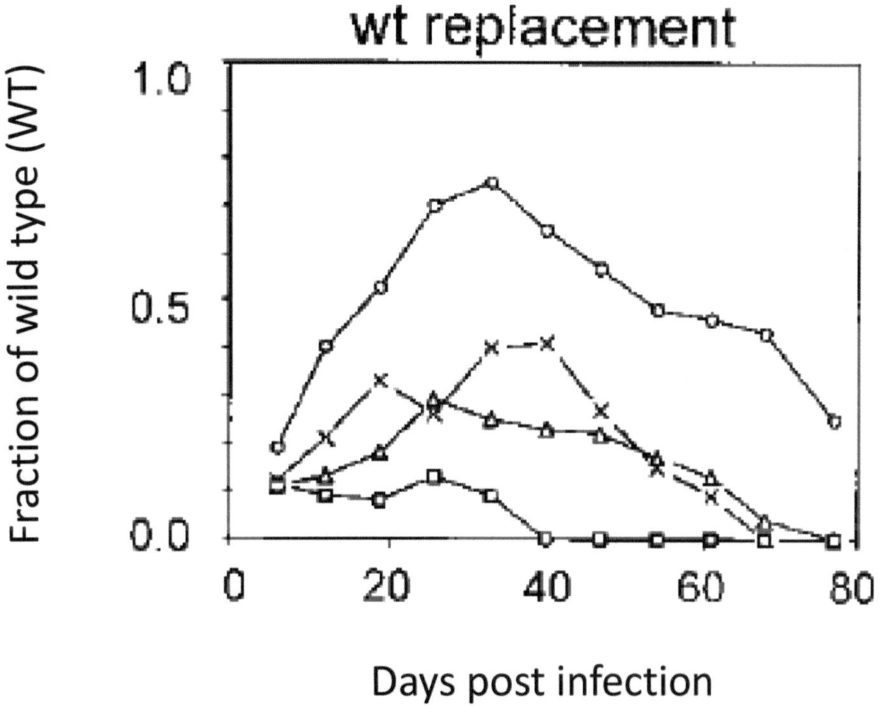

Figure 6. WT DHBV was being replaced over time. The fraction of WT DHBV DNA in serum of four DHBV-infected ducks was determined by PCR sequencing assay and plotted against the time postinfection. The kinetics of replacing WT DHBV infection suggests DHBV infection in fully infected livers remains dynamic and featured with clearing WT and new rounds of infection with MT.

These conclusions are supported by clinical HBV infection data.

It is well known that WT HBV infection is frequently replaced with mutant (MT) infection [25, 57–82] in untreated chronic HBV-infected patients. For instance, naturally occurring pre-core, core, pre-S and S mutants became only or dominant viral population following the WT was being eliminated from infected livers during natural course of chronic HBV infection. The data strongly imply that WT or early HBV infection is frequently cleared at cccDNA level during chronic HBV infection. It is notable that such cccDNA clearance naturally occurs without intervention. This understanding is consistent with cccDNA clearance in adult patients with acute HBV infection in which HBV infection is naturally resolved, and no antiviral treatment is needed.

Available data also suggest that HBV WT is replaced with HBV MT in NAs-treated chronic HBV-infected patients as evidenced by emergence of drug resistant mutant infection [25, 82]. The drug mutant infection that may not bear drug resistant phenotypes was also frequently detected in new generation of NAs-treated patients. A recent report shows that approximately 50% of patients treated with tenofovir (TDF) who remained viremic, developed pol/RT mutant infection though none of patients showed the drug resistance phenotypes [83]. The frequency of mutant infection in this report may be still underestimated because only the pol/RT sequence was analyzed. The observation that drug-related mutants spread following elimination of WT during NAs treatment suggests frequent viral clearance at cccDNA level and new rounds of infection with mutants.

3. New strategy and therapeutics for treating HBV infection guided by the viral infection biology

We propose a new strategy for treating HBV infection. This strategy directly aims to establish HBsAg seroconversion as early as possible through administrating sufficient amount of specific neutralizing antibodies, which will constantly and completely neutralize extracellular viruses to block repeated rounds of infection. This new strategy represents a paradigm shift in treating HBV infection, which has been treated primarily by inhibiting viral replication.

3.1. Directly dealing with the huge pool of HBsAg in chronic HBV infection

As the evidence points out, chronic HBV infection is not a simple extension of the initial infection, but is established and maintained by new rounds of infection. A unique situation in HBV infection is that it produces a huge pool of subviral particles (HBsAg) that are 1000–10,000 fold higher than virions [84]. The HBsAg primarily depletes the limited amount of endogenous neutralizing antibodies and leaves virions unneutralized and infectious. Current treatment strategy and approved antivirals are not designed to deal with new rounds of infection, almost impossibly deliver HBsAg seroconversion, and this is why current treatment rarely cures chronic HBV infection. The key to curing chronic HBV infection is to establish HBsAg seroconversion and to interrupt the infection course as early as possible by providing and maintaining high level of HBV neutralizing antibodies until the amount of endogenous HBV neutralizing antibodies exceeds the amount of HBV particles or all infected cells cleared HBV.

Advantages of the new strategy:

1. It directly immediately targets extracellular viruses and blocks the spread of infection;
2. It facilitates permanent and complete viral clearance in the liver;

3. It significantly reduces side effects of treating HBV infection. Unlike NAs and interferon that function intracellularly, the neutralizing antibody is to replenish a normal component of the immunity, which is relatively deficient in face of a huge pool of HBsAg, and it mainly functions extracellularly;

4. Neutralizing efficacy does not depend on efficiency of viral replication in infected cells.

4. Conclusions

In this paper, we analyze the deficiencies of current HBV treatment strategy and antivirals and the reason why they cannot cure chronic HBV infection. We also review the viral infection biology to fresh our understanding of general phases and natural course of HBV infection. We conclude that a full-blown HBV infection is established and maintained through multiround infection. We propose a new strategy for treating HBV infection. The core of this new strategy is that we must achieve HBsAg seroconversion naturally or interventionally to effectively clear HBV infection. Under the proposed strategy, a main target of the treatment is extracellular viruses, and an effective therapeutics is specific neutralizing antibodies.

Author details

Yong-Yuan Zhang

Address all correspondence to: yongyuanzhang@hbvtech.com

HBVtech, Frederick Innovative Technology Center, Frederick, MD, USA

References

[1] Hepatitis B [Internet] 2015. Available from: http://www.who.int/mediacentre/factsheets/fs204/en/.

[2] Franco E, Bagnato B, Marino MG, Meleleo C, Serino L, Zaratti L. Hepatitis B: epidemiology and prevention in developing countries. World Journal of Hepatology. 2012;4(3): 74–80. doi:10.4254/wjh.v4.i3.74. PubMed PMID: 22489259; PMCID: 3321493.

[3] Beasley RP, Trepo C, Stevens CE, Szmuness W. The e antigen and vertical transmission of hepatitis B surface antigen. American Journal of Epidemiology. 1977;105(2):94–8. PubMed PMID: 835566.

[4] Okada K, Kamiyama I, Inomata M, Imai M, Miyakawa Y. e antigen and anti-e in the serum of asymptomatic carrier mothers as indicators of positive and negative trans-

mission of hepatitis B virus to their infants. The New England Journal of Medicine. 1976;294(14):746–9. doi:10.1056/NEJM197604012941402. PubMed PMID: 943694.

[5] Stevens CE, Beasley RP, Tsui J, Lee WC. Vertical transmission of hepatitis B antigen in Taiwan. The New England Journal of Medicine. 1975;292(15):771–4. doi:10.1056/NEJM197504102921503. PubMed PMID: 1113797.

[6] Fattovich G, Brollo L, Giustina G, Noventa F, Pontisso P, Alberti A, Realdi G, Ruol A. Natural history and prognostic factors for chronic hepatitis type B. Gut. 1991;32(3):294–8. PubMed PMID: 2013423; PMCID: 1378837.

[7] Liaw YF, Tai DI, Chu CM, Chen TJ. The development of cirrhosis in patients with chronic type B hepatitis: a prospective study. Hepatology. 1988;8(3):493–6. PubMed PMID: 3371868.

[8] Beasley RP. Hepatitis B virus. The major etiology of hepatocellular carcinoma. Cancer. 1988;61(10):1942–56. PubMed PMID: 2834034.

[9] Lozano R, Naghavi M, Foreman K, Lim S, Shibuya K, Aboyans V, Abraham J, Adair T, Aggarwal R, Ahn SY, Alvarado M, Anderson HR, Anderson LM, Andrews KG, Atkinson C, Baddour LM, Barker-Collo S, Bartels DH, Bell ML, Benjamin EJ, Bennett D, Bhalla K, Bikbov B, Bin Abdulhak A, Birbeck G, Blyth F, Bolliger I, Boufous S, Bucello C, Burch M, Burney P, Carapetis J, Chen H, Chou D, Chugh SS, Coffeng LE, Colan SD, Colquhoun S, Colson KE, Condon J, Connor MD, Cooper LT, Corriere M, Cortinovis M, de Vaccaro KC, Couser W, Cowie BC, Criqui MH, Cross M, Dabhadkar KC, Dahodwala N, De Leo D, Degenhardt L, Delossantos A, Denenberg J, Des Jarlais DC, Dharmaratne SD, Dorsey ER, Driscoll T, Duber H, Ebel B, Erwin PJ, Espindola P, Ezzati M, Feigin V, Flaxman AD, Forouzanfar MH, Fowkes FG, Franklin R, Fransen M, Freeman MK, Gabriel SE, Gakidou E, Gaspari F, Gillum RF, Gonzalez-Medina D, Halasa YA, Haring D, Harrison JE, Havmoeller R, Hay RJ, Hoen B, Hotez PJ, Hoy D, Jacobsen KH, James SL, Jasrasaria R, Jayaraman S, Johns N, Karthikeyan G, Kassebaum N, Keren A, Khoo JP, Knowlton LM, Kobusingye O, Koranteng A, Krishnamurthi R, Lipnick M, Lipshultz SE, Ohno SL, Mabweijano J, MacIntyre MF, Mallinger L, March L, Marks GB, Marks R, Matsumori A, Matzopoulos R, Mayosi BM, McAnulty JH, McDermott MM, McGrath J, Mensah GA, Merriman TR, Michaud C, Miller M, Miller TR, Mock C, Mocumbi AO, Mokdad AA, Moran A, Mulholland K, Nair MN, Naldi L, Narayan KM, Nasseri K, Norman P, O'Donnell M, Omer SB, Ortblad K, Osborne R, Ozgediz D, Pahari B, Pandian JD, Rivero AP, Padilla RP, Perez-Ruiz F, Perico N, Phillips D, Pierce K, Pope CA, 3rd, Porrini E, Pourmalek F, Raju M, Ranganathan D, Rehm JT, Rein DB, Remuzzi G, Rivara FP, Roberts T, De Leon FR, Rosenfeld LC, Rushton L, Sacco RL, Salomon JA, Sampson U, Sanman E, Schwebel DC, Segui-Gomez M, Shepard DS, Singh D, Singleton J, Sliwa K, Smith E, Steer A, Taylor JA, Thomas B, Tleyjeh IM, Towbin JA, Truelsen T, Undurraga EA, Venketasubramanian N, Vijayakumar L, Vos T, Wagner GR, Wang M, Wang W, Watt K, Weinstock MA, Weintraub R, Wilkinson JD, Woolf AD, Wulf S, Yeh PH, Yip P, Zabetian A, Zheng ZJ, Lopez AD, Murray CJ, AlMazroa MA, Memish ZA. Global and regional mortality from 235 causes of death for 20 age groups in 1990 and

2010: a systematic analysis for the Global Burden of Disease Study 2010. Lancet. 2012;380(9859):2095–128. doi:10.1016/S0140-6736(12)61728-0. PubMed PMID: 23245 604.

[10] Liao B, Wang Z, Lin S, Xu Y, Yi J, Xu M, Huang Z, Zhou Y, Zhang F, Hou J. Significant fibrosis is not rare in Chinese chronic hepatitis B patients with persistent normal ALT. PLoS One. 2013;8(10):e78672. doi:10.1371/journal.pone.0078672. PubMed PMID: 24205292; PMCID: 3808379.

[11] Wang H, Xue L, Yan R, Zhou Y, Wang MS, Cheng MJ, Hai-Jun H. Comparison of histologic characteristics of Chinese chronic hepatitis B patients with persistently normal or mildly elevated ALT. PLoS One. 2013;8(11):e80585. doi:10.1371/journal.pone.0080585. PubMed PMID: 24260428; PMCID: 3832452.

[12] Lai M, Hyatt BJ, Nasser I, Curry M, Afdhal NH. The clinical significance of persistently normal ALT in chronic hepatitis B infection. Journal of Hepatology. 2007;47(6):760–7. doi:10.1016/j.jhep.2007.07.022. PubMed PMID: 17928090.

[13] Gui HL, Wang H, Yang YH, Wu YW, Zhou HJ, Guo SM, Lin LY, Wang L, Cai W, Chen R, Guo Q, Zhou XQ, Bao SS, Xie Q. Significant histopathology in Chinese chronic hepatitis B patients with persistently high-normal alanine aminotransferase. Journal of Viral Hepatitis. 2010;17(Suppl 1):44–50. doi:10.1111/j.1365-2893.2010.01270.x. PubMed PMID: 20586933.

[14] Lok AS, McMahon BJ. Chronic hepatitis B: update 2009. Hepatology. 2009;50(3): 661–2. doi:10.1002/hep.23190. PubMed PMID: 19714720.

[15] European Association For The Study Of The L. EASL clinical practice guidelines: management of chronic hepatitis B virus infection. Journal of Hepatology. 2012;57(1):167–85. doi:10.1016/j.jhep.2012.02.010. PubMed PMID: 22436845.

[16] Kwon H, Lok AS. Hepatitis B therapy. Nature Reviews Gastroenterology and Hepatology. 2011;8(5):275–84. doi:10.1038/nrgastro.2011.33. PubMed PMID: 21423 260.

[17] Trepo C, Chan HL, Lok A. Hepatitis B virus infection. Lancet. 2014;384(9959): 2053–63. doi:10.1016/S0140-6736(14)60220-8. PubMed PMID: 24954675.

[18] Lok AS, Lai CL. Acute exacerbations in Chinese patients with chronic hepatitis B virus (HBV) infection. Incidence, predisposing factors and etiology. Journal of Hepatology. 1990;10(1):29–34. PubMed PMID: 2307827.

[19] Liaw YF, Tai DI, Chu CM, Pao CC, Chen TJ. Acute exacerbation in chronic type B hepatitis: comparison between HBeAg and antibody-positive patients. Hepatology. 1987;7(1):20–3. PubMed PMID: 2433203.

[20] Sarin S, Kedarisetty C, Abbas Z, Amarapurkar D, Bihari C, Chan A, Chawla Y, Dokmeci AK, Garg H, Ghazinyan H, Hamid S, Kim D, Komolmit P, Lata S, Lee G, Lesmana L, Mahtab M, Maiwall R, Moreau R, Ning Q, Pamecha V, Payawal D, Rastogi A, Rahman S, Rela M, Saraya A, Samuel D, Saraswat V, Shah S, Shiha G, Sharma B, Sharma M,

Sharma K, Butt A, Tan S, Vashishtha C, Wani Z, Yuen M-F, Yokosuka O. Acute-on-chronic liver failure: consensus recommendations of the Asian Pacific Association for the Study of the Liver (APASL) 2014. Hepatology International. 2014;8(4):453–71.

[21] Olson J, Kamath P. Acute-on-chronic liver failure: concept, natural history, and prognosis. Current Opinion in Critical Care. 2011;17(2):165–9.

[22] Elbaz T, El-Kassas M, Esmat G. New era for management of chronic hepatitis C virus using direct antiviral agents: a review. Journal of Advanced Research. 2015;6(3):301–10. doi:10.1016/j.jare.2014.11.004. PubMed PMID: 26257927; PMCID: PMC4522579.

[23] Mishra P, Murray J, Birnkrant D. Direct-acting antiviral drug approvals for treatment of chronic hepatitis C virus infection: scientific and regulatory approaches to clinical trial designs. Hepatology. 2015;62(4):1298–303. doi:10.1002/hep.27880. PubMed PMID: 25953139.

[24] Lau DT, Khokhar MF, Doo E, Ghany MG, Herion D, Park Y, Kleiner DE, Schmid P, Condreay LD, Gauthier J, Kuhns MC, Liang TJ, Hoofnagle JH. Long-term therapy of chronic hepatitis B with lamivudine. Hepatology. 2000;32(4 Pt 1):828–34. doi:10.1053/jhep.2000.17912. PubMed PMID: 11003630.

[25] Ghany MG, Doo EC. Antiviral resistance and hepatitis B therapy. Hepatology. 2009;49(5 Suppl):S174–84. doi:10.1002/hep.22900. PubMed PMID: 19399794; PMCID: 2707848.

[26] Luo J, Li X, Wu Y, Lin G, Pang Y, Zhang X, Ao Y, Du Z, Zhao Z, Chong Y. Efficacy of entecavir treatment for up to 5 years in nucleos(t)ide-naive chronic hepatitis B patients in real life. International Journal of Medical Sciences. 2013;10(4):427–33. doi:10.7150/ijms.5472. PubMed PMID: 23471472; PMCID: 3590603.

[27] Pan CQ, Tong M, Kowdley KV, Hu KQ, Chang TT, Lai CL, Yoon SK, Lee SS, Cohen D, Tang H, Tsai N. High rates of viral suppression after long-term entecavir treatment of Asian patients with hepatitis B e antigen-positive chronic hepatitis B. Clinical Gastroenterology and Hepatology. 2012;10(9):1047–50 e1. doi:10.1016/j.cgh.2012.03.016. PubMed PMID: 22475742.

[28] Lok AS, Trinh H, Carosi G, Akarca US, Gadano A, Habersetzer F, Sievert W, Wong D, Lovegren M, Cohen D, Llamoso C. Efficacy of entecavir with or without tenofovir disoproxil fumarate for nucleos(t)ide-naive patients with chronic hepatitis B. Gastroenterology. 2012;143(3):619–28 e1. doi:10.1053/j.gastro.2012.05.037. PubMed PMID: 22643350.

[29] Heathcote EJ, Marcellin P, Buti M, Gane E, De Man RA, Krastev Z, Germanidis G, Lee SS, Flisiak R, Kaita K, Manns M, Kotzev I, Tchernev K, Buggisch P, Weilert F, Kurdas OO, Shiffman ML, Trinh H, Gurel S, Snow-Lampart A, Borroto-Esoda K, Mondou E, Anderson J, Sorbel J, Rousseau F. Three-year efficacy and safety of tenofovir disoproxil fumarate treatment for chronic hepatitis B. Gastroenterology. 2011;140(1):132–43. doi:10.1053/j.gastro.2010.10.011. PubMed PMID: 20955704.

[30] Zhu Y, Yamamoto T, Cullen J, Saputelli J, Aldrich CE, Miller DS, Litwin S, Furman PA, Jilbert AR, Mason WS. Kinetics of hepadnavirus loss from the liver during inhibition of viral DNA synthesis. Journal of Virology. 2001;75(1):311–22. doi:10.1128/JVI.75.1.311-322.2001. PubMed PMID: 11119601; PMCID: 113925.

[31] Wursthorn K, Lutgehetmann M, Dandri M, Volz T, Buggisch P, Zollner B, Longerich T, Schirmacher P, Metzler F, Zankel M, Fischer C, Currie G, Brosgart C, Petersen J. Peginterferon alpha-2b plus adefovir induce strong cccDNA decline and HBsAg reduction in patients with chronic hepatitis B. Hepatology. 2006;44(3):675–84. doi: 10.1002/hep.21282. PubMed PMID: 16941693.

[32] Werle-Lapostolle B, Bowden S, Locarnini S, Wursthorn K, Petersen J, Lau G, Trepo C, Marcellin P, Goodman Z, Delaney WE 4th, Xiong S, Brosgart CL, Chen SS, Gibbs CS, Zoulim F. Persistence of cccDNA during the natural history of chronic hepatitis B and decline during adefovir dipivoxil therapy. Gastroenterology. 2004;126(7):1750–8. PubMed PMID: 15188170.

[33] Tseng TC, Kao JH. Clinical utility of quantitative HBsAg in natural history and nucleos(t)ide analogue treatment of chronic hepatitis B: new trick of old dog. Journal of Gastroenterology. 2013;48(1):13–21. doi:10.1007/s00535-012-0668-y. PubMed PMID: 23090000; PMCID: 3698422.

[34] Dahari H, Shudo E, Ribeiro RM, Perelson AS. Modeling complex decay profiles of hepatitis B virus during antiviral therapy. Hepatology. 2009;49(1):32–8. doi:10.1002/hep.22586. PubMed PMID: 19065674; PMCID: 3712859.

[35] Perelson AS, Guedj J. Modelling hepatitis C therapy—predicting effects of treatment. Nature Reviews Gastroenterology and Hepatology. 2015;12(8):437–45. doi:10.1038/nrgastro.2015.97. PubMed PMID: 26122475; PMCID: PMC4692721.

[36] Rivadeneira PS, Moog CH, Stan GB, Brunet C, Raffi F, Ferre V, Costanza V, Mhawej MJ, Biafore F, Ouattara DA, Ernst D, Fonteneau R, Xia X. Mathematical modeling of HIV dynamics after antiretroviral therapy initiation: a review. Bioresearch Open Access. 2014;3(5):233–41. doi:10.1089/biores.2014.0024. PubMed PMID: 25371860; PMCID: PMC4215334.

[37] Warren TK, Jordan R, Lo MK, Ray AS, Mackman RL, Soloveva V, Siegel D, Perron M, Bannister R, Hui HC, Larson N, Strickley R, Wells J, Stuthman KS, Van Tongeren SA, Garza NL, Donnelly G, Shurtleff AC, Retterer CJ, Gharaibeh D, Zamani R, Kenny T, Eaton BP, Grimes E, Welch LS, Gomba L, Wilhelmsen CL, Nichols DK, Nuss JE, Nagle ER, Kugelman JR, Palacios G, Doerffler E, Neville S, Carra E, Clarke MO, Zhang L, Lew W, Ross B, Wang Q, Chun K, Wolfe L, Babusis D, Park Y, Stray KM, Trancheva I, Feng JY, Barauskas O, Xu Y, Wong P, Braun MR, Flint M, McMullan LK, Chen SS, Fearns R, Swaminathan S, Mayers DL, Spiropoulou CF, Lee WA, Nichol ST, Cihlar T, Bavari S. Therapeutic efficacy of the small molecule GS-5734 against Ebola virus in rhesus monkeys. Nature. 2016;531(7594):381–5. doi:10.1038/nature17180. PubMed PMID: 26934220.

[38] Gish RG, Lok AS, Chang TT, de Man RA, Gadano A, Sollano J, Han KH, Chao YC, Lee SD, Harris M, Yang J, Colonno R, Brett-Smith H. Entecavir therapy for up to 96 weeks in patients with HBeAg-positive chronic hepatitis B. Gastroenterology. 2007;133(5): 1437–44. doi:10.1053/j.gastro.2007.08.025. PubMed PMID: 17983800.

[39] Bernuau J, Goudeau A, Poynard T, Dubois F, Lesage G, Yvonnet B, Degott C, Bezeaud A, Rueff B, Benhamou JP. Multivariate analysis of prognostic factors in fulminant hepatitis B. Hepatology. 1986;6(4):648–51. PubMed PMID: 3732998.

[40] Oren I, Hershow RC, Ben-Porath E, Krivoy N, Goldstein N, Rishpon S, Shouval D, Hadler SC, Alter MJ, Maynard JE, et al. A common-source outbreak of fulminant hepatitis B in a hospital. Annals of Internal Medicine. 1989;110(9):691–8. PubMed PMID: 2930106.

[41] Tsang SW, Chan HL, Leung NW, Chau TN, Lai ST, Chan FK, Sung JJ. Lamivudine treatment for fulminant hepatic failure due to acute exacerbation of chronic hepatitis B infection. Alimentary Pharmacology and Therapeutics. 2001;15(11):1737–44. PubMed PMID: 11683687.

[42] McMahon BJ, Alward WL, Hall DB, Heyward WL, Bender TR, Francis DP, Maynard JE. Acute hepatitis B virus infection: relation of age to the clinical expression of disease and subsequent development of the carrier state. The Journal of Infectious Diseases. 1985;151(4):599–603. PubMed PMID: 3973412.

[43] Parry MF, Brown AE, Dobbs LG, Gocke DJ, Neu HC. The epidemiology of hepatitis B infection in housestaff. Infection. 1978;6(5):204–6. PubMed PMID: 730389.

[44] Sherlock S. The natural history of hepatitis B. Postgraduate Medical Journal. 1987;63(Suppl 2):7–11. PubMed PMID: 3317361.

[45] Zhang YY, Summers J. Rapid production of neutralizing antibody leads to transient hepadnavirus infection. Journal of Virology. 2004;78(3):1195–201. PubMed PMID: 14722274; PMCID: 321410.

[46] McMichael AJ, Rowland-Jones SL. Cellular immune responses to HIV. Nature. 2001;410(6831):980–7.

[47] Bertoletti A, Gehring AJ. The immune response during hepatitis B virus infection. The Journal of General Virology. 2006;87(Pt 6):1439–49. doi:10.1099/vir.0.81920-0. PubMed PMID: 16690908.

[48] Guidotti LG, Rochford R, Chung J, Shapiro M, Purcell R, Chisari FV. Viral clearance without destruction of infected cells during acute HBV infection. Science. 1999;284(5415):825–9. PubMed PMID: 10221919.

[49] Liaw YF, Sheen IS, Chen TJ, Chu CM, Pao CC. Incidence, determinants and significance of delayed clearance of serum HBsAg in chronic hepatitis B virus infection: a prospective study. Hepatology. 1991;13(4):627–31. PubMed PMID: 2010157.

[50] Liu J, Yang HI, Lee MH, Lu SN, Jen CL, Wang LY, You SL, Iloeje UH, Chen CJ, Group R-HS. Incidence and determinants of spontaneous hepatitis B surface antigen seroclearance: a community-based follow-up study. Gastroenterology. 2010;139(2):474–82. doi:10.1053/j.gastro.2010.04.048. PubMed PMID: 20434450.

[51] Barker LF, Murray R. Relationship of virus dose to incubation time of clinical hepatitis and time of appearance of hepatitis-associated antigen. The American Journal of the Medical Sciences. 1972;263(1):27–33. PubMed PMID: 5057849.

[52] Liang TJ. Hepatitis B: the virus and disease. Hepatology. 2009;49(5 Suppl):S13–21. doi:10.1002/hep.22881. PubMed PMID: 19399811; PMCID: 2809016.

[53] Chisari FV, Ferrari C. Hepatitis B virus immunopathology. Springer Seminars in Immunopathology. 1995;17(2–3):261–81. PubMed PMID: 8571172.

[54] Chisari FV, Isogawa M, Wieland SF. Pathogenesis of hepatitis B virus infection. Pathologie-Biologie. 2010;58(4):258–66. doi:10.1016/j.patbio.2009.11.001. PubMed PMID: 20116937; PMCID: 2888709.

[55] Zhang YY, Summers J. Enrichment of a precore-minus mutant of duck hepatitis B virus in experimental mixed infections. Journal of Virology. 1999;73(5):3616–22. Epub 1999/04/10. PubMed PMID: 10196253; PMCID: 104136.

[56] Pult I, Abbott N, Zhang YY, Summers J. Frequency of spontaneous mutations in an avian hepadnavirus infection. Journal of Virology. 2001;75(20):9623–32. doi:10.1128/JVI.75.20.9623-9632.2001. PubMed PMID: 11559794; PMCID: 114533.

[57] Brunetto MR, Giarin MM, Oliveri F, Chiaberge E, Baldi M, Alfarano A, Serra A, Saracco G, Verme G, Will H, et al. Wild-type and e antigen-minus hepatitis B viruses and course of chronic hepatitis. Proceedings of the National Academy of Sciences USA. 1991;88(10):4186–90. Epub 1991/05/15. PubMed PMID: 2034663; PMCID: 51623.

[58] Carman WF, Jacyna MR, Hadziyannis S, Karayiannis P, McGarvey MJ, Makris A, Thomas HC. Mutation preventing formation of hepatitis B e antigen in patients with chronic hepatitis B infection. Lancet. 1989;2(8663):588–91. PubMed PMID: 2570285.

[59] Karasawa T, Shirasawa T, Okawa Y, Kuramoto A, Shimada N, Aizawa Y, Zeniya M, Toda G. Association between frequency of amino acid changes in core region of hepatitis B virus (HBV) and the presence of precore mutation in Japanese HBV carriers. Journal of Gastroenterology. 1997;32(5):611–22. Epub 1997/11/14. PubMed PMID: 9349986.

[60] Lin CL, Liao LY, Liu CJ, Chen PJ, Lai MY, Kao JH, Chen DS. Hepatitis B genotypes and precore/basal core promoter mutants in HBeAg-negative chronic hepatitis B. Journal of Gastroenterology. 2002;37(4):283–7. Epub 2002/05/08. PubMed PMID: 11993512.

[61] Funk ML, Rosenberg DM, Lok AS. World-wide epidemiology of HBeAg-negative chronic hepatitis B and associated precore and core promoter variants. Journal of Viral Hepatitis. 2002;9(1):52–61. Epub 2002/02/20. PubMed PMID: 11851903.

[62] Okamoto H, Tsuda F, Akahane Y, Sugai Y, Yoshiba M, Moriyama K, Tanaka T, Miyakawa Y, Mayumi M. Hepatitis B virus with mutations in the core promoter for an e antigen-negative phenotype in carriers with antibody to e antigen. Journal of Virology. 1994;68(12):8102–10. Epub 1994/12/01. PubMed PMID: 7966600; PMCID: 237274.

[63] Omata M, Ehata T, Yokosuka O, Hosoda K, Ohto M. Mutations in the precore region of hepatitis B virus DNA in patients with fulminant and severe hepatitis. The New England Journal of Medicine. 1991;324(24):1699–704. Epub 1991/06/13. doi:10.1056/NEJM199106133242404. PubMed PMID: 2034246.

[64] Tur-Kaspa R, Klein A, Aharonson S. Hepatitis B virus precore mutants are identical in carriers from various ethnic origins and are associated with a range of liver disease severity. Hepatology. 1992;16(6):1338–42. PubMed PMID: 1446889.

[65] Shiraki K, Hamada M, Sugimoto K, Ito T, Yamanaka T, Wagayama H, Shimizu A, Makino Y, Takase K, Nakano T, Tameda Y. Detection of precore-mutant hepatitis B virus genome in patients with acute and fulminant hepatitis using mutation site-specific assay (MSSA). Hepatogastroenterology. 2002;49(47):1352–6. Epub 2002/09/21. PubMed PMID: 12239941.

[66] Chu CM, Yeh CT, Chiu CT, Sheen IS, Liaw YF. Precore mutant of hepatitis B virus prevails in acute and chronic infections in an area in which hepatitis B is endemic. Journal of Clinical Microbiology. 1996;34(7):1815–8. Epub 1996/07/01. PubMed PMID: 8784599; PMCID: 229124.

[67] Santantonio T, Jung MC, Miska S, Pastore G, Pape GR, Will H. Prevalence and type of pre-C HBV mutants in anti-HBe positive carriers with chronic liver disease in a highly endemic area. Virology. 1991;183(2):840–4. PubMed PMID: 1853582.

[68] Santantonio T, Jung MC, Miska S, Pastore G, Pape GR, Will H. High prevalence and heterogeneity of HBV preC mutants in anti-HBe-positive carriers with chronic liver disease in southern Italy. Journal of Hepatology. 1991;13(Suppl 4):S78–81. Epub 1991/01/01. PubMed PMID: 1822518.

[69] Manzin A, Paolucci S, Lampertico P, Menzo S, Rumi MG, Colombo M, Clementi M. Direct detection of HBV preC mutants in heterogeneous viral populations by a modified DNA sequencing method. Research in Virology. 1993;144(4):303–6. Epub 1993/07/01. PubMed PMID: 8210713.

[70] Chan HL, Leung NW, Hussain M, Wong ML, Lok AS. Hepatitis B e antigen-negative chronic hepatitis B in Hong Kong. Hepatology. 2000;31(3):763–8. doi:10.1002/hep.510310330. PubMed PMID: 10706570.

[71] Brunetto MR, Stemler M, Bonino F, Schodel F, Oliveri F, Rizzetto M, Verme G, Will H. A new hepatitis B virus strain in patients with severe anti-HBe positive chronic hepatitis B. Journal of Hepatology. 1990;10(2):258–61. Epub 1990/03/01. PubMed PMID: 2332598.

[72] Okamoto H, Yotsumoto S, Akahane Y, Yamanaka T, Miyazaki Y, Sugai Y, Tsuda F, Tanaka T, Miyakawa Y, Mayumi M. Hepatitis B viruses with precore region defects

prevail in persistently infected hosts along with seroconversion to the antibody against e antigen. Journal of Virology. 1990;64(3):1298–303. Epub 1990/03/01. PubMed PMID: 2304145; PMCID: 249247.

[73] Raimondo G, Schneider R, Stemler M, Smedile V, Rodino G, Will H. A new hepatitis B virus variant in a chronic carrier with multiple episodes of viral reactivation and acute hepatitis. Virology. 1990;179(1):64–8. PubMed PMID: 2219740.

[74] Tong SP, Li JS, Vitvitski L, Trepo C. Active hepatitis B virus replication in the presence of anti-HBe is associated with viral variants containing an inactive pre-C region. Virology. 1990;176(2):596–603. PubMed PMID: 2345966.

[75] Li J, Tong S, Vitvitski L, Zoulim F, Trepo C. Rapid detection and further characterization of infection with hepatitis B virus variants containing a stop codon in the distal pre-C region. The Journal of General Virology. 1990;71 (Pt 9):1993–8. Epub 1990/09/01. PubMed PMID: 2212990.

[76] Raimondo G, Stemler M, Schneider R, Wildner G, Squadrito G, Will H. Latency and reactivation of a precore mutant hepatitis B virus in a chronically infected patient. Journal of Hepatology. 1990;11(3):374–80. Epub 1990/11/01. PubMed PMID: 2290029.

[77] Lindh M, Furuta Y, Vahlne A, Norkrans G, Horal P. Emergence of precore TAG mutation during hepatitis B e seroconversion and its dependence on pregenomic base pairing between nucleotides 1858 of 1896. Journal of Infectious Diseases. 1995;172(5):1343–7. Epub 1995/11/01. PubMed PMID: 7594674.

[78] Brunetto MR, Giarin M, Saracco G, Oliveri F, Calvo P, Capra G, Randone A, Abate ML, Manzini P, Capalbo M, et al. Hepatitis B virus unable to secrete e antigen and response to interferon in chronic hepatitis B. Gastroenterology. 1993;105(3):845–50. PubMed PMID: 7689519.

[79] Lok AS, Akarca U, Greene S. Mutations in the pre-core region of hepatitis B virus serve to enhance the stability of the secondary structure of the pre-genome encapsidation signal. Proceedings of the National Academy of Sciences United States of America. 1994;91(9):4077–81. Epub 1994/04/26. PubMed PMID: 8171038; PMCID: 43726.

[80] Locarnini S, Zoulim F. Molecular genetics of HBV infection. Antiviral Therapy. 2010;15(Suppl 3):3–14. Epub 2010/11/10. doi:10.3851/IMP1619. PubMed PMID: 21041899.

[81] Zoulim F, Locarnini S. Hepatitis B virus resistance to nucleos(t)ide analogues. Gastroenterology. 2009;137(5):1593–608 e1–2. doi:10.1053/j.gastro.2009.08.063. PubMed PMID: 19737565.

[82] Locarnini S, Bowden S. Drug resistance in antiviral therapy. Clinics in Liver Disease. 2010;14(3):439–59. Epub 2010/07/20. doi:10.1016/j.cld.2010.05.004. PubMed PMID: 20638024.

[83] Kitrinos KM, Corsa A, Liu Y, Flaherty J, Snow-Lampart A, Marcellin P, Borroto-Esoda K, Miller MD. No detectable resistance to tenofovir disoproxil fumarate after 6 years of therapy in patients with chronic hepatitis B. Hepatology. 2014;59(2):434–42.

[84] Ganem D, Prince AM. Hepatitis B virus infection--natural history and clinical consequences. The New England Journal of Medicine. 2004;350(11):1118–29. doi:10.1056/NEJMra031087. PubMed PMID: 15014185.